The Central Nervous System

THE CENTRAL NERVOUS SYSTEM

Structure and Function

Fourth Edition

PER BRODAL, MD, PhD
Institute of Basic Medical Sciences
University of Oslo
Oslo, Norway

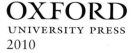
UNIVERSITY PRESS
2010

OXFORD
UNIVERSITY PRESS

Oxford University Press, Inc., publishes works that further
Oxford University's objective of excellence
in research, scholarship, and education.

Oxford New York
Auckland Cape Town Dar es Salaam Hong Kong Karachi
Kuala Lumpur Madrid Melbourne Mexico City Nairobi
New Delhi Shanghai Taipei Toronto

With offices in
Argentina Austria Brazil Chile Czech Republic France Greece
Guatemala Hungary Italy Japan Poland Portugal Singapore
South Korea Switzerland Thailand Turkey Ukraine Vietnam

Copyright © 1992, 1998, 2004, 2010 by Oxford University Press, Inc.

Published by Oxford University Press, Inc.
198 Madison Avenue, New York, New York 10016
www.oup.com

Oxford is a registered trademark of Oxford University Press

Library of Congress Cataloging-in-Publication Data
Brodal, Per.
  The central nervous system : structure and function / Per Brodal. — 4th ed.
    p. ; cm.
  Includes bibliographical references and index.
  ISBN-13: 978-0-19-538115-3 (alk. paper)
  ISBN-10: 0-19-538115-7 (alk. paper)
  1. Central nervous system. I. Title.
  [DNLM: 1. Central Nervous System—physiology. WL 300 B8645c 2010]
  QP370.B76 2010
  612.8'2—dc22
                                                    2009028992

3 5 7 9 8 6 4 2

Printed in China

Preface

This book is intended primarily for use by students of medicine, physical therapy, and psychology—that is, for use in neuroscience or neuroanatomy courses by students who need knowledge of the nervous system as a basis for later clinical study and practice. This fourth edition has been thoroughly revised and renewed. In addition to the updated and rewritten text, all figures have been redrawn and printed in full color to improve their impact, and many new ones have been added. The number of chapters has been increased to facilitate reading and grasp of the material. Further, each chapter begins with a short overview, setting the stage for what to come and emphasizing salient points.

My intentions remain the same as those of my father, Alf Brodal, when he wrote the Norwegian forerunner of this book more than 60 years ago: to stimulate understanding rather than memorization of isolated facts, while at the same time fostering a realistic attitude toward our still-limited ability to explain the marvels of the human brain.

The book aims to present the difficult subject of neuroscience so that those approaching it for the first time can understand it. Therefore, many details are left out that might be of great interest to the specialist but would merely obscure the essentials for the beginner. Everyday experiences and clinical examples are integrated throughout the text to help students link the new material with their prior knowledge and future profession. The nervous system, however, is exceedingly complex, both structurally and functionally, and much remains to be learned before we can answer many fundamental questions. Thus, while an undergraduate course can provide only partial insights, no one is served by a presentation that avoids controversial issues and areas of ignorance. Indeed, pointing out what we do not know is sometimes better than presenting an oversimplified version. For this reason I have also discussed how the data were obtained and the limitations inherent in the various methods.

The main challenge—for both the student and the scientist—is to understand how the nervous system solves its multifarious tasks. This requires an integrated approach, drawing on data from all fields of neurobiology, as well as from psychology and clinical research.

Textbooks sharing this goal nevertheless differ markedly in how they present the material and where they put the emphasis. Perhaps because my own field of research is the wiring patterns of the brain, I strongly feel that knowledge of how the nervous system is built—in particular, how the various parts are interconnected to form functional systems—is a prerequisite for proper understanding of data from other fields. A fair knowledge of brain anatomy is especially important for sound interpretations of the symptoms of brain disease. Textbooks of neuroanatomy often overwhelm the reader with details that are not strictly relevant for either functional analysis or clinical thinking. Neither does a strong emphasis on cellular mechanisms at the expense of the properties of neural systems seem the right choice if the aim is to help readers understand how the brain performs its tasks and how the site of a disease process relates to a patient's symptoms. Therefore, neither anatomical nor cellular and molecular details are included in this book if they cannot in some way be related to function. My hope is that the book presents a balance of cellular and neural systems material that is right for students.

In-depth sections and more advanced clinical material are clearly marked so that they should not disturb reading of the main text. Because the needs of readers differ, however, they are encouraged to read selectively and pick the material they find most relevant and interesting from their perspective, regardless of whether it is placed in the main text or in boxes. The frequent subheadings should facilitate such selective reading.

During the preparation of the former and the present editions, I have received help from several colleagues, for which I am truly grateful. Jan Bjaalie, Niels Christian Danbolt, Paul Heggelund, Jan Jansen, Harald Kryvi, Kirsten Osen, Ole Petter Ottersen, Eric Rinvik, and Jon Storm-Mathisen have all provided constructive criticism and advice. I also gratefully acknowledge the expert help of Gunnar Lothe and Carina Knudsen, who produced the photographic work.

Per Brodal, MD, PhD
Oslo, Norway

Contents

Introduction

A BIRD'S EYE VIEW OF THE NERVOUS SYSTEM

What are the main tasks of the nervous system? This question is not easily answered—our brains represent most of what we associate with being a human. At a superior level, the brain creates our reality: it selects, sorts, and interprets the overwhelming amount of information we receive from our bodies and the environment, and it controls behavior in accordance with its interpretations of reality. This control concerns behavior in a wide sense: one aspect is control and maintenance of the body and its inner milieu; another is our interaction with our surroundings and other human beings through actions and speech. A third aspect is our inner, subjective, mental reality that others can only partially know. In early childhood, the brain must create order and predictability so that we learn to relate successfully to ourselves and our environment.

The essential building block of the nervous system is the **neuron** (nerve cell), specialized for rapid conveyance of signals over long distances and in a very precise manner. Together, billions of neurons in the brain form complicated and highly organized networks for **communication** and **information processing.**

The nervous system receives a wealth of information from an individual's surroundings and body. From all this information, it extracts the essentials, stores what may be needed later, and emits a command to muscles or glands if an answer is appropriate. Sometimes the answer comes within milliseconds, as a **reflex** or automatic response. At other times it may take considerably longer, requiring cooperation among many parts of the brain and involving **conscious processes.** In any case, the main task of the nervous system is to ensure that the organism adapts optimally to the environment.

The nervous system is equipped with sense organs, **receptors,** that react to various forms of sensory information or stimuli. Regardless of the mode of stimulation (the form of energy), the receptors "translate" the energy of the stimulus to the language spoken by the nervous system, that is, **nerve impulses.** These are tiny electric discharges rapidly conducted along the nerve processes. In this way signals are conveyed from the receptors to the regions of the nervous system where information processing takes place.

The nervous system can elicit an external response only by acting on **effectors,** which are either muscles or glands. The response is either **movement** or **secretion.** Obviously, muscle contraction can have various expressions, from communication through speech, facial expression, and bodily posture to walking and running, respiratory movements, and changes of blood pressure. But one should bear in mind that the nervous system can only act on muscles and glands to express its "will." Conversely, if we are to judge the activity going on in the brain of another being, we have only the expressions produced by muscle contraction and secretion to go by.

On an anatomic basis we can divide the nervous system into the **central nervous system** (CNS), consisting of the brain and the spinal cord, and the **peripheral nervous system** (PNS), which connects the CNS with the receptors and the effectors. Although without sharp transitions, the PNS and the CNS can be subdivided into parts that are concerned primarily with the regulation of visceral organs and the internal milieu, and parts that are concerned mainly with the more or less conscious adaptation to the external world. The first division is called the **autonomic** or **visceral nervous system;** the second is usually called the **somatic nervous system.** The second division, also called the cerebrospinal nervous system, receives information from sense organs capturing events in our surroundings (vision, hearing, receptors in the skin) and controls the activity of voluntary muscles (made up of cross-striated skeletal muscle cells). In contrast, the autonomic nervous system controls the activity of involuntary muscles (smooth muscle and heart muscle cells) and gland cells. The autonomic system may be further subdivided into the **sympathetic system,** which is mainly concerned with mobilizing the resources of the body when demands are increased (as in emergencies), and the **parasympathetic system,** which is devoted more to the daily maintenance of the body.

The **behavior** of a vertebrate with a small and—comparatively speaking—simple brain (such as a frog) is dominated by fairly fixed relationships between stimuli and their response. Thus, a stimulus, produced for example by a small object in the visual field, elicits a stereotyped pattern of goal-directed movements. Few neurons are intercalated between the sense organ and the effector, with correspondingly limited scope of response adaptation. Much of the behavior of the animal is therefore instinctive and automatic, and not subject to significant change by learning. In mammals with relatively small brains compared with their body weights (such as rodents) a large part of their brain is devoted to fairly direct sensorimotor transformations. In primates, the relative brain weight has increased dramatically during some million years of evolution. This increase is most marked in humans with relative brain weight double that of the chimpanzee. In humans, there are few fixed relationships between sensations and behavior (apart from a number of vital reflexes). Thus, a certain stimulus may cause different responses depending on its context and the antecedents. Consequently, we often can choose among several responses, and the response can be changed on the basis of experience. Such flexibility requires, however, increased "computational power" in terms of number of neurons available for specific tasks. The more an animal organizes its activities on the basis of previous experience, and the more it is freed from the dominance of immediate sensations, the more complex are the processes required of the central nervous system. The behavior of humans cannot be understood merely on the basis of what happened immediately before. The British neuropsychologist Larry Weiskrantz (1992) puts it this way: "We are controlled by predicted consequences of our behavior as much as by the immediate antecedents. We are goal-directed creatures."

The higher processes of integration and association—that is, what we call **mental processes**—are first and foremost a function of the **cerebral cortex**. It is primarily the vast number of neurons in this part of the brain that explains the unique adaptability and learning capacity of human beings. Indeed, the human brain not only permits adaptation to extremely varied environments, it also enables us to change our environment to suit our needs. This entails enormous possibilities but also dangers, because we produce changes that are favorable in the short run but in the long run might threaten the existence of our species.

STUDYING THE STRUCTURE AND FUNCTION OF THE NERVOUS SYSTEM

Some of the many methods used for the study of the nervous system are described in the following chapters—that is, in conjunction with discussion of results produced by the methods. Here we limit ourselves to some general features of neurobiological research.

Many approaches have been used to study the structure and function of the nervous system, from straightforward observations of its macroscopic appearance to determination of the function of single molecules. In recent years we have witnessed a tremendous development of methods,

so that today problems can be approached that were formerly only a matter of speculation. The number of neuroscientists has also increased almost exponentially, and they are engaged in problems ranging from molecular genetics to behavior. Although the mass of knowledge in the field of neurobiology has increased accordingly, more importantly, the understanding of how our brains work has improved considerably. Nevertheless, the steadily expanding amount of information makes it difficult for the scientist to have a fair knowledge outside his or her specialty. It follows that the scientist may not be able to put findings into the proper context, with danger of drawing erroneous conclusions

Traditionally, methods used for neurobiological research were grouped into those dealing with **structure** (neuroanatomy) and those aiming at disclosing the **function** of the structures (neurophysiology, neuropsychology). The borders are far from sharp, however, and it is typical of modern neuroscience that anatomic, physiological, biochemical, pharmacological, psychological, and other methods are combined. Especially, cell biological methods are being applied with great success. Furthermore, the introduction of modern computer-based imaging techniques has opened exciting possibilities for studying the relation between structure and function in the living human brain. More and more of the methods originally developed in cell biology and immunology are being applied to the nervous system, and we now realize that neurons are not so different from other cells as was once assumed.

Animal Experiments Are Crucial for Progress

Only a minor part of our present knowledge of the nervous system is based on observations in humans; most has been obtained in experimental animals. In humans we are usually limited to a comparison of symptoms that are caused by naturally occurring diseases, with the findings made at postmortem examination of the brain. Two cases are seldom identical, and the structural derangement of the brain is often too extensive to enable unequivocal conclusions.

In animals, in contrast, the experimental conditions can be controlled, and the experiments may be repeated, to reach reliable conclusions. The properties of the elements of neural tissue can be examined directly—for example, the activity of single neurons can be correlated with the behavior of the animal. Parts of the nervous system can also be studied in isolation—for example, by using tissue slices that can be kept viable in a dish (*in vitro*) for hours. This enables recordings and experimental manipulations to be done, with subsequent structural analysis of the tissue. Studies in invertebrates with a simple nervous system have made it possible to discover the fundamental mechanisms that underlie synaptic function and the functioning of simple neuronal networks.

When addressing questions about functions specific to the most highly developed nervous systems, however, experiments must be performed in higher mammals, such as cats and monkeys, with a well-developed cerebral cortex. Even from such experiments, inferences about the human nervous system must be drawn with great caution. Thus, even though the nervous systems in all higher mammals show striking similarities with regard to their basic principles of organization, there are important differences in the relative development of the various parts. Such anatomic differences indicate that there are functional differences as well. Thus, results based on the study of humans, as in clinical neurology, psychiatry, and psychology, must have the final word when it comes to functions of the human brain. But because clinicians seldom can experiment, they must often build their conclusions on observations made in experimental animals and then decide whether findings from patients or normal volunteers can be explained on such a basis. If this is not possible, the clinical findings may raise new problems that require studies in experimental animals to be solved. Basically, however, the methods used to study the human brain are the same as those used in the study of experimental animals.

Ethics and Animal Experiments

Experiments on animals are often criticized from an ethical point of view. But the question of whether such experiments are acceptable cannot be entirely separated from the broader question of whether mankind has the right to determine the lives of animals by using them for food, by taking over their territories, and so forth. With regard to using animals for scientific purposes, one has to realize that a better understanding of human beings as thinkers, feelers, and actors requires, among other things, further animal experiments. Even though cell cultures and computer models may replace some of them, in the foreseeable future we will still need animal experiments. Computer-based models of the neuronal interactions taking place in the cerebral cortex, for example, usually require further animal experiments to test their tenability.

Improved knowledge and understanding of the human brain is also mandatory if we want to improve the prospects for treatment of the many diseases that affect the nervous system. Until today, these diseases—most often leading to severe suffering and disability—have only occasionally been amenable to effective treatment. Modern neurobiological research nevertheless gives hope, and many promising results have appeared in the last few years. Again, this would not have been possible without animal experiments.

Yet there are obviously limits to what can be defended ethically, even when the purpose is to alleviate human suffering. Strict rules have been made by government authorities and by the scientific community itself to ensure that only properly trained persons perform animal experiments and that the experiments are conducted so that discomfort and pain are kept at a minimum. Most international neuroscience journals require that the experiments they publish have been conducted in accordance with such rules.

Sources of Error in All Methods

Even though we will not treat systematically the sources of error inherent in the various methods discussed in this book, certainly all methods have their limitations. One source of error when doing animal experiments is to draw premature conclusions about conditions in humans. In general, all experiments aim at isolating structures and processes so that they can be observed more clearly. However necessary this may be, it also means that many phenomena are studied out of their natural context. Conclusions with regard to how the parts function in conjunction with all of the others must therefore be speculative.

Purely anatomic methods also have their sources of error and have led to many erroneous conclusions in the past about connections between neuronal groups. In turn, such errors may lead to misinterpretations of physiological and psychological data. The study of humans also entails sources of error—for example, of a psychological nature. Thus, the answers and information given by a patient or a volunteer are not always reliable; for example, the patient may want to please the doctor and answer accordingly.

Revising Scientific "Truths" from Time to Time

That our methods have sources of error and that our interpretations of data are not always tenable are witnessed by the fact that our concepts of the nervous system must be revised regularly. Reinterpretations of old data and changing concepts are often made necessary by the introduction of new methods. As in all areas of science, conclusions based on the available data should not be regarded as final truths but as more or less probable and preliminary interpretations. Natural science is basically concerned with posing questions to nature. How understandable and unequivocal the answers are depends on the precision of our questions and how relevant they are to the problem we are studying: stupid questions receive stupid answers. It is furthermore fundamental to science—although not always easy for the individual scientist to live up to—that conclusions and interpretations be made without any bias and solely on the strength of the facts and the arguments. It should be irrelevant whether the scientist is a young student or a Nobel laureate.

The Central Nervous System

I | MAIN FEATURES OF STRUCTURE AND FUNCTION

GENERAL information about the structure and function of the nervous system forms a necessary basis for treatment of the specific systems described in subsequent parts of this book. **Chapters 1** and **2** describe the structure of nervous tissue and some basic features of how neurons are interconnected, while **Chapters 3, 4,** and **5** deal with the functional properties of neurons as a basis for understanding communication between nerve cells. **Chapter 6** provides an overview of the macroscopic (and, to some extent, the microscopic) structure of the nervous system with brief descriptions of functions. **Chapter 7** treats the membranes covering the central nervous system, the cavities within the brain, and the cerebrospinal fluid produced in these. Finally, **Chapter 8** describes the blood supply of the brain and the spinal cord.

1 | Structure of the Neuron and Organization of Nervous Tissue

OVERVIEW

The nervous system is built up of nerve cells, **neurons**, and special kinds of supporting cells, **glial cells** (discussed in Chapter 2). The nerve cells are responsible for the functions that are unique to the nervous system, whereas the glial cells are non-neuronal cells that primarily support and protect the neurons. Neurons are composed of a cell body called the **soma** (plural somata) and several processes. Multiple short **dendrites** extend the receiving surface of the neuron, while a single **axon** conducts nerve impulses to other neurons or to muscle cells. Neurons are characterized by their ability to respond to stimuli with an electrical discharge, a **nerve impulse**, and, further, by their fast **conduction** of the nerve impulse over long distances. In this way, signals can be transmitted in milliseconds from one place to another, either within the central nervous system (CNS) or between it and organs in other systems of the body. When the nerve impulse reaches the **synapse**, which is the site of contact between the axon and the next neuron, a substance called a **neurotransmitter** is released from the **axon terminal** that conveys a chemical signal from one neuron to the next.

Neurons are classified into two broad groups: **projection neurons** that transmit signals over long distances and **interneurons** that mediate cooperation among neurons that lie grouped together. Many axons are surrounded with a **myelin sheath** to increase the speed of impulse propagation. Nervous tissue contains some areas that look gray—**gray matter**—and others that look whitish—**white matter**. White matter consists of axons and no neuronal somata, and the color is due to the whitish color of myelin. Gray matter consists mainly of somata and dendrites, which have a gray color. Neuronal somata are collected in groups sharing connections and functional characteristics. In the CNS, such a group is called a **nucleus** and in the peripheral nervous system (PNS), a **ganglion**. A bundle of axons that interconnect nuclei is called a **tract**. A nerve connects the CNS with peripheral organs. Groups of neurons that are interconnected form complex **neuronal networks** that are responsible for performing the tasks of the CNS. A fundamental principle of the CNS is that each neuron influences many others (**divergence**) and receives synaptic contacts from many others (**convergence**). A neuron contains a cytoskeleton consisting of various kinds of neurofibrils. They are instrumental in forming the neuronal processes and in transport of substances along them. By **axonal transport**, building materials and signal substances can be brought from the cell soma to the nerve terminals (anterograde transport), and signal substances are carried from the nerve terminal to the soma (retrograde transport).

NEURONS AND THEIR PROCESSES

Neurons Have Long Processes

Like other cells, a neuron has a **cell body** with a nucleus surrounded by cytoplasm containing various organelles. The nerve cell body is also called the perikaryon or **soma** (Figs. 1.1, 1.2, and 1.3). Long processes extend from the cell body. The numbers and lengths of the processes can vary, but they are of two main kinds: **dendrites** and **axons** (Fig. 1.1). The dendrites usually branch and form dendritic "trees" with large surfaces that receive signals from other nerve cells. Each neuron may have multiple dendrites, but has only one axon, which is specially built to conduct the nerve impulse from the cell body to other cells. The axon may have many ramifications, enabling its parent cell to influence many other cells. Side branches sent off from the parent axon are termed **axon collaterals** (Fig. 1.1). The term **nerve fiber** is used synonymously with "axon."

Neurons Are Rich in Organelles for Oxidative Metabolism and Protein Synthesis

When seen in a microscopic section, the nucleus of a neuron is characterized by its large size and light staining (i.e., the chromatin is extended, indicating that much of the genome is in use). There is also a prominent nucleolus (Figs. 1.2 and 1.3). These features make it easy to distinguish a neuron from other cells (such as glial cells), even in sections in which only the nuclei are clearly stained. The many **mitochondria** in the neuronal cytoplasm are an indication of the high metabolic activity of nerve cells. The mitochondria depend entirely on

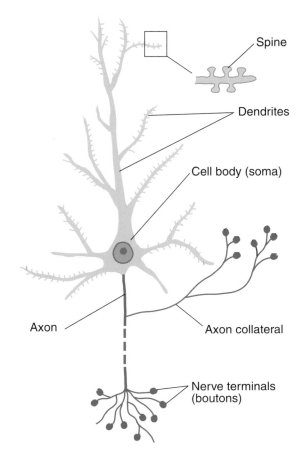

FIGURE 1.1 *A neuron.* Half-schematic to illustrate the neuron's main parts. The axon is red.

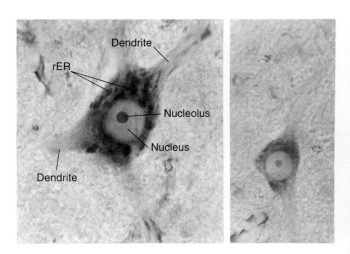

FIGURE 1.2 *Neuronal somata (cell bodies).* Two motor neurons, one small and one large, are shown. The large, pale nucleus has a distinct nucleolus. Only the cell body and the proximal parts of the dendrites are visible with the staining method used here. The stain (thionine) binds primarily to nucleic acids (DNA in the nucleus and RNA in the cytoplasm and nucleolus). The deeply stained clumps in the cytoplasm represent aggregates of rough endoplasmic reticulum (rER). Photomicrographs taken with a light microscope of a 20 μm thick section of the spinal cord. Magnification, ×800.

aerobic adenosine triphosphate (ATP) production and, unlike those in most other cell types, cannot utilize anaerobic ATP synthesis. **Glucose** is the substrate for ATP production in the mitochondria of nerve cells, which cannot, unlike in muscle cells, for example, use fat.

Neuronal somata also contain conspicuous amounts of free ribosomes and **rough endoplasmic reticulum** (**rER**) for synthesis of proteins. Large clumps of rER are seen via light microscopy in the cytoplasm of neurons greater than a certain size (Figs. 1.2 and 1.3). These were called tigroid granules or Nissl bodies long before their true nature was known. There are also as a rule several Golgi complexes, which modify proteins before they are exported or inserted in membranes. The large neuronal production of proteins probably reflects the enormous neuronal surface membrane, which contains many protein molecules that must be constantly renewed. Membrane proteins, for example, form ion channels and receptors (binding sites) for neurotransmitters, are constantly being recycled.

Dendrites Are Equipped with Spines

To study the elements of nervous tissue, it is necessary to use thin sections that can be examined microscopically.

Different staining methods make it possible to distinguish the whole neuron or parts of it from the surrounding elements (Figs. 1.2 and 1.4). It then becomes evident that the morphology of neurons may vary, with regard to both the size of the cell body and the number, length, and branching of the dendrites (Fig. 1.2; see also Figs. 33.5–6). The size of the dendritic tree is related to the number of contacts the cell can receive from other nerve cells. Dendrites often have small spikes, **spinae** (sing. spina) or **spines**, which are sites of contact with other neurons (Figs. 1.1, 1.7, and 1.8). The axons also vary, from those that ramify and end close to the cell body to those that extend for more than 1 meter (see Fig. 1.10; see also Figs. 21.3, 33.5, and 33.6). These structural differences are closely connected to functional differences.

Most Neurons Are Multipolar

Most neurons have several processes and are therefore called **multipolar** (Fig. 1.5). Special kinds of neurons, however, may have a different structure. Thus, neurons that conduct sensory signals from the receptors to the CNS have only one process that divides close to the cell body. One branch conducts impulses from the receptor toward the cell soma; the other conducts impulses toward and into the CNS. Such neurons are called **pseudounipolar** (Fig. 1.5). In accordance with the usual definition, the process conducting signals toward the cell body should be termed a dendrite. In terms of both structure and function, however, this process must be regarded as an axon. Some neurons have two processes, one conducting

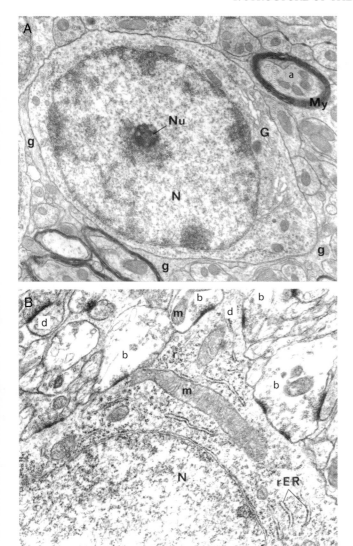

FIGURE 1.3 *Ultrastructure of the neuron*. Electron micrograph showing the cell body of a small neuron (**A**) and parts of a larger neuron (**B**). The nucleus (N) is light, due to extended chromatin, and contains a nucleolus (Nu). The cytoplasm contains rough endoplasmic reticulum (rER) and a Golgi complex (G)—that is, organelles involved in protein synthesis. The presence of many mitochondria (m) reflects the high oxidative metabolism of neurons. Nerve terminals, or boutons (b), forming axosomatic and axodendritic synapses are also seen. Glial processes (g) follow closely the surface of the cell body and the dendrites (d). a, axon; My, myelin. Magnifications, ×9000 (top) and ×15,000 (bottom).

toward the cell body, the other away from it (Fig. 1.5). Such neurons, present in the retina (see Fig. 16.7) and the inner ear (see Fig. 17.5B), are called **bipolar**. Also in these neurons both processes function as axons.

Communication between Nerve Cells Occurs at Synapses

The terminal branches of an axon have club-shaped enlargements called **boutons** (Figs. 1.1 and 1.6).

The term **terminal bouton** is used when the bouton sits at the end of an axon branch, and we also use the term **nerve terminal**. In other instances, the bouton is only a thickening along the course of the axon, with several such **en passage boutons** along one terminal branch (Fig. 1.8). In any case, the bouton lies close to the surface membrane of another cell, usually on the dendrites or the cell body. Such a site of close contact between a bouton and another cell is called a **synapse**. In the PNS, synapses are formed between boutons and muscle cells. The synapse is where information is transmitted from one neuron to another. This transmission does not occur by direct propagation of the nerve impulse from one cell (neuron) to another, but by liberation of signal molecules that subsequently influence the other cell. Such a signal molecule is called a **neurotransmitter** or, for short, a **transmitter** (the term "transmitter substance" is also used). The neurotransmitter is at least partly located in small vesicles in the bouton called **synaptic vesicles** (Figs. 1.6 and 1.7). How the synapse and the transmitters work is treated in Chapters 4 and 5. Here we restrict ourselves to the structure of the synapse.

The membrane of the nerve terminal is separated from the membrane of the other nerve cell by a narrow cleft approximately 20 nm wide (i.e., 2/100,000 mm). This **synaptic cleft** cannot be observed under a light microscope. Only when electron microscopy of nervous tissue became feasible in the 1950s could it be demonstrated that neurons are indeed anatomically separate entities. In the electron microscope, one can observe that the membranes facing the synaptic cleft are thickened (Figs. 1.6 and 1.7), due to accumulation of specific proteins that are of crucial importance for transmission of the synaptic signal. Many of these protein molecules are receptors for neurotransmitters; others form channels for passage of charged particles. The membrane of the bouton facing the cleft is called the **presynaptic membrane**, and the membrane of the cell that is contacted is called the **postsynaptic membrane** (Fig. 1.6). We also use the terms pre- and postsynaptic neurons.

The **postsynaptic density** (Fig. 1.6; see also Fig. 4.17) connects to the cytoskeleton with actin filaments and other proteins. This connection probably anchors the postsynaptic receptors to the site of neurotransmitter release. In addition, certain proteins in the postsynaptic density, such as **cadherins**, bind to corresponding proteins in the presynaptic membrane to keep the nerve terminal in place (cadherins are present also in many other cell-to-cell contacts, e.g., in adherence contacts between epithelial cells). Other proteins in the postsynaptic density have modulatory actions on synaptic function, for example, by changing receptor properties. Synaptic modifications associated with learning involve structural and functional changes of the postsynaptic density.

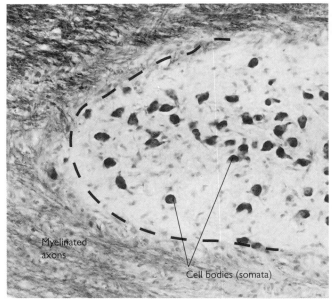

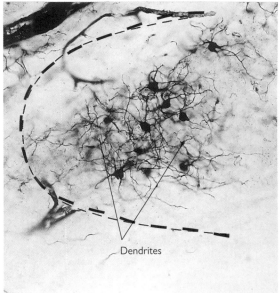

FIGURE 1.4 *Neurons*. Photomicrographs of sections stained with two different methods. **Left:** Only the cell bodies (somata) of a group of neurons are stained and visible in the section. The dark region surrounding the group of neurons contains myelinated fibers that are also stained. **Right:** The same cell group, but treated via the Golgi method so that the dendrites and the cell bodies are visualized. Magnification, ×150.

Synapses formed on the cell soma are called **axosomatic**, while synapses on dendrites are called **axodendritic** (Figs. 1.3 and 1.8). Where dendrites are equipped with spines, one or two **axospinous** synapses are always formed with the spine head (Figs. 1.7B, 1.8, and 1.9). The functional role of spines is not fully understood (see Chapter 4). Boutons may also form a synapse with an axon (usually close to a terminal bouton of that axon), and such synapses are called **axoaxonic** (Fig. 1.8 and 1.9B). This enables selective control of one terminal only without influencing the other terminals of the parent axon. Axoaxonic synapses thus increase the precision of the signal transmission.

There are many more axodendritic than axosomatic synapses because the dendritic surface is so much larger. Every neuron has many thousands of synapses on its surface, and the sum of their influences determines how active the postsynaptic neuron will be at any moment.

Two Main Kinds of Nerve Cell: Projection Neurons and Interneurons

Some neurons influence cells that are at a great distance, and their axons are correspondingly long (more than a meter for the longest). They are called **projection neurons**, or Golgi type 1 (Fig. 1.10). Neurons that convey signals from the spinal cord to the muscles are examples of projection neurons; other examples are neurons in the cerebral cortex with axons that contact cells in the brain stem and the spinal cord (see Fig. 33.5). As a rule, the axons of projection neurons send out branches, or **collaterals**, in their course (Figs. 1.1 and 1.11; see also Fig. 33.5). Thus, one projection neuron may send signals to neurons in various other parts of the nervous system.

FIGURE 1.5 *Neurons exemplifying three different arrangements of processes*. Multipolar (**A**), pseudounipolar (**B**), bipolar (**C**). Arrows show the direction of impulse conduction.

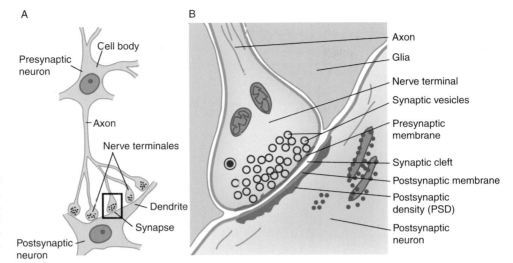

FIGURE 1.6 *The synapse.* **A:** Schematic overview of pre- and postsynaptic neurons **B:** The main structural elements of a typical synapse. Based on electron micrographs. Compare with Figs. 1.3 and 1.7.

The other main type of neuron is the **interneuron**, or Golgi type 2 (Fig. 1.10, see also Fig. 33.6), characterized by a short axon that branches extensively in the vicinity of the cell body. Its name implies that an interneuron is intercalated between two other neurons (Fig. 1.12). Even though, strictly speaking, all neurons with axons that do not leave the CNS are thus interneurons, the term is usually restricted to neurons with short axons that do not leave one particular neuronal group. The interneurons thus mediate communication between neurons within one group. Because interneurons may be switched on and off, the possible number of interrelations among the neurons within one group increases dramatically. The number of interneurons is particularly high in the cerebral cortex, and it is the number of interneurons that is so much higher in the human brain than in that of any other animal. The number of typical projection neurons interconnecting the various parts of the nervous system, and linking the nervous system with the rest of the body, as a rule varies more with the size of the body than with the stage of development.

The distinction between projection neurons and interneurons is not always very clear, however. Many neurons previously regarded as giving off only local branches have been shown via modern methods also to give off long axonal branches to more distant cell groups. Thus, they function as both projection neurons and interneurons. In contrast, many of the "classical" projection neurons, for example, in the cerebral cortex (Fig. 33.5), give off collaterals that end within the cell group in which the cell body is located.

Tasks of Interneurons

Figure 1.12 shows how an interneuron (b) is intercalated in an impulse pathway. One might perhaps think that the simpler direct pathway shown below from neuron A to neuron C would be preferable. After all, the

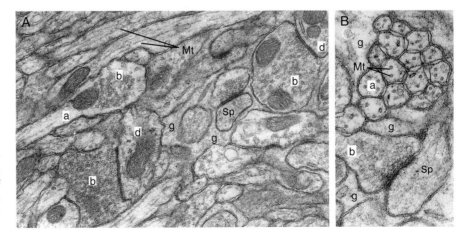

FIGURE 1.7 *Synapses.* **A, B:** Electron micrographs showing boutons (b) in synaptic contacts with dendrites (d), and dendritic spines (Sp). Note how processes of glia (g) cover the dendrites and nerve terminals except at the site of synaptic contact. Note bundle of unmyelinated axons (a) in **B.** Microtubules (Mt) are responsible for axonal transport. Magnifications, ×20,000 (**A**) and ×40,000 (**B**).

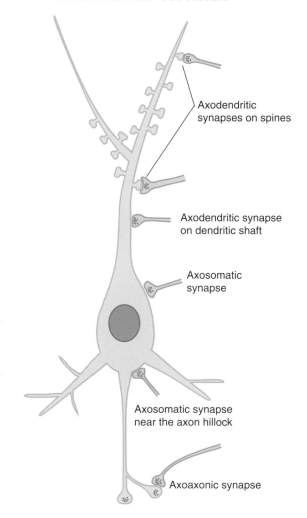

Axodendritic
synapses on spines

Axodendritic synapse
on dendritic shaft

Axosomatic
synapse

Axosomatic synapse
near the axon hillock

Axoaxonic synapse

FIGURE 1.8 *The placement of synapses.* The position of a synapse determines (together with other factors) its effect on the postsynaptic neuron. A synapse close to the exit of the axon, for example, has much greater impact that a synapse located on a distal dendrite.

interneuron leads to a delay in the propagation of the signal from A to C, and this would be a disadvantage. Most important, however, is that the interneuron provides added **flexibility**. Thus, whether the signal is transmitted from a to c can be controlled by other synaptic inputs to interneuron b. Identical synaptic inputs to a neuron a may in one situation be propagated further by neuron c but in another situation not, depending on the state of interneuron b. This kind of arrangement may partly explain why, for example, identical stimuli may cause pain of very different intensity: interneurons along the pathways conveying sensory signals are under the influence of other parts of the brain (e.g., neurons analyzing the meaning of the sensory stimulus).

Figure 1.13 illustrates another important task performed by interneurons. Interneuron B enables neuron A to act back on itself and reduce its own firing of impulses. The arrangement acts to prevent neuron A from becoming excessively active. Thus, the **negative feedback** provided by the interneuron would stop the firing of neuron A. Such an arrangement is present, for example, among motor neurons that control striated muscle contraction (see Fig. 21.14).

Many Axons Are Isolated to Increase the Speed of Impulse Propagation

The velocity with which the nerve impulse travels depends on the diameter of the axon, among other factors. In addition, how well the axon is insulated is of crucial importance. Many axons have an extra layer of insulation (in addition to the axonal membrane) called a **myelin sheath**. Such axons are therefore called **myelinated**, to distinguish them from those without a myelin sheath, which are called **unmyelinated** (see Figs. 2.6 and 2.7).

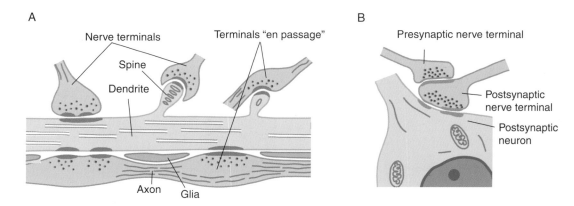

A

Nerve terminals

Spine

Dendrite

Terminals "en passage"

Axon   Glia

B

Presynaptic nerve terminal

Postsynaptic
nerve terminal

Postsynaptic
neuron

FIGURE 1.9 **A:** *Axodendritic synapses.* A nerve terminal (bouton) may form a synapse directly on the shaft of the dendrite or on a spine. The axon may also have several boutons en passage. **B:** *Axoaxonic* synapse. The presynaptic nerve terminal influences—by usually inhibiting—the release of neurotransmitter from the postsynaptic nerve terminal.

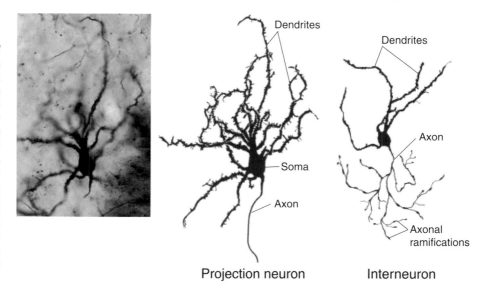

FIGURE 1.10 *Projection neuron and interneuron.* A projection neuron sends its axon to neurons in other nuclei (cell groups), often at a long distance. The axon of an interneuron ramifies and makes synaptic contacts in its vicinity (within the same nucleus). Examples from the brain stem of a monkey, based on sections treated via the Golgi method, which impregnate the whole neuron with silver salts. The photomicrograph to the left is from the Golgi-stained section containing the drawn projection neuron. The depth of field is only a fraction of the thickness of the section (100 µm). Therefore, only part of the projection neuron is clearly visible in the photomicrograph.

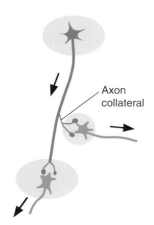

FIGURE 1.11 *Collateral of a projection neuron.* By sending off collaterals, a projection neuron may establish synapses in different cell groups (nuclei). Arrows show the direction of impulse conduction.

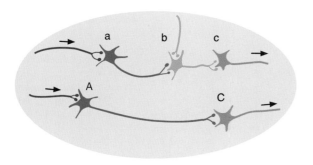

FIGURE 1.12 *An interneuron (b) intercalated in a pathway from neuron a to neuron c.* This arrangement increases the flexibility, as compared with the direct pathway from neuron A to C shown below. Arrows show the direction of impulse conduction.

Many of the tasks performed by the nervous system require very rapid conduction of signals. If unmyelinated axons were to do this, they would have to be extremely thick. Nerves bringing signals to the muscles of the hand, for example, would be impossibly thick, and the brain would also have to be much larger. Insulation is thus a very efficient way of saving space and expensive building materials. Efficient insulation of axons is, in fact, a prerequisite for the dramatic development of the nervous system that has taken place in vertebrates as compared with invertebrates.

Myelin and how it is formed is treated in Chapter 2, while the conduction of nerve impulses is discussed Chapter 3.

White and Gray Matter

The surfaces made by cutting nervous tissue contain some areas that are whitish and others that have a gray color. The whitish areas consist mainly of myelinated axons, and the myelin is responsible for the color; such regions are called **white matter**. The gray regions, called **gray matter**, contain mainly cell bodies and dendrites (and, of course, axons passing to and from the neurons). The neurons themselves are grayish in color. Owing to this difference in color, one can macroscopically identify regions containing cell bodies and regions that contain only nerve fibers in brain specimens (Fig. 1.14).

Neurons Are Collected in Nuclei and Ganglia

When examining sections from the CNS under the microscope, one sees that the neuronal cell bodies are not diffusely spread out but are collected in groups.

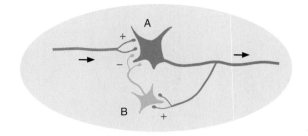

FIGURE 1.13 *An interneuron (B) mediates negative feedback to the projection neuron (A).* Arrows show the direction of impulse conduction.

Such a group is called a **nucleus** (Figs. 1.14, 1.15, and 1.16). Neurons collected in this manner share connections with other nuclei and constitute in certain respects a **functional unit**; thus, the neurons in a nucleus receive the same kind of information and act on the same (or similar) target. In the PNS, a corresponding collection of cell bodies is called a **ganglion**.

Axons that end in a nucleus are termed afferent, whereas axons that leave the nucleus are efferent. We also use the terms afferent and efferent for axons conducting toward and away from the CNS, respectively. Thus, sensory axons conveying information from sense organs are afferent, while the motor axons innervating muscles are efferent.

Axons Form Tracts and Nerves

Axons from the neurons of one nucleus usually have common targets and therefore run together, forming bundles. Such a bundle of axons connecting one nucleus with another is called a **tract** (tractus; Figs. 1.15 and 1.16). In the PNS, a collection of axons is called a **nerve** (nervus; Fig. 1.16, see also Figs. 11.1 and 28.3). We also use the term **peripheral nerve** to emphasize that a nerve is part of the PNS. Tracts form white matter of the CNS, and likewise, peripheral nerves containing myelinated axons are whitish.

Schematically, the large tracts of the nervous system are the main routes for nerve impulses—to some extent, they are comparable to highways connecting big cities. In addition, there are numerous smaller pathways often running parallel to the highways, and many smaller bundles of axons leave the big tracts to terminate in nuclei along the course. The number of smaller "footpaths" interconnecting nuclei is enormous, making possible, at least theoretically, the spread of impulses from one nucleus to almost any part of the nervous system. Normally, the spread of impulses is far from random but, rather, is highly ordered and patterned. As a rule, the larger tracts have more significant roles than the smaller ones in the main tasks of the nervous system. Consequently, diseases affecting such tracts usually produce marked symptoms that can be understood only if one has a fair knowledge of the main features of the wiring patterns of the brain.

COUPLING OF NEURONS: PATHWAYS FOR SIGNALS

In addition to the properties of synapses, which determine the transfer of signals among neurons, the function of the nervous system depends on how the various neuronal groups (nuclei) are interconnected (often called

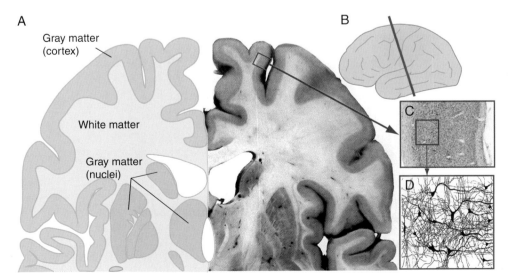

FIGURE 1.14 *Gray and white matter.* **A:** Drawing and photograph of an unstained frontal section through the human brain. **B:** The white matter consists only of axons and glial cells, whereas the gray matter contains the cell bodies, dendrites, and nerve terminals. **C:** Low-power photomicrograph of a section through the cerebral cortex (frame in A) stained so that only neuronal somata are visible (as small dots) **D:** Drawing of neurons in a section through the cerebral cortex (Golgi method). Only a small fraction of the neurons present in the section are shown.

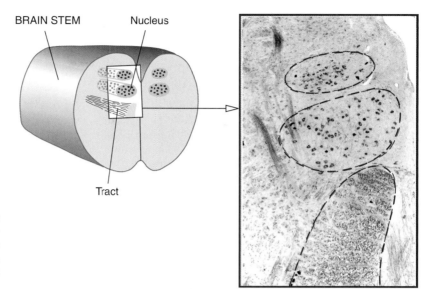

FIGURE 1.15 *Nucleus and tract.* **Left:** Schematic of part of the brain stem, showing the three-dimensional shape of two nuclei and a tract. **Right:** Photomicrograph showing the same structures in a section stained to visualize somata and myelinated axons. Magnification, ×75.

the **wiring pattern** of the brain). This pattern determines the pathways that signals may take and the possibilities for cooperation among neuronal groups. Thus, although each neuron is to some extent a functional unit, it is only by proper cooperation that neurons can fulfill their tasks. We will describe here some typical examples of how neurons are interconnected, as such general knowledge is important for understanding the specific examples of connections dealt with in later chapters.

Divergence and Convergence

A fundamental feature of the CNS is that each neuron influences many—perhaps thousands—of others; that is, information from one source is spread out. This phenomenon is called **divergence** of connections. Figure 1.17 shows schematically how a sensory signal (e.g., from a fingertip) is conducted by a sensory neuron to the spinal cord and there diverges to many spinal neurons. Each of the spinal neurons acts on many neurons at higher levels.

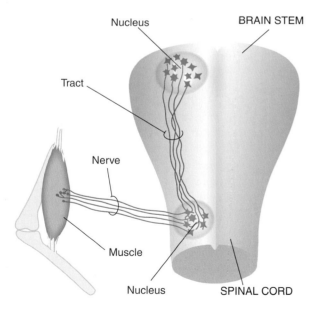

FIGURE 1.16 *Nucleus, tract, and nerve.* Three-dimensional schematic of parts of the brain stem, spinal cord, and a muscle in the upper arm. Axons from a nucleus in the brain stem form a tract destined for a nucleus in the spinal cord. The axons of the neurons in the spinal nucleus leave the CNS and form a nerve passing to the muscle.

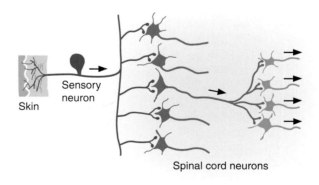

FIGURE 1.17 *Divergence of neural connections.* Highly simplified diagram. The axon collaterals of one sensory neuron contact many neurons in the spinal cord (red). Each of the spinal neurons contacts many other neurons (blue) in the cord or in the brain stem. In this way, the signal spreads from one neuron to many others. Arrows show the direction of impulse conduction.

Another equally ubiquitous feature, **convergence** of connections, is shown schematically in Fig. 1.18. It means that each neuron receives synaptic contacts from many other neurons. The motor neuron in Fig. 1.18 controls the contraction of a number of striated muscle cells (but could have been almost any neuron in the CNS). The motor neuron receives synaptic contacts from many sources (peripheral sense organs, motor neurons in the cerebral cortex that initiate voluntary movements, and so forth). In this case, the motor neuron represents the **final common pathway** of all the neurons acting on it.

The nerve impulses may not necessarily follow all the available pathways shown in Figs. 1.17 and 1.18 because, as a rule, many synapses must be active almost simultaneously to make a neuron fire impulses. Thus, more than one of the blue neurons in Fig. 1.18 must be active at the same time to bring the motor neuron to fire impulses and make the muscle contract. This phenomenon is termed summation and is exemplified further in Fig. 1.19. The many synapses axon a makes on neuron A brings the latter to fire a series of nerve impulses whenever axon a is active. But because of fewer synapses, the impact of axon a on neurons B and C is too weak to make them fire impulses. If, however, axons b and c are active simultaneously with a, their effects are summated so that neurons B and C may fire impulses. Summation is discussed further in Chapter 4.

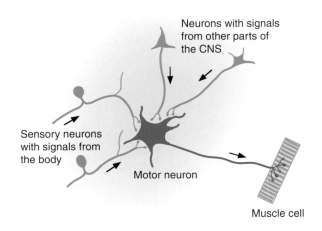

FIGURE 1.18 *Convergence of neural connections.* Synaptic inputs from many neurons (blue) converge onto one neuron (red). In this example, the red neuron is motor and sends its axon to striated muscle cells. The sum of all converging synaptic inputs determines the frequency of impulses sent from the motor neuron to the muscle cells—and thus their strength of contraction. Arrows show the direction of impulse conduction.

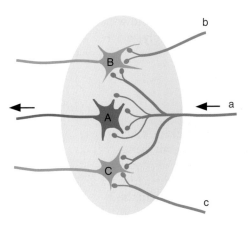

FIGURE 1.19 *Summation.* Many synapses must act on a neuron at the same time to make it fire impulses. Axon a makes many synaptic contacts with neuron A, and their effects summate so that the neuron A fires impulses. In contrast, axon a forms only few synapses with neurons B and C and is not able on its own to fire these neurons. If, however, also axons b and c send impulses at the same time as a, summation ensures that neurons B and C fire impulses. Arrows show the direction of impulse conduction.

Parallel Pathways and Reciprocal Connections

Figure 1.20 illustrates common types of connections among neuronal groups (nuclei). Figure 1.20A shows the principle of **parallel pathways**. There is one direct pathway from nucleus N1 to N2, and one indirect pathway that is synaptically interrupted in other nuclei (n1 and n2). Thus, some of the information reaching N2 is a direct consequence of the activity in N1, whereas information passing through n1 and n2 is modified by other connections acting on these nuclei (not shown). The abundance of such parallel pathways in the human cerebral cortex is one of the factors that explain its enormous flexibility and capacity for information processing (Fig. 1.23). Parallel pathways may, further, be of practical importance after partial **brain injury**. If, for example, the direct pathway between N1 and N2 is interrupted, the indirect one may at least partly take over the tasks formerly performed by the direct one (examples of this are discussed in Chapter 11, under "Restitution of Function").

Reciprocal connections represent another common arrangement, in which a nucleus receives connections from the nuclei to which it sends axons (Fig. 1.20B). In many cases, such back-projections serve as **feedback**, whereby the first nucleus is informed of the outcome of the impulses emitted to the second one. If the influence was too strong, the feedback may serve to reduce activity, and vice versa if the influence was too weak. Among other actions, such feedback connections serve to stabilize the functioning of the nervous system. Thus, many of the symptoms appearing in neurological diseases are due to the failure of feedback mechanisms. Often, however, it is not obvious which one should be regarded as a feedback connection and which one as a **feed-forward** connection. Presumably, a single pathway may serve both purposes.

Couplings Contributing to Continuous Neuronal Activity

There is always electric activity in the CNS, because numerous neurons are firing impulses at any given time. In the cerebral cortex, for example, even during sleep there is considerable neuronal activity. How is this activity sustained, even in the absence of sensory inputs? In early embryonic life, groups of neurons become spontaneously active—that is, they fire impulses without any external influence (this is caused by development of special membrane properties). As the nervous system matures, neuronal behavior is governed more and more by synaptic connections with other neurons; nevertheless, some neurons remain spontaneously active. Another feature contributing to continuous activity is that, when activated, most neurons fire a train of impulses, not just one. Further, interneurons contribute to prolongation of activity, as schematically exemplified in Fig. 1.21. Impulses in axon a make neuron A fire impulses, propagated along its axon. At the same time, axon a makes interneuron 1 fire impulses, which act on neuron A and interneuron 2. The latter acts on neuron A to produce impulses. Owing to a delay of a few milliseconds at each synapse and the time for conducting the impulse in the axons, neuron A receives synaptic inputs over a prolonged period. This kind of coupling (in reality far more elaborate than shown in Fig. 1.21) can translate a brief synaptic input to long-lasting neuronal firing in a neuronal network. Working memory, that is, the ability to keep task-relevant information in mind for a while, depends on neurons that continue firing after a stimulus has stopped.

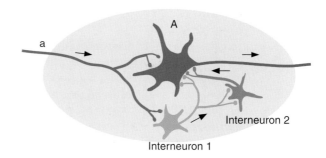

FIGURE 1.21 *Interneurons that prolong the activity of a projection neuron (A) when activated by impulses in axon a.* Arrows show the direction of impulse conduction.

Connections between the Two Halves of the Central Nervous System

Another important general feature of the CNS is that many nuclei have connections with both sides of the brain—so-called **bilateral connections** (Fig. 1.22A). Some tracts supply both sides with approximately the same number of axons (i.e., equal numbers of crossed and uncrossed axons), whereas other tracts are predominantly crossed (contralateral), with only a few axons supplying the same (ipsilateral) side. Although the functional significance of such bilateral connections may not always be clear, they can contribute to recovery of function after partial brain damage.

That the two sides of the CNS cooperate extensively is witnessed by the vast number of **commissural connections**—that is, direct connections between corresponding parts in the two brain halves (Fig. 1.22B). Such connections occur at all levels of the CNS, but the most prominent one connects the two halves of the cerebral hemispheres (corpus callosum; see Figs. 3.26 and 3.27). In humans, this pathway contains approximately 200 million axons.

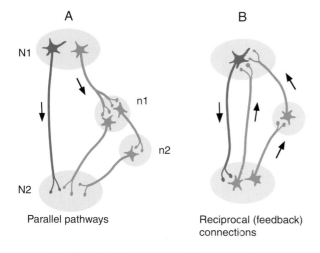

FIGURE 1.20 *Examples of organization of neuronal pathways.* Arrows show the direction of impulse conduction; N1, N2, n1, and n2 are nuclei in different parts of the CNS.

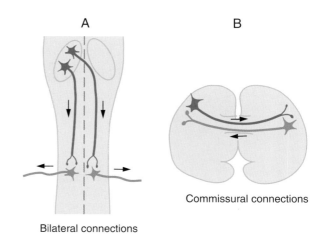

FIGURE 1.22 *Examples of organization of neuronal pathways.* Arrows show the direction of impulse conduction.

Single Neurons Are Parts of Neural Networks

The tasks of a neuron can be understood only in conjunction with the thousands of neurons with which it is synaptically interconnected. Further, functions of the brain are very seldom the responsibility of one neuronal group or "center" but, rather, the result of cooperation among many neuronal groups. Such cooperating groups or nuclei often lie far apart. For example, proper voluntary movements require cooperation among specific neuronal groups in the cerebral cortex, the cerebellum, and the basal ganglia deep in the cerebral hemispheres. Today we use the term **distributed system** rather than **center** when referring to the parts of the brain that are responsible for a specific function. Such a distributed system is a complicated **neural network** of spatially separate but densely interconnected neuronal groups. Figure 1.23 gives a very simplified example of such a network that could be dedicated to, for example, the subjective sensation of pain. Owing to the abundance of reciprocal connections, the signal traffic can take various routes within the network, and each neuronal group has connections outside the network. This means that a variety of inputs can activate the network—all presumably giving the same functional result (the sensation of pain, a specific memory, an emotion, and so forth). Nevertheless, it should not be surprising that each group, or **node**, might participate in several different, function-specific networks. Thus, as a rule one neuronal group participates in several tasks.

The organization of the brain in distributed systems is particularly clear with regard to **higher mental functions**. Language is a good example: there is not one center for language but specific neuronal groups in many parts of the cerebral cortex that cooperate. Other networks are responsible for attention, spatial orientation, object identification, short-term memory, and so forth.

Data-based models of neural networks have provided new insight into the workings of the cerebral cortex and how symptoms arise from partial destruction of networks.

Injuries of Neural Networks

An important feature of distributed systems is that **partial damage** can degrade their performance but seldom eliminate it. Sometimes partial damage may become evident only in situations with very high demands, for example, with regard to the speed and accuracy of movements, the capacity of short-term memory, and so forth. If the number of neurons participating in the network undergoes further reduction, however, performance may deteriorate severely. In such cases, symptoms may occur rather abruptly, even though the disease process responsible for the cell loss may have been progressing slowly for years. This is typical of degenerative brain diseases such as Parkinson's disease and Alzheimer's disease.

THE CYTOSKELETON AND AXONAL TRANSPORT

The cell bodies and processes of neurons contain thin threads called **neurofibrils**, which can be observed in specially stained microscopic sections (Fig. 1.24). The neurofibrils are of different kinds, but together they form the **cytoskeleton**—the name refers to its importance for development and maintenance of **neuronal shape**. The fact that neurons have very different shapes—with regard to dendrites, cell bodies, and axons—is due to cytoskeletal specializations. For example, the neurofibrils have a decisive role when axons grow for long distances, and the cytoskeleton serves to anchor synaptic elements at the postsynaptic density (see Fig. 4.6).

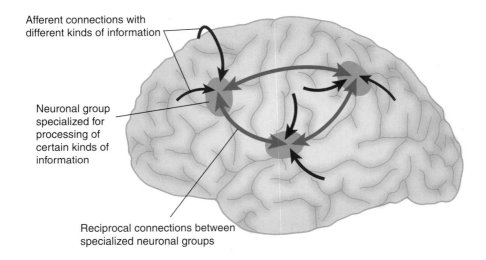

Afferent connections with different kinds of information

Neuronal group specialized for processing of certain kinds of information

Reciprocal connections between specialized neuronal groups

FIGURE 1.23 *Distributed neural networks.* Simplified. Three regions (groups of neurons) in the cerebral cortex are interconnected by reciprocal connections (red arrows). The collective activity of all parts of the network is responsible for its "product"— for example, the sensation of pain.

The neurofibrils of the cytoskeleton are also responsible for another important cellular function: the transport of **organelles** and **particles** in the neuronal processes. Although such transport takes place in both dendrites and axons, **axonal transport** (Fig. 1.25) has been most studied (mainly because, for technical reasons, transport in dendrites is much harder to study). It is obvious that neurons need direction-specific transport mechanisms. Thus, the organelles necessary for protein synthesis and degradation of particles are present almost exclusively in the cell body. Nevertheless, dendrites contain small amounts of mRNA located at the base of dendritic spines, which may enable a limited amount of protein synthesis important for synaptic changes related to learning and memory.

Transport from the cell body toward the nerve terminals is called **anterograde** axonal transport (Fig. 1.25). Examples of particles transported anterogradely are mitochondria, synaptic vesicles, proteins to be inserted in the axonal membrane, and enzymes for transmitter synthesis and degradation in the nerve terminals. Growth factors, synthesized in the cell body but liberated far away at the synapses, also require efficient anterograde axonal transport. Transport toward the cell body from the nerve terminals is called **retrograde** axonal transport. Retrograde transport brings signal molecules of various kinds that are taken up by the nerve terminals to the cell body (Fig. 1.25). Often such molecules are produced by postsynaptic cells and released to the extracellular space. In the cell body (nucleus) the signal molecules can influence genetic expressions—that is, they can change protein synthesis. In this way, the properties of the neuron can be changed transiently or in some instances permanently. This is a form of **feedback**: ensuring that the neuron is informed of its effects on other cells and of the state of its target cells. In some instances, neurons even require this kind of feedback to survive. Retrograde transport also moves "worn-out" organelles to the cell body for degradation in lysosomes.

Components of the Cytoskeleton

Electron microscopic and biochemical analyses have shown that the cytoskeleton consists of various kinds of fibrillary proteins, making threads of three main kinds:

1. **Actin filaments** (microfilaments) and associated protein molecules (approximately 5 nm thick)
2. **Microtubules** (narrow tubes) and associated proteins (approximately 20 nm thick)
3. **Intermediary filaments** or neurofilaments (approximately 10 nm thick)

Actin (microfilaments) is present in the axon, among other places. There it has an important role during development. When the axon elongates, actin together with microtubules serves to produce movements of the **growth cone** (Fig. 9.16) at the tip of the axon (in general, actin is present in cells capable of movement, such as muscle cells). The growth cone continuously sends out thin fingerlike extensions (filopodia) in various directions. These probably explore the environment for specific molecules that mark the correct direction of growth. In addition, actin is probably important in maintaining the shape of the fully grown axon.

Microtubules and **microtubule-associated proteins** (MAPs) are present in all kinds of neuronal processes and are most likely important for their shape (Figs. 1.7 and 2.7). Of special interest is the relation of microtubules to the transport of substances in the neuronal processes. As mentioned, there is a continuous movement of organelles, proteins, and other particles in the axons and dendrites. Destruction of microtubules by drugs (such as colchicine) stops axonal transport.

The functional role of the **intermediary filaments** (neurofilaments) is uncertain, although they make up about 10% of axonal proteins. One function might be to maintain the diameter of thick myelinated axons, as internal scaffolding. Whatever their normal role is, it is noteworthy that neurofilaments are altered in several degenerative neurological diseases. In Alzheimer's disease, for example, a characteristic feature is disorganized

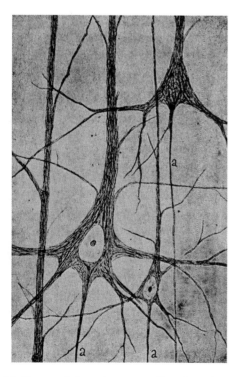

FIGURE 1.24 *The cytoskeleton in neurons.* Drawing of neurons from the cerebral cortex, as appearing in sections stained with heavy metals to visualize neurofibrils. Both dendrites and axons (a) contain numerous neurofibrils. (From Cajal 1952.)

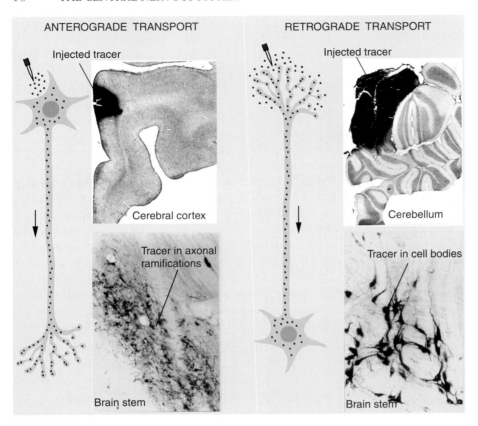

ANTEROGRADE TRANSPORT

Injected tracer

Cerebral cortex

Tracer in axonal ramifications

Brain stem

RETROGRADE TRANSPORT

Injected tracer

Cerebellum

Tracer in cell bodies

Brain stem

FIGURE 1.25 *Axonal transport.* The photomicrographs illustrate the use of axonal transport for tract tracing, that is, to map the connections in the CNS. A cat received injections of an enzyme (horse-radish peroxidase, HRP) in the cerebellum and in the cerebral cortex (0.2 μL in each). The enzyme was taken up by endocytosis of neuronal cell bodies and terminals. Vesicles with enzyme were then transported anterogradely from the cerebral cortex to the brain stem (**left**) and retrogradely from the cerebellum to the brain stem (**right**). A black reaction product in the upper photomicrographs shows the extension of the tracer at the injection site. The anterogradely labeled terminal ramifications of the axons appear as black dust in the left lower photomicrograph, while retrogradely labeled cell bodies are seen in the right lower photomicrograph. Magnifications, ×8 (**upper**) and ×150 (**lower**)

tangles of intermediary filaments in the cerebral cortex (neurofibrillary tangles).

More about Axonal Transport and Its Machinery

The injection of radioactively labeled substances taken up by neurons has shown that axonally transported material moves in at least **two phases**. One phase is **rapid**, with particles moving up to half a meter per day; the other is **slow**, with movement of between 1 and 3 mm per day. The rapid phase carries mainly organelles and vesicles, that is, membrane-bound structures. The slow phase carries primarily enzymes and components of the cytoskeleton. As mentioned, microtubules are of particular importance for axonal transport. Each microtubule is composed of smaller building blocks of the protein **tubulin**. **MAPs** help the formation of tubes from many tubulin molecules. MAPs also anchor the microtubules to the cell membrane and to other parts of the cytoskeleton, such as neurofilaments. Two kinds of MAPs found only in neurons—**MAP2** and **tau**—stiffen the microtubules. Specific kinds of MAPs perform

anterograde and retrograde transport, respectively, serving as the "motors" of axonal transport. These MAPs are ATPases (enzymes that split ATP), and the released energy alters their form, thus producing movement. The transported particles, such as vesicles and mitochondria, move by temporarily binding to MAPs protruding from the microtubule, so that they appear to "walk" along the microtubule. One microtubule can transport in both directions, depending on the kind of motor to which a particle binds. Proteins belonging to the **kinesin** family are responsible for anterograde movement. Different varieties of kinesin appear to transport different "cargo"; for example, one variety transports mitochondria and another transports precursors of synaptic vesicles. **Dynein**, which is a more complex protein than kinesin, is responsible for the bulk of retrograde transport, although certain kinesins probably also contribute.

Injections into nervous tissue of substances that are transported axonally and later can be detected in tissue sections are widely used for tract tracing, that is, to reveal the "wiring pattern" of the brain (Fig. 1.25).

2 | Glia

OVERVIEW

Glial cells are the most numerous cells in the brain and are indispensable for neuronal functioning. Glial cells are of three kinds that differ structurally and functionally. **Astrocytes** have numerous processes that contact capillaries and the lining of the cerebral ventricles. They serve important **homeostatic functions** by controlling the concentrations of ions and the osmotic pressure of the extracellular fluid (water balance), thereby helping to keep the neuronal environment optimal. Astrocytes also take part in **repair processes**. **Oligodendrocytes** insulate axons by producing **myelin sheaths** in the central nervous system (CNS). **Microglial** cells are the **macrophages** of nervous tissue. **Schwann cells** are a specialized form of glial cells that form myelin sheaths in the peripheral nervous system (PNS). Apart from these specific functions, glial cells are involved in the prenatal **development** of the nervous system, for example, by providing surfaces and scaffoldings for migrating neurons and outgrowing axons.

TYPES OF GLIAL CELLS

Although they do not take part in the fast and precise information processing in the brain, glial cells are nevertheless of crucial importance to proper functioning of neurons. In fact, the number of glial cells in the brain is much higher than the number of neurons. The name *glia* derives from the older notion that glial cells served as a kind of glue, keeping the neurons together. Although improved methods have revealed hitherto unknown properties of glial cells, much still remains to be understood about their functional roles in the nervous system.

It is customary to group glial cells into three categories: **astrocytes**, or astroglia; **oligodendrocytes**, or oligodendroglia; and **microglial cells**, or microglia. Each is structurally and functionally different from the others. Astrocytes have numerous processes of various shapes whereas oligodendrocytes have relatively few and short processes (*oligo* means few, little). In routinely stained sections, glial cells can be distinguished from neurons by their much smaller nuclei. The identification of the various types, however, requires immunocytochemical methods to identify proteins that are specific to each type.

Specialized Forms of Glial Cells

In addition to the three main kinds, there are other, specialized forms of glial cells. The surface of the cavities inside the CNS is lined with a layer of cylindrical cells called **ependyma** (Fig. 2.3; see also Fig. 9.6). There are also special types of glial cells in the retina (**Müller cells**), the cerebellum (**Bergman cells**), and the posterior pituitary gland (**pituicytes**).

GLIAL CELLS AND HOMEOSTASIS

Astrocytes Contact Capillaries, Cerebrospinal Fluid, and Neurons

Astrocytes have structural features that make them well suited to control the extracellular environment of the neurons:

1. They have numerous short or long processes that extend in all directions (Figs. 2.1 and 2.2). Thus, the astrocytes have a very **large surface area** that enables efficient exchange of ions and molecules with the extracellular fluid (ECF).

2. Some processes contact the surface of **capillaries** with expanded **end "feet"** and cover most of the capillary surface (Figs. 2.3 and 2.4).

3. Some processes form a continuous, thin sheet (membrana limitans, also called glia limitans) where nervous tissue borders the **cerebrospinal fluid** (CSF), that is, in the cavities inside the CNS and against the connective tissue membranes on its exterior (Fig. 2.3).

4. Other processes contact **neuronal surfaces**; in this manner, parts not contacted by boutons are covered by glia (Figs. 2.3 and 2.5). Glial processes usually enclose the nerve terminal (see Figs. 1.6 and 1.7).

5. Numerous **gap junctions** (nexus) couple astrocytes, allowing free passage of ions and other small particles among them (Fig. 2.4). Thus, apart from allowing electric currents to spread, astrocytes form continuous, large fluid volumes for distribution of substances removed from the ECF.

Glial Cells Communicate with Electric Signals and Influence Cerebral Blood Flow

Although glial cells do not send precise signals over long distances, they can produce brief electric impulses

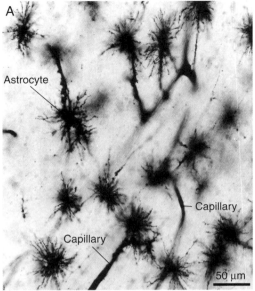

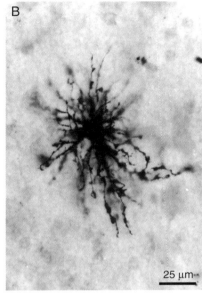

FIGURE 2.1 *Astrocytes.* Photomicrographs of Golgi-stained sections from the cerebral cortex. No neurons are visible. Note the close relationship between astrocytic processes and capillaries.

(currents) by opening of membrane **channels for Ca^{2+}**. Such an opening can be evoked by binding of neurotransmitters (e.g., glutamate) to G-protein–coupled receptors in the glial cell membrane. Thus, neuronal activity can directly influence the astrocytes, whereas the latter affects neuronal activity. Owing to the electric coupling (nexus) of the astrocytes, the "calcium signal" can presumably spread rapidly in networks of astroglial cells, and thus influence many neurons almost simultaneously, which, among other roles, can help synchronize the activity of neurons in a group. In light of the electric coupling among astrocytes, one might expect the population of neurons influenced by an astrocytic network to be quite large. Recent data, however, indicate that the population can be surprisingly small, enabling spatially precise interactions among neurons and astrocytes. Thus, although it is well known that a specific sensory input (e.g., from a small spot in the visual field) activates neurons in a precisely defined, small part of the cortex, recent experiments (Schummers et al. 2008) suggest that astroglial cells are activated in a similarly precise manner (although a few seconds later than the neurons). Presumably, inputs from the periphery activate neurons that in turn activate astrocytes in their immediate vicinity. When activated, the astrocytes increase local **blood flow** (see Chapter 8, under "Regional Cerebral Blood Flow and Neuronal Activity").

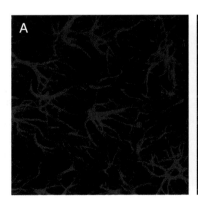

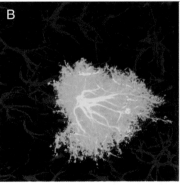

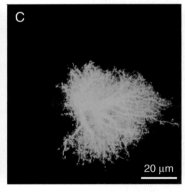

FIGURE 2.2 *Astrocytes.* **A:** Astrocytic processes visualized using an antibody against glial fibrillary acidic protein (GFAP) present in intermediary filaments. The antibody was labeled with a substance with red fluorescence. **B:** One of the astrocytes in A has been filled completely with intracellular injection of a substance with green fluorescence (Lucifer yellow), and reconstructed three-dimensionally. It is obvious that the astrocytic processes are much more abundant and of finer caliber than in **A. C:** View of the injected astrocyte in **B** in isolation, showing to advantage its dense and bushy halo of processes. (Reproduced with permission from Wilhelmsson et al. (2004) and *The Journal of Neuroscience.*)

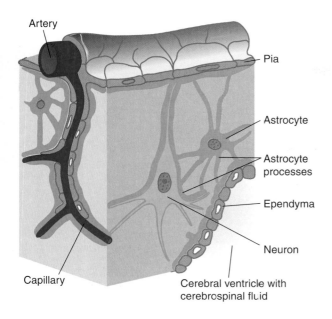

FIGURE 2.3 *The relationship between astroglia and neurons, blood vessels and the CSF.* The astrocytes cover the surface of the neurons and are also closely related to vessels, ependymal cells, and the innermost part of the cerebral meninges (pia).

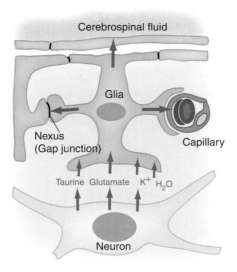

FIGURE 2.4 *Astroglia and the homeostasis of nervous tissue.* Schematic shows the close contacts between astroglial cells on the one hand and neurons, capillaries, and the CSF on the other. The astroglial cells are coupled by nexus (gap junctions), and thus form a large fluid volume for distribution of substances. Some important substances handled by astroglia are indicated (the transport is not always in the direction of the arrows). Surplus of water, K^+ ions, and the amino acid taurine can be transported to the blood and the CSF, thereby preventing their accumulation in the ECF. Next to glutamate, taurine is the amino acid with the highest concentration in the CNS and therefore significantly contributes to the osmolarity of the ECF. Taurine does not appear to function as a neurotransmitter, but its transport in and out of astroglia may be a mechanism for controlling the volume of the neurons. The neurotransmitter glutamate is treated differently, however. Glutamate is transformed to glutamine after uptake in glia, and thus loses its transmitter actions and becomes neutral to the neurons. Glutamine can therefore be returned to the ECF for subsequent uptake into neurons where it is used for resynthesis of glutamate. Because the neurons need large amounts of glutamate, this is an economic means to ensure a sufficient supply. (Based on Nagelhus 1998.)

Astroglia and the Control of Neuronal Homeostasis

Their intimate contact with neurons, capillaries, and the CSF places astroglial cells in a unique position to control the environment of the neurons, that is, the extracellular (interstitial) fluid of the brain (see Fig. 1.28). Such control is vitally important for three main reasons. First, neurons are exquisitely sensitive to changes in extracellular concentrations of ions and neurotransmitters. Second, the osmotic pressure (the water concentration) must be tightly controlled because the brain cannot expand in the skull. Third, adding even minute amounts of a substance may produce a substantial increase in its extracellular concentration, owing to the very limited extracellular space in the brain (less than 20% of total volume), as illustrated in electron micrographs showing only narrow slits between the cellular elements (see Figs. 1.3 and 1.7). Further, the tortuous shape of the extracellular space hampers free diffusion of particles.

With regard to extracellular **ions**, the control of K^+ (potassium ions) is particularly important. Thus, neuronal excitability is strongly influenced even by small changes in the amount of K^+ ions extracellularly, and as neurons fire impulses, K^+ ions pass out of the cell (Fig. 2.4). Prolonged or intense neuronal activity would therefore easily produce dangerously high extracellular levels of K^+ ions were it not for their efficient removal by glia. Further, astrocytes contribute to **extracellular pH** control by removing CO_2.

Extracellular **neurotransmitter concentration** must be tightly controlled, because proper synaptic functioning requires that their extracellular concentrations be very low, except during the brief moments of synaptic release. Most neurotransmitters are indeed removed from the ECF near the synapses by **transporter proteins** in the membranes of neurons and astrocytes. Specific transporters have been identified for several neurotransmitters (discussed further in Chapter 5). Figure 2.5 gives an impression of the abundance of a specific kind of transporter proteins (for the ubiquitous neurotransmitter glutamate, which is neurotoxic in abnormally high concentrations).

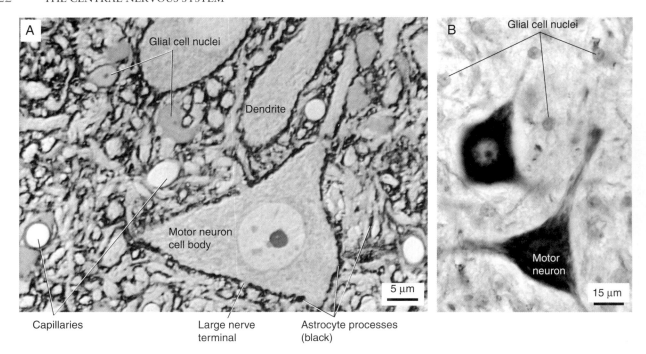

FIGURE 2.5 *Astroglial processes in nervous tissue*. **A:** Photomicrograph showing the distribution of a glutamate-transporter protein, as visualized via an immunocytochemical technique. In this 1 μm thick section from the spinal cord, the dark spots and bands are astrocytic processes expressing glutamate transporters. They outline the somata, dendrites, and capillaries. The picture illustrates both the capacity of astroglia to take up glutamate from the ECF and the enormous astroglial surface facing neurons and capillaries. The contours of dendrites and neuronal somata are uneven because of synaptic contacts (thin arrow) breaking the otherwise continuous layer of astroglia. Capillaries are marked with asterisks. The cell body of an astroglial cell is marked with a thick arrow. (Courtesy of Drs. J. Storm-Mathisen and N.C. Danbolt, Department of Anatomy, University of Oslo.) **B:** For comparison, a photomicrograph of a thionine-stained section from the same part of the spinal cord as in **A**.

As mentioned, astrocytes are also involved in the control of the extracellular osmotic pressure, that is, in controlling the **water balance** of the brain (Fig. 2.4). Of particular interest in this respect are channels for transport of water—**aquaporins**—that are present in the membranes of astrocytes. Aquaporins were first described in kidney tubular systems, where they were shown to increase significantly the capacity for water passage. Interestingly, in the brain they are most abundant on the glial processes that are in close contact with capillaries and the CSF, that is, where one would expect them to be if they were involved in brain water balance. Exchange by astroglial cells of small neutral molecules, such as the amino acid **taurine**, may be another mechanism to control extracellular osmolarity.

Finally, the layer of astrocytic processes surrounding brain capillaries helps to prevent many potentially harmful substances from entering the brain (see Chapter 7, under "The Blood–Brain Barrier").

Aquaporins in Health and Disease

Two varieties of aquaporin are present in the brain. **AQP4** is located in the astrocyte membrane, and particularly concentrated in the end-feet region close to capillaries and in glial processes bordering the CSF. **AQP1** is present in epithelial cells of the choroid plexus (which produces the CSF; see Chapter 7). In general, aquaporins increase water permeability of the cell membrane, thus allowing water to follow active ion transport. A function of AQP4 in the normal brain is probably to export water. Thus, AQP4-deficient mice have increased ECF volume compared to normal mice. Further, in so-called **vasogenic brain edema**, wherein water accumulates extracellularly, AQP4 contributes to removal of excess water. This kind of edema arises when the brain capillaries become leaky due to, for example, traumatic brain injury. On the other hand, when water accumulates intracellularly, as typically occurs in cerebral ischemia or hypoxia (e.g., in stroke), the presence of AQP4 seems to *increase* the edema by allowing more water to enter the astrocytes. Such **cytotoxic brain edema** is caused by failure of energy-dependent ion pumping, which reduces the ability of the cells to maintain osmotic stability. Brain edema is a serious and often life-threatening complication in many brain disorders, such as stroke and traumatic brain injuries. Therefore, the discovery of a relationship between aquaporins and brain edema led to an intensive search for drugs that can modulate the activity of aquaporins.

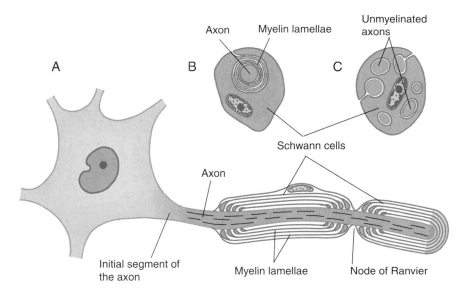

FIGURE 2.6 *Myelin sheath, myelination, and unmyelinated axons.* Schematics based on electron microscopic observations. **A:** Cell body with proximal parts of the dendrites and myelinated axon. The myelin sheath consists of lamellae formed by the membrane of glial cells (oligodendroglia, or Schwann cells). Each cell produces one segment of myelin. The node of Ranvier is the site of contact between two segments of myelin. The nerve impulse usually starts in the initial segment of the axon, and then "jumps" from one node of Ranvier to the next. **B:** Cross section of an axon in the process of becoming myelinated. The myelin sheath is formed when a glial cell wraps itself around the axon. **C:** Unmyelinated axons in the peripheral nervous system are surrounded by Schwann cell cytoplasm.

In animal experiments, inhibitors of AQP4 can reduce cytotoxic edema whereas they seem to worsen vasogenic edema. This complicates the search for the ideal drug because in human brain disorders the two kinds of brain edema usually coexist (although one may dominate depending on the specific disorder).

INSULATION AND PROTECTION OF AXONS

Oligodendrocytes and Schwann Cells

The myelin sheaths, which insulate axons, are formed by oligodendrocytes[1] in the CNS and by Schwann cells in the PNS. Although the structure and function of the myelin sheaths they produce are the same,[2] oligodendrocytes and Schwann cells are not identical. One difference is that a single oligodendrocyte usually sends out processes to produce myelin segments for several axons (up to 40), whereas each Schwann cell forms a myelin segment for only one axon (Fig. 2.6). A particularly interesting difference concerns their differential influence on **regeneration** of damaged axons. In the PNS, a cut axon can regenerate under favorable conditions, provided that viable Schwann cells are present. In the CNS, however, such regeneration of axons does not normally occur, mainly because of inhibiting factors produced by oligodendrocytes.

In addition to forming myelin sheaths, oligodendrocytes and Schwann cells are important for survival of the axons. Thus, diseases affecting oligodendrocytes or Schwann cells produce axonal loss in addition to loss of myelin. In addition, oligodendrocytes and Schwann cells influence axonal thickness and axonal transport.

The Myelin Sheath

The **myelin sheath** forms an insulating cylinder around the axons (Fig. 2.6), reducing the loss of current from the axon to the surrounding tissue fluid during impulse conduction. This contributes to the much higher conduction velocity in myelinated axons than in unmyelinated axons (discussed further in Chapter 3 under "Impulse Conduction in Axons"). The thickest myelinated axons conduct at approximately 120 m/sec (versus less than 1 m/sec in unmyelinated axons).

The myelin sheath consists almost exclusively of numerous layers of cell membrane, as evident from electron micrographs (Figs. 2.6 and 2.7). The layers, or **lamellae**, are formed when a glial cell wraps itself around the axon (Fig. 2.6B). During this process, the cytoplasm of the glial cell is squeezed away so that the layers of cell membrane lie closely apposed. The composite of material ensheathing the axons is called **myelin**. Myelin is whitish in color because of its high lipid content.

The cell membrane forming the myelin has a unique lipid and protein composition. Among other components, myelin has a high content of cholesterol and various **glycolipids**. The glycolipids appear to be crucial

---

1 We do not know whether *all* oligodendrocytes form myelin. Thus, their cell bodies are often closely apposed to neuronal cell bodies, suggesting that they may have other tasks in addition to myelination.

2 Even though the myelin sheaths produced by oligodendroglial cells and by Schwann cells look the same, they differ significantly in their lipid and protein composition. For example, myelin basic protein (MBP) makes up a much larger fraction of the total myelin protein in the CNS than in the PNS, whereas **peripheral myelin protein-22** (PMP-22) is absent in the CNS. Another example is **myelin-oligodendrocyte glycoprotein** (MOG), which is expressed in the CNS only. Such differences may help explain why some diseases affect only myelinated axons in the CNS (e.g., multiple sclerosis), whereas others are restricted to peripheral axons.

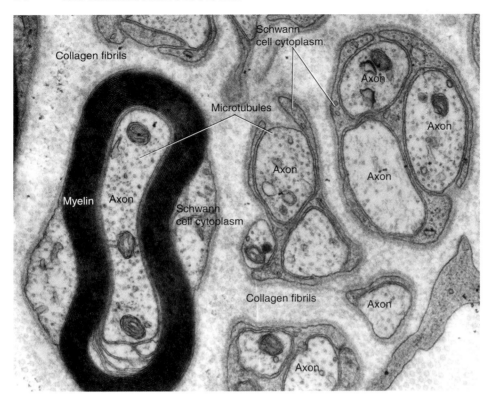

FIGURE 2.7 *Myelinated and unmyelinated axons.* (Detail from Fig. 2.8.) An axon is surrounded by myelin. The myelin lamellae are seen as dark stripes, arranged concentrically. The cytoplasm of the Schwann cell that is responsible for producing the myelin is seen externally. The unmyelinated axons are completely surrounded by Schwann cells. Between the axons are numerous collagen fibrils. Magnification, ×30,000.

for the insulating properties of myelin. Certain **membrane proteins** related to the immunoglobulins bind the external (apposing) sides of the membranes tightly together. Another membrane protein, **myelin basic protein** (MBP), seals the cytoplasmic sides of the membranes in the myelin lamellae so that very little cytoplasm (with poor insulating properties) takes up space in the myelin sheath. Mice with a mutation of the *MBP* gene make abnormal myelin and develop serious movement disorders.

Myelination of the axons starts prenatally, but many neural pathways in the human are not fully myelinated until 2 years after birth (see Chapter 9, under "Myelination"). The process of myelination is closely related to functional maturation of the brain.

Nodes of Ranvier

Longitudinal views of axons show that the myelin sheath is interrupted at intervals, forming the **nodes of Ranvier** (Fig. 2.6A). The nodes of Ranvier exist because the glial cells forming myelin lie in a row along the axon, each cell making myelin only for a restricted length, or segment, of the axon. When viewed in the electron microscope, the axolemma (the axonal membrane) is "naked" at the node; that is, it is exposed to the ECF. Thus, only at the node of Ranvier can current in the form of ions pass from the axon to the ECF (and

in the opposite direction). This arrangement makes it possible for the nerve impulse to "jump" from node to node, thus increasing the speed of impulse propagation (discussed further in Chapter 3). The distance between two nodes of Ranvier in the PNS may be 0.5 mm or greater.

Multiple Sclerosis

In demyelinating diseases of the nervous system, the myelin sheaths degenerate. The most common of these diseases is **multiple sclerosis** (MS), which typically manifests in young adults and usually has a long course of increasing disability. Its cause is still unknown, but most likely environmental factors precipitate an inflammatory process in individuals with a certain inherited susceptibility. Histopathologically, isolated and apparently randomly distributed regions of inflammation and demyelination are characteristic. In these regions, called **plaques**, impulse conduction in the axons is severely slowed or halted, and usually the symptoms are ascribed to the loss of myelin. For some reason, the optic nerve is often the first to be affected, resulting in reduced vision. Later symptoms that usually occur in varying proportions are muscle weakness, incoordination, and sensory disturbances. In most patients, exacerbations of the symptoms occur episodically in the beginning, associated with fluctuation in the inflammatory process.

Thus, periods of marked symptoms (such as paresis of extremities) are followed by periods of partial recovery. The improvement of symptoms is ascribed to partial remyelination of the affected regions. After a variable time (often many years), the disease becomes progressive, with a steady deterioration of the patient's condition.

There is not always a clear relationship between degree of demyelination and symptoms, suggesting that the disease process also directly harms axonal conductance and axonal viability. Indeed, it is now well established that in MS not only myelin sheets but also axons degenerate from the beginning of the disease. Presumably, the number of axons lost at early stages is modest and brain plasticity may compensate for their loss. As the disease progresses, however, the axon loss becomes so large that permanent and steadily progressing disability ensues.

Intense research activity is devoted to clarifying the etiology and pathogenesis of MS. Although clearly the disease process includes both inflammation and degeneration, it was long held that inflammation was the primary phenomenon (perhaps evoked by autoimmunity), and that loss of nervous tissue was secondary. This is now being questioned, however. Thus, it seems possible that "... people who develop multiple sclerosis will be shown to have a (genetically determined) diathesis [disease disposition] that does indeed predispose to neurodegeneration ... but the exposure of that vulnerability requires an inflammatory insult without which the degenerative component does not manifest" (Compston, 2006, p. 563).

With regard to the inflammatory process, **T lymphocytes, microglial cells, brain endothelial cells,** and numerous **immune mediators** are involved, but their relative contributions are not fully understood. The role of microglia illustrates the complexity: they may contribute both to destruction of myelin and axons and to regenerative processes (such as remyelination), presumably depending on the local situation.

Unmyelinated Axons

As mentioned, unmyelinated axons conduct much more slowly (at less than 1 m/sec) than myelinated ones, because they are thinner and lack the extra insulation provided by the myelin sheath. In the CNS, unmyelinated axons often lie in closely packed bundles without any glial cells separating them (see Fig. 1.7). In the PNS, however, unmyelinated axons are always ensheathed in Schwann cells that do not make layers of myelin

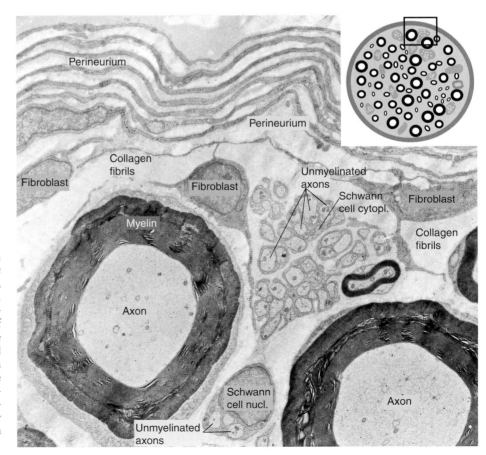

FIGURE 2.8 *Peripheral nerve.* Electron micrograph of cross section of the sciatic nerve. The picture shows a small, peripheral part of a nerve fascicle. The perineurium surrounding the fascicle, is formed by several lamellae of flattened cells. Note the large difference in diameter among various myelinated axons. The thickness of the myelin sheath increases apace with the increase in axonal diameter. Between the myelinated axons are numerous unmyelinated ones. Collagen fibrils, produced by fibroblasts, fill most of the space between the axons. Magnification, ×4000.

(Figs. 2.6–2.8). During early development, several axons become embedded in the cytoplasm of the Schwann cells by invagination of the Schwann cell membrane. This arrangement probably serves to protect the axon from harmful substances in the interstitial fluid. Such protection may not be necessary in the CNS, as the composition of the interstitial fluid is governed by astroglia cells and by the blood–brain barrier.

Peripheral Nerves Are Built for Protection of the Axons

Fresh nervous tissue is soft, almost jellylike, with virtually no mechanical strength in itself. Protection of the CNS against external mechanical forces is afforded by its location within the skull and the vertebral canal and by its "wrapping" in membranes of connective tissue (see Fig. 6.1). For peripheral parts of the nervous system, the situation is different. Often located superficially, the peripheral bundles of axons and groups of nerve cells are exposed to various mechanical stresses. They are also subject to considerable stretching forces by movements of the body. Axons can be stretched only slightly before their impulse conduction suffers, and they may even break. To prevent this, peripheral nerves contain large amounts of dense connective tissue with numerous collagen fibers arranged largely longitudinally (Fig. 2.7). The collagen fibers, specialized to resist stretching, protect the axons effectively. The presence of connective tissue in peripheral nerves is the reason that the nerves become much thicker where they leave the skull or the vertebral canal.

The connective tissue components of peripheral nerves form distinctive layers. The **epineurium** is an external thick layer of mostly longitudinally running collagen fibers. Internal to this layer, the axons are arranged into smaller bundles, or **fascicles**, which are wrapped in the perineural sheath **or perineurium** (Fig. 2.8). The collagen fibers and fibroblasts within the fascicles constitute the **endoneurium**. The perineurium is special in that it contains several layers of flattened cells. The cells, which in some respects resemble epithelial cells, interconnect by various kinds of junctions. In addition, the capillaries within the endoneurium are unusually tight and prevent passage of many substances from reaching the axons, consistent with experimental data showing that the perineurium constitutes a **blood–nerve barrier** preventing certain substances from reaching the interior of the fascicles with the axons. It is not surprising that PNS tissue also needs extra protective mechanisms to ensure that its environment is kept optimal for conducting impulses. The protection is not as efficient as in the CNS, however, and may perhaps explain why peripheral nerves are often subject to diseases that affect their conductive properties.

MICROGLIA AND REACTIONS OF THE CNS TO INJURY

Microglial Cells Are Phagocytes

The third kind of glial cell, **microglia,** is so named because of its small size. Studies with immunocytochemical identification of specific membrane proteins show unequivocally that microglial cells constitute a distinct kind. Estimates indicate that microglia may constitute 5% to 20% of all glial cells, being fairly evenly distributed through all parts of the CNS. Microglial cells are of **mesodermal** origin. Thus, animal experiments indicate that **monocytes** invade the nervous system from the bone marrow during embryonic development and perhaps shortly after birth. This may correspond with periods of high rate of cell death (a surplus of neurons is formed in early embryonic life, with subsequent elimination of a large number). After invading nervous tissue, the monocytes undergo changes—such as development of processes—that transform them to microglial cells, as identified in the adult. Nevertheless, microglial cells retain the typical phagocytic capacity of monocytes. Further, several surface markers (antigens) are common to blood monocytes and microglia, and cells that express such antigens first occur in the CNS (of rodents) in late embryonic development.

The number of microglial cells is relatively stable after the prenatal invasion. Under normal conditions, the stock of microglial cells does not appear to be supplemented from the bloodstream. After **injury**, the number of cells with phagocytic activity (macrophages) increases in the CNS. The increase appears to be due both to invasion of monocytes from the bloodstream and to activation of local microglial cells. The invasion of monocytes after injury probably depends on damage to the blood–brain barrier (i.e., brain capillaries allow passage of elements of the blood they normally restrict).

In the **normal brain**, microglial cells are probably not solely in a "resting: state in anticipation of challenges (e.g., intruding microorganisms, trauma, ischemia, and so forth). Thus, their processes are steadily moving and renewed, and are therefore believed to constantly "scan" their immediate environment for foreign material and sick or dead cellular elements. In addition, microglial cells are equipped with receptors for several neurotransmitters, suggesting that they also may sense the state of neuronal activity in their vicinity. If they detect something unusual, more microglial cells move quickly to the site. They release inflammatory mediators and phagocytose foreign or dead material. These responses of microglial cells generally serve to minimize damage and protect neurons; that is, microglial cells serve to conserve **homeostasis**. For example, animal experiments show that the presence of microglial cells reduces ischemic brain damage (after loss of blood supply). Removal of dead material by microglia seems to be necessary for regeneration of neuronal processes to occur. Nevertheless, in certain diseases with strong activation of microglial cells (and astrocytes) they promote tissue injury rather than repair. Activation of microglial cells in the spinal cord also seems to contribute to persistence of **pain** after nerve damage.

Reaction of Nervous Tissue to Injury and Inflammation

Tissue damage leads to an inflammatory reaction in which the invasion and activation of immunocompetent cells have a central role. The purpose of the invasion is to kill microorganisms, remove debris, and aid reparative processes. However, the inflammatory reaction is different in the CNS than in other tissues. Thus, there is often no invasion of neutrophil granulocytes, and the activation of microglia and invading monocytes to macrophages may take several days. Overall, immune reactions are weaker and slower in the CNS than elsewhere. This may be explained—at least in part—by the lack of lymphatic drainage from the CNS. The immune system, therefore, does not possess much information about nervous tissue conditions, in contrast to tissues of most other organs. Normally, only a small number of T lymphocytes, entering from the bloodstream, patrol the CNS.[3] Perhaps these special conditions are necessary to prevent neuronal damage from the potent substances that are liberated from granulocytes and activated macrophages. For example, edema—a central component of inflammation—may become harmful and even life threatening when it occurs in the brain (because of the limited possibilities of expansion within the skull). Nevertheless, immune reactions *do* occur in the brain, sometimes with serious consequences, as in multiple sclerosis.

The main task of **astrocytes** after injury is probably to strengthen their normal function of keeping the ECF composition constant. Tissue damage—regardless of whether it is caused by bleeding, contusion, or circulatory arrest—increases the flow of ions and transmitters from the neurons to the ECF. Astrocytes increase their uptake to counteract such disturbances of the neuronal environment. Because the substances taken up are osmotically active, the astrocytes may swell quickly: seconds or minutes after the damage (if the normal uptake capacity is surpassed). This may contribute to brain edema, a dangerous complication of head injuries. In the long term, astrocytes produce a kind of scar tissue at sites where neurons are lost.

In Chapters 9 and 11, we discuss the plastic processes of the nervous system that permit functional recovery after injuries (such as stroke).

Diseases of Peripheral Nerves

Diseases involving degeneration of peripheral nerves are called **neuropathies** and in humans can have various causes. In any case, the symptoms are due to transitory or permanent loss of impulse conduction. Neuropathy is a well known complication of metabolic diseases such as diabetes but can also be caused by toxic substances (e.g., lead). Some neuropathies are due to attacks of the immune system on axons or myelin. This sometimes occurs after an infectious disease or in the course of cancer, probably because the immune system produces antibodies that cross-react with normal antigens expressed by axonal or Schwann cell membranes. Axons express some antigens that are specific to whether the axons are motor or sensory, thick or thin, and so forth. Thus, it may be understandable why neuropathies often affect certain nerves only or certain kinds of axons only. Thus, when motor axons are affected, the patient presents with pareses in certain muscles, while affection of sensory axons might produce loss of cutaneous sensation and joint sense. Neuropathies may also affect subgroups of sensory axons, for example, affecting only the very thin axons mediating sensations of pain and temperature but sparing axons related to touch. In other cases only axons mediating joint sense are affected, whereas cutaneous sensation is spared (examples are described in Chapter 13, under "Clinical Examples of Loss of Sensory Information").

A large group of neuropathies is **inherited**, among them, **Charcot–Marie–Tooth disease** (peroneal muscle atrophy). In most cases, the disease is inherited dominantly. The disease usually starts before the age of 20 years and leads to gradually increasing pareses and sensory loss, starting distally in the legs. Loss of myelin and degeneration of axons cause the symptoms. Most patients with Charcot–Marie–Tooth disease have a doubling of the gene coding for the peripheral myelin protein (PMP-22). Animal models with overexpression of PMP-22 suggest that this defect alone can cause deficient myelination and symptoms corresponding to Charcot–Marie–Tooth disease in humans.

---

3 **HIV** (human immune deficiency virus) can enter the CNS via infected T lymphocytes. Microglial cells then become infected because they express surface receptors that bind the virus. After being infected, microglial cells secrete toxic substances that kill neurons, thus producing the neurological symptoms occurring in AIDS (acquired immune deficiency syndrome).

3 | Neuronal Excitability

OVERVIEW

In Chapter 1 we considered some of the characteristic properties of neurons, such as their excitability and their ability to conduct impulses. The term **excitability** means that when a cell is sufficiently stimulated, it can react with a brief electrical discharge, called an action potential. The **action potential** (the nerve impulse) travels along the axon and is a major component in the communication among nerve cells and between nerve cells and other cells of the body. The action potential results from movement of charged particles—ions—through the cell membrane. A prerequisite for such a current across the membrane is an electric potential—the **membrane potential**—between the interior and the exterior of the cell, and the presence of **ion channels** that are more or less selective for the passage of particular ions. The opening of ion channels is controlled by neurotransmitters binding to the channel (**transmitter or ligand-gated channels**) or by the magnitude of the membrane potential (**voltage-gated channels**). The membrane potential results from an unequal distribution of positively and negatively charged particles on either side of the membrane.[1] Energy-requiring **ion pumps** are responsible for maintaining the membrane potential. The **resting potential**, that is, the membrane potential when the neuron is not receiving any stimulation, is due mainly to unequal distribution of K^+ ions and the fact that the membrane is virtually impermeable to all ions other than K^+ in the resting state. The resting potential, with the interior of the cell negative compared with the exterior, is typically approximately –60 mV. The **action potential** is a brief change of the membrane potential, caused by opening of channels that allow cations (especially Na^+) to enter the neuron, followed by an outward flow of K^+ ions. A net influx of cations reduces the membrane potential by making the interior less negative. This is called **depolarization**, and if it is sufficiently strong, an action potential is elicited due to opening of voltage-gated Na^+ channels. After the brief depolarization caused by influx of Na^+ ions, the membrane potential is restored by the outward flow of K^+ ions. Restoration of the membrane potential is called **repolarization**. An increase of the membrane potential—hyperpolarization—makes the neuron less excitable (more depolarization is necessary to elicit an action potential). In a short period after an action potential, the membrane is in a **refractory state**, which means that another action potential cannot be elicited. This ensures that neurons can maintain the correct ion concentration balance. Once an action potential is elicited, it is conducted along the axon. This is not merely a passive movement of charged particles in the fluid inside the axon. Because axons are poor conductors (compared with a metal thread), the action potential has to be renewed along the axonal membrane by cycles of depolarization and repolarization. In **unmyelinated** axons, these cycles move along the axon as a continuous wave, while in **myelinated** axons renewal of the action potential occurs only at the **nodes of Ranvier**. Because the process of depolarization–repolarization takes some time, the speed of conduction is very much slower in unmyelinated axons than in myelinated ones. The action potential, when first elicited, is of the same magnitude. Neurons are nevertheless able to vary their messages because of the varying frequency and pattern of action potentials. Generally, the more synaptic inputs depolarize a neuron, the higher will be the frequency of axonal action potentials.

BASIS OF EXCITABILITY

Cell Membrane Permeability Is Determined by Ion Channels

Ions cross the cell membrane almost exclusively through specific, water-filled channels because their electrical charges prevent them from passing through the lipid bilayer (Figs. 3.1 and 3.2). The channels are more or less **selective** for particular ions, that is, some ions pass more easily through a channel than others. Some channels are very selective, allowing passage of only one kind of ion (e.g., Na^+ ions), whereas other channels are less selective (e.g., letting through several cations such as Na^+, K^+, and Ca^{2+}). It follows that the ease with which an ion can pass through the membrane—that is,

---

1 Neither membrane potentials nor action potentials are properties unique to nerve cells. All cells have a membrane potential, although usually of less magnitude than that of neurons. Muscle cells and endocrine gland cells also produce action potentials in relation to contraction and secretion, respectively.

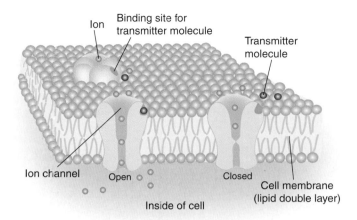

FIGURE 3.1 *Ion channels.* Schematic of a small part of the lipid bilayer of the cell membrane with interspersed ion channels. Binding of a transmitter molecule alters the opening state of the ion channel.

the **membrane permeability**[2] to that particular kind of ion—depends on (1) the presence of channels that let the ion through, (2) how densely these channels are distributed in the membrane, and (3) their opening state.

The current of ions through the membrane, however, does not depend solely on the density and opening of channels; an additional important factor is the **concentration gradient** across the membrane for the ion. That is, the steeper the gradient, the greater the flow of ions will be from high to low concentration (provided that the membrane is not totally impermeable to the ion). Further, because ions are electrically charged particles,

the **voltage gradient** across the membrane (i.e., the membrane potential) will also be important (Fig. 3.3). This means that if the interior of the cell is negative in relation to the exterior, the **cations** (positively charged ions) on the exterior will be exposed to a force that attracts them into the cell, while the interior cations will be subjected to forces that tend to drive them out. The strength of these attractive and expulsive forces depends on the magnitude of the membrane potential. Therefore, the concentration gradient and the membrane potential together determine the flow of a particular ion through the membrane (Fig. 3.3).

The Membrane Potential

In a typical nerve cell, the potential across the cell membrane is stable at approximately 60 mV (millivolts) in the resting state, that is, as long as the cell is not exposed to any stimuli. We therefore use the term **resting potential**

2 The term **conductance** expresses the membrane permeability of a particular kind of ion more precisely. The conductance is the inverse of the membrane resistance. In an electrical circuit the current is $I = V/R$, where V is the voltage and R is the resistance (Ohm's law). This may be rewritten by using conductance (g) instead of R, as $I = g \cdot V$. In this way, one may obtain quantitative measures of membrane permeability under various conditions. For our purpose, however, it is sufficient to use the less precise term permeability.

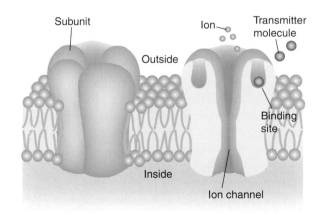

FIGURE 3.2 *Ion channels.* Five protein subunits are arranged around a central opening that can admit ions. At the outer side, the channel proteins are equipped with receptor sites for neurotransmitter molecules that regulate the opening of the channel. The figure shows the probable appearance of an acetylcholine receptor. (Based on Changeux 1993.)

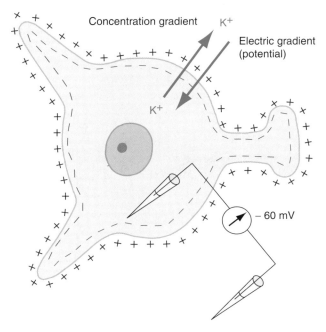

FIGURE 3.3 *Forces acting on the K⁺ ions.* At the resting potential there is equilibrium between the inward and outward forces (large arrows) acting on the K⁺ ions. One intracellular and one extracellular electrode (cones) measure the membrane potential.

in this situation (in different kinds of nerve cells, the resting potential may vary from about 45 mV to approximately 75 mV). The resting potential is due to a small surplus of negatively charged ions, **anions**, inside the cell versus the outside, and it has arbitrarily been decided to define the resting potential as negative, for example, –60 mV (Fig. 3.3).

The resting potential is caused primarily by two factors:

1. The **concentration of K⁺ ions** is about 30 times higher inside than outside the cell (Figs. 3.4 and 3.5).

2. The cell membrane is **selectively permeable** to K⁺ ions in the resting state (Fig. 3.5), that is, no other ions pass the membrane with comparable ease (the membrane, e.g., is about 50 times more permeable to K⁺ than to Na⁺).

Although the concentration differs greatly inside and outside the cell for ions other than K⁺ (Fig. 3.4), the membrane is, as mentioned, almost impermeable to them (there are, e.g., very few open Na⁺ channels in the resting state). Other ions therefore influence the resting membrane potential only slightly. Therefore, to explain the membrane potential we can, for the time being, ignore ions other than K⁺. The concentration gradient will tend to drive K⁺ out of the cell, and further, K⁺ ions can pass the membrane with relative ease through a particular kind of potassium channel that is open in the resting state. This means that positive charges are lost

from the interior of the cell, making the interior negative compared to the exterior, thereby creating a membrane potential. The membrane potential reaches only a certain value, however, because it will oppose the movement of K⁺ ions out of the cell. Two opposite forces are at work: the concentration gradient tending to drive K⁺ out of the cell and the electrical gradient (the membrane potential) tending to drive K⁺ into the cell (Fig. 3.3). When the membrane potential is about –75 mV, these two forces are equally strong: that is, the flow of K⁺ into the cell equals the flow out. This is therefore called the **equilibrium potential for K⁺**, and its magnitude is determined by the concentration gradient for K⁺ ions (the concentration gradient varies somewhat among neurons). The resting potential in most neurons, however, is lower than the equilibrium potential for K⁺ because the cell membrane is slightly permeable to Na⁺ (about 1/50th of the permeability to K⁺). Therefore, some positive charges (Na⁺) pass into the cell, driven by both the concentration gradient and the membrane potential, making the interior of the cell less negative than the equilibrium potential for K⁺. The membrane potential is consequently changed somewhat in the direction of the **equilibrium potential for Na⁺**: that is, +55 mV. In the resting state, the inflow of positive charges is equal to their outflow, and the membrane potential is therefore stable. Even though the two opposite currents of K⁺ and Na⁺ are small, over time they would eliminate the concentration gradients across the membrane. This is prevented, however, by energy-requiring "pumps" in the cell membrane that actively transport ions through the membrane against a concentration gradient. This **sodium–potassium pump** expels Na⁺ ions from the

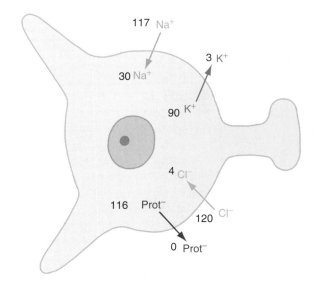

FIGURE 3.4 *Distribution of ions of particular importance for the membrane potential.* The exact concentrations depend on the resting potential (in this case –85 mV). Concentrations in mM.

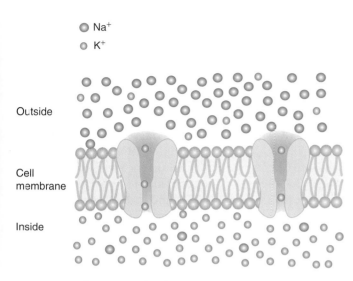

○ Na⁺
○ K⁺

Outside

Cell membrane

Inside

FIGURE 3.5 *The unequal distribution of K⁺ and Na⁺ ions, together with open K⁺ channels, largely explain the resting membrane potential.*

interior, in exchange for K⁺, at the same rate that the ions leak through the membrane. In this way, the concentration gradients across the cell membrane are maintained.

Normally, the extracellular K⁺ concentration is under tight control, as discussed in Chapter 2 ("Astroglia and the Control of Neuronal Homeostasis"). Such control is necessary because even small alterations in K⁺ concentration influence the excitability of neurons significantly. For example, increased extracellular concentration moves more K⁺ ions into the cell, thus depolarizing the neuron (making the membrane potential less negative) and lowering the threshold for eliciting action potentials.

Recording of Single-Cell Activity

Microelectrodes, with tips less than 1 μm thick, can be used to record the activity of single neurons and their processes (single units) intracellularly. Among other things, this has made it possible to study in detail the electrical events at the synapses and how they are influenced by various experimental manipulations. The effects of different concentrations of intra- and extracellular ions have been studied, as have the synaptic effects of various transmitter candidates and drugs. The **voltage clamp** technique, which permits manipulation of the membrane potential, has been instrumental to our understanding of the properties of synapses and the basic mechanisms underlying their operations. Likewise, great progress has been made with the **patch clamp technique**, making possible measurements of ion currents limited to even a single ion channel. The study of the properties of ion channels and membrane receptors is today highly interdisciplinary. **Implanted extracellular**

electrodes can be used to record the activity of single neurons in relation to specific stimuli or behavioral tasks. This method has, for example, provided new insight into functional specializations within various areas of the cerebral cortex. By combining anatomic and physiological techniques, it has been possible to determine the functional properties of structurally defined cell types. After an intracellular recording has been made from a neuronal cell body or its axon, it can be filled with a tracer substance through the same pipette. Afterward, the neuron with all its processes can be visualized in sections.

Anions Are Also Unevenly Distributed

For simplicity, we have so far dealt with only two cations, K⁺ and Na⁺, because they are the most important ones for the membrane potential and also for the action potential (discussed later in this chapter). Nevertheless, there are as many anions as cations. Chloride ions (Cl⁻) and negatively charged protein molecules (Prot⁻) are the major anions (Fig. 3.4). These ions are also unevenly distributed across the cell membrane: the concentration of Cl⁻ is 20 to 30 times higher outside than inside the cell, whereas the opposite situation exists for Prot⁻. Therefore, **chloride** is the major extracellular anion, whereas **proteins** are the major intracellular ones. The proteins are so large that they cannot pass through the membrane; the membrane is impermeable to protein molecules. The membrane is somewhat permeable to Cl⁻, however. The concentration gradient tends to drive chloride into the cell, whereas the membrane potential tends to drive it out, making the net flow of Cl⁻ small. In fact, the **equilibrium potential** for Cl⁻, –65 mV, is close to the resting potential of most nerve cells. Therefore, no active mechanism for pumping of chloride is needed.

The Sodium–Potassium Pump and Osmotic Equilibrium

All cells depend on the sodium–potassium pump to maintain the membrane potential and osmotic equilibrium between the intracellular and extracellular fluid compartments. Particular to neurons is their need for increased pumping in association with the firing of action potentials, which arise because of a current of Na⁺ into the cell and of K⁺ out of it. The speed of pumping increases with increasing intracellular Na⁺ concentration. A significant part of our energy in the form of ATP is spent on driving the sodium–potassium pump. In the resting state of nerve cells, this may constitute approximately one-third of the total energy requirement, whereas after high-frequency trains of action potentials it may increase to two-thirds.

The unequal distribution of ions is of fundamental importance also for the ability of neurons to maintain

osmotic equilibrium. The distribution of ions must be such that the total concentrations of water-dissolved particles are equal inside and outside the cell. In other words, osmotic equilibrium means that the **water concentration** is equal inside and outside the cell (osmosis is the movement of water molecules from sites of high to sites of low water concentration). In case of osmotic imbalance, the cell will either swell or shrink (depending on whether the water concentration is lower inside or outside, respectively). An essential condition for osmotic balance is the low resting membrane permeability to Na^+, as both the concentration gradient and the membrane potential tend to drive Na^+ into the cell. This situation changes dramatically when the cells fire action potentials, because the membrane then becomes highly permeable to Na^+. Long trains of high-frequency action potentials may threaten the osmotic balance because more Na^+ ions enter the cell than can be pumped out. Fortunately, neurons have properties that limit their maximal firing rate and the duration of active periods. Under pathological conditions, however, these safeguards may fail. In severe **epileptic seizures**, for example, neurons fire with abnormal frequency for long periods, and this may probably contribute to cell damage by causing osmotic imbalance. Further, in situations with insufficient blood supply (ischemia), for example, after a **stroke**, ATP production suffers, resulting in slowing of the sodium–potassium pump. This, in turn, leads to osmotic imbalance and swelling of neurons. Such swelling is dangerous because neurons may be injured directly but also because swelling of the brain inside the skull (brain edema) reduces the blood supply.

Transmitter-Gated Ion Channels

Neurotransmitters control neuronal excitability by changing the opening state of ion channels (Figs. 3.1 and 3.2). A channel that is controlled by neurotransmitters (or other chemical substances) is called **transmitter-gated** or **ligand-gated** (the term "transmitter-activated" is also used). A large number of ion channels are now characterized that differ with regard to ion selectivity and transmitter specificity, that is, the ions that can pass a channel and the transmitter that controls it. The transmitter can either bind **directly** to the channel polypeptides (proteins) or act **indirectly** via chemical intermediates. In most known cases, the transmitter opens the channel to increase the permeability of the relevant ions. We consider here only the effects of directly acting neurotransmitters (indirect effects are discussed later in this chapter). Binding of a transmitter molecule to a specific **receptor site** at the external face of a channel polypeptide may change the form of the polypeptides, thereby changing the diameter of the channel (Figs. 3.1 and 3.2). Usually, the channel is open only briefly after binding of a transmitter molecule, allowing a brief current of ions to pass through the membrane. In this way, a chemical signal from a presynaptic neuron—the neurotransmitter—elicits an electric current through the postsynaptic membrane.

As mentioned, ion channels are more or less **selectively permeable**, that is, they let certain kinds of ions pass through more easily than others. Some channels are highly selective, allowing the passage of one kind only (such as Ca^{2+} ions), whereas others are less selective and will allow passage of, for example, most cations. Channels that are permeable for anions in general are usually termed chloride (Cl^-) channels because Cl^- is the only abundant anion that can pass through the membrane. Size and charge of the ion influence its permeability. For example, the Na^+ ions are more hydrated (bind more water molecules) than the K^+ ion and therefore are larger (Fig. 3.5). This may explain some of their differences in permeability. By regulating the channel opening, the transmitter controls the flow of ions through the postsynaptic membrane. However, the transmitter only alters the **probability** of the channel being in an open state; it does not induce a permanent open or closed state.

Voltage-Gated Ion Channels

Many channels are not controlled primarily by chemical substances but by the magnitude of the membrane potential and are therefore called **voltage-gated.** Voltage-gated Na^+ and K^+ channels, for example, are responsible for the action potential and therefore also for the propagation of impulses in the axons. There are also several kinds of voltage-gated Ca^{2+} channels, which control many important neuronal processes, for example, the release of neurotransmitters. Voltage-gated channels are responsible for the activation of nerves and muscles by external electrical stimulation. Electrical stimulation of a peripheral nerve may produce muscle twitches by activating motor nerve fibers, as well as sensations due to activation of sensory nerve fibers.

The Structure of Ion Channels

The structure of several **ligand-gated** ion channels has now been determined. They consist of five polypeptide subunits arranged around a central pore. Three **families** of ligand-gated channels have been identified: the nicotinic receptor superfamily ($GABA_A$, glycine, serotonin, and nicotinic acetylcholine receptors), the glutamate receptor family, and the ionotropic ATP receptors. The subunits span the membrane and extend to the external and internal faces of the membrane (Fig. 3.2). Therefore, signal molecules inside the cell may also influence the opening of ion channels. As an example, members of the nicotinic receptor family consist of five equal subunits (Fig. 3.2), all contributing to the wall of the channel.

The subunits are large polypeptides with molecular masses of approximately 300,000. The transmitter binds extracellularly at the transition between two subunits but it is still unknown how the rapid binding (in less than 1 msec) produces conformational change in parts of the channel located, relatively speaking, far away.[3]

Voltage-gated channels resemble ligand-gated ones; they consist of four subunits arranged around a central pore. The amino-acid sequence has been determined for several of the subunits, although lack of three-dimensional data has prevented clarification of the mechanisms that control their opening and ion selectivity. Presumably, subtle differences between the subunits forming the channel explain their high selectivity to particular ions.

Inherited Channelopathies

Many different genes code for channel proteins. Because ion channels determine the excitability of neurons, it is not surprising that **mutations** of such genes are associated with dysfunctions of neurons and muscle cells. Common to many such **channelopathies** is that the symptoms occur in bouts. Of particular clinical interest is that many of the channelopathies affecting neurons are associated with **epilepsy**. Although channelopathies may not be the primary cause in the majority of patients with epilepsy, they may increase the susceptibility to other factors. For example, mutations associated with epilepsy affect ligand-gated channels that are receptors for the neurotransmitters γ-aminobutyric acid (**GABA**) and **acetylcholine**. Mutations affecting channels gated by **glycine** (an inhibitory transmitter) are associated with abnormal startle reactions. This may probably be related to the fact that glycine is preferentially involved in inhibition of motor neurons. Patients with a certain kind of headache—**familial hemiplegic migraine**—have a mutation of the gene coding for a specific Ca^{2+}-channel protein. Other mutations of the same gene are associated with other rare nervous diseases, for example, some that affect the cerebellum and lead to ataxic movements. Mutations of a kind of **voltage-gated potassium channel** ($K_V \alpha 1.1$)—expressed in highest density around the initial segment of axons—produce abnormal repolarization of motor axons and lead to repetitive discharges. This may explain the muscle cramps of such patients. Their episodes of ataxic movements are presumably caused by abnormal excitability of cerebellar neurons. Mutations of voltage-gated sodium channels (among other factors) cause bursts of intense pain (see also Chapter 15, under "Nociceptors, Voltage-Gated Sodium Channels, and Channelopathies"). A number of mutations affect channels in **striated muscle** membranes, many of them associated with **myotonia** (inability to relax after a voluntary muscle contraction).

Different mutations of one gene can give different **phenotypes**, such as reduced density of channels or reduced opening probability. It is noteworthy, however, that the same mutation can produce different symptoms in different individuals, even within the same family. This strongly suggests that the genes coding for the proteins of a channel do not alone determine its final properties. Additional factors, such as the products of other genes and environmental factors, must also contribute. Many features of channelopathies are still unexplained—that they tend to occur episodically, that the symptoms often start at a certain age (in spite of the defect being present from birth), and that some forms remit spontaneously.

Alteration of the Membrane Potential: Depolarization and Hyperpolarization

As previously mentioned, in the resting state the membrane permeability for Na^+ is low. If for some reason Na^+ channels are opened so that the permeability is increased, Na^+ ions will flow into the cell and thereby reduce the magnitude of the membrane potential. Such a reduction of the membrane potential is called **depolarization**. The membrane potential is made less negative by depolarization. Correspondingly, one may predict that when the membrane permeability for K^+ is increased, more positive charges will leave the cell and the membrane potential will become more negative than the resting potential. This is called **hyperpolarization**. The same would be achieved by opening channels for chloride ions, enabling negative charges (Cl^-) to flow into the cell, provided that the membrane potential is more negative than the resting potential of Cl^-.

In conclusion, the membrane potential is determined by the **relative permeability** of the various ions that can pass through the membrane. At rest, the membrane is permeable primarily to K^+, and the resting potential is therefore close to the equilibrium potential of K^+. Synaptic influences can change this situation by opening Na^+ channels, thereby making the permeability to Na^+ dominant. This changes the membrane potential toward the equilibrium potential of Na^+ (at 55 mV). As shown in the following discussion, the action potential is caused by a further, sudden increase in the Na^+ permeability.

Markers of Neuronal Activity

Several methods can be used to visualize the activity of neurons. One method involves intracellular injection of a **voltage-sensitive fluorescent dye**. The intensity of fluorescence (as recorded with fluorescence microscopy

---

3 The binding of the transmitter most likely elicits a wave of conformational change in specific parts of the channel polypeptides. The actual opening of the channel may be caused by conformational change of just one, specific amino acid.

and advanced computer technology) gives an impression of neuronal activity at a given time. Thus, this (indirect) measure of activity can be correlated with experimental manipulation of a specific transmitter, the execution of specific tasks, and so forth. Another method takes advantage of the fact that **optic properties** of nervous tissue change with the degree of neuronal activity. This enables the recording of slow as well as rapid changes in neuronal activity in relation to experimental influences (it has been applied, e.g., in conscious persons during neurosurgery that necessitates exposure of the cerebral cortex). Other methods enable mapping of variations in neuronal activity at the time of death in experimental animals. Intravenously injected radiolabeled **deoxyglucose** is taken up by cells in the same way as glucose. It is not broken down, however, and therefore accumulates in the cells. Because glucose is the substrate for oxidative metabolism in the neurons, its uptake correlates with degree of neuronal activity. After exposing an animal to certain kinds of stimulation or eliciting certain behaviors, one can afterwards determine with autoradiography which neuronal groups were particularly active during stimulation or at the time of certain actions. Another method utilizes the fact that a few minutes with excitatory synaptic input induces expression of so-called **immediate early-genes** in many neurons. Most studied among such genes is **c-*fos***. Without extra stimulation, C-*fos* mRNA and its protein product are present in only minute amounts in most neurons. Detection of increased levels of *c-fos* mRNA in tissue sections is therefore used as a marker of neurons that were particularly active in a certain experimental situation. This method is also used to determine where in the brain a drug exerts its effect. The method has its limitations, however. Thus, *c-fos* expression may be caused by nonspecific influences, and not all neurons express *c-fos* even when properly activated.

THE ACTION POTENTIAL

Voltage-Gated Sodium Channels Are Instrumental in Evoking an Action Potential

The basis of the action potential is found in the presence of **voltage-gated Na^+ channels**, which are opened by depolarization of the membrane (Fig. 3.6). Depolarization may be induced in several ways; for example, under artificial conditions by direct electrical stimulation. Normally, however, it is caused by neurotransmitters acting on transmitter-gated channels. The opening of transmitter-gated Na^+ channels often starts depolarization. Opening of the voltage-gated channels requires that the membrane be depolarized to a certain **threshold** value, that is, the threshold for

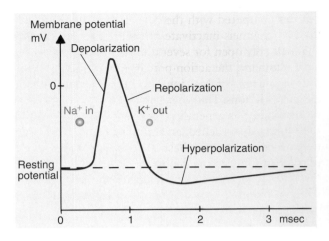

FIGURE 3.6 *The action potential.*

producing an action potential (Fig. 3.6). When voltage-gated channels are opened, the permeability to Na^+ is increased beyond what was achieved by the opening of transmitter-gated channels, and Na^+ flows into the cell driven by both the concentration gradient and the membrane potential. The membrane becomes more depolarized; in turn, this opens more voltage-gated channels, and so on. In this way, as soon as the membrane is depolarized to the threshold value, the permeability to Na^+ increases in an explosive manner. Even with all sodium channels fully open, however, the inward current of Na^+ ions stops when the membrane is depolarized to +55 mV; at that value the inward concentration force is equal to the outward electrical force (the membrane potential). As mentioned, +55 mV is the equilibrium potential of Na^+. Figure 3.6 shows how, during an action potential, the membrane potential quickly changes to positive values and then returns almost as rapidly to approximately the resting value. This occurs because the membrane again becomes impermeable to Na^+; the Na^+ channels are closed or **inactivated**.[4] Therefore, at the peak of the action potential and for a short time afterward, no Na^+ can pass through the membrane. In this situation with a positive membrane potential, K^+ is driven out by both the concentration gradient and the membrane potential (electrical force). Because no Na^+ can enter the cell, there is a net outward flow of positive charges, again making the interior of the cell negative. We say that the membrane is **repolarized**. The speed of repolarization is increased by the presence of **voltage-gated K^+ channels**, which open when the membrane is sufficiently depolarized. The opening of the voltage-gated K^+ channels is somewhat

---

4 **Inactivation** and **closure** involve different parts of the voltage-gated Na^+ channel. This is indicated by, among other findings, that whereas closure of the channel lasts as long as the membrane potential remains below threshold, inactivation is transitory and lasts only some milliseconds.

delayed compared with the Na⁺ channels, but whereas the Na⁺ channels inactivate after about 1 msec, the K⁺ channels stay open for several milliseconds.

In summary, the action potential is caused by a brief inward current of Na⁺ ions, followed by an outward current of K⁺ ions. The whole sequence of depolarization–repolarization is generally completed in 1 to 2 msec. If the threshold is reached, an action potential of a certain magnitude arises, regardless of the strength of the stimulus that produced the depolarization.

Where Does the Action Potential Arise?

The action potential usually arises in the first part of the axon, the **initial segment** (Fig. 3.7; see also Fig. 2.6), where the density of voltage-gated Na⁺ channels is higher than in the membrane of the dendrites and the cell soma. The current spreads electrotonically (passively) from dendritic and somatic synapses toward the initial segment. If the depolarization is sufficiently strong (reaches threshold), voltage-gated Na⁺ and K⁺ channels open and produce an action potential that is propagated along the axon. Although action potentials can be elicited in dendrites, their threshold is usually much higher than in the initial segment owing to lower density of voltage-gated channels.

The Action Potential and Changes of Ion Concentrations

One might think that an action potential would cause significant changes in the concentrations of Na⁺ and K⁺ on the two sides of the membrane, but this is not the case. The number of ions actually passing through the membrane during an action potential is extremely small compared with the total number inside the cell and in its immediate surroundings. Even in an axon with a diameter of about 1 μm, with a very small intracellular volume compared to the membrane surface area, only 1 of 3000 K⁺ ions moves out during the action potential. In addition, active pumping (the sodium–potassium pump) ensures that Na⁺ is moved out and K⁺ is moved in between each action potential and during periods of rest. Even when the sodium–potassium pump is blocked experimentally, a nerve cell can produce several thousand action potentials before concentration gradients are reduced so much that the cell loses its excitability.

The Refractory Period

After an action potential, some time must elapse before the neuron can again produce an action potential in response to a stimulus. The cell is said to be in a **refractory state**. This ensures at least a minimal rest for the cell between each action potential and thereby puts an upper limit on the frequency with which the cell can fire. The length of the refractory period, and therefore also the maximal frequency of firing, varies considerably among different kinds of nerve cells.

Two conditions are responsible for the refractory period. One is the aforementioned inactivation of the voltage-gated Na⁺ channels, and the other is the fact that the membrane is hyperpolarized immediately after the action potential (Fig. 3.6). The inactivation of Na⁺ channels means that they cannot be opened, regardless of the strength of the stimulus and the ensuing depolarization. Hyperpolarization occurs because the K⁺ channels remain open longer than required just to bring the membrane potential back to resting value. These two different mechanisms can account for why the refractory period consists of two phases. During the first phase, the **absolute refractory period**, the cell cannot be made to discharge, however strong the stimulus may be; during the **relative refractory period**, stronger depolarization than normal is needed to produce an action potential.

Calcium and Neuronal Excitability

A cation other than Na⁺—namely, Ca²⁺—may also contribute to the rising phase of the action potential. For Ca²⁺, as for Na⁺, the extracellular concentration is much higher than the intracellular one, and there are voltage-gated calcium channels in the membrane.

Cellular influx of calcium can be visualized after intracellular injection of a substance that fluoresces when Ca²⁺ binds to it. During the action potential, calcium enters the cell—partly through Na⁺ channels and partly through voltage-gated calcium channels, which have a more prolonged opening–closing phase than the sodium channels. There are also transmitter-gated calcium channels. In most neurons, the contribution of Ca²⁺ to the action potential is nevertheless small compared with that of Na⁺. In certain other cells such as

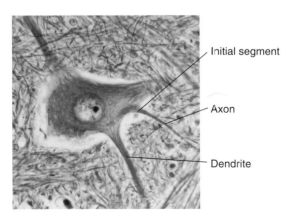

Initial segment

Axon

Dendrite

FIGURE 3.7 *The initial segment of the axon is where the action potential usually arises.* Photomicrograph of a motoneuron from the spinal cord stained with a silver-impregnation method.

heart muscle, however, calcium is the ion largely responsible for the action potential. Because the calcium channels open and close more slowly than the Na^+ channels, an action potential produced by calcium currents lasts longer than one produced by flow of Na^+.

Another aspect of the functional role of calcium is that the extracellular calcium concentration influences the membrane excitability, which is most likely mediated through effects on the Na^+ and K^+ channels. Reducing the calcium concentration in the blood and interstitial fluid—**hypocalcemia**—lowers the threshold for evoking action potentials in neurons and muscle cells, whereas increasing the concentration—**hypercalcemia**—has the opposite effect. A typical symptom of hypocalcemia is muscle spasms—**tetany**—due to hyperexcitability of nerves and muscles. Severe hypercalcemia can cause drowsiness, nausea, and anorexia.

IMPULSE PROPAGATION

Electrical Properties of Axons

We now consider how the action potential moves along the axon. The ability of the axon to conduct electrical current depends on several conditions, some of which are given by the physical properties of axons, which are very different from, for example, those of copper wire. In addition, some conditions vary among axons of different kinds. An axon is a poor conductor compared with electrical conductors made of metal because the axoplasm through which the current has to pass consists of a weak solution of electrolytes (i.e., low concentrations of charged particles in water). In addition, the diameter of an axon is small (from <1 to 20 μm) with a correspondingly enormous **internal resistance** to the current in the axoplasm. Further, the axonal membrane is not a perfect insulator, so that charged particles are lost from the interior of the axon as the current passes along its length. The amount of current being lost is determined by the degree of **membrane resistance** (i.e., the resistance of the membrane to charged particles trying to pass). Finally, the axonal membrane (like all cell membranes) has an **electrical capacity**; that is, it can store a certain number of charged particles in the same way a battery does. This further contributes to the rapid attenuation of a current that is conducted along an axon: the membrane has to be charged before the current can move on.

The Action Potential Is Regenerated as It Moves Along the Axon

From the foregoing it can be concluded that how well the current is conducted in an axon depends on its internal

resistance (its diameter), the membrane resistance (how well insulated it is), and the capacity of the axonal membrane. If the propagation of the action potential along the axon occurred only by passive, electrotonic movement of charged particles, the internal resistance and loss of charges to the exterior would cause the action potential to move only a short distance before it "died out." The solution to this problem is that the action potential is **regenerated** as it moves along the axon. Therefore, it is propagated with undiminished strength all the way from the cell body to the nerve terminals. As discussed, the strength of the action potential—that is, the magnitude of the changes of the membrane potential taking place—is the same regardless of the strength of the stimulus that produced it (as long as the stimulus depolarizes the membrane to threshold). Thus, increasing the strength of the stimulus increases the frequency of action potentials, whereas the magnitude of each action potential remains constant.

When the cell membrane at the initial segment (Fig. 3.7) is depolarized to threshold, an action potential is produced and is conducted passively a short distance along the axon. From then on, what occurs differs somewhat in myelinated and unmyelinated axons (Figs. 3.8 and 3.9).

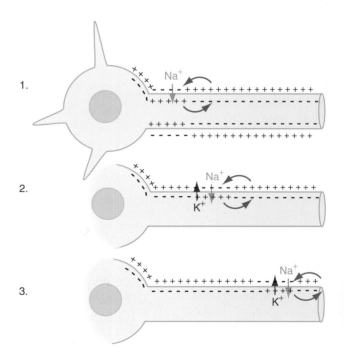

FIGURE 3.8 *Impulse conduction in unmyelinated axons.* Arrows show direction of movement of charged particles. The action potential is renewed continuously along the axonal membrane by a wave of depolarization–repolarization.

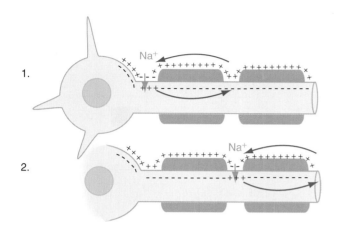

1.

2.

FIGURE 3.9 *Impulse conduction in myelinated axons.* Arrows show direction of movement of charged particles. The current moves electrotonically in the myelinated part of the axons, and the action potential is renewed only at the node of Ranvier, causing a small delay in impulse propagation.

Impulse Conduction in Unmyelinated Axons

The action potential is produced by positive charges penetrating to the interior of the axon, which at that point becomes positive relative to more distal parts along its length (Fig. 3.8). Positive charges then start moving in the distal direction (along the electrical gradient that has been set up). Outside the axon, a corresponding current of positive charges moves in the opposite direction, so that an **electrical circuit** is established. Movement of positive charges in the distal direction inside the axon means that the membrane is depolarized as the charges move along. This depolarization leads to the opening of enough voltage-gated Na$^+$ and K$^+$ channels to produce a "new" action potential. In this manner, the action potential moves along the axon at a speed that depends on the speed with which the charged particles (i.e., ions) move inside the axon and on the time needed for full opening of the ion channels. The membrane capacity represents a further factor slowing the propagation because the membrane has to be charged before there can be a net flow of charges through it.

In essence, the action potential is propagated as a wave of depolarization, followed closely by a corresponding wave of repolarization. When the membrane has just completed this cycle, it is in the refractory state for some milliseconds. This delay prevents the action potential from spreading "backward" toward the cell body (**antidromic** impulse conduction), and ensures that under normal conditions the impulse conduction is unidirectional. If, however, the axon is artificially stimulated (e.g., electrically) at some distance from the cell

body, the action potential spreads toward both the cell body and the end ramifications (**orthodromic** impulse conduction). Antidromic impulse conduction may occur in branches of peripheral sensory axons on natural stimulation and may play a part in certain disease symptoms (see Chapter 29, "Antidromic Impulses and the Axonal Reflex").

Impulse Conduction in Myelinated Axons

In myelinated axons, the action potential is also regenerated along the axon (Fig. 3.9). However, in contrast to that in unmyelinated axons, the action potential is regenerated only at each **node of Ranvier**—that is, where the axon membrane lacks a myelin covering and is in direct contact with the extracellular fluid (see Fig. 2.6). As in unmyelinated axons, the action potential arises in the initial segment of the axon. The current then spreads passively (electrotonically) to the first node of Ranvier. Here, the depolarization of the membrane leads to opening of voltage-gated channels and a "new" action potential. The density of voltage-gated sodium channels is particularly high in the axonal membrane at the node of Ranvier. The current can flow electrotonically as far as the first node of Ranvier (and probably sometimes farther) because the axon is so well insulated by myelin, preventing loss of charges from the interior of the axon. (Myelin dramatically increases the resistance across the membrane and also reduces the membrane capacity.) In addition, the axonal diameter is larger in myelinated than in unmyelinated axons, thus reducing the internal resistance.

In conclusion, in myelinated axons the action potential does not move smoothly and slowly along, as in unmyelinated axons, but instead "jumps" from one node of Ranvier to the next. Although the impulse propagation is very rapid between nodes, at each node there is a delay due to the time required for opening of channels and establishment of sufficient flow of current.

Conduction Velocities in Myelinated and Unmyelinated Axons

The main reason myelinated axons conduct so much more rapidly than unmyelinated ones is that the action potential needs to be regenerated only at certain sites. A figure for conduction velocity (expressed in meters per second) in myelinated axons is obtained by multiplying the axonal diameter (in micrometers) by 6. An axon of 20 µm (the maximal diameter) therefore conducts at approximately 120 m/sec, whereas the thinnest myelinated axons of about 3 µm conduct at 18 m/sec. In comparison, a typical unmyelinated axon of about 1 µm conducts at less than 1 m/sec.

HOW NERVE CELLS VARY THEIR MESSAGES

Frequency Coding and Firing Patterns

So far we have treated the action potential as a unitary phenomenon. As mentioned, the strength of each action potential of a neuron does not vary: whenever depolarized to the threshold, the cell fires action potentials of constant magnitude. Therefore, the action potential is an **all-or-none** phenomenon, and one might think that each neuron would only be able to tell whether or not a stimulus occurs. We know, however, that the individual nerve cell can communicate to others about the strength of the stimulation it receives—such as the intensity of light or a sound, of something touching the skin, and so forth. It does so by varying the frequency and pattern of action potentials. To understand this, we need to know that a neuron is more or less continuously influenced by impulses from many other neurons. A sustained synaptic input that is strong enough to depolarize the cell to threshold does not merely produce one action potential but rather several in succession. The stronger the depolarization, the shorter the time required reaching the threshold after each action potential. Consequently, the firing frequency depends on the strength of depolarization (Fig. 3.10). We say that the neuron uses a **frequency code** to tell how strongly it has been stimulated. The **maximal frequency** of action potentials in some neurons is more than 100 per second (100 Hz), whereas in others it is much lower.

The average firing frequency is not the only way by which the neuron can alter its message. The **firing pattern** also carries information, and each neuronal type has its characteristic firing pattern that is caused by differences in membrane properties and synaptic

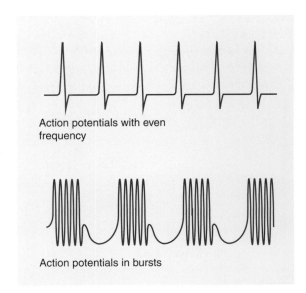

Action potentials with even frequency

Action potentials in bursts

FIGURE 3.11 *Different patterns of nerve impulses provide neurons with an additional means to vary the information they send to other neurons and muscle cells.*

inputs (see earlier, "The Refractory Period"). Two neurons may both fire with an average frequency of, for example, 10 per second but nevertheless influence a postsynaptic cell differently. So-called **burst neurons** produce trains of action potentials with a high frequency and then pause for a while before a new train (burst) of impulses arises. Other neurons—so-called **single-spike neurons**—produce action potentials with regular intervals (Fig. 3.11).

Some neurons can switch between these two modes of firing. In such cases, the relationship is not linear between the strength of synaptic input and the firing frequency. The transition between the different firing patterns is evoked by a specific neurotransmitter, which does not in itself produce action potentials in the postsynaptic cell but changes its reactions to other inputs. For example, the neuron may change from burst to single-spike patterns or from a high firing frequency to no firing at all.

In conclusion, because the strength of action potential is constant, the code for the information carried by an axon is the frequency and pattern of action potentials.

Plateau Potentials

In some neurons, the occurrence of so-called plateau potentials causes the switch from low-frequency firing to high-frequency or bursting firing pattern. This has been shown for many neurons that control rhythmic muscle contractions. Plateau potentials are produced by a slow, depolarizing current, for example, by certain

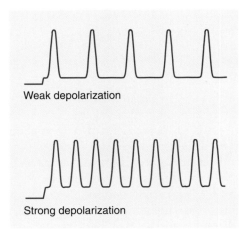

Weak depolarization

Strong depolarization

FIGURE 3.10 *The frequency of action potentials depends on the magnitude of depolarization.* Therefore, the frequency of action potentials reflects the total synaptic input to a neuron.

voltage-gated Ca^{2+} channels that are open in a limited range of membrane potentials. Such a neuron can therefore change abruptly between two entirely different behaviors. The neurotransmitter **serotonin** can evoke plateau potentials in groups of spinal motor neurons (see Chapter 21, under "Muscle Cramps and Plateau Potentials," and Chapter 22, under "Monoaminergic Pathways from the Brain Stem to the Spinal Cord"). Release of this transmitter relates to motivation and attention rather than to specific information.

4 | Synaptic Function

OVERVIEW

In Chapter 3, we discussed the basis of nerve impulses and their conduction in axons. This chapter deals with the properties of synapses. We discuss mainly **chemical synapses**: synapses in which the signal is mediated by a neurotransmitter. Synapses with direct **electric coupling** (gap junctions) are common among glial cells but occur infrequently among neurons. The key events underlying signal transfer at chemical synapses are as follows: First, an action potential reaches the nerve terminal (bouton) and **depolarizes** it. This depolarization opens Ca^{2+} **channels**, enabling Ca^{2+} to enter the nerve terminal. Increase in intracellular Ca^{2+} concentration is a signal for release of **neurotransmitter** from vesicles by exocytosis. This produces a high concentration of neurotransmitter in the synaptic cleft. The released transmitter binds briefly to **receptors** in the **postsynaptic membrane**. After activation of the receptor, the transmitter must be **inactivated** quickly to reestablish a low background activity of the receptors, that is, to ensure a high **signal-to-noise ratio** at the synapse. Inactivation occurs partly by diffusion of the transmitter, partly by **enzymatic degradation**, and partly by specific uptake mechanisms (**transporter proteins**).

There are two main kinds of transmitter receptors. **Ionotropic receptors** are parts of ion channels and therefore influence the functional state of the channel directly. Therefore, transmitter actions elicited by ionotropic receptors are fast and precise. **Metabotropic receptors** are coupled indirectly (via intracellular second messengers) to ion channels. Their effects are therefore slower to start and longer lasting than effects mediated by ionotropic receptors. We also use the term **modulatory** of the synaptic effects of metabotropic receptors, because they adjust the excitability of the postsynaptic neuron so that it responds more or less vigorously to the precise effects of ionotropic receptors (in addition, metabotropic receptors may have effects on the growth and survival of the postsynaptic neuron).

The change of the membrane potential arising as a result of synaptic influence is called a **synaptic potential**. If the synaptic influence depolarizes the postsynaptic cell, the probability that the cell will fire action potentials is increased. This synaptic effect is called an **excitatory postsynaptic potential (EPSP)**. If the synaptic potential hyperpolarizes the cell, it is called an inhibitory postsynaptic potential (IPSP) because the probability of the cell's firing is diminished. If the transmitter produces an EPSP, we use the terms **excitatory synapse** and **excitatory transmitter**. Likewise, an **inhibitory transmitter** produces an IPSP at an **inhibitory synapse**.

Because the depolarization caused by one EPSP is small, **summation** of many EPSPs is usually needed to reach a threshold for eliciting an action potential. This enables the neuron to integrate information from often many thousand synapses.

Synapses are **plastic**; that is, they can change their properties by use. This implies that certain kinds of activity can enhance or reduce the subsequent effect of a synapse on the postsynaptic neuron for a variable period (from milliseconds to years). Most likely, such **use-dependent** synaptic plasticity is the neuronal basis for **learning** and **memory**.

Unusual Synapses: Electrotonic and Dendrodendritic Transmission

Although it is rare, the pre- and postsynaptic elements are electrically rather than chemically coupled at some synapses. Electron microscopically, such electronic synapses differ from chemical synapses in that the synaptic cleft is only 2 nm compared to about 20 nm. This kind of cell contact is called a **nexus** or **gap junction**; it consists of channels that span the synaptic cleft. Through these channels ion currents can pass directly and quickly from one cell to another with no synaptic delay. In invertebrates and lower vertebrates, electrotonic synapses are formed between neurons mediating short-latency responses to stimuli (e.g., escape reactions). Electrotonic synapses may also provide electrical coupling between many neurons in a group, so that their activity may be **synchronized**. Chemical synapses may occur close to electrical ones and serve to uncouple the electrical synapse so that these apparently can be switched on and off. Even a small number of gap junctions between nerve cells—too small to produce efficient electric coupling—may be important by enabling transfer of small signal molecules, such as Ca^{2+}, cyclic AMP, and inositol triphosphate (IP_3). In this way, one neuron may alter the properties of another without ordinary synaptic contact. Electrical coupling by gap junctions is much more common among glial cells than among neurons, and it occurs regularly among cardiac, smooth-muscle, and epithelial cells. There are also other unusual types of synapses. Contacts between dendrites with all the morphological characteristics of synapses have been observed in several places in the central nervous system (CNS). Such dendrodendritic synapses are often part of more complex synaptic arrangements. Through dendrodendritic synapses, adjacent neurons can influence each other without being connected with axons. The function of such synapses, however, is not fully understood.

NEUROTRANSMITTER HANDLING AT THE SYNAPSE

Release of Neurotransmitters

We have previously described transmitter-containing synaptic vesicles, aggregated near the presynaptic membrane of boutons (Figs. 4.1 and 5.9). Depolarization of the presynaptic membrane by an action potential is the normal event preceding transmitter release. The depolarization opens voltage-gated calcium channels and allows a flow of Ca^{2+} ions into the bouton. The rise in Ca^{2+} concentration triggers the release of transmitter by exocytosis of vesicles (Fig. 4.1). The more calcium that enters, the more transmitter is released. By exocytosis, the membrane of synaptic vesicles fuses with the presynaptic membrane. The fusion opens the vesicle so that its content flows quickly into the cleft (Figs. 4.1 and 4.2). It takes only 0.1 to 0.2 msec from calcium inflow to the occurrence of release, which means that only vesicles already attached to the presynaptic membrane empty their contents. Further, although voltage-gated Ca^{2+} channels are present in all parts of the nerve terminal membrane, only those situated in the presynaptic membrane can influence the fusion of the vesicle with the presynaptic membrane.[1] The part of the synapse where the vesicles attach to the presynaptic membrane is called the active zone, and is characterized by cytoskeletal components that probably bind the vesicles to the calcium channels. That fusion really occurs during release is supported by, among other data, electron microscopic observations showing that the number of vesicles drops with long-term stimulation (trains of action potentials), while the number increases after a period of rest.

Exocytosis of vesicles is controlled by a large number of regulatory proteins that appear to be the same in all kinds of cells. Two features are nevertheless specific to exocytosis in neurons as compared with that in other cells: one is the speed of the process (<1 msec from arrival of the action potential to release); the other is that the release is restricted to a specific site (the synapse).

---

1 This is because the fusion requires a very high concentration of Ca^{2+}, which occurs only close to the intracellular opening of the channel. In fact, there is evidence that the calcium channel constitutes a part of the protein complex that binds the vesicle to the presynaptic membrane. This ensures maximal Ca^{2+} concentration around the vesicle.

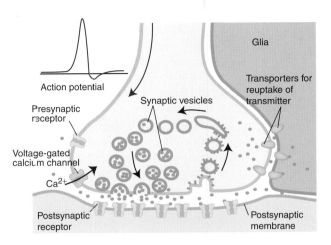

FIGURE 4.1 *Signal transmission at the synapse.* Schematic of some important features: calcium-dependent transmitter release, reuptake of transmitter by glia and neurons, and recycling of synaptic vesicles.

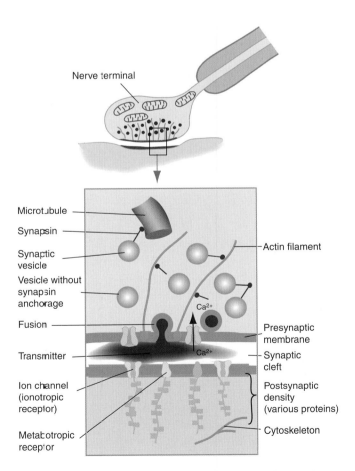

FIGURE 4.2 *Transmitter release and some of its machinery.* Calcium channels are located close to where the vesicles fuse with the presynaptic membrane. (Based on Walmsey et al. 1998.)

This indicates that some proteins are specific to the control of exocytosis in neurons. The fusion requires specific binding of vesicle-surface receptors to receptors in the presynaptic membrane. In addition, during fusion, various proteins dissolved in the cytoplasm participate by binding to the membrane-bound receptors, thus forming large complexes.

New, empty vesicles are formed by the opposite process of exocytosis, **endocytosis**. The endocytotic vesicles are **coated** with proteins (among them **clathrin** and **dynamin**) that are thought to help in budding of the vesicles from the membrane and in selecting their content. The recycled vesicles undergo a series of regulated steps until they are again filled with neurotransmitter (Fig. 4.1).

Several of the proteins involved in vesicle transport and fusion alter their activity in a use-dependent manner; that is, they may be involved in **synaptic plasticity** during development, recovery after brain damage, and learning in general. Some are also targets of drugs and toxins.

Mechanisms for Vesicle Transport and Fusion

Specific **transporter proteins** in the vesicle membrane fill the vesicles with neurotransmitter. After filling, the vesicles are moved toward the presynaptic membrane by a regulated process (Fig. 4.2). While some vesicles empty their contents, others move toward the presynaptic membrane and prepare for fusion. The synaptic vesicles can therefore be divided into two main groups: those situated close to the membrane that are ready for release when the Ca^{2+} concentration rises around them, and those that must move to the membrane before they can release their contents. The movement of vesicles requires the presence of **actin** filaments, and **microtubules** may also play a role. A group of proteins, **synapsins**, bind the vesicles to the actin filaments (Fig. 4.2), which probably serves to assemble the vesicles in positions for further movement and is triggered by the rise in the calcium concentration. Certain **protein kinases** (phosphorylating proteins) regulate the activity of the synapsins. Phosphorylation of synapsins increases mobility of the vesicles and is most likely another way of controlling the amount of transmitter released by an action potential, for example, in response to altered use of the synapse. Several proteins take part in the **docking** of the vesicle at the presynaptic membrane, and they probably also prepare the vesicles for fusion. Vesicle-bound receptors, such as **synaptobrevin/VAMP** (vesicle-associated membrane protein), mediate attachment to receptors in the presynaptic membrane (**syntaxin** is one such receptor). These receptors interact with several others—among them, **SNAP-25** that is free in the cytoplasm—thus forming large protein complexes that anchor the vesicles to the presynaptic membrane. The fusion appears to require that the complex include **synaptotagmin**, which binds Ca^{2+} with low affinity (i.e., the concentration of Ca^{2+} must be high for bonding to occur). According to one hypothesis, synaptotagmin acts as a brake on fusion, and the binding of Ca^{2+} releases the brake. Mice lacking the gene for synaptotagmin have only reduced transmitter release, however, suggesting that other factors also play a role.

Neurotransmitters Are Released in Quanta

There is convincing evidence that transmitters are released in packets, or **quanta,** corresponding to the transmitter content of one vesicle. For synapses between motor nerve terminals and striated muscle cells, one vesicle contains on average 10,000 transmitter molecules. Only a few thousand molecules of each quantum are likely to bind to a receptor before they diffuse away or are removed by other means. Release of one quantum elicits a tiny excitatory postsynaptic potential (EPSP)—a **miniature EPSP**. If stimulation is increased, so that more transmitter is released, the depolarization of the muscle cell membrane increases in steps corresponding to one miniature EPSP. In the CNS, each bouton probably releases from none to a few quanta for each presynaptic action potential. This means that an action potential does not necessarily elicit transmitter release; it merely increases the **probability of release.** As discussed later, many presynaptic action potentials must coincide to fire a postsynaptic neuron.

Transmitters Act on Ionotropic and Metabotropic Receptors

The effects of a neurotransmitter depend primarily on the properties and localization of the receptors it can activate. There are two main kinds of transmitter receptors: ionotropic and metabotropic. **Ionotropic receptors** are parts of ion channels (Fig. 4.3A). Ionotropic receptors that are parts of Na^+ or Ca^{2+} channels evoke fast and brief **depolarizations** of the postsynaptic membrane, thus exerting **excitatory** actions. Ionotropic receptors coupled to Cl^- channels as a rule **hyperpolarize** the postsynaptic membrane and **inhibit** the postsynaptic neuron. Synapses equipped with ionotropic receptors mediate **fast** and **precise information**—for example, about "when," "what," and "where" concerning a sensory stimulus.

The other main kind—**metabotropic receptor**—is not coupled directly to ion channels but acts indirectly by way of **G proteins** and intracellular second messengers (Fig. 4.3B). G proteins may be regarded as universal translators, translating various kinds of extracellular signals to a cellular response (e.g., the "translation" of light and of gaseous and watery chemical substances to nerve impulses).

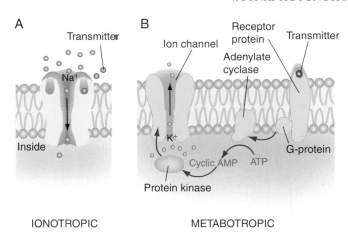

FIGURE 4.3 *Two kinds of transmitter receptors.* **A:** Ionotropic receptor with direct action on the ion channel. Note that the receptor is part of the channel proteins. **B:** Metabotropic receptor with indirect action on ion channels. Schematic. All indirectly coupled receptors act via G proteins, whereas other elements of the intracellular signal pathway may vary among different receptors. In this example cyclic AMP serves as the second messenger.

Most neurotransmitters act on both ionotropic and metabotropic receptors. That is, a neurotransmitter can exert both fast, direct synaptic effects and slow, indirect ones (at the same or different synapses). **Glutamate** and **GABA** (γ-aminobutyric acid) are by far the most abundant and ubiquitous transmitters acting on ionotropic receptors, although they also act on several kinds of metabotropic receptors. Several important neurotransmitters, such as **norepinephrine, dopamine,** and **serotonin,** exert their main actions on metabotropic receptors. We can conclude that to predict the actions of a neurotransmitter on a neuronal group, we must know the repertoire of receptors expressed by those neurons. Further, because the distribution of receptors differs, one transmitter may exert different actions in different parts of the brain.

Toxins Can Prevent Transmitter Release

Some of the proteins necessary for fusion are degraded by **tetanus toxin** and **botulinum toxin** (produced in certain foods if not treated properly). Both toxins are produced by anaerobic bacteria (i.e., they only grow in the absence of oxygen) and produce violent muscle spasms and paralysis, respectively. The toxins are proteases acting on the proteins that are involved in docking and fusion of synaptic vesicles. While tetanus toxin and some botulinum toxins degrade synaptobrevin, other botulinum toxins destroy SNAP-25, or syntaxin. Even extremely small amounts of the toxins produce muscle spasms (tetanus toxin) or paralysis (botulinum toxins) by preventing transmitter release. They evoke opposite effects because they act on different kinds of synapses: the tetanus toxin affects primarily a type of inhibitory synapse, whereas botulinum toxin acts at the neuromuscular junction, preventing release of the excitatory transmitter acetylcholine.

Inactivation of Neurotransmitters

Synaptic signal transfer is characterized by a precisely timed start and stop. We have looked into the mechanisms responsible for precise timing of transmitter release. It is also necessary, however, that the transmitter, once released, be quickly removed from the synaptic cleft after receptor activation. Simple **diffusion** of the transmitter seems to play an important part, especially during the first few milliseconds after release. Some transmitters (acetylcholine and neuropeptides) are degraded extracellularly by specific enzymes. The majority of transmitters, however, are removed from the extracellular fluid by **uptake** into glial cells or neurons (see also Chapter 2, under "Astroglia and the Control of Neuronal Homeostasis"). Specific transporter proteins in the cell membrane (see Figs. 2.5, 4.1, and 5.5) carry out the transmitter uptake. The transmitter transporters are driven by ion-concentration gradients across the cell membrane. There are two **families** of such transporter proteins. One is driven by the concentration gradients of Na$^+$ and Cl$^-$ and transports the transmitters **GABA, glycine, dopamine, norepinephrine,** and **serotonin.** The other comprises five different transporters for **glutamate** and is driven by the concentration gradients of Na$^+$ and K$^+$.

The task of the transporters is not to remove all traces of neurotransmitters from the extracellular fluid. Because both number and activity of the transporters are regulated, they rather serve to modulate up or down a certain baseline extracellular transmitter concentration. Even a small alteration of transporter activity can cause changes of transmitter–receptor activation. In areas with a high density of transporters, they also influence the ease by which neurotransmitters may activate receptors outside the synaptic cleft (on nerve terminals, dendrites, and cell bodies). In this way, the transmitter transporters participate in the control of synaptic transmission and neuronal excitability.

Because the transporter proteins have important physiological roles, they are also interesting from a pharmacological aspect. Drugs that alter their function can be used therapeutically (such as **antidepressants** that are selective serotonin reuptake inhibitors), but some also have potential for abuse (such as **cocaine**, which inhibits the dopamine-reuptake transporter).

SYNAPTIC POTENTIALS AND TYPES OF SYNAPSES

Mechanisms of Postsynaptic Potentials (EPSPs and IPSPs)

Synaptic potentials arise when neurotransmitters activate ion channels. An **excitatory postsynaptic potential** (**EPSP**) arises at synapses where the transmitter **depolarizes** the postsynaptic membrane. An **inhibitory postsynaptic potential** (**IPSP**) arises at synapses where the transmitter **hyperpolarizes** the membrane.

Opening of cation channels allowing Na^+ to enter and K^+ to leave the cell produces an EPSP. Because the cations outside the cell are driven inward, by both the concentration gradient and the membrane potential, whereas K^+ inside the cell is driven out only by its concentration gradient, at first the inward current is largest (see Figs. 3.3, 3.4, and 3.5). As the membrane becomes more and more depolarized, however, the outward flow of K^+ increases and counteracts further depolarization (Fig. 4.4). Transmitter-gated channel opening is not subject to self-reinforcement, unlike the voltage-gated channels that produce the action potential. This means that the synaptic potentials rise and fall gradually (Fig. 4.4 and 4.5) and last longer than the action potential. We use the term **graded potential**, as opposed to the all-or-none behavior of the action potential. The current spreads passively (electrotonically) from the synapse outward in all directions along the cell membrane. In this way, the potential becomes gradually weaker, unlike the action potential that is constantly regenerated. Because typical EPSPs in neurons are small (<1 mV), and the membrane has to be depolarized at about 10 mV near the initial segment to reach **threshold** for an action potential, it follows that many EPSPs must be summated to fire the neuron. We return to summation of EPSPs later.

The mechanism behind an **IPSP** is usually the opening of transmitter-gated K^+ or Cl^- channels. This results in an outward flow of K^+ or an inward flow of Cl^-. In both cases, the inside of the cell becomes more negative, that is, the membrane is hyperpolarized. This is only true if the membrane potential is less negative than the equilibrium potentials of the ions in question, however. Although this is the normal situation for K^+ (equilibrium potential −90 mV), the equilibrium potential of

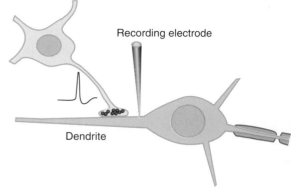

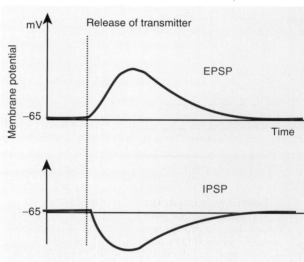

FIGURE 4.4 *Synaptic potentials.* Alterations of the membrane potential evoked by a single presynaptic action potential that releases a transmitter into the synaptic cleft. An EPSP (excitatory postsynaptic synaptic potential) is evoked by an excitatory transmitter (typically glutamate), while an inhibitory transmitter (typically GABA) produces an IPSP (inhibitory postsynaptic synaptic potential).

Cl^- is close to the resting potential in many neurons. If the resting potential is equal to the equilibrium potential of Cl^-, there is no net flow of Cl^- ions and, consequently, no IPSP is evoked.[2] Even in this case, however, opening of chloride channels can counteract the effects of excitatory transmitters. Thus, as long as the chloride channels remain open, even the slightest depolarization will cause Cl^- ions to flow into the cell and thereby minimize the change of the membrane potential. In this case, opening of chloride channels by an inhibitory transmitter **short-circuits** the depolarizing currents at nearby excitatory synapses.

---

2 If the resting potential is more negative than the equilibrium potential of Cl^-, opening of chloride channels causes a net outward flow of chloride ions and the cell is depolarized. This is the case in early embryologic development; the transmitter GABA, which is inhibitory in the adult nervous systems, has excitatory actions in the immature brain.

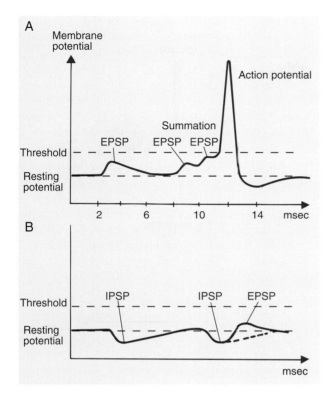

FIGURE 4.5 *Synaptic potentials.* **A:** The time course and polarity of an excitatory postsynaptic synaptic potential (EPSP). In this example, one EPSP alone does not depolarize the membrane to threshold for eliciting an action potential (AP), but if one EPSP (or more) follows shortly after the first one, the threshold is reached (summation). **B:** The time course and polarity of an inhibitory postsynaptic synaptic potential (IPSP) and how the hyperpolarization is reduced when an EPSP is added to an IPSP.

Summation of Stimuli Is Necessary to Evoke an Action Potential

One or a few presynaptic action potentials leading to transmitter release do not evoke an action potential in the postsynaptic cell. As previously mentioned, the membrane has to be depolarized to a **threshold** value (Fig. 4.5A) for an action potential to be evoked. Usually, the threshold is approximately 10 mV more positive than the resting potential, and the size of an EPSP is probably in most cases less than 1 mV. As previously mentioned, to produce an action potential the current produced at synaptic sites must be strong enough to reach the initial segment and depolarize the membrane to threshold (by opening voltage-gated Na^+ channels).

A subthreshold depolarization may nevertheless be of functional significance. If the synaptic potential is followed by another depolarization before the membrane potential has returned to resting value, the second depolarization is added to the first one so that threshold is reached. This phenomenon is called **summation** (Fig. 4.5A). The summation may be in time, as in the example above, and is then called **temporal summation**,

or it may be in space, and is then called **spatial summation**. In temporal summation, impulses may follow one another in rapid succession in one terminal, whereas in spatial summation, nerve terminals at different places on the cell surface release transmitter and depolarize the cell almost simultaneously. In addition, IPSPs are subject to spatial and temporal summation.

An EPSP increases the **probability** that the postsynaptic neuron produce an action potential: for a moment the neuron is more responsive to other inputs. Likewise, an IPSP decreases this probability.

Slow Synaptic Effects Modulate the Effect of Fast Ones

Because neurons are equipped with both ionotropic and metabotropic transmitter receptors, we may safely assume that every neuron receives both fast (direct) and slow (indirect) synaptic inputs. The slow effects modulate the effects of the fast ones, and we therefore use the term **modulatory transmitter actions**. A modulatory transmitter (when binding to an indirectly acting receptor) does not by itself evoke action potentials but alters the response of a neuron to fast, ionotropic transmitter actions. Usually, modulatory synaptic effects are mediated by altering opening states of K^+ or Ca^{2+} channels, thereby modulating both the membrane potential and the refractory period. The effects are nevertheless much more varied because there are several kinds of potassium and calcium channels, and several transmitters may influence each channel.

A brief train of impulses in axons releasing a transmitter that binds to indirectly acting receptors may keep the membrane depolarized or hyperpolarized for seconds after the train of impulses ends (slow EPSP or IPSP; Fig. 4.6). More intense stimulation may produce depolarization that lasts minutes in some neurons.

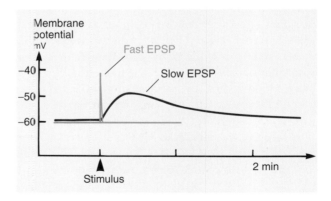

FIGURE 4.6 *Fast and slow synaptic actions.* Schematic. A fast EPSP lasts milliseconds and is caused by binding of transmitter molecules directly to channel proteins. A slow EPSP may last seconds or minutes and is due to activation of receptors indirectly coupled to ion channels.

An example may make this clearer: motor neurons in the cord receive fast, excitatory synaptic input from the cerebral cortex. These signals mediate the precise, voluntary control of muscle contraction. In addition, the motor neurons receive slow, modulatory synaptic inputs from cell groups in the brain stem whose activity is related to the degree of motivation for a particular movement. The modulatory input influences the strength of the response (frequency of action potentials) to signals from the cerebral cortex, that is, how fast the movement will be. However, the modulatory input does not initiate movements on its own.

Mechanisms of Modulatory Synaptic Effects

Slow EPSPs may be mediated by transmitters closing a kind of voltage-gated K^+ channel that is open at the resting membrane potential. This leads to lowered K^+ permeability and reduced flow of K^+ out of the cell, which results in depolarization. Because the membrane potential is shifted toward the threshold, fast depolarization is more likely to elicit an action potential. In addition, the effect on this kind of channel makes a fast EPSP larger and longer-lasting because the fast transmitter opens the K^+ channel during the repolarization phase of the EPSP. When the modulatory transmitter counteracts the opening of the channel in this phase, the depolarization becomes stronger, and the repolarization phase is prolonged. In this way the fast transmitter, rather than eliciting one, may produce a train of action potentials.

Modulatory synaptic effects may not change the resting membrane potential, if they are confined to channels that are not open at the resting potential. A kind of K^+ channel—closed at the resting potential—is opened by Ca^{2+} entering the cell during the action potential. This produces a relatively long-lasting hyperpolarization (the refractory period). A modulatory transmitter that reduces the opening of the K^+ channel would shorten the refractory period. As in the preceding example, a fast excitatory input might produce a train of impulses rather than only one, or the frequency of impulses during a train might be higher than without the modulatory influence.

Slow, long-lasting hyperpolarizing synaptic effects (slow IPSPs) are usually mediated by the indirect opening of K^+ channels. As we discussed later, the ubiquitous inhibitory transmitter GABA can act on receptors with such effect.

A Neuron Integrates Information from Many Others

We have seen that as a rule many impulses must reach a neuron almost simultaneously to make it fire, that is, to send an action potential through its axon. In other words, summation of excitatory synaptic effects is necessary. The stronger the sum of excitatory effects, the shorter the time necessary to depolarize the cell to the threshold for eliciting another action potential. This means that the frequency of action potentials, or **firing frequency**, is an expression of the **total synaptic input** to a neuron. Total synaptic input here means the sum of both excitatory and inhibitory synaptic influences. Most neurons receive thousands of synapses; for example, large neurons in the motor cortex of the monkey may receive as many as 60,000 synapses. Often a neuron is strongly influenced (many synaptic contacts) by one neuronal group and weakly influenced by many others. This means that while such a neuron primarily transmits signals from one nucleus to another, many other cell groups facilitate or inhibit the efficiency of signal transmission.

Examples of Synaptic Integration

We will provide two examples of the integration of different synaptic inputs. The first concerns **motor neurons** of the spinal cord. Such a neuron—sending its axon to innervate hundreds of striated muscle cells in a particular muscle—is synaptically contacted by neurons in many parts of the nervous system. It may receive around 30,000 synapses, distributed over its dendrites and cell body. Some synapses inform the cell about sensory stimuli that are important for the movement produced by the muscle, others about the posture of the body, others about how fast an intended movement should be, and so forth. The sum of all these synaptic inputs—some of them excitatory, others inhibitory—determines the frequency of action potentials sent to the muscle and by that means the force of muscle contraction (each muscle, however, is governed by many such neurons, so that their collective activity determines the behavior of the whole muscle).

The other example concerns neurons in the spinal cord that mediate information about **painful stimuli**. Although such a neuron receives its strongest synaptic input (most synapses) from sensory organs reacting to painful stimuli, it is also contacted by thousands of synapses from other sources, such as cell groups that are active when the person is anxious. This means that the final firing frequency of this "pain-transmitting" neuron depends not only on the actual stimuli reaching the receptors but also on the activity within the CNS itself. This correlates well with the everyday experience that the pain we feel depends not only on the strength of the peripheral painful stimulus (such as dental drilling) but also on our state of mind. Although the main task of the neuron is to convey sensory information to the brain, this information is integrated in the spinal cord with signals from other sources conveying information the salience of the sensory information.

The Placement of Synapses Has Functional Significance

Where a synapse is located on the neuronal surface is obviously not a matter of chance (Fig. 1.8). There are several examples of axons arising from different cell groups that end on different parts: for example, some end only on proximal dendrites, others on distal dendrites or a particular segment of the dendrite. Further, **inhibitory** synapses are often located on or near the soma of the nerve cell, whereas **excitatory** ones are most abundant on dendrites. The placement can be of functional importance, because synapses close to the **initial segment** of the axon would be expected to have a greater chance of eliciting (or preventing) an action potential than synapses far out on the dendrites. (This is due to the loss of current during electrotonic spread of the synaptic potential over long distances.) In some neurons, powerful inhibitory synapses are even located on the initial segment itself, thereby forming a very efficient "brake" on neuronal firing.

In general, a synapse far out on a dendrite would be expected to exert a weaker effect on the excitability of the neuron than one placed close to the soma, and, consequently, that more summation would be needed for distal synapses than for proximal ones to fire the neuron. New findings suggest that this may not always hold true, however. Studies of pyramidal neurons (in the hippocampus) indicate that an EPSP recorded in the soma is of about equal magnitude regardless of whether it is evoked by a synapse that is proximal or distal on a dendrite. This means that a stronger depolarizing action at distal synapses compensates for their greater loss of current by electrotonic spread.

Another important point regarding the placement of synapses is that most excitatory synapses are located on dendritic **spines** (Figs. 1.1, 1.7, and 1.9). Most of the neurons in the cerebral cortex conform to this arrangement. Because cortical neurons constitute a large proportion of all neurons in the human brain, suggestions that about 90% of all excitatory synapses are located on spines may be realistic.

Spines: Crucial for Learning?

The functional significance of dendritic spines is still under debate. It is not simply a matter of increasing the receiving surface of the neuron because the dendritic membrane between spines may be virtually free of synapses. A spine typically consists of a narrow neck and an expanded part called the spine head (see Fig. 1.9). Since their microscopic identification more than 100 years ago, spines have been implicated in **learning** and **memory,** and recent animal experiments support this hypothesis. For example, the density of spines in the cerebral cortex is higher in rats that live in a challenging environment than in those that are confined to standard laboratory cages. Further, the density of spines in the cerebral cortex is markedly reduced in individuals with severe mental retardation. Animal experiments with electric stimulation indicate that long-term increases in synaptic efficacy (long-term potentiation, LTP) are associated with changes of spine morphology and number. This effect is observed only among synapses affected by the increased stimulation and may be directly related to learning and memory.

An important function of spines may be to facilitate **local synaptic changes.** The narrow neck of the spines may ensure that the concentration of signal molecules responsible for LTP induction, such as Ca^{2+}, reach much higher levels in the spine head than in the dendrite. This would facilitate changes in those synapses contacting a particular spine, leaving other synapses unaffected.[3] Spatial restriction of increased Ca^{2+} concentration may also serve a **protective role** since high intracellular Ca^{2+} concentration may damage the neuron.

Axoaxonic Synapses Enable Presynaptic Control of Transmitter Release

In axoaxonic synapses, the presynaptic bouton makes synaptic contact with a postsynaptic bouton, which, in turn, contacts a cell body or a dendrite (Fig. 4.7). Release of transmitter from the presynaptic bouton serves to regulate the amount of transmitter released by the postsynaptic bouton. This enables inhibition or facilitation of a subset of synaptic inputs to a neuron. The excitability of the postsynaptic neuron is unaltered, in contrast to the situation described above with postsynaptic inhibition by IPSPs.

In the best-studied kind of axoaxonic contacts, action potentials in the presynaptic bouton lead to reduced transmitter release from the postsynaptic bouton; that is, the effect is inhibitory with regard to the neuron contacted by the postsynaptic bouton (the postsynaptic bouton usually has an excitatory action). A prerequisite for this inhibitory effect to occur, however, is that the presynaptic bouton be depolarized (by an action potential) at the same time as or immediately before an action potential reaches the postsynaptic bouton. This phenomenon is termed **presynaptic inhibition** to distinguish it from postsynaptic inhibition. Presynaptic inhibition has been found most frequently among fiber systems that transmit sensory information; for example, sensory fibers entering the spinal cord are subject to

---

3 Indeed, experiments performed in slices of tissue from the hippocampus (a region involved in learning and memory)—enabling stimulation of single axospinous synapses—suggest that enduring changes (LTP) may be limited to the stimulated synapse. However, it seems that nearby synapses (10–20 synapses within a distance of 10 μm along the dendrite) have lowered thresholds for induction of LTP for some minutes after the stimulation. Such "crosstalk" among nearby synapses is presumably caused by dendritic spread of a diffusible substance produced in the stimulated spine.

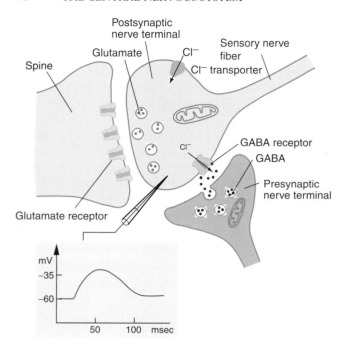

FIGURE 4.7 *Presynaptic inhibition is mediated by axoaxonic synapses.* The example is from the spinal cord where an inhibitory interneuron contacts the terminal of a sensory nerve fiber (from a spinal ganglion cell). The interneuron releases GABA that opens Cl⁻ channels and thereby depolarizes the postsynaptic nerve terminal (frame). This leads to release of less transmitter. See text for further explanations. (Based on Alvarez 1998.)

powerful presynaptic inhibition. In this way, signals to a sensory neuron from pain receptors can be selectively inhibited, while signals from other receptors are passed on unaltered.

Mechanisms of Presynaptic Inhibition and Facilitation

Several mechanisms may be involved in **presynaptic inhibition**. The phenomenon has been most studied in the spinal cord dorsal horn, where axoaxonic synapses are formed by inhibitory interneurons as they contact terminals of primary sensory afferents (Fig. 4.7). The transmitter released from the interneuron (usually GABA) opens chloride channels in the postsynaptic terminal (bouton). In most neurons, opening of chloride channels either hyperpolarizes or short-circuits the membrane, as described. In the sensory terminals in the cord, however, opening of chloride channels **depolarizes** the membrane, due to an unusually high intracellular chloride concentration. (To uphold this concentration gradient, these sensory neurons are equipped with a special transport mechanism for chloride coupled to the sodium–potassium pump). In this way, the equilibrium potential of Cl⁻ is more positive (−30 mV) than the resting potential (−65 mV) and, consequently, chloride ions move *out* of the nerve terminal

when chloride channels open. But how can depolarization of the presynaptic terminal reduce transmitter release? The answer seems to be that depolarization reduces the amplitude of action potentials as they invade the postsynaptic terminal; in turn, this leads to opening of fewer voltage-gated calcium channels. Because the amount of transmitter released is proportional to the influx of Ca²⁺, less transmitter will be released. It remains to be explained why depolarization of the postsynaptic terminal reduces the amplitude of the action potential. The most likely explanation is that depolarization inactivates some voltage-gated sodium channels in the postsynaptic terminal. In addition, direct influence on Ca²⁺ channels by the transmitter released from the presynaptic terminal may also contribute to presynaptic inhibition.

Presynaptic facilitation can be elicited by axoaxonic synapses by increasing Ca²⁺ influx in the postsynaptic bouton. Closure of K⁺ channels by the presynaptic transmitter prolongs the action potential by slowing the repolarization phase, thereby allowing more Ca²⁺ to enter the postsynaptic bouton.

Why Do We Need Inhibitory Synapses?

Inhibitory synapses are present everywhere in the CNS and are of vital importance for its proper functioning. For example, inhibition is necessary to suppress irrelevant **sensory information**, thereby enabling us to concentrate on certain events and leave others out. Inhibitory synapses also serve to increase the precision of sensory information by, for example, enhancing contrast between regions with different light intensity in visual images.

Inhibition is also necessary for another reason—namely, to interrupt or **dampen excitation**, which might otherwise lead to cell damage. As mentioned earlier, ions have to be pumped through the cell membrane in order to maintain osmotic equilibrium. If many neurons fire continuously with high frequency, even maximal pumping may be insufficient in this respect. Increased extracellular potassium concentration depolarizes neurons, thereby increasing further the neuronal excitation; this leads to more potassium extracellularly, and so on. **Epileptic seizures** are due to uncontrolled firing of groups of neurons, and drugs reducing the tendency for seizures generally increase the effect of inhibitory transmitters. Figure 4.8 shows how an excitatory neuron can limit its firing by way of an **inhibitory interneuron**. Although not shown in the figure, the interneuron is influenced by many other neurons that serve to adjust the brake, as it were. Such arrangements are common, for example, among the motor neurons that control muscle contractions (see Fig. 21.14). In general, inhibitory interneurons increase the **flexibility** of the nervous system.

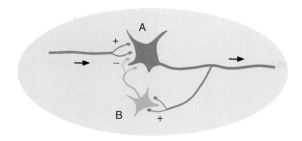

FIGURE 4.8 *Inhibitory interneuron (B) mediating negative feedback to the projection neuron (A). Arrows show the direction of impulse conduction.*

Signaling by Disinhibition

In some instances, inhibitory synaptic couplings may lead to increased rather than decreased excitation. This occurs when inhibitory neurons inhibit other inhibitory neurons that in their turn act on excitatory ones (Fig. 4.9). With such an arrangement, firing of the first inhibitory interneuron (green) inhibits the next inhibitory interneuron, which thereby reduces its activity. Thereby, the excitatory neuron (red) receives less inhibition and increases its firing. This is called **disinhibition**, and it plays an important role in diverse structures such as the retina and the basal ganglia (Fig. 23.14). If an inhibitory interneuron contacts both excitatory and inhibitory neurons, it might produce both inhibition and disinhibition at the same time in different neurons. By controlling the firing of such interneurons, central command centers—such as the motor cortex—can direct the signals in the desired direction. This occurs, for example, in the spinal cord where inhibitory interneurons serve to select the muscles that are best suited for a particular task.

SYNAPTIC PLASTICITY

Basis of Learning and Memory?

There is much evidence that synapses can alter their structure and function in an **activity-dependent** or **use-dependent** manner: that is, they are **plastic**. This means

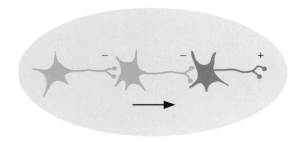

FIGURE 4.9 *Disinhibition.* Two inhibitory neurons (green) coupled in series increases the activity of an excitatory neuron (red).

that for a shorter or longer period, the postsynaptic action may be enhanced or reduced, as evidenced by altered amplitude of the postsynaptic potentials. Further, much experimental evidence supports the hypothesis that synaptic plasticity is the cellular basis of learning and memory. Martin, Grimwood, and Morris (2000, p. 650) express the hypothesis as follows: "Activity-dependent synaptic plasticity is induced at appropriate synapses during memory formation, and is both necessary and sufficient for the information storage underlying the type of memory mediated by the brain area in which that plasticity is observed." When we learn, most likely numerous synapses change their efficacy within distributed neural networks; when we later can recall what we learned, it must mean that synaptic changes have been retained. When we forget, one reason may be the decay of learning-related synaptic changes. Obviously, the most difficult part of the hypothesis to prove is a causal relationship between specific synaptic changes and memory in behavioral terms.

Under Which Conditions do Synaptic Changes Occur?

Only a minute fraction of all the information reaching the brain is retained in memory, and correspondingly, use of a synapse does not always change its subsequent behavior. To induce a change, the presynaptic influences must conform to certain patterns. In general, plastic changes are likely to occur when the presynaptic activity is particularly strong and coincide in time with the postsynaptic neuron firing an action potential.[4] This makes sense, as the immediate firing of an action potential after a synaptic input might be regarded as a sign of success. This situation is likely to arise only when several excitatory synaptic inputs reach the neuron at the same time. Looking for the functional meaning of simultaneous inputs, a crucial point may be the ability of neurons to detect **coincidences**. For example, a sensory input is significant only in a certain **context**, and only then should it be remembered. Accordingly, synaptic changes would occur only when information about the sensory event and its context coincide. However, contextual information should lead to synaptic change only if it signals that the sensory stimulus is important or unexpected. Indeed, in many situations, it appears that synaptic change depends on the coincidence of a specific input mediated by activation of ionotropic receptors and a modulatory input mediated by metabotropic receptors (Fig. 4.10). The first input provides fast and precise information—for example,

4 This was postulated by the Canadian psychologist Donald Hebb in 1949 (p. 62) in an influential attempt to explain the cellular basis of learning: "when an axon of cell A is near enough to excite a cell B and repeatedly or persistently takes part in firing it, some growth process or metabolic change takes place in one or both cells such that A's efficiency, as one of the cells firing B, is increased."

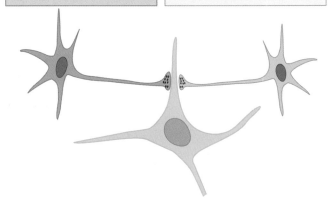

Precise information about "what", "where", and "when"	Modulating information about motivation, attention, emotions
Transmitters: Glutamate (excitatory) GABA (inhibitory)	Transmitters: Norepinephrine, dopamine, acetylcholine, serotonin, and others

FIGURE 4.10 *Synaptic plasticity.* Learning—that is, synaptic change—depends in this example on simultaneous action of a specific synaptic input and a modulatory one. The latter provides a signal about the salience of the specific stimulus.

about the nature of a sensory stimulus—the other about the **salience** of the stimulus.

Mechanisms for Synaptic Plasticity

Broadly speaking, a change of synaptic efficacy may arise because:

- The **presynaptic** terminal releases more or less neurotransmitter in response to an action potential.
- The **postsynaptic** neuron has increased or reduced its response to the transmitter.

We have discussed the complex cellular processes that link an action potential to transmitter release (see, e.g., Figs. 4.1 and 4.2), and many of the factors involved have been shown experimentally to change their activity in a use-dependent manner. For example, there may be changes in the amount and activity of intracellular second messengers and protein kinases (among other things, regulating ion channels and receptor proteins). The properties, number, and distribution of transmitter receptors are also subject to activity-dependent modifications. Nevertheless, in spite of the large number of molecular mechanisms involved in induction and maintenance of synaptic plasticity, increased intracellular **calcium concentration** appears as a rule to **initiate** the process. The further pathways from a calcium signal to altered synaptic efficacy are multifarious and only partly known. With regard to structural correlates of synaptic plasticity, we mentioned above that **spines** undergo changes of size and form that are

correlated with altered synaptic efficacy. Further, the **formation** of new synapses (synaptogenesis) and **elimination** of old ones is very prominent during pre- and postnatal development but occur throughout adult life.

Enduring changes in neurons—at either a molecular or a structural level—require altered **protein synthesis.**[5] Proteins have a restricted lifetime, however, and long-term change would therefore require long-term (in many instances life-long) alteration of **gene expression**. We now have much evidence that even synaptic activity lasting for minutes or less may produce altered expression of certain genes that encode for transcription factors (see Chapter 3, under "Markers of Neuronal Activity"). The experimental evidence so far mainly concerns transitory changes of gene expression; nevertheless, a number of genes have been shown to alter their expression in long-term synaptic changes. Although the complex signaling pathways that link neuronal activity to gene expression are thus starting to be revealed, many questions remain. It is not clear, for example, how the altered gene expression can be directed to certain synapses (those subjected to a "memorable" input) and not to others.

Kinds of Synaptic Plasticity

Several kinds of synaptic plasticity have been described on the basis of animal experiments, and more are probably yet to be discovered. It is customary to distinguish between short-term and long-term synaptic plasticity, without a sharp transition. **Short-term plasticity** lasts from less than a second to some minutes, whereas **long-term plasticity** can last for at least several weeks. For practical reasons it is not feasible to study the phenomenon for longer periods in experimental animals. Nevertheless, if synaptic plasticity underlies memories, we know from our own experience that some synaptic changes must last for a lifetime.

The ability of synapses to express plastic changes is subject to regulation by various signal substances. This phenomenon is called **metaplasticity**. Generally, metaplasticity may serve **homeostatic** purposes, by keeping plastic changes within certain limits. However, plasticity may probably also be up- or down-regulated by environmental challenges ("enriched" environment, stress), and in neurological diseases (e.g., Alzheimer's disease, stroke, and Parkinson's disease).

---

5 Brain-derived neurotrophic factor (BDNF) is an example of a growth factor that appears to be instrumental for induction of certain forms of long-term synaptic plasticity. Interestingly, BDNF plays a role in many brain processes in which synaptic plasticity plays a prominent role (from brain development to mental diseases).

Short-Term Plasticity

When action potentials reach the nerve terminal at relatively brief intervals, the amplitude of the ensuing postsynaptic potentials often increases gradually. This phenomenon is called **facilitation** and is due to increased transmitter release by each presynaptic action potential. The postsynaptic effect increases for each action potential until reaching a steady state after about 1 sec and then decays rapidly when stimulation stops. Further, at some synapses a series of presynaptic action potentials produce increased synaptic efficacy for minutes after the stimulation ends. This is called (synaptic) **potentiation**, and like facilitation, it is due to increased transmitter release from the nerve terminal. Potentiation can be particularly strong and long lasting after tetanic stimulation (action potentials with maximal frequency). This is called **posttetanic potentiation**. The presynaptic terminal "remembers" that it recently received unusually intense stimulation and alters its behavior accordingly. Facilitation and posttetanic potentiation are examples of short-term plasticity that are important for the nervous system's capacity for storage of information. **Short-term depression**—that is, a weaker postsynaptic response with repeated presynaptic action potentials—is probably due to insufficient renewal of the releasable synaptic pool (Fig. 4.2).

Long-Term Plasticity: LTP and LTD

Long-term plasticity means changes of synaptic efficacy lasting for hours to weeks (years). **Long-term potentiation (LTP)** and **long-term depression (LTD)** can somewhat arbitrarily be defined as activity-dependent increases or decreases of synaptic efficacy that lasts for more than 1 hour. Presumably, LTP and LTD represent storage of information that is in some way meaningful to the individual (or interpreted as such). With these forms of long-term plasticity, cellular changes occur presynaptically and postsynaptically (not only presynaptically, as do facilitation and posttetanic potentiation). Different forms of both LTP and LTD have been described; they differ with regard to duration, the kind of activity that induces them, and molecular mechanisms. One important mechanism seems to be the **insertion of new receptors** in the postsynaptic membranes, which increases the receptor density and the effect of each quanta of transmitter released from the presynaptic terminal (see "Silent Synapses" later). Regardless of molecular mechanisms involved in the expression of LTP and LTD, the end results are input-specific alterations of synaptic efficacy (see also Chapter 32, under "LTP and Memories").

LTP and LTD are evoked by different patterns of synaptic inputs. Whereas high-frequency firing or two simultaneous inputs induces LTP, low-frequency firing or two inputs that are out of phase induces LTD. It seems reasonable that intense activity and synchronization of specific inputs strengthens connections within a network, whereas low activity or desynchronized inputs reduce strength of connectivity—the latter being interpreted as "noise" rather than meaningful information. Further, it appears that LTP is induced if a presynaptic action potential repeatedly precedes firing of the postsynaptic cell, whereas LTD occurs if the postsynaptic firing precedes the presynaptic action potential. In this way, inputs that cause postsynaptic firing (that is, "successful" ones) are strengthened, whereas inputs that do not contribute to postsynaptic firing are weakened.

It may seem paradoxical that the opposite phenomena—LTP and LTD—are both induced by an increase in intracellular Ca^{2+}. There is evidence, however, that intracellular responses to calcium transients can vary depending on their magnitude, time course, and site of origin.

Silent Synapses

It might seem unlikely that the brain contains a large number of synapses that are not in use. Nevertheless, there is now strong evidence that some synapses do not transmit a signal, even though the nerve terminal is invaded by action potentials (this is mainly studied in

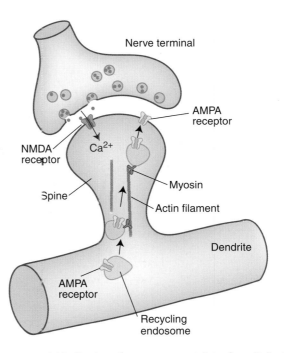

FIGURE 4.11 *Getting silent synapses to "speak up."* Activation of NMDA receptors leads to rapid influx of Ca^{2+} ions into the spine. This induces transport of so-called recycling endosomes—containing AMPA receptors—from the dendrite to the spine head. The transport depends on interaction between actin filaments and a special form of myosin molecules in the spine shaft.

the cord and the hippocampus). This is not just a case of low release probability, because even repeated presynaptic firing is without effect (the probability that a presynaptic action potential releases the content of a synaptic vesicle varies enormously in the CNS). Further, in some areas stimulation of an axon evokes a weaker response than expected from the number of terminals. The reason for synapses being silent can be lack of either transmitter release or a postsynaptic response to the transmitter (due to lack of receptors or that the receptors are blocked). There is evidence of both mechanisms. For example, some glutamatergic synapses in the hippocampus lack the ionotropic amino-methylisoxazole-propionic acid (AMPA) receptors, while expressing voltage-dependent N-methyl-D-aspartate (NMDA) receptors (these are further described in Chapter 5, under "Glutamate Receptors"). Such synapses are silent because "normal" presynaptic glutamate release does not activate them. This is because the opening of NMDA receptors requires a certain magnitude of depolarization in addition to binding of glutamate. If NMDA receptors are opened by particularly strong depolarization of the postsynaptic membrane, however, this may, in turn, lead to the insertion of AMPA receptors in the postsynaptic membrane (Fig. 4.11). The receptors are transported rapidly from endosomes to the postsynaptic density, as shown with fluorescence labeling methods. Afterward, the synapse is no longer silent but "speaks up" when glutamate is released. In many instances, LTP may be caused by silent synapses being activated by insertion of AMPA receptors. The finding that silent synapses appear to be most numerous shortly after birth (in rats) supports their possible role in learning and memory.

5 | Neurotransmitters and Their Receptors

OVERVIEW

Certain general properties of neurotransmitters were outlined in the preceding chapters. We recall that a signal is conveyed from one neuron to the next by release of a **neurotransmitter** (transmitter). "Conventional" or "classical" neurotransmitters are small molecules, such as amino acids and amines. Another important group of signal substances, released at synapses, are peptide molecules, called neuropeptides. Although the "typical" transmitter is released and acts at receptors in a synapse, many transmitter receptors are found **extrasynaptically**, that is, without connection to a synapse. Indeed, many transmitters act both at synapses and extrasynaptically. The latter action is called **volume transmission**, and is obviously less precise than synaptic transmission. Many receptors are located presynaptically on nerve terminals. Some of them are **autoreceptors** (binding the transmitter released from the terminal), and others are **heteroreceptors** (binding other transmitters released from neurons in the vicinity). Many nerve terminals contain more than one transmitter; often a classical transmitter is **colocalized** with one or more neuropeptides.

Synthesis of a transmitter usually depends on the activity of a **key enzyme**, which controls the amount of transmitter available at a synapse. Transmitter receptors far outnumber the transmitters; thus each transmitter usually acts on several **ionotropic** and **metabotropic** receptors. The effects of a transmitter on a certain neuron therefore depend on which receptors the neuron expresses. Both the amount of transmitter available for release and the postsynaptic receptors are subject to use-dependent plasticity.

The most important **amino acid transmitters** are **glutamate** and γ-aminobutyric acid (**GABA**). Both are present in virtually all parts of the central nervous system (CNS), and are responsible for most of the fast and precise synaptic transmission, by acting on ionotropic receptors. Glutamate is the dominant excitatory transmitter, whereas GABA is inhibitory. These transmitters mediate most of the spatially and temporally precise excitation and inhibition needed for perception, movements, and cognition. Glutamate binds to three families of receptors (amino-methylisoxazole propionic acid [AMPA], N-methyl-D-aspartate [NMDA], and metabotropic glutamate receptors). The **AMPA** receptors are typical ionotropic receptors with fast excitatory action, whereas the **NMDA** receptors have properties that make them especially suited to detect coincidences and induce long-term potentiation (LTP). GABA acts on ionotropic **GABA$_A$** receptors and metabotropic **GABA$_B$** receptors.

Acetylcholine is used as transmitter by a limited number of neurons in the brain stem and basal forebrain, while axonal ramifications of the neurons occur in most parts of the brain. Acetylcholine acts on ionotropic **nicotinic** receptors and metabotropic **muscarinic** receptors. The latter type dominates in the CNS, and the actions of acetylcholine are especially related to motivation, sleep–wakefulness, and memory. The group of **biogenic amines** includes the monoamines **dopamine, norepinephrine** (epinephrine), and **serotonin** (and in addition histamine). Like acetylcholine, these transmitters are produced in a small number of neurons but nevertheless act in most parts of the brain. They bind mostly to metabotropic receptors, with actions related to arousal, mood (emotions), and synaptic plasticity. In general, acetylcholine and the biogenic amines have **modulatory** actions that serve to regulate the excitability of neurons, thus determining the magnitude of response to fast-acting transmitters such as glutamate and GABA. **Adenosine triphosphate** (ATP) and **nitric oxide** (NO) function as signal substances with transmitter-like actions in the CNS.

A large number of **neuropeptides** have modulatory and metabolic actions in the brain, and influence a variety of processes, from basic homeostasis to complex behaviors.

GENERAL ASPECTS

How to Prove that a Substance Functions as a Neurotransmitter

Many signal substances present in the brain are small molecules, including the **amino acids** glutamate, glycine, and GABA, and the **amines** norepinephrine, dopamine, serotonin, and histamine. Acetylcholine and ATP also belong to this group. Other signal substances are peptides and therefore fairly large. Such **neuropeptides** are chains of 5 to 30 amino acids. In general, the functions of the neuropeptides are far less clarified than those of the small-molecule transmitters. To prove that a substance present in a neuron actually functions as a neurotransmitter is not easy. It is not sufficient that neurons express specific **binding sites** for a substance; hormones, growth factors, and other molecules also bind to neuronal membrane receptors. Neither are there clear-cut chemical differences between neurotransmitters and other intercellular signal molecules. Indeed, the same molecule may function in several roles; for example, norepinephrine is both a neurotransmitter and a hormone. Further, some molecules—such as glutamate and glycine—are intercellular signal molecules and have a role in cellular metabolism (e.g., as building blocks for proteins).

To **prove** that a substance functions as a signal molecule, one must show the presence of corresponding receptors and that the substance is released in sufficient amounts (under physiological conditions) to activate the receptors. Additional criteria must be met to classify such a signal substance as a neurotransmitter, however. The substance must be **produced** by neurons, it must be **stored** in nerve terminals and **released** by depolarization, and the release must be **calcium dependent**. In addition, the released substance must be directly responsible for the postsynaptic changes. Finally, there must exist mechanisms for **inactivation** of the transmitter after release. Only a few signal substances have met all of these criteria when tested experimentally. For several others, the probability that they function as transmitters is nevertheless high, and they are often described as transmitters without reservation. Strictly speaking, however, they should be termed "transmitter candidates" or "putative transmitters." Acetylcholine was the first substance to be classified with certainty as a transmitter. The excitatory action of glutamate was discovered in the 1950s, but only toward 1990 was the neurotransmitter status of this ubiquitous amino acid verified.

Determination of Neuronal Content of Neurotransmitters and Distribution of Receptors

With biochemical methods, the content of transmitters in parts of the brain and in subcellular fractions can be determined. To obtain further knowledge, however, it is also necessary to link the transmitters to specific neurons with known connections and physiological properties. The first possibilities of studying the anatomy of neurons with known transmitters arose in the 1960s, when it was discovered that monoamine-containing neurons could be made fluorescent by a special treatment with formalin. This marked the beginning of intense investigations, with other methods as well, to characterize neurons with regard to connections and at the same time with regard to their transmitters. The introduction of immunological methods, such as **immunocytochemistry**, to localize substances in nervous tissue has been of particular importance. By purifying a potentially interesting substance present in nervous tissue, **antibodies** may be raised against it. The antibodies bind antigens where they are exposed in the tissue sections, and the antibodies can be visualized subsequently with the use of secondary antibodies. The secondary antibodies may be labeled with a fluorescent molecule, or they may be identified in other ways. Such methods have been widely used to demonstrate the localization of enzymes that are critical for synthesis or degradation of certain transmitters, such as tyrosine hydroxylase, which is necessary for the synthesis of dopamine and norepinephrine (Fig. 5.1A), choline acetyltransferase (ChAT) for synthesis of acetylcholine (Fig. 5.1B), and glutamic acid decarboxylase (GAD) for GABA. Even transmitter molecules that are themselves too small to serve as antigens can be specifically identified in tissue sections via immunocytochemical methods when conjugated to tissue proteins (with glutaraldehyde). This is the case for GABA (Fig. 5.1C), glutamate, and glycine. Immunocytochemical methods can also be applied to **ultrastructural** analysis, in order to determine the transmitter accumulated at specific synapses and also whether the transmitter is localized to certain organelles, such as presynaptic vesicles (Fig. 5.2). Combination of axonal transport methods and immunocytochemical procedures makes it possible to determine the connections, as well as the transmitter candidates and other neuroactive substances of specific neuronal groups.

Even though the determination of the transmitter candidates present in a neuron is of great importance, it is not always possible to know whether the substance has been synthesized in the cell or whether it has merely been taken up. Further, the concentration of a transmitter in parts of a neuron may be so low that it cannot be reliably detected with immunocytochemical methods. The use of *in situ* **hybridization** techniques helps to overcome this kind of problem. By these methods, it is not the neuropeptides or enzymes related to transmitter metabolism that are demonstrated but the presence of the corresponding **mRNA**.

Volume Transmission: Extrasynaptic Transmitter Release and Actions

A neurotransmitter (transmitter) is usually defined as a chemical substance that is released at a synapse and transmits a signal from one neuron to another (or to muscle cells or glandular cells). However, not all substances, otherwise behaving as neurotransmitters, are released at synapses (Fig. 5.3). In some places, neurotransmitters are released from **axonal varicosities** that do not form synapses. Further, many transmitter receptors are present **extrasynaptically**—that is, in the neuronal membrane outside synapses (Fig. 5.3). Therefore, some neurotransmitters act both at typical

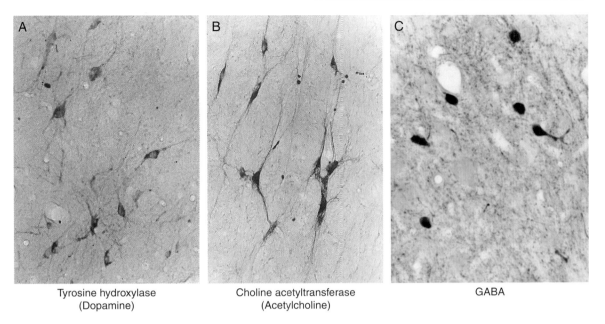

Tyrosine hydroxylase
(Dopamine)

Choline acetyltransferase
(Acetylcholine)

GABA

FIGURE 5.1 *Immunocytochemical demonstrations of neurotransmitters.* **A:** Dopaminergic neurons (substantia nigra) are visualized with an antibody against the enzyme tyrosine hydroxylase, which is involved in the synthesis of dopamine (Fig. 5.7). Neurons in between the black, labeled ones—not containing the enzyme—are not visible. Note that the method does not demonstrate the transmitter itself. **B:** Cholinergic neurons (basal nucleus) are visualized with an antibody against the enzyme choline acetyltransferase **C:** GABAergic neurons are visualized with an antibody that binds to a GABA–protein complex in the section. The brown cell bodies, showing GABA-like immunoreactivity, are interneurons in a brain stem nucleus (monkey). The small brown dots are partly dendrites, partly axons and nerve terminals.

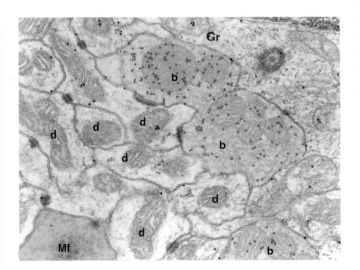

FIGURE 5.2 *Electron microscopic, immunocytochemical demonstration of neurotransmitters.* The small black dots represent gold particles bound in the tissue where GABA is present. The gold particles are conjugated to an antibody directed against a GABA–protein complex. The gold particles are concentrated over a particular kind of bouton (b), whereas dendrites (d) and part of a cell body (Gr) are not labeled. Another kind of nerve terminal (Mf) is also unlabeled and most likely contains a neurotransmitter other than GABA. Rat cerebellum. (Courtesy of Prof. O. P. Ottersen, Department of Anatomy, University of Oslo.)

synapses and more diffusely like local hormones—that is, on all receptors with the proper specificity within a certain distance from its release site. The distance depends on how quickly the transmitter is inactivated and how easily it diffuses. It appears that the effective distance is in the range of a few micrometers from the release site. We use the term **volume transmission** to distinguish this kind of transmitter action from the spatially precise action at synapses. The narrow definition of transmitters, focusing on their actions at synapses, fits well for transmitters such as glutamate and GABA with spatially and temporally precise actions. Other transmitters with mainly modulatory actions, such as norepinephrine, dopamine, and serotonin, act also by volume transmission. These different forms of transmitter actions complicate the analysis of how neurotransmitters control neurons and human behavior.

Colocalization of Transmitters

It was formerly assumed that each neuron releases only one transmitter. Recent studies have shown, however, that nerve terminals often contain more than one transmitter. Such **colocalization** of transmitters appears to be the rule rather than an exception. In most cases described so far, a small-molecule, "**classical" transmitter** is colocalized with one or several **neuropeptides**. In such cases, the terminal can evoke both fast synaptic

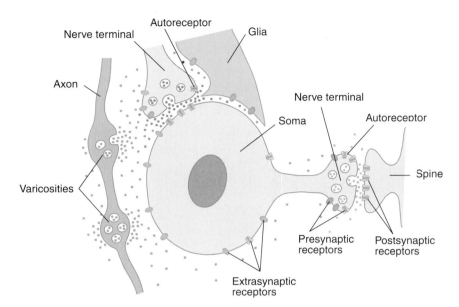

FIGURE 5.3 *Extrasynaptic receptors and transmitter release outside synapses.* Extrasynaptic receptors are localized both at the nerve terminals and on the somatic and dendritic surfaces of the neuron. Autoreceptors bind the transmitter released by the neuron itself. Note the release of transmitter from varicosities that do not form typical synaptic contacts.

actions mediated by ionotropic receptors and slow effects mediated by metabotropic receptors. Colocalization of two "classical" transmitters such as GABA and glycine—both acting on ionotropic receptors—has also been reported. GABA and glycine are both inhibitory, and it seems reasonable that colocalized transmitters exert similar postsynaptic actions. Even this may not be universally true, however. For example, certain spinal interneurons and neurons in the hypothalamus release ATP (excitatory) together with GABA (inhibitory); this means that both act on ionotropic receptors but apparently with opposite effects.

The widespread occurrence of colocalization complicates the interpretation of one particular transmitter's contribution to synaptic effects, and accordingly, its contribution to certain behaviors. Hypotheses about neural functions and disease symptoms have often been based on the erroneous belief that a particular neuronal group or fiber system uses only one transmitter (the one that was first discovered).

Transmitter Receptors in General

The many transmitters and transmitter candidates (more than 50, including the neuropeptides) have an even larger variety of receptor types to act on. More than 200 different metabotropic (G protein–coupled) receptors have been identified in the CNS. (Not all bind neurotransmitters, however; many bind hormones and a variety of growth factors.)

Several requirements have to be met to conclude that a binding site for a transmitter functions as a receptor. The "final proof" requires that the amino-acid sequence of the receptor site has been determined. After cloning of the protein, one can then determine whether it binds the transmitter (and agonists and antagonists) and produces the expected physiological effects.

As discussed in Chapter 3 (under "The Structure of Ion Channels"), all the **directly** acting, **ionotropic**, receptors—being part of ion channel proteins—are similarly built, with several subunits arranged around a central pore (see Fig. 3.2). In addition, the **indirectly** acting, **metabotropic** receptors share several structural features, although they are quite different from the ionotropic receptors. The metabotropic receptors usually consist of one large protein that makes several turns through the membrane with hydrophilic (water-soluble) groups on the interior and exterior of the membrane. The receptors mediate their effects via **G proteins** (see Fig. 4.2). Several receptor types with different postsynaptic actions have been identified for each of the best-known transmitters.

The most abundant transmitters, such as glutamate and GABA, act on both ionotropic and metabotropic receptors. The link between a neurotransmitter and its actions is made even more complex by the existence of subtypes of each main kind of receptor. Subtypes of the ionotropic (directly acting) GABA receptor (GABA$_A$) exemplify this. Each of the protein subunits forming the receptor (and the ion channel) comes in several varieties, and different combinations of them produce numerous subtypes of the GABA$_A$ receptor. These subtypes are differently distributed in the brain. This may explain why drugs acting on different subtypes of the GABA$_A$ receptor have different physiological and behavioral effects: they act on different neuronal networks.

Regulation of Receptor Density

The transmitter receptors are not static, immutable elements of the nervous system. We have discussed how changes in receptor density and activity may mediate **synaptic plasticity**. This means that learning would be expected to be associated with receptor changes. In animal experiments, for example, stressful psychological experiences leading to altered behavior also alter the activity of specific transmitter receptors. Drugs that interfere with transmitter actions often induce changes in the receptors. A drug that blocks the effect of a transmitter on a particular receptor type (antagonist) may indirectly produce increased postsynaptic receptor density. The reverse may occur with drugs that mimic the transmitter (agonist). Probably such **up- or down-regulation** of receptors represents an adaptive response: an abnormally high concentration of the transmitter (or an agonist) is counteracted by reduced receptor activity to maintain normal synaptic transmission. Down-regulation of receptors may explain many of the dramatic **withdrawal symptoms** that occur when an addicted individual abruptly discontinues a narcotic drug.

Presynaptic Transmitter Receptors

Transmitter receptors are also localized to the presynaptic membrane and can thereby modulate transmitter release (Fig. 5.3). We have discussed the axoaxonic synapses that mediate presynaptic inhibition by acting on receptors in the presynaptic membrane (see Fig. 4.7). In addition, the presynaptic membrane can express receptors for the transmitter released by the nerve terminal itself (see Fig. 4.1). Here we use the term **autoreceptors**. Often, autoreceptors inhibit transmitter release as a kind of **negative feedback**. Some neurons, for example, dopaminergic ones, are equipped with autoreceptors also on the cell body and dendrites. In addition to autoreceptors, nerve terminals may express **heteroreceptors**, that is, receptors for transmitters other than those they release themselves (often released by nearby terminals). Nerve terminals releasing **norepinephrine** can exemplify the complexity of presynaptic modulation. Such terminals can express α_2 adrenergic autoreceptors and muscarinic (acetylcholine), opiate, and dopamine receptors that inhibit release of norepinephrine from the terminal. In addition, the terminals also express β_2 adrenergic autoreceptors and nicotinic (acetylcholine) receptors that facilitate transmitter release. Thus, the amount of transmitter released by such a nerve terminal depends not only on the presynaptic activity of the neuron but also on the **local milieu** of the terminal (the concentration of various transmitters and other signal substances, as well as the presence of drugs or toxic substances). It should not come as a surprise that the functional roles of presynaptic receptors are not fully understood.

Synthesis of Neurotransmitters

The small-molecule, "classical" neurotransmitters (Table 5.1) are synthesized in the nerve terminals, the synthesis being catalyzed by enzymes transported axonally from the cell body. As a rule, the rate of transmitter synthesis is determined by the activity of one **key enzyme**. Up- or down-regulation of the enzymatic activity represents one way of changing the properties of nerve cells—with regard to learning, for example. Activation of enzymes often requires that they be phosphorylated, and this may be a result of external stimuli that, via membrane receptors, induce increased intracellular concentration of second messengers (such as Ca^{2+} or cyclic AMP).

As the organelles necessary for protein synthesis are present almost exclusively in the cell body, the **neuropeptides** must be synthesized in the cell body and subsequently transported to the terminals. Accordingly, substances that block axonal transport, such as **colchicine**, lead to accumulation of neuropeptides in the cell body. Usually, the neuropeptides are produced as larger polypeptides (prepropeptides) that most likely are split into smaller units on their way to the terminals.

SPECIFIC NEUROTRANSMITTERS

Excitatory Amino Acid Transmitters: Glutamate and Aspartate

The amino acid group contains the ubiquitous excitatory transmitter, **glutamate** (Fig. 5.4). Neurons that release glutamate at their synapses are called **glutamatergic**. The dominant effect of glutamate in the CNS is fast excitation by direct action on ion channels, although it also acts on metabotropic receptors. Glutamate is responsible for fast and precise signal transmission in the majority (all?) of the large sensory and motor tracts, as well as in the numerous connections between various parts of the cerebral cortex that form the networks responsible for higher mental functions. The total concentration of glutamate in the brain is very high, although the distribution is uneven. Notably, effective uptake mechanisms keep the extracellular concentration very low (about 1/1000 of intracellular concentration). This is a prerequisite for glutamate's function as a neurotransmitter—acting only on specific receptors after controlled release from nerve terminals. Low extracellular concentration is also mandatory because even a small increase is toxic to the neurons. Transporter proteins in astroglial membranes maintain the concentration gradient (probably with a

TABLE 5.1 *The Best-Known Small-Molecule (Classical) Neurotransmitters*

Transmitter	Chemical	Receptor Name Mechanism, Ion Permeability*	Synaptic Action	Distribution of Receptors in the CNS†	Localization of Neurons Synthesizing the Transmitter in the CNS†	Localization of Neurons in the PNS
Glutamate	Amino acid	AMPA, ionotropic, Na^+; NMDA, ionotropic, Ca^{2+}; MGluR1-5, metabotropic	Fast, excitation; Fast, excitation; Slow, excitation or inhibition, metabolic effects	"Everywhere"	"Everywhere"	Spinal ganglion cells
GABA	Amino acid	GABA ionotropic, Cl^-; $GABA_B$, metabotropic, K^+, Ca^{2+}	Fast, inhibition; Slow, inhibition	"Everywhere"	"Everywhere"	Gut, ganglia
Glycine	Amino acid	Ionotropic, Cl^-	Fast, inhibition		Brain stem, spinal cord, cerebellum	
Acetylcholine	Quaternary amine	Nicotinic, ionotropic, Na^+	Fast, excitation	Cerebral cortex, spinal cord (and other places)	Motoneurons, preganglionic autonomic neurons, basal nucleus, septal nuclei, nuclei in the reticular formation of the brain stem (and other places)	Parasympathetic ganglia
		Muscarinic, metabotropic K^+, Ca^{2+}	Slow, excitation or inhibition	Cerebral cortex, hippocampus, thalamus (and other places)		
Norepinephrine	Amine	α (α_1–α_2), metabotropic; β (β_1–β_2), metabotropic	Slow; Slow	"Everywhere"	Locus coeruleus and diffuse cell groups in the reticular formation	Sympathetic ganglia
Dopamine	Amine	D_1(D_1, D_5), metabotropic, increase cyclic AMP; D_2(D_2, D_3, D_4), metabotropic, decrease cyclic AMP	Slow; Slow	"Everywhere" (especially basal ganglia and pre-frontal cortex)	Mesencephalon (Substantia nigra and ventral tegmental area)	
Serotonin (5-HT)	Amine	$5\text{-}HT_{1A}$, metabotropic, K^+; $5\text{-}HT_2$, metabotropic; $5\text{-}HT_3$, ionotropic, Na^+	Slow, inhibition; Slow, excitation; Fast, excitation	"Everywhere"	Raphe nuclei (brain stem)	

*There are more receptor subtypes than shown here.

†The table is not complete regarding distribution of neurons and receptors.

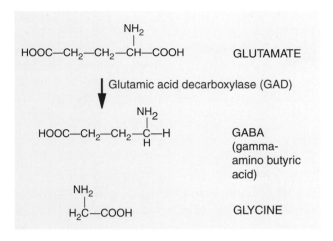

FIGURE 5.4 *Amino acid transmitters.* The enzyme glutamic acid decarboxylase (GAD) is specific for neurons that synthesize GABA.

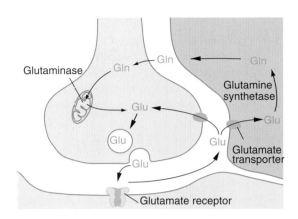

FIGURE 5.5 *The glutamate–glutamine "circuit."* The enzyme glutamine synthetase converts glutamate (Glu) to glutamine (Gln) after uptake by glial cells. In contrast to glutamate, glutamine is neutral to neurons. Glutamine is transferred to nerve terminals where it is used to synthesize new glutamate that is concentrated in vesicles for release, and so forth.

smaller contribution from transporters in neuronal membranes). In situations with poor energy supply, such as reduced blood flow or low blood sugar, glutamate leaks from the cells because the uptake mechanisms fail. The ensuing rise in extracellular glutamate concentration contributes significantly to the rapid occurrence of neuronal damage—for example, in cases of cardiac arrest (see also Chapter 11, under "Ischemic Cell Damage").

The amino acid **aspartate** is also highly concentrated in the CNS. It exerts an excitatory action by binding to glutamate receptors. Although decisive evidence is still lacking, recent studies speak in favor of aspartate being a neurotransmitter. For example, aspartate was found to be colocalized with glutamate in synaptic vesicles and released by exocytosis. Nevertheless, the distribution of possible aspartatergic synapses seems to be very limited in the brain. Therefore, with regard to excitatory synaptic transmission, aspartate must play a minor role compared with glutamate.

Synthesis of Glutamate

Glutamate is synthesized from two sources in the nerve terminals: **glucose** (via the Krebs cycle) and **glutamine** that is synthesized in glial cells and thereafter transported into the neurons (Fig. 5.5). Glutamine is converted in mitochondria to glutamate by the enzyme **glutaminase**. Specific transport proteins in the vesicle membrane fill the synaptic vesicles with glutamate. Glutamate is released as other transmitters by calcium-dependent exocytosis. Released glutamate is taken up by glia and converted to glutamine by the enzyme **glutamine synthetase**. Glutamine is then transported to nerve terminals, converted to glutamate, and so forth. Figure 5.5 shows the "glutamate–glutamine circuit," which ensures reuse of the transmitter. Another advantage with the

circuit is that glutamine, unlike glutamate, does not influence neuronal excitability, and is not toxic in high concentrations. Therefore, its concentration need not be strictly controlled.

Glutamate Receptors

As mentioned, the dominant action of glutamate in the CNS is fast excitation by direct binding to ionotropic receptors. In the early 1980s, however, additional kinds of glutamate receptors (**GluRs**) were found. We now recognize three groups or families of receptors that glutamate can bind to: **AMPA/kainate receptors,**[1] **NMDA receptors,** and **metabotropic glutamate receptors** (**mGluRs**). The two first groups are glutamate-gated ion channels (ionotropic receptors). The metabotropic glutamate receptors are G protein–coupled, like other metabotropic receptors. The various glutamate receptors were discovered via use of glutamate analogs that turned out to act only on certain kinds of receptors. The receptors were named after the analog that activated them selectively (amino-methylisoxazole propionic acid [AMPA]; N-methyl-D-aspartate [NMDA]). Cloning of the receptor proteins in the early 1990s showed that AMPA, NMDA, and metabotropic receptors belonged to different protein families. To date, 10

---

1 **Kainate receptors** belong to the same family of ionotropic receptors as AMPA receptors. They have been identified in many parts of the CNS and can be localized both pre- and postsynaptically. The concentration of kainate receptors is low in most areas, and they have not been as extensively studied as AMPA and NMDA receptors. Their total contribution to fast excitation—as compared to that of AMPA receptors—is therefore still not clarified. Kainate receptors are expressed in spinal ganglion cells (sensory neurons), and animal experiments suggest that blockage of these receptors may alleviate chronic pain.

varieties of AMPA/kainate receptors, 5 NMDA receptors, and 8 metabotropic receptors have been cloned.[2]

AMPA receptors are ion channels admitting Na^+ (and K^+), which is typical of fast, excitatory synapses. The current view is that AMPA receptors are responsible for the majority of the fast excitatory signals in the CNS (mediating, e.g., precise sensory information and motor commands).

NMDA receptors have properties that distinguish them from other ionotropic receptors. They have attracted much interest due to their role in long-term potentiation (LTP), and, therefore, most likely in learning and memory. They have a much slower synaptic action than the AMPA receptors and are engaged in other tasks. One important feature of NMDA-gated ion channels is that they are much more permeable to Ca^{2+} than to Na^+ (in contrast to AMPA-gated channels). This makes possible many postsynaptic effects of glutamate binding in addition to depolarization, because Ca^{2+} can trigger a number of intracellular processes (e.g., related to synaptic plasticity). Another special feature of NMDA receptors is that they are **voltage-dependent** and remain closed at resting membrane potential. Binding of glutamate (or NMDA) to the receptor opens it only if the membrane is already depolarized—for example, by the opening of AMPA receptors in the vicinity. Depolarization removes Mg^{2+} ions that otherwise block the channel. A final characteristic feature is that when the NMDA channel is opened, the flow of Ca^{2+} through it lasts much longer than an ordinary EPSP (which is produced by opening the AMPA channels).

Metabotropic glutamate receptors (mGluRs) are located both postsynaptically and presynaptically.[3] They fall into three groups, differing with regard to which intracellular signal pathway they activate. As to postsynaptic effects, it appears that **group I mGluRs** produce a long-lasting depolarization (slow EPSP), whereas **group II** has the opposite effect (slow IPSP). Obviously, the existence of glutamate receptors with inhibitory actions further complicates the analysis of glutamate as a transmitter. In addition, mGluRs have

metabolic effects that influence various neuronal processes—among them, the induction of LTP and LTD. As mGluRs are thought to be involved in a several brain diseases (e.g., epilepsy, schizophrenia, and stroke), drugs modulating the function mGluRs are being developed and tested in animal models of human diseases.

NMDA Receptors: Mediators of Both Learning and Neuronal Damage

Long-term potentiation (LTP) was described in Chapter 4. The transmission at an excitatory synapse can be changed for a long time when the synapse is active simultaneously with other excitatory synapses in the vicinity (associative LTP). In many areas in the CNS, the induction of LTP depends on activation of NMDA receptors, and the NMDA receptors appear to have just the right properties for this task because they require both postsynaptic depolarization and glutamate binding. (Not all LTP depends on NMDA receptors, however.) NMDA receptors have binding sites for substances other than glutamate, also. The amino acid **glycine** (otherwise acting as an inhibitory transmitter) binds to the NMDA receptor, and such binding is necessary for glutamate to open the NMDA channel. Other substances that occur naturally in the brain also influence the activity of the NMDA receptors, and thereby presumably determine how plastic many synapses are (**metaplasticity**). Changes in the concentrations of such substances might be relevant for learning and memory in general and for recovery after brain damage.

The NMDA receptor is also one among several candidates for mediating **cell damage** after abnormal excitatory activation (see also Chapter 11, under "Ischemic Cell Damage"). This occurs when nervous tissue receives insufficient oxygen (hypoxia), as in severely reduced blood pressure, stroke, cerebral bleeding, and so forth. Abnormally intense excitation may also occur during **epileptic seizures**. In such circumstances, extracellular glutamate concentration rises steeply and presumably, all kinds of glutamate receptors are activated (see later, "Glutamate Transporters"). Activation of NMDA receptors may nevertheless be especially important because it can lead to a rapid increase of the intracellular Ca^{2+} concentration. There is evidence that increased calcium concentration is crucial for cell death, among other things by increasing depolarization and initiating a vicious cycle that activates proteolytic enzymes and induces large concentration changes of ions. In turn, this causes osmotic imbalance with cell swelling and potential destruction. If activation of glutamate receptors has a crucial role for cell death after a stroke, blockage of glutamate receptors might be effective in reducing the damage (if started within 1–2 hours after onset of the symptoms).

2 Glutamate receptors are expressed also in **peripheral tissues** such as bone (osteoblasts and osteoclasts), in taste cells, in some ganglion cells, and in insulin-producing cells in the pancreas where they modulate insulin secretion. NMDA receptors (and other kinds of glutamate receptors) are expressed in the membrane of unmyelinated axons that lead from nociceptors (pain receptors) in the skin. The functions of glutamate receptors in peripheral tissues are less understood than in the brain.

3 Studies with immunogold labeling indicate that **metabotropic glutamate receptors** (mGluR1) are located at the periphery of synapses, whereas AMPA receptors occupy the central region. In addition, mGluRs are found without relation to synapses (enabling extrasynaptic transmission, see Fig. 5.1). Such segregation might allow the receptors to respond differentially to glutamate: the AMPA receptors would be activated by normal presynaptic stimulation (low frequency of action potentials), whereas mGluRs would be activated only by high-frequency stimulation that releases large amounts of glutamate at the synapse, or by spillover of glutamate from nearby synapses.

Animal experiments have yielded positive results, but so far they have not been confirmed in humans. Excitatory amino acid transmitters and the NMDA receptor may also be involved in the cell damage that occurs in various **neurodegenerative disorders** of the nervous system, such as amyotrophic lateral sclerosis (ALS) and Huntington's disease.

While excessive NMDA-receptor activation can harm neurons, **blockage** can also produce dramatic symptoms. This is exemplified by the drugs **ketamine** (Ketalar, used as a short-acting anesthetic) and **phencyclidine** (PCP, or "angel dust") that block NMDA receptors. Both drugs influence consciousness and disturb thought processes. Side effects of ketamine used for anesthesia are nightmares and hallucinations during awakening. The thought disturbances resemble those occurring in schizophrenia, and this led to the "**glutamate hypothesis**" for this disease. Ketamine in low doses may be effective for treating chronic pain, probably by blocking NMDA receptors on sensory neurons in the cord. **Alcohol** (ethanol) also influences NMDA receptors (besides many other actions in the nervous system; see later, "GABA Receptors Are Influenced by Drugs, Alcohol, and Anesthetics").

Glutamate Transporters

Five structurally different glutamate transporter proteins are identified, which also differ with regard to their distribution in the brain. The quantitatively dominant transporters are concentrated in glial membranes apposing neurons, particularly around synapses (see Fig. 4.1; see also Fig. 2.5). It is not unexpected that the concentration of transporters is highest in parts of the brain with a high density of glutamatergic nerve terminals.

The transport of glutamate into glial cells is driven by concentration gradients of Na^+ and K^+. That is, the electrochemical gradient is crucial for the activity of the transporters. Other factors also influence their activity, however. Thus, the expression of transporter proteins increases with activation of glutamate receptors, while the expression decreases after removal of glutamatergic innervation.

Glutamate Transporters and Brain Damage

Under pathologic conditions with insufficient energy supply (e.g., low blood flow) the electrochemical gradient cannot be maintained. Because of the high intracellular concentration of glutamate, the transporters reverse their direction of transport so that glutamate is released into the extracellular space instead of being removed from it. In this way, the extracellular glutamate concentration can reach levels several hundred times that of the normal resting level. This leads to massive receptor activation and high flow of Na^+ and Ca^{2+}

into the neurons, probably initiating a vicious cycle leading to cell death (see also earlier, "NMDA Receptors: Mediators of Both Learning and Neuronal Damage," and Chapter 11, under "Ischemic Cell Damage").

Inhibitory Amino Acid Transmitters: GABA and Glycine

GABA is the dominant inhibitory transmitter, being present in nearly all parts of the CNS (Figs. 5.1 and 5.2). As many as 20% of all synapses in the CNS may be GABAergic. GABA is used as a transmitter mainly by **interneurons** (most projection neurons are glutamatergic). It is synthesized from glutamic acid in a single step by the enzyme **glutamic acid decarboxylase** (**GAD**, Fig. 5.4). GABA acts on ionotropic **GABA$_A$** receptors, and metabotropic **GABA$_B$** receptors. GABA is removed from the extracellular space by high-affinity transporters (GAT), which are mainly localized to neuronal membranes (differing in this respect from glutamate transporters).

GABA appears to play an important role during **development** of the nervous system, and occurs very early—even before synapses are established. When synapses start to occur, GABA acts as an excitatory transmitter because it depolarizes rather than hyperpolarizes the postsynaptic neuron (by acting on GABA$_A$ receptors).[4] GABA is possibly the first excitatory transmitter to shape neuronal networks (before glutamate has taken over as the dominant excitatory transmitter). In addition, GABA influences proliferation, migration, and maturation of neurons.

Glycine (Fig. 5.4) is also an inhibitory transmitter, although with a much more limited distribution than GABA. Glycine is used as transmitter by a population of spinal interneurons and by some brain stem and cerebellar neurons. **Glycine receptors** are parts of chloride channels and have fast excitatory actions. **Strychnine** blocks glycine receptors (thereby blocking inhibition of spinal and brain stem motor neurons), and this explains why strychnine poisoning produces muscle cramps. Likewise, the **tetanus toxin** provokes violent muscle spasms because it inhibits synaptic release of glycine.

GABA Receptors

In most areas, GABA acts by opening **chloride channels**, thereby producing a brief hyperpolarizing current (IPSP) or short-circuiting excitatory currents (see Chapter 3, "Mechanisms of Postsynaptic Potentials (EPSPs and IPSPs)"). The receptor that forms the

---

4 This is probably due to high intracellular chloride concentration in embryonic neurons. The equilibrium potential for Cl⁻ is therefore more negative than in mature neurons, so that opening of chloride channels leads to net flow of Cl⁻ *out* of the neuron. The same situation appears to arise in the adult spinal cord in certain conditions with chronic pain, that is, GABAergic interneurons may lose their normal inhibitory action on pain transmission.

Cl⁻ channel is termed **GABA$_A$**; it consists of five membrane-spanning subunits (similar to the acetylcholine receptor shown in Fig. 4.2). There are several subtypes of the GABA$_A$ receptor, as mentioned (see earlier, "Transmitter Receptors in General"). Besides the binding site for GABA, the GABA$_A$ receptor has several others, which are targets of alcohol and several common drugs. GABA is normally present in low concentrations extracellularly, and may bind to **extrasynaptic** GABA$_A$ receptors (Fig. 5.3). This would mediate a tonic, fairly diffuse inhibition (in addition to the phasic one produced at GABAergic synapses). Although the function of this tonic inhibition is unknown, it is modulated by anesthetics, certain drugs, and alcohol.

GABA can also produce **slow IPSP** (long-lasting hyperpolarization) by indirectly opening K⁺ channels or blocking Ca²⁺ channels. The receptors producing these effects are termed **GABA$_B$**, and are G protein–coupled, metabotropic receptors. GABA$_B$ receptors are found both presynaptically and postsynaptically.[5] GABA$_B$ receptors inhibit several **reflexes**, such as the spinal stretch reflex (contraction in response to rapid stretch of a muscle) and the cough reflex. Although GABA$_B$ receptors are present in many parts of the CNS, the concentration in most places is much lower than that of GABA$_A$. Accordingly, blockage of GABA$_B$ receptors produces fewer behavioral effects than does blockage of GABA$_A$. It is possible that GABA$_B$ receptors are activated only under special circumstances, whereas GABA$_A$ receptors are more continuously active.

GABA Receptors Are Influenced by Drugs, Alcohol, and Anesthetics

Benzodiazepines, barbiturates, and some anesthetics bind to different sites at the GABA$_A$ receptor, but all potentiate the synaptic effect of GABA. The **benzodiazepines** (e.g., diazepam) act by increasing the opening frequency of the Cl⁻ channels, whereas the barbiturates prolong their opening time. Benzodiazepines are used to reduce anxiety and provide muscle relaxation, and some derivatives are used as hypnotics. The **barbiturates** have similar effects and were formerly widely used as sedatives and hypnotics (they are now mainly used to induce general anesthesia and to treat epilepsy). Another drug, **baclofen** (Lioresal), binds selectively to the GABA$_B$ receptor and potentiates the effect of GABA. It is used to reduce abnormal muscle tension occurring after damage to descending motor pathways (see Chapter 22,

under "Spasticity").[6] Certain steroid hormones, among them the female sex hormone **progesterone**, also bind to GABA$_A$ receptors and produce actions similar to barbiturates. An anesthetic drug (alphaxalone) was developed on this basis.

The central nervous effects of both **alcohol** and **inhalation anesthetics** (i.e., gases used for general anesthesia, such as halothane) were formerly ascribed to unspecific membrane influences. It now seems, however, that they act mainly by way of receptor binding. Both alcohol and gaseous anesthetics bind to (among others) GABA$_A$ receptors and increase their activity by increasing inhibition. Chronic alcohol consumption down-regulates GABA$_A$ receptors, and this may contribute to the development of tolerance (i.e., the dose must be increased to achieve the same effect) and the heightened excitability by abstinence. As mentioned, alcohol also binds to **NMDA receptors**. There is evidence that chronic alcohol intake leads to up-regulation of NMDA receptors in the frontal lobes, probably because alcohol inhibits NMDA-receptor activation. Alcohol also increases the amount of the transmitter **dopamine** in parts of the brain (especially in the nucleus accumbens), perhaps as a consequence of reduced NMDA-receptor activation (glutamate is believed to reduce dopamine release). Other transmitters, such as serotonin and neuropeptides, as well as several intracellular signal pathways, are influenced by alcohol. Genetic variations in transmitter receptors and enzyme systems may at least partly explain why people react so differently to alcohol.

Acetylcholine

The actions of acetylcholine in the CNS are especially important with regard to **attention**, **learning**, and **memory** (see Fig. 4.10; see also Chapter 26 under "Multiple Pathways and Transmitters Are Responsible for Cortical Activation").[7] In **Alzheimer's disease**—with memory impairment as a key feature—acetylcholine and acetylcholine receptors in the cerebral cortex are severely reduced (see also Chapter 10, under "Alzheimer's Disease and Frontotemporal Dementia [Pick's Disease]," and Chapter 31, under "Cholinergic Neurons Projecting to the Cerebral Cortex").

---

5 Some **sensory neurons** express GABA$_B$ receptors in their peripheral ramifications, where GABA inhibits release of other transmitters. Peripheral release of neuropeptides can cause increased local blood flow, edema, and stimulation of pain receptors (see Chapter 13, under "Release of Neuropeptides from Peripheral Branches of Sensory Neurons").

6 It was initially assumed that **baclofen** reduces muscle tension by increasing presynaptic inhibition of sensory nerve terminals in the spinal cord, thereby reducing the depolarization of motor neurons. Recent data indicate that axoaxonic synapses on sensory terminals act mainly on GABA$_A$ receptors, however, and that baclofen acts directly on the motor neurons and interneurons rather than presynaptically.

7 Acetylcholine also influences the **microcirculation** of the brain, by producing vasodilatation via muscarinic receptors and release of nitric oxide (see later, "Nitric Oxide and Blood Vessels"). The cholinergic fibers innervating brain vessels arise in the basal forebrain and not in the peripheral parts of the autonomic nervous system.

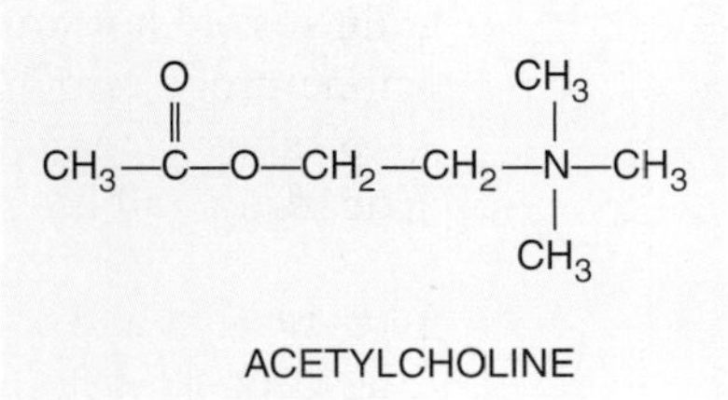

$$CH_3-\overset{\overset{\displaystyle O}{\|}}{C}-O-CH_2-CH_2-\overset{\overset{\displaystyle CH_3}{|}}{\underset{\underset{\displaystyle CH_3}{|}}{N}}-CH_3$$

ACETYLCHOLINE

FIGURE 5.6 *Structure of the neurotransmitter acetylcholine.*

Acetylcholine is a quaternary amine (Fig. 5.6) **synthesized** through the binding of choline to acetyl-coenzyme A by the enzyme **choline acetyltransferase** (ChAT). The presence of this enzyme is characteristic of **cholinergic neurons** (neurons containing acetylcholine, Fig. 5.1). Acetylcholine is present in somatic and autonomic motor neurons in the spinal cord and brain stem and in autonomic (parasympathetic) ganglia. In addition, cholinergic neurons make up several diffusely organized cell groups in the brain stem (parabrachial nucleus) and in the basal forebrain (the basal nucleus and the septal nuclei; see Fig. 10.1).

After release, acetylcholine is broken down to choline and acetate by the enzyme **acetylcholine esterase** (AchE). The enzyme is very efficient: one molecule can hydrolyze 5000 molecules of acetylcholine per second. Choline (but not acetylcholine) is taken up into nerve terminals by high-affinity transporter proteins. Uptake of choline appears to be the most important factor in regulating the synthesis of acetylcholine.

An important feature of cholinergic neurons with axon ramifications within the CNS is that they to only a limited extent release transmitter at typical synapses. In the cerebral cortex, for example, axons from cholinergic neurons form widespread ramifications with **varicosities** (Fig. 5.3). Only about 10% of the varicosities were estimated to form typical synapses when examined via serial sections and electron microscopy. Therefore, acetylcholine must be expected to act rather diffusely on all neurons in the vicinity equipped with the appropriate receptors--that is, it acts mainly via **volume transmission**. This fits with the fact that both nicotinic and muscarinic receptors in the cerebral cortex are localized extrasynaptically on dendrites, neuronal somata, and nerve terminals (presynaptically). The same arrangement holds for other cell groups with widespread axon ramifications that release modulatory transmitters (such as monoaminergic ones, discussed later).

Acetylcholine Receptors (AchRs)

Acetylcholine can bind to two kinds of receptors: ionotropic **nicotinic receptors** (nAchR; see Fig. 4.2), and metabotropic **muscarinic receptors** (mAchR). The names

derive from the early observations that nicotine and muscarine mimicked the effects of acetylcholine (nicotine and muscarine are plant alkaloids; muscarine is present in certain kinds of poisonous mushrooms). The nicotinic receptors produce fast, excitatory synaptic actions, whereas the muscarinic receptors mediate indirect, modulatory effects on neuronal excitability. Depending on the subtype of muscarinic receptor present, the effect may be inhibitory or excitatory. Nicotinic and muscarinic receptors are distributed differently in the nervous system, and there are several subtypes of both (which can be distinguished pharmacologically by use of different agonists and antagonists). For example, different subtypes of nicotinic receptors are expressed in striated muscle cells, in autonomic ganglia, and in the CNS.

Seven **subtypes** of the **nicotinic receptor** have been identified. There are three main groups: receptors in skeletal muscle, in autonomic ganglia, and in the CNS. The functional role of nicotinic receptor in the CNS is not well understood, but they are present in many places and are localized both presynaptically and postsynaptically. They therefore may influence neuronal excitability both directly and indirectly by modulating release of other transmitters (e.g., glutamate). Much better known are the actions of acetylcholine at the cholinergic synapses between motor neurons and **skeletal muscle** cells (see Figs. 21.4 and 21.5). Binding of acetylcholine opens the channel for cations, but the permeability is largest for Na^+. Opening of such channels elicits an action potential that spreads out in all directions to reach all parts of the muscle cell membrane. This is the signal that leads to muscle contraction. (Whereas skeletal muscle cells contain only nicotinic receptors, **smooth muscle cells** are equipped only with muscarinic receptors.)

Muscarinic receptors are quantitatively the dominant acetylcholine receptors in the CNS. So far, five subtypes (**m1–m5**) have been cloned (all are blocked by atropine) but m1 and m2 are the quantitatively most important ones. Whereas m1 receptors are located postsynaptically, m2 receptors are found predominantly presynaptically. In the **cerebral cortex**, which receives many cholinergic nerve terminals, a major effect of acetylcholine is to reduce the permeability of a K^+ channel by acting on m1 receptors. This makes the neurons more susceptible to other excitatory inputs so that, for example, a neuron will react more easily to a specific sensory stimulus. Another kind of muscarinic receptor opens a K^+ channel, thereby producing long-lasting hyperpolarization, while a third type closes a Ca^{2+} channel.

Blockers of Acetylcholine Receptors

Curare is an antagonist (blocker) of the nicotinic receptors and was used as an arrow poison by South American natives to paralyze victims. Derivatives of curare are used to achieve muscle relaxation during surgery. **Atropine** and **scopolamine** are relatively unselective antagonists of muscarinic receptors (i.e., they block all subtypes). The snake venom α-**bungarotoxin** binds specifically to muscle nicotinic receptors and blocks the effect of acetylcholine (and kills the victim by paralyzing all skeletal muscles). The French neuroscientist Jean-Pierre Changeux and coworkers achieved the first isolation and characterization of a transmitter receptor by use of α bungarotoxin. To obtain sufficient amounts of the receptor, **electric eels** (*Torpedo*) were chosen for study because they are equipped with electric organs that produce strong electric shocks by activating nicotinic receptors.

Nicotine Addiction

Genetic variability among AchR subunits appears to be related to nicotine dependence; that is, persons with genes for a certain subunit might have an increased risk of becoming nicotine dependent. The development of addictive behavior depends, at least partly, on nicotine-receptor-mediated stimulation of **dopaminergic** neurons (that release dopamine in the nucleus accumbens; see Chapter 23, under "The Ventral Striatum, Psychosis, and Drug Addiction"). However, the relation between nicotine and addictive behavior is complex and several transmitters other than dopamine are involved (e.g., glutamate and GABA). Further, chronic nicotine consumption induces plastic changes in several neuronal groups. At the cerebral cortical level, a region called **insula** (see Chapter 34 under "The Insula") may be particularly important. For example, activation of neuronal groups in the insula was found in a brain imaging study to increase in relation to the person feeling an urge for a drug. Further, smokers suffering a stroke that damaged the insula were much more likely to quit smoking than were smokers suffering lesions in other parts of the brain.

Biogenic Amines

The **biogenic amines** constitute a subgroup of the small-molecule transmitters. The group includes the **monoamines** norepinephrine, epinephrine, dopamine, and serotonin (one amine group), and in addition **histamine** (two amine groups). Neurons that use monoamines as transmitters are called **monoaminergic**. The monoamines are **synthesized** by enzymatic removal of the carboxylic group from an aromatic amino acid (Figs. 5.7 and 5.8). Norepinephrine, epinephrine, and dopamine are **catecholamines**.[8] Neurons that contain the monoamines

---

8 Catecholamines: Compounds consisting of a catechol group (benzene ring with two hydroxyl groups) with an attached amine group.

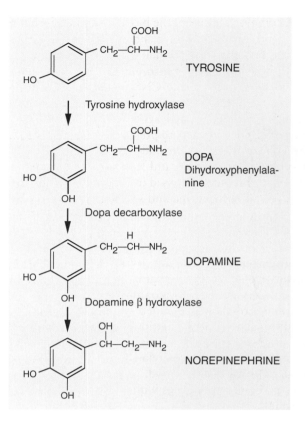

FIGURE 5.7 *The catecholamines dopamine and norepinephrine and the key enzymes in their synthesis.*

norepinephrine, dopamine, serotonin, and histamine are said to be noradrenergic, dopaminergic, serotonergic, and histaminergic, respectively (the same terminology is used for the receptors corresponding to these transmitters).

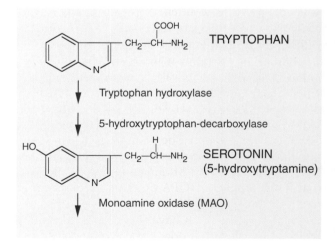

FIGURE 5.8 *Serotonin.* This neurotransmitter synthesized from tryptophan in two enzymatic steps. It is broken down by monoamine oxidase in the nerve terminals.

A common feature of the biogenic amines is that they are synthesized only in a small number of neurons, which, however, have widely branching axons. In this way, these few neurons ensure that the transmitters can act in most parts of the CNS. Like acetylcholine, the biogenic amines are to a large extent released from varicosities without typical synaptic contacts (Fig. 5.3); therefore, their effects are presumably mainly mediated by **volume transmission** and binding to extrasynaptic receptors. Localization and functions of monoaminergic cell groups are discussed in Chapters 23 (dopamine) and 26 (norepinephrine and serotonin).

Actions of the Biogenic Amines

The biogenic amines act (with one exception) on **metabotropic receptors**; that is, they exert mainly slow, **modulatory** actions. Monoaminergic (like cholinergic) neurons are therefore suited to modulate simultaneously the specific information processing mediated by glutamate and GABA in many anatomically separate neuronal groups. This is related to regulation of **attention, motivation,** and **mood.** In addition, the monoamines play important roles with regard to **plasticity** and **learning.**

Drugs used to treat diseases such as schizophrenia, Parkinson's disease, and depression alter the functioning of monoamines.

Synthesis of Biogenic Amines

Norepinephrine (noradrenaline), epinephrine (adrenaline), and dopamine are all synthesized from the amino acid tyrosine (Fig. 5.7). Tyrosine is taken up from the bloodstream by active transport mechanisms and concentrated in the nervous tissue. The synthesis of catecholamines goes through several enzymatic steps. The first is the conversion of tyrosine to dihydroxyphenylalanine (DOPA) by the enzyme tyrosine hydroxylase (Fig. 5.7), which appears to be rate limiting for the synthesis of catecholamines under most conditions. The activity of tyrosine hydroxylase is regulated by negative feedback from released catecholamines by way of presynaptic autoreceptors (other factors also influence the activity, however). DOPA is converted to dopamine by the enzyme aromatic amino acid decarboxylase (DOPA decarboxylase). The reaction is so rapid that very little DOPA can be detected in the brain normally. Therefore, the synthesis of dopamine can be increased by artificial supply of DOPA (in the form of levodopa, Sinemet, Parcopa), as done in Parkinson's disease in which parts of the brain have very low levels of dopamine. (Dopamine itself does not pass the blood–brain barrier and therefore cannot be used therapeutically.) Norepinephrine is synthesized from dopamine by the enzyme dopamine β-hydroxylase (Fig. 5.7). The detection of this enzyme in tissue sections is used to identify noradrenergic neurons.

Serotonin (5-hydroxytryptamine [5-HT]) is synthesized from the amino acid **tryptophan** (Fig. 5.8). The reaction is catalyzed by the enzyme **tryptophan hydroxylase** (and the same aromatic amino acid decarboxylase that catalyzes DOPA to dopamine). Tryptophan hydroxylase is rate limiting for the synthesis of serotonin, although other factors also contribute.[9] The serotonin concentration is much higher in certain cell types peripherally than in the brain (blood platelets, mast cells, chromaffin cells in the gut, and others). It is therefore mandatory that serotonin—like other transmitters—cannot pass the blood–brain barrier. Peripherally, serotonin produces contraction of **smooth muscle cells,** among other effects.

Histamine hardly passes the blood–brain barrier, and is synthesized in the brain from the amino acid **histidine.**

Monoamine Receptors

Like the other neurotransmitters discussed so far, each of the monoamines bind to several different receptors (see Table 5.1). Monoamine receptors are found both presynaptically and postsynaptically (as mentioned, the majority are most likely localized extrasynaptically). Their effects are correspondingly diverse: some monoaminergic receptors inhibit transmitter release, others increase it; some produce slow EPSPs, others produce slow IPSPs. Consequently, each monoamine can have diverse effects, depending on the receptor repertoire of the target neurons.

Norepinephrine (and epinephrine, which mainly functions as a hormone) binds to two main receptor types, α- and β-**adrenergic receptors.** Their effects are often opposite, and they are differentially distributed (these receptors are treated in more detail in Chapter 28). In the cerebral cortex, norepinephrine produces a slow depolarization by binding to β receptors (by indirect, G protein–coupled closure of a K^+ channel).

Dopamine acts on two main types of receptors—D_1 and D_2—with different properties and different distribution in the CNS. Common to the dopamine receptors in the D_1 group is that they act by increasing the synthesis of cyclic AMP, whereas the D_2 receptors decrease it. Usually, one uses the terms D_1-like (D_1 and D_5) and D_2-like receptors (D_2, D_3, and D_4). Dopamine receptors are discussed further in Chapter 23 (under "Actions of Dopamine in the Striatum").

Serotonin receptors fall into seven groups—5-HT_1 to 5-HT_7—with further subtypes of each (see Table 5.1).

---

[9] In contrast to catecholamines, the synthesis of serotonin appears not be regulated by negative feedback by way of autoreceptor stimulation; that is, increased extracellular transmitter concentration does not inhibit the synthesis.

All of the serotonin receptors are metabotropic except the 5-HT$_3$ receptor, which is ionotropic (belonging to the same protein family as the other ion channel receptors). The metabotropic serotonin receptors act through different intracellular signal pathways and can have either excitatory or inhibitory effects (evoking slow EPSPs and IPSPs). For example, activation of 5-HT$_1$ receptors causes inhibition by opening certain K$^+$ channels. The same neurons may also be equipped with another kind serotonin receptor that closes K$^+$ channels, making it difficult to sort out the total effect of serotonin. Serotonin is further discussed in Chapter 13 (under "Nociceptors"), Chapter 22 ("Monoaminergic Pathways to the Brain Stem and Spinal Cord"), and Chapter 26 (under "The Raphe Nuclei" and "Pathways and Transmitters Responsible for Cortical Activation").

Histamine Receptors—Homeostasis and Wakefulness?

Histamine receptors occur extrasynaptically and on varicosities in many parts of the CNS. In the **thalamus** and the **cerebral cortex**, histamine actions appear to be involved in **arousal** and **wakefulness**. Histamine receptors in the **hypothalamus** are most likely involved in **homeostatic processes** (e.g., food and water intake, temperature regulation, and hormone secretion). The axon ramifications releasing histamine contact not only neurons but also **glial cells** and small **blood vessels**. Presumably, this also relates to homeostatic control.

Three varieties of the histamine receptor—H$_1$-H$_3$—have been identified in the CNS; all acting indirectly via G proteins. H$_1$ receptors mediate the effect of histamine on wakefulness, partly directly on neurons in the cerebral cortex, partly on subcortical cholinergic and monoaminergic neurons, which in their turn influence the cerebral cortex. The **antihistamines** used against travel sickness and allergy are H$_1$ antagonists, and this probably explains why drowsiness is a frequent side effect of such drugs. Activation of H$_1$ receptors in the hypothalamus reduces food intake in experimental animals. Many psychoactive drugs have antihistaminergic side effects, which may be one reason why weight gain is common among patients with long-term treatment with such drugs.

Monoamine Removal

Transporter proteins in the membrane of nerve terminals end the transmitter action and control the extracellular concentration of monoamines. Glial cells do not appear to play an important part in uptake of monoamines (in contrast to glutamate). There are specific transporters for norepinephrine, dopamine, and serotonin—all belonging to the same protein family (called NAT, DAT, and SERT/5-HTT, respectively). The two catecholamine transporters have low selectivity, however, so that, for example, the dopamine transporter also can take up norepinephrine, if it is present in the vicinity. After uptake into nerve terminals, the monoamines are partly transported into vesicles, partly broken down by the enzyme **monoamine oxidase (MAO)**.

Monoamine Oxidase, Serotonin Transporters, and Behavior

There are two varieties of monoamine oxidase (MAO). **MAO-A** has the highest affinity to the monoamine transmitters and is particularly concentrated in catecholaminergic neurons. **MAO-B** is concentrated in serotonergic and histaminergic neurons and in glia. Mutation of the gene coding for MAO-A (located on the X chromosome) was found in a Dutch family with lack of MAO-A, and abnormal aggressiveness among the male members. Correspondingly, knockout mice that lack the *MAO-A* gene behave aggressively and have increased brain levels of monoamines. These and other findings have led some to suggest that individual variations among the genes for monoamine oxidase may dispose for excessive aggressiveness and violent behaviors.

Individual differences in personality and behavior have also been associated with genetic **polymorphism** in monoamine metabolism. For example, certain varieties of the gene coding for the **serotonin transporter** are associated with high levels of anxiety and depression. These traits appear to be associated with a heritable reduced functioning of the serotonin transporter (not increased as one might have expected, because antidepressants inhibit reuptake of monoamines).[10] Further, animal experiments indicate that symptoms in adult animals depend on reduced transporter activity during a short period after birth. Only animals with genetic vulnerability *plus* experience of psychological trauma in this period (such as separation from the mother) developed behavioral disturbances as adults. Therefore, it seems that normal serotonin transmission in early postnatal development is necessary for the development of neuronal networks handling emotions and stress. This assumption is further supported by other animal experiments showing that the presence of the 5-HT$_{1A}$ receptor in early development is necessary and sufficient for normal anxiety-related behavior as an adult, regardless of whether or not the receptor is expressed in the adult animals.

When interpreting findings such as those described here, one should bear in mind that they say more about

---

10 This seeming paradox can probably be explained by complex compensatory processes initiated by inhibition of the transporter, such as up- and down-regulation of receptors, enzymes, and feedback loops. Therefore, reduced transporter activity does not necessarily lead to increased transmitter activity.

the behavior of a brain with disturbed monoamine functions than about the normal functions of monoamines. Serotonin is, for example, certainly not the substrate of aggression but may—together with many other transmitters—be necessary for normal signal processing in the complex networks that generate and control certain emotions and their behavioral expressions. Further, genetic vulnerability of the kind described above increases the probability of developing certain mental disorders or personality traits, but does not determine their development. How easily a person becomes mentally disturbed as an adult depends on how certain brain networks developed in early childhood. This, in turn, depends on a complex interaction between inherited traits (e.g., variety of the serotonin transporter) and the environment.

Localization of Monoaminergic Neurons

Neurons that synthesize **catecholamines** are largely restricted to some small cell groups in the brain stem, hypothalamus, and peripheral nervous system. Most **noradrenergic neurons** in the CNS occur in somewhat diffuse cell groups in the brain stem reticular formation, the **locus coeruleus** being the largest and most distinct one (see Fig. 26.7). The majority of **dopaminergic neurons** are localized to the mesencephalon, in one large nucleus called the **substantia nigra** (see Fig. 23.5) and more diffuse cells groups in the vicinity (**ventral tegmental area, VTA**). In addition, smaller numbers of dopaminergic neurons are found in the retina, in the olfactory bulb, and the hypothalamus.

Serotonergic neurons lie almost exclusively in a group of nuclei near the midline of the brain stem reticular formation, called the **raphe nuclei** (see Fig. 26.1).

Histamine is synthesized only in the small **tuberomammillary nucleus** in the hypothalamus.

Modulatory Transmitter "Systems"

We described some features shared by monoaminergic and cholinergic neuronal groups (with the exception of cholinergic motor neurons). First, a small number of neurons send axons to large parts of the CNS—that is, the cell bodies producing the enzymes necessary for transmitter synthesis are very restricted in distribution, whereas the transmitters and their receptors are present almost everywhere. Second, each axon ramifies extensively, and the terminal branches are equipped with numerous **varicosities** (Fig. 5.3). As mentioned, these varicosities only infrequently form typical synapses but release transmitters more diffusely (**volume transmission**), presumably by acting largely on extrasynaptic receptors. Finally, the transmitters act predominantly via **metabotropic** receptors—exerting slow, modulatory effects on neuronal excitability.

These anatomic and physiological features imply that the monoaminergic and cholinergic cell groups do not mediate precise temporal or spatial information. They are well suited, however, to modulate the functions of specific glutamatergic and GABAergic systems, for example, by improving the **signal-to-noise** ratio. In this way, they may increase the precision of information handling in many parts of the brain—for example, in the cerebral cortex during processing of complex cognitive tasks. Their widespread connections furthermore ensure that many neuronal groups receive a similar modulatory input, as would be important for control of consciousness, awareness, different phases of sleep, emotions, motivation, and so forth. Monoamines furthermore set the level of excitability of spinal neurons to control voluntary movements and of neurons that are transmitting specific sensory information. For example, brain stem serotonergic neurons with axonal ramifications in the cord appear to both facilitate movement and inhibit sensory transmission.

Trying to bind together seemingly disparate actions, one might speculate that the modulatory transmitter "systems" ensure that sensory, motor, and cognitive processes are coordinated toward a common goal. The modulatory transmitters would do this by mediating a signal about the **value** of specific events. These speculations are supported by the well-established roles of monoamines and acetylcholine in **synaptic plasticity** (Fig. 4.10).

In spite of their homogeneities, it is an oversimplification to regard each transmitter-specific group as a functional entity and to use terms such as "the serotonin system," "the dopamine system," and so on. First, the large number of receptors for each transmitter, with different distributions and effects in the brain, indicate that each transmitter-specific cell group has complex relations to behavior. For example, dopaminergic neurons influence neuronal networks engaged in quite different behavioral tasks. Second, even if localizations are not sharp, each transmitter-specific group contains subgroups that differ in where they send their axons, and from where they receive afferents. For example, the various serotonergic raphe nuclei (see Fig. 26.6) send axons to different parts of the CNS. Third, most or all monoaminergic neurons also contain one or more neuropeptides. The effects obtained by stimulation of one of these cell groups therefore cannot be ascribed to one transmitter alone.

Adenosine Triphosphate and Adenosine

The purines adenosine triphosphate (ATP) and adenosine can exert marked effects on neuronal excitability, both in the CNS and peripherally. Only ATP, however, appears to act as a transmitter (it is, e.g., concentrated in vesicles and its release is calcium dependent).

The effects are mediated by purinoceptors, localized both pre- and postsynaptically. (Many other cell types than neurons express purinoceptors—e.g., smooth muscle cells.) P_1 receptors bind adenosine, while P_2 receptors bind ATP. After release, ATP is enzymatically degraded. The transmitter role of ATP is best known in the autonomic nervous system, where it is usually colocalized with acetylcholine or norepinephrine and. ATP and the "classic" transmitter are found in the same vesicles, and they are released together (see Chapter 28, under "Noncholinergic and Nonadrenergic Transmission in the Autonomic Nervous System"). As a rule, ATP excites neurons and smooth muscle cells by acting on ionotropic receptors. There are, however, examples of inhibitory effects of ATP (probably by way of metabotropic receptors) on smooth muscle cells—for example, in the longitudinal muscle layer of the large intestine. In the inner ear, efferent nerve fibers to the sensory cells (hair cells) release ATP together with acetylcholine, and modulate the sensitivity of the sensory cells.

So far, little is known with certainty about the transmitter role of ATP in the CNS, in spite of the wide distribution of purinoceptors. Some brain stem neuronal groups appear to use ATP as transmitter (notably **locus coeruleus**, where it colocalizes with norepinephrine). It is probably also used as transmitter in a subgroup of **spinal ganglion cells**—that is, sensory neurons conducting impulses from peripheral receptors to the spinal cord (see Chapter 13, under "Primary Sensory Fibers and Neurotransmitters"). A population of **spinal interneurons** seems to release ATP in parts of the cord that receives signals from pain receptors (laminae I and II; see Fig. 6.10). Ionotropic P_2 receptors increase the release of glutamate and substance P from terminals of spinal ganglion cells in the dorsal horn. This may contribute to the heightened excitability of spinal neurons, which is typical of chronic pain conditions.

ATP and purinoceptors mediate signals between neurons and **glial cells**, and may participate in the interaction between the immune system and neurons.

As mentioned, **adenosine** has marked effects on neurons, even though it is unlikely to act as a transmitter. Injection of minute amounts of adenosine inhibits spinal cord neurons that mediate signals from **pain** receptors to the brain. Adenosine also appears to be involved—in some yet unknown way—with the analgesic effects of morphine and the morphine-like substances produced in the brain (opioids).

Purinoceptors

There are two main groups of P_2 **receptors**. One group (P_{2X}) consists of six **ionotropic** receptors with fast, excitatory action. The channels are most permeable to Ca^{2+} and have a longer opening time than, for example AMPA receptors (but much shorter than NMDA receptors). The other group (P_{2Y}) consists of seven **metabotropic** receptors. Both groups are widely distributed in the CNS, although the transmitter role of ATP is reasonably certain only in a few areas. The study of ATP as a neurotransmitter has so far been hampered by the lack of specific receptor antagonists. P_1 **receptors** are blocked by **xanthenes**, such as **caffeine** and **theophylline**. Theophylline inhibits bronchial smooth muscle cells and is used therapeutically in **asthma**.

Nitric Oxide

Nitric oxide (NO) is a gas that diffuses freely through biologic membranes. It functions as a signal molecule in many organs of the body, among them the nervous system. Its functional role in the nervous system is only partly clear, however. Even though NO often is called an "unconventional neurotransmitter," it does not meet the criteria used to define a transmitter: it is not stored in vesicles, it is not released by calcium-dependent exocytosis, and it does not bind to membrane-bound receptors.

In the **peripheral nervous system**, autonomic nerve fibers release NO that acts on smooth muscle cells. In the **CNS**, NO has a number of cellular effects and appears to take part in the control of various systems; it also influences behavior. It has quite different effects in the brain depending on its concentration, however: in low concentrations, it functions as a signal molecule that modulates neuronal behavior, whereas it is toxic in higher concentrations (which is perhaps not surprising because NO is a free radical and as such very reactive).

NO is **synthesized** from the amino acid **arginine** by specific enzymes, **NO synthases**, of which there are several different types. Synthesis of NO in nerve terminals is probably induced by the increase of intracellular Ca^{2+} concentration that is triggered by a presynaptic action potential. After synthesis, NO diffuses freely in all directions. It is not only delivered into the synaptic cleft but also enters all cells that are near the nerve terminal. Calculations from the cerebral cortex indicate that NO can diffuse more than 100 μm from its release site and reach about 2 million synapses. The most abundant **NO receptor** is a water-soluble, cytoplasmic enzyme, **guanylyl cyclase**, which controls synthesis of cyclic GMP. This is an intracellular messenger with various effects, such as activating protein kinases and acting directly on ion channels. In this way NO can modulate neuronal excitability and firing frequency.

NO synthases are present in neurons in several parts of the central and peripheral nervous system. In the cerebral cortex, they are found in GABAergic neurons, which, in addition, contain neuropeptides (substance P and somatostatin). In other parts of the brain, NO synthases occur in cholinergic and monoaminergic neurons. Although we do not know the functions of

NO liberated from such neurons, there is some evidence that NO is one of numerous factors that are involved in the induction of **LTP**, and therefore presumably also in neuronal **plasticity**. NO also appears to play a special role in neurons with **rhythmic** firing—such as the brain stem and thalamic neurons that regulate sleep–wakefulness, and the hypothalamic neurons that control bodily functions with daily variations (circadian rhythms). Presumably, NO, due to its fast and wide diffusion, is particularly suited to **synchronize** the activity of many neurons.

In situations with insufficient energy supply (most often due to reduced blood flow), increased intracellular Ca^{2+} concentration leads to increased NO synthesis. This seems likely to contribute to the neuronal damage in such situations (see Fig. 10.2). On the other hand, release of NO might improve the blood supply by producing local vasodilatation.

NO and Blood Vessels

NO was first discovered in endothelial cells and named **endothelium-derived relaxing factor**. In fact, its main effect in most organs is relaxation of smooth muscle cells, causing vasodilatation and increased blood flow. NO released from autonomic (parasympathetic) nerve fibers, for example, is responsible for penile erection. **Nitroglycerin** and similar drugs give vasodilatation by inducing synthesis of NO.

Vessels in the CNS are also affected by NO. There is evidence that NO, together with other signal molecules, mediates the increased **local blood flow** associated with increased neuronal activity (e.g., the blood flow in the cortical motor area increases when the neurons increase their firing during execution of voluntary movements).

Neuropeptides

A large number of neuroactive peptides have so far been identified in the CNS, but many of them were first found in the peripheral nervous system and in the gut. Although there is firm evidence of a transmitter function for only a few neuropeptides, many of them have marked effects on physiological processes and behavior when administered locally in the CNS. Several of the neuropeptides elicit slow inhibitory or excitatory synaptic potentials when administered in minute amounts close to neurons, suggesting a **modulatory** transmitter role. This assumption is supported by the identification of several G protein–coupled neuropeptide receptors. Neuropeptides can also elicit intracellular responses related to **growth** and **development**. Normally, the concentrations of neuropeptides are low in neurons. The synthesis increases, however, when the homeostasis of the nervous system is challenged (e.g., in infections, stroke, trauma). The way neuropeptides are released

may perhaps fit an "emergency" role: it seems that neuropeptide release requires a high firing frequency or burst firing, whereas low-frequency firing suffices to release small molecule (classical) transmitters.

The duration of action appears to be longer for neuropeptides than for other neuromodulators (in spite of the presence of extracellular peptidases). Thus, the half-life after release can be very long (about 20 minutes for vasopressin, for example)—giving ample time for extracellular diffusion. In addition, at least some neuropeptides are released from dendrites. Thus, it seems that the actions of the neuropeptides are, as a rule, rather diffuse. Some of the neuropeptides may thus function more like local hormones than like neurotransmitters, as also suggested by a mismatch between the distribution of receptors for a neuropeptide and nerve terminals containing the neuropeptide.

A characteristic feature of neuropeptides is that they are **colocalized** in nerve terminals with small-molecule (classical) transmitters. Whereas small-molecule transmitters are stored in small, electron-lucent vesicles, neuropeptides are found in larger vesicles with an electron-dense center (**dense-core vesicles**; Fig. 5.9). Two or more peptides may also coexist, and there may be more than one small-molecule transmitter together with the peptides.

Several neuropeptides will be mentioned in subsequent chapters in relation to various cell groups and neuronal systems.

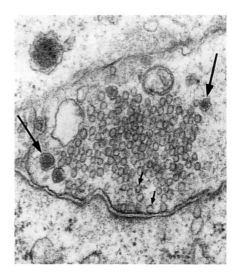

FIGURE 5.9 *Nerve terminal containing both a "classical" transmitter and neuropeptides.* Large arrows show the dense-core vesicles that contain neuropeptides with transmitter actions. Small arrows show the small, clear vesicles that contain small molecule "classical" transmitters.

Examples of Colocalization of Neuropeptides and Small-Molecule Transmitters

Terminals of nerve fibers innervating **salivary glands** contain both **acetylcholine** and the neuropeptide **vasoactive intestinal polypeptide** (**VIP**). Both substances are released when the nerves are stimulated, but they act on different target cells: acetylcholine elicits secretion from glandular cells, whereas VIP produces vasodilatation by relaxing smooth muscle cells, thereby increasing blood flow to the organ at the same time as its secretion is increased. Another example concerns **primary sensory neurons** (spinal ganglion cells; see Figs. 6.9 and 13.16) mediating information from peripheral sense organs to the spinal cord. Some of these—particularly those related to painful stimuli—contain both **glutamate** and the peptides **substance P** and **calcitonin gene-related peptide**. When released with glutamate, these peptides appear to have several actions: they can bind to specific postsynaptic receptors, they can act presynaptically to increase their own release and the release of glutamate, and they can sensitize the postsynaptic glutamate receptors to enhance the effect of glutamate.

Spinal interneurons that receive sensory information exhibit different transmitter combinations. One group of interneurons contains **GABA** and the peptide **enkephalin**. Another group contains both **enkephalin** and **substance P** in combination with (most likely) **glutamate**. Therefore, one neuropeptide (enkephalin) may be colocalized with either an inhibitory or an excitatory transmitter with fast synaptic actions. Apparently, spinal interneurons may express a variety of transmitter combinations with correspondingly complex synaptic actions. When we also think of the variety of receptors each neuron expresses, it is easy to understand why unraveling the functional role of a single transmitter can be difficult.

ACTIONS OF DRUGS ON THE NERVOUS SYSTEM

Most Drugs Influence Synaptic Function

Several drugs have been mentioned in connection with discussions of synaptic function and neurotransmitters. Most drugs acting on the nervous system do so by influencing synaptic transmission directly or indirectly, regardless of whether their aim is to alleviate disorders of mood, cognition, movements, memory, or behavior. The drugs may interfere presynaptically in the synthesis, release, degradation, or reuptake of transmitters or postsynaptically in the activity, numbers, or localization of receptors. Certain drugs have one or more of these actions regarding one or several transmitters. Some drugs also seem to influence synaptic functions indirectly by changing the expression of neurotrophic factors that (among other tasks) govern synaptic plasticity.

Examples: Drugs Altering Monoamine Activity in the Brain

The most common **antipsychotic drugs** (neuroleptics) all block **dopamine receptors**. Their therapeutic effects are primarily related to altering the transmitter functions of dopamine, although they also influence other transmitters (they exhibit, for example, more or less anticholinergic and antihistaminergic effects). In addition, dopamine receptors are present in neuronal groups related to movement control and muscle tone, and this explains why motor dysfunctions are common side effects of antipsychotics. Conversely, patients with Parkinson's disease who are treated with levodopa to increase dopamine levels in the brain may develop psychotic symptoms during treatment. Nevertheless, the "dopamine hypothesis of schizophrenia," which states that the symptoms can be explained as a result of dopaminergic overactivity, is too simplistic. Not all symptoms can be explained in this way, and dopaminergic overactivity does not appear to be present in all patients. Further, psychotic symptoms can also be treated effectively with drugs that block serotonin receptors (so-called atypical antipsychotic drugs, such as **clozapine**, have higher affinity for serotonin receptors than for dopamine receptors). **MAO inhibitors** were the first drugs with significant effects on major **depressions**. Later, **tricyclic antidepressants** (TCAs) were introduced, which inhibit relatively selectively the norepinephrine transporter. The new antidepressants, such as **fluoxetine** (Prozac), inhibit rather selectively the serotonin transporter (**selective serotonin-uptake inhibitors** [**SSRIs**]). Although the clinical effects of antidepressants may appear to be caused simply by increased levels of monoamines available at the synapses, this cannot be the whole story. For example, while inhibition of the transporters occurs immediately, the clinical effect comes after days or weeks with treatment. Therefore, clinical effects were sought in compensatory processes, such as up- and down-regulation of receptors. Recent research has revealed a number of effects of antidepressants other than altering monoamine levels—for example, on expression of **neurotrophins** and neuronal **plasticity**. The fact that antidepressants, in spite of acting on different monoamine transporters, have similar clinical effects prompted the hypothesis that they act by regulating **transcription** of the same set of genes. This has received some experimental support. For example, one study identified gene transcripts that were equally regulated by treatment with different classes of antidepressants.

Cocaine inhibits the dopamine transporter very selectively; that is, its affinity to the dopamine transporter is much higher than to other monoamine transporters. The dopamine transporter has even been called a "cocaine receptor." **Amphetamine** inhibits the dopamine transporter but also other monoamine transporters, although relatively weakly compared with cocaine. In addition, amphetamine increases the release of catecholamines and has other synaptic effects as well.

Drug Effects Are Often Multifarious

Most transmitters are present in several parts of the nervous system, which differ anatomically and physiologically. Therefore, it should not be surprising that even drugs that apparently influence the actions of only one transmitter nevertheless have multifarious effects. Some of these are desired therapeutic effects, whereas others are disturbing or even dangerous side effects. Development of more specific drugs—for example, drugs acting on only one receptor subtype—may reduce the side effects but will hardly eliminate them. This is because each receptor type (even one among several subtypes for one transmitter) occurs in functionally different parts of the nervous system.

Drugs Interact with Dynamic Processes in the Brain

Another important point is that storage, release, and uptake of transmitters, as well as the expression of receptors, are **dynamic processes**. The acute perturbations caused by a drug are usually counteracted quickly by feedback loops that up- or down-regulate the transmitter release, the transporters, the receptors, and so forth. For example, when the activity of **tryptophan hydroxylase** (the rate-limiting enzyme in serotonin synthesis) is reduced, the neurons respond by increasing synthesis of the enzyme and its axonal transport to the nerve terminals.[11] Finally, we should keep in mind that alteration of one transmitter's activity as a rule leads to alterations of other transmitters as well. One mechanism behind this is the action on presynaptic receptors: a cholinergic terminal in the cerebral cortex may be equipped with serotonin receptors, so that a drug with specific action on serotonergic transmission may nevertheless also alter cholinergic transmission. Another mechanism is postsynaptic: many dopaminergic neurons receive glutamatergic synapses, so that drugs altering the action of glutamate will change dopamine release as well.

---

11 **Lithium**, used prophylactically for major bipolar disorder (manic depression), increases tryptophan uptake and initially increases serotonin synthesis (this is only one of several cellular effects of lithium). After 2 to 3 weeks with treatment, however, the tryptophan uptake is still increased, but the tryptophan hydroxylase activity is reduced so that the rate of serotonin synthesis is normal. It is possible that the therapeutic effect of lithium is due to stabilization of serotonin metabolism, which makes it less vulnerable to psychological stress or spontaneous chemical changes in the brain.

6 | Parts of the Nervous System

OVERVIEW

In this chapter, we describe the main features of the anatomy of the central nervous system (CNS), with brief mention of the functional significance of the various parts. We will treat structure and function of many of these parts in more depth in later chapters dealing with functional systems. It will then be assumed, however, that the reader is familiar with the names and the locations of the major cell groups and tracts of the CNS.

The CNS can be subdivided anatomically into different parts. The **spinal cord** lies in the vertebral canal, whereas the **brain** is located in the cranial cavity. The brain is further subdivided into the **brain stem**, which constitutes the upward continuation of the spinal cord, the **cerebellum** ("little brain"), and the **cerebrum** or **cerebral hemispheres**. The cerebellum and cerebrum largely cover the brain stem and constitute the major part of the brain in higher mammals and particularly in humans.

The **spinal cord** consists of a central region with gray matter surrounded by white matter. The **gray matter** contains neurons that may be subdivided based on where they send their axons. **Motor neurons** send their axons out of the cord to reach muscles and glands. **Sensory neurons** receive signals from sense organs in the body and transmit this information to the brain. The spinal **interneurons** or **propriospinal** neurons ensure communication among neurons in the spinal cord. The **white matter** contains ascending tracts carrying signals to higher levels, and descending tracts enabling the brain to control spinal cord neurons (e.g., motor neurons). In addition, many propriospinal axons interconnect neurons in different parts of the cord. The cord consists of **segments**, each giving rise to a pair of **spinal nerves**. The spinal nerves and their peripheral branches transmit sensory signals from the tissues of the body and motor signals to muscles and glands. Each spinal nerve connects with the cord through a dorsal and a ventral **nerve root**. The **dorsal roots** carry only sensory nerve fibers, and the cell bodies of the sensory neurons of each root form a **spinal ganglion**, which appears as an ovoid enlargement of the dorsal root. Functionally, the cord enables fast, automatic responses to signals from the body (e.g., withdrawal of the hand from a hot object). Nevertheless, most tasks carried out by the cord are controlled or modulated by higher levels of the CNS.

The **brain stem** is a rostral continuation of the spinal cord but has a more complex internal organization. On a purely anatomical basis, the brain stem is divided (starting caudally) into the **medulla oblongata**, the **pons**, the **mesencephalon**, and the **diencephalon** (often, however, we do not include the diencephalon). Twelve **cranial nerves** emanate from the brain stem being numbered from rostral to caudal. With some exceptions, the cranial nerves innervate structures in the head ("spinal nerves of the head") and contain sensory and motor nerve fibers. The first cranial nerve—the **olfactory nerve**—serves the sense of smell. The second—the **optic nerve**—transmit signals from the retina, while the third (**oculomotor**), fourth (**trochlear**), and sixth (**abducens**) nerves control the movements of the eye ball. The fifth nerve—the **trigeminal**—emanates from the pons and brings sensory signals from the face as well as motor signals to the masticatory muscles. The seventh nerve—the **facial**—innervates the mimic muscles of the face. The eighth nerve—the **vestibulocochlear**—carries signals from the vestibular apparatus (recording movements and positions of the head in space) and the cochlea (recording sound waves). The ninth nerve—the **glossopharyngeal**—is concerned mainly with sensations and movements of the pharynx, including taste impulses from the back of the tongue. The tenth nerve—the **vagus** nerve—participates in the innervation of the pharynx but in addition innervates the larynx, and sends (autonomic) motor signals to the heart, the lungs, and the most of the gastrointestinal tract. The eleventh nerve—the **accessory**—innervates two muscles in the neck (the trapezius and the sternocleidomastoid). The twelfth nerve—the **hypoglossal**—is the motor nerve of the tongue. The cranial nerves arise in **cranial nerve nuclei**; some of which are sensory, others are motor.

Diffuse collections of neurons in between the cranial nerve nuclei are collectively termed the **reticular formation**. The reticular formation consists of neuronal groups with different tasks. Some groups are concerned with control of **circulation** and **respiration**; some regulate **sleep** and **wakefulness**, while others control **eye movements**.

The thalamus and the hypothalamus make up the bulk of the **diencephalon**. The **thalamus** is a large, egg-shaped collection of nuclei in the centre of the cerebral hemispheres. The thalamic nuclei transmit sensory information (of all kinds except smell) to the cerebral cortex. In addition, thalamic nuclei transmit information to the cerebral cortex from subcortical motor regions, notably the basal ganglia and the cerebellum. The **hypothalamus** is concerned mainly with the control of autonomic and endocrine functions that serve to maintain bodily homeostasis (e.g., circulation, digestion, and temperature control).

The **cerebral cortex** is a folded sheet of gray matter covering the cerebral hemispheres. It consists of six layers of neurons, each layer characterized by the morphology and connectivity of its neurons. In addition, the cortical mantle is divided into many **areas**, differing with regard to, among other things, their thalamic connections. Even though each area is to some extent specialized, most tasks of the cerebral cortex—whether they are motor, sensory, or cognitive—are carried out by **distributed networks** interconnecting neurons in many areas of the cerebral cortex. Among the many descending tracts from the cerebral cortex, **the pyramidal tract** targets motor neurons in the spinal cord and brain stem. The **corpus callosum**, consisting of commissural fibers, enables cooperation between the two cerebral hemispheres.

The **basal ganglia** consist of several large nuclei in the interior of the cerebral hemispheres. The **striatum** consists of **putamen** and the **caudate nucleus**, and receive its main afferents from the cerebral cortex. The striatum send efferents to the **globus pallidus** and the **substantia nigra**. From these, signals are directed to the brain stem, and back to the cerebral cortex via the thalamus. By influencing motor neuronal groups in the frontal lobe of cerebral cortex (and in the brain stem), the basal ganglia contribute to the **control of movements**. Connections with other frontal areas in cerebral cortex (and certain subcortical nuclei) enable the basal ganglia to influence **cognitive functions**.

The **cerebellum**, situated dorsal to the brain stem in the posterior cranial fossa, consists of a thin sheet of highly folded gray matter, and a group of centrally located, **deep cerebellar nuclei**. The cerebellum is divided anatomically into a narrow middle part called the **vermis**, and more bulky lateral parts called the cerebellar **hemispheres**. In addition, a deep fissure divides the cerebellum into an **anterior lobe** and a **posterior lobe**. These anatomic subdivisions correspond largely to differences with regard to connections. Thus, the vermis has reciprocal connections with the spinal cord and motor nuclei in the brain stem, whereas the cerebellar hemispheres are reciprocally connected with the cerebral cortex. These connections enable the cerebellum to play a decisive role in **coordination** of voluntary movements by acting on motor neurons in the cerebral cortex, the brain stem, and the spinal cord.

Some Anatomic Terms Used in this Book

The terms **medial**, toward the midline, and **lateral**, away from the midline, are used to describe the relative position of structures in relation to a midsagittal plane of the body. The terms **cranial** (or **rostral**), toward the head or nose, and **caudal**, toward the tail, are used to describe the relative position of structures along a longitudinal axis of the body. Thus, for example, nucleus A in the brain stem lies medial to and rostral to nucleus B, which in turn lies lateral to and caudal to A. The terms **ventral** and **dorsal** are used to describe the relative position of structures in relation to the front (*venter* means belly) and the back (*dorsum*) of the body, respectively. **Anterior** (front) and **posterior** (rear) are used interchangeably with ventral and dorsal, except for the human forebrain, where anterior means toward the nose and ventral means toward the base of the skull.

The Living Human Brain Can Be Studied with Computer-Based Imaging Techniques: CT, MRI, and DWI

Techniques for computer-based image analysis of the living human brain have revolutionized the possibilities for localizing disease processes in the brain and for studying normal structure and function.

The first of the imaging techniques that enabled us to identify smaller parts of the living brain is **computer tomography** (**CT**). This method makes it possible to see X-ray pictures of thin slices through the brain. The examiner may choose the plane of sectioning. CT affords much more precise visualization of brain structures than conventional X-ray examination, which includes all tissue between the X-ray tube and the film. It also provides good visualization of the ventricular system, which previously could be visualized only by replacing the cerebrospinal fluid with air and then making an X-ray examination. CT can also visualize the distribution of a radioactive substance in the living brain, enabling the study of the distribution of neuroactive substances and also the comparison of blood flow in different parts the brain.

Magnetic resonance imaging (**MRI**) represents a further technical development. This technique is based not on X-rays but on signals emitted by protons when they are placed in a magnetic field. Depending on the proton concentration in different tissue components, the pictures may show clearly, for example, the contrast between gray and white matter (Figs. 6.1 and 6.28). The bone of the skull gives very little or no signal and is seen as black in the pictures. With this technique, the brain can be visualized in slices with a resolution not far from that of a corresponding section through a fixed brain. Areas with changes in the tissue—for example, infarction, bleeding, or tumor—can be identified. In addition, blood vessels can be visualized to advantage (see Fig. 8.3 and 8.8). Apart from the diagnostic advantages, the MRI technique also improves the correlation of the functional disturbances with the actual damage

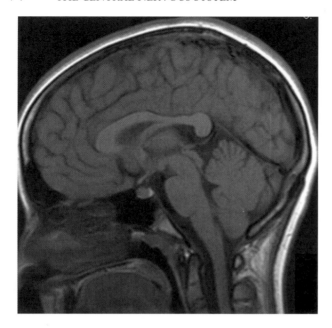

FIGURE 6.1 *Magnetic resonance image (MRI).* This is taken at a level corresponding to the drawing in Fig. 3.1. Most of the structures seen in Fig. 3.1 can be identified in this picture. (Courtesy of Dr. S. J. Bakke, Rikshospitalet University Hospital, Norway.)

of the brain. MRI can also be used to study dynamic processes in the brain (see Chapter 14, under "Methods to Study Neuronal Activity and Metabolism in the Living Human Brain").

Further developments of the MRI technology have added new applications. For example, with **diffusion-weighted imaging (DWI)** a region devoid of blood supply can be detected only minutes after occlusion of an artery (much earlier than with conventional functional [fMRI]). Further, DWI also enables study of myelination during normal brain development, and even the visualization of major fiber tracts.

THE SPINAL CORD

In humans, the spinal cord is a 40 to 45 cm-long cylinder of nervous tissue of approximately the same thickness as a little finger. It extends from the lower end of the brain stem (at the level of the upper end of the first cervical vertebra) down the vertebral canal (Figs. 6.2 and 6.3) to the upper margin of the second lumbar vertebra (L$_2$). Here the cord has a wedge-shaped end called the **medullary conus** (or simply conus). In **children**, the spinal cord extends more caudally, however, and reaches to the third lumbar vertebra in the newborn. This difference between the position of the lower end of the spinal cord in adults and infants is caused by the vertebral column growing more rapidly than the spinal cord. In early embryonic life, the neural tube and the

primordium of the vertebral column are equally long (see Fig. 9.12).

The spinal cord is somewhat flattened in the antero-posterior direction and is not equally thick along its length. In general, the thickness decreases caudally, but there are two marked **intumescences** (Fig. 6.3): the **cervical** and **lumbar enlargements** (intumescentia cervicalis and lumbalis). The intumescences supply the extremities with sensory and motor nerves, hence the increased thickness.

In the midline along the anterior aspect of the cord, there is a longitudinal furrow or fissure, the **anterior (ventral) median fissure** (Fig. 6.4). Some of the vessels of the cord enter through this fissure and penetrate deeply into the substance of the cord. At the posterior aspect of the cord, there is a corresponding, but shallower, furrow in the midline—the **posterior (dorsal) median fissure**. In addition, on each side there are shallow, longitudinal sulci anteriorly and posteriorly—the **anterior** and **posterior lateral sulci**. These laterally

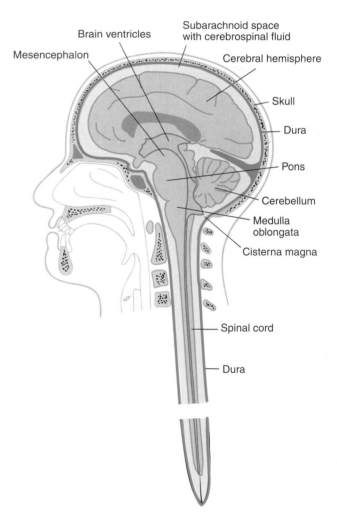

FIGURE 6.2 *The central nervous system, as viewed in a midsagittal section.*

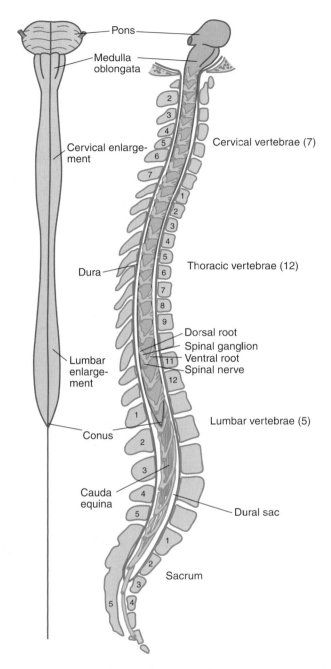

FIGURE 6.3 *The spinal cord*. **Left:** The cord from the ventral side, with the cervical and lumbar enlargements. **Right:** The cord and the vertebral column from the side, but the right halves of the vertebrae have been removed to expose the vertebral canal with its contents. Below the first and second lumbar vertebrae, the vertebral canal contains only nerve roots (the cauda equina), which then unite to form the spinal nerves.

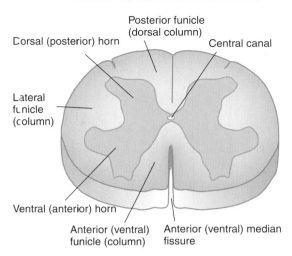

FIGURE 6.4 *Cross section of the spinal cord at a lumbar level*. There is a central H-shaped region of gray matter, and the surrounding white matter is subdivided into funiculi.

Spinal Nerves Connect the Spinal Cord with the Body

Axons mediating communication between the CNS and other parts of the body make up the **peripheral nerves**. The axons (nerve fibers) leave and enter the cord in small bundles called **rootlets** (Fig. 6.5). Several adjacent rootlets unite to a thicker strand, called a root or **nerve root**. In this manner, rows of roots are formed along the dorsal and ventral aspects of the cord: the **ventral (anterior) roots** and the **dorsal (posterior) roots**, respectively. Each dorsal root has a swelling, the **spinal ganglion**, which contains the cell bodies of the sensory axons that enter the cord through the dorsal root (Figs. 6.3 and 6.5). A dorsal and a ventral root unite to form a **spinal nerve**. The spinal ganglion lies in the

placed sulci mark where the spinal nerves connect with the cord.

The **color** of the spinal cord is whitish because the outer part consists of axons, many of which are myelinated. The **consistency** of the cord, as of the rest of the CNS, is soft and jellylike.

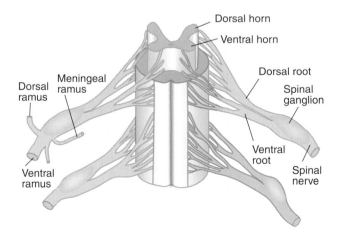

FIGURE 6.5 *Two segments of the spinal cord, as viewed from the ventral aspect*. In the upper part, the white matter has been removed. The dorsal and ventral roots emerge from the posterior and anterior lateral sulci, respectively, and unite to form spinal nerves. The spinal ganglion is located at the site where the roots unite.

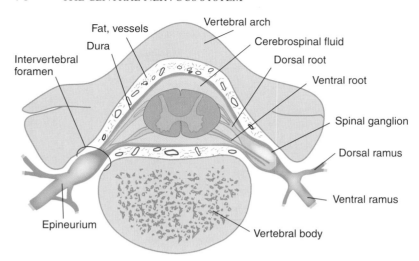

FIGURE 6.6 *Cross section of the vertebral column showing the positions of the spinal cord and the spinal nerves.* The spinal ganglion is located in the intervertebral foramen. The spinal cord is surrounded by the cerebrospinal fluid contained within the dura. Outside the dura there is fat and a venous plexus, which also serve as soft padding for the cord and the spinal nerves.

intervertebral foramen just where the dorsal and ventral roots unite (Fig. 6.6). There is an important functional difference between the ventral and dorsal roots: the ventral roots consist of efferent (motor) fibers, and the dorsal roots of afferent (sensory) fibers.

In total, 31 spinal nerves are present on each side, forming symmetrical pairs (Fig. 6.3). They all leave the vertebral canal through the intervertebral foramina on each side. As mentioned, the ventral and dorsal roots unite at the level of the intervertebral foramen to form the spinal nerves. The spinal nerves are numbered (as a general rule) in accordance with the number of vertebrae above the nerve. We therefore have 12 pairs of **thoracic nerves**, 5 pairs of **lumbar nerves**, and 5 pairs of **sacral nerves**. In humans, there is only 1 pair of coccygeal nerves. There are seven cervical vertebrae but 8 pairs of **cervical nerves** because the first cervical nerve leaves the vertebral canal above the first cervical vertebra (Fig. 6.3). Therefore, the numbering of the cervical nerves differs from the numbering of the other spinal nerves.

The spinal cord extends caudally only to the level of between the first and the second lumbar vertebrae. Whereas the upper spinal nerves pass approximately horizontally from the cord to the intervertebral foramen, the lower ones have to run obliquely downward in the vertebral canal to reach the corresponding intervertebral foramen, and the distance between the site of exit from the cord and the site of exit from the canal increases steadily (Fig. 6.3). Below the conus, the vertebral canal contains only spinal nerve roots running longitudinally. This collection of dorsal and ventral roots is called the **cauda equina** (the horsetail).

The Spinal Cord Is Divided into Segments

The part of the spinal cord that gives origin to a pair of spinal nerves is called a **spinal segment**. There are,

therefore, as many segments as there are pairs of spinal nerves. They are numbered accordingly, the first cervical segment giving origin to the first cervical nerves, and so on. There are no surface markings of the cord to indicate borders between the segments, but the rootlets nevertheless outline them rather precisely (Fig. 6.5).

The cervical **enlargement** (intumescence) corresponds to the fourth cervical (C_4) segment through the second thoracic (T_2) segment, the lumbar enlargement to the

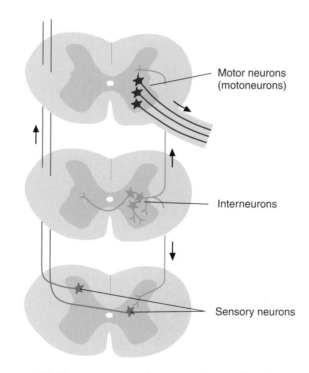

FIGURE 6.7 *Three main types of neurons in the spinal cord.* Schematic of neuronal types classified in accordance with where their axons terminate: *Motor neurons* supply skeletal muscles, smooth muscles, and glands. The *interneurons* ensure communication among neurons in the cord, and the *sensory neurons* send their axons to higher levels of the central nervous system. (See also Fig. 6.9.)

first lumbar (L_1) segment through the second sacral (S_2) segment.

The difference in rostrocaudal level between the spinal segments and the exit from the vertebral canal of the spinal nerves is of practical importance. Thus, identical symptoms may be provoked by a process close to the cord at one level and by one close to the intervertebral foramen at a considerably lower level (as should be clear from the preceding description; however, this does not concern the nerves in the cervical region).

The Spinal Cord Consists of Gray and White Matter

When cut transversely, the fresh spinal cord can be seen to consist of an outer zone of white matter and a central, H-shaped region of **gray matter**. The arms of the H, extending dorsally and ventrally, are called the **dorsal horn** and **ventral horn**, respectively (Figs. 6.4 and 6.8). The gray matter extends as a column through the length of the spinal cord (Fig. 6.5). The **central canal** is seen as a narrow opening in the center of the cord (Fig. 6.4). The central canal ends blindly in the caudal end of the cord, whereas it continues rostrally into the ventricular system of the brain (Fig. 6.1).

The **white matter** of the cord contains axons running longitudinally. Some of these axons convey signals from the cord to higher levels of the CNS; others, from higher levels to the cord. Finally, a large proportion of the fibers serve the signal traffic, and hence cooperation, between the segments of the cord. Because the first two groups of axons become successively more numerous in the rostral direction, the proportion of white to gray matter increases from caudal to rostral.

The white matter is divided into **funicles**, or **columns**, by drawing lines in the transverse plane from the sulci on the surface of the cord to the center (Fig. 6.4). Thus, in each half of the cord, the white matter is divided into a **ventral** or **anterior funicle** (funiculus), a **lateral funicle**, and a **dorsal** or **posterior funicle**. For the latter, the term **dorsal column** is used most frequently.

The Spinal Gray Matter Contains Three Main Types of Neurons

Among neurons in the gray matter of the spinal cord, there are both morphological and functional differences. Three main types may be identified according to where they send their axons (Fig. 6.7):

1. Neurons sending their axons out of the CNS
2. Neurons sending their axons to higher levels of the CNS (such as the brain stem)
3. Neurons sending their axons to other parts of the spinal cord

Often neurons of the same kind lie together in the gray matter of the cord. We will now consider in some detail each of these three groups.

Efferent Fibers from the Cord Control Muscles and Glands

The cell bodies of the first kind of neuron listed above are located in the ventral horn and at the transition between the dorsal and ventral horns. The **somatic motor neurons** or **motoneurons** have large, multipolar cell bodies and are located in the ventral horn proper (Fig. 6.8; see also Figs. 1.2 and 21.3). The dendrites extend for a considerable distance in the gray matter (Fig. 6.12). The axons leave the cord through the ventral root, follow the spinal nerves, and end in skeletal muscles (muscles that are controlled voluntarily). The motoneurons are discussed further in Chapter 21.

There is also another group of neurons that sends its axons out of the cord through the ventral root—the **autonomic motor neurons**. These supply smooth muscles and glands with motor signals. They belong to the autonomic nervous system, which controls the vascular smooth muscles and visceral organs throughout the body. These neurons are termed **preganglionic** because they send their axons to a ganglion (see Figs. 28.1 and 28.2). The cell bodies lie in the **lateral horn** (Fig. 6.8). Most of them form a long, slender column, the **intermediolateral cell column**. This column is present only in the thoracic and upper two lumbar segments of the cord and belongs to the sympathetic part of the autonomic nervous system. A corresponding, smaller group of neurons is present in the sacral cord (S_3–S_4) and

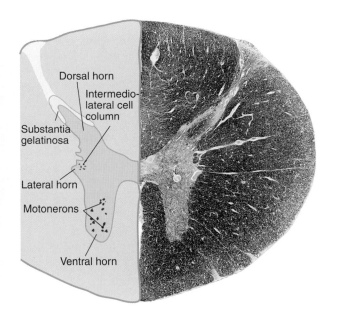

FIGURE 6.8 *Cross section of the spinal cord at the thoracic level.* Photomicrograph of a section stained so that myelinated axons appear dark. The large motoneurons in the ventral horn have also been stained (Nissl staining) and are just visible. Owing to shrinkage, the motoneurons are surrounded by a clear zone.

belongs to the parasympathetic part of the autonomic nervous system.

Both the somatic and the autonomic motor neurons are under synaptic influence from higher levels of the CNS.

Sensory Neurons in the Cord Are Influenced from the Dorsal Roots and Convey Signals to the Brain

The second main type of spinal neuron sends axons to higher levels of the CNS. Their cell bodies lie mainly in the dorsal horn and in the transition zone between the dorsal and ventral horn (Figs. 6.7 and 6.9). Their job is to inform the brain of the activities of the spinal cord, and especially about what is going on in the body. To fulfill the latter task, the neurons must receive signals from **sense organs**—receptors—in various parts of the body (in the skin, muscles, viscera, and so on). **Sensory**, or **afferent**, nerve fibers conducting impulses from the receptors enter the spinal cord through the dorsal roots and ramify, forming terminals in the gray matter of the cord (Fig. 6.9; see also Fig. 13.12). The sensory neurons have their cell bodies in the **spinal ganglia** (Fig. 6.5; see also) and are therefore called **spinal ganglion cells** (see Fig. 13.13). These are morphologically special, as they have only one process, which divides shortly after leaving the cell body: One peripheral process connects with the sense organs, and the other extends centrally and enters the spinal cord (pseudounipolar neuron; see Fig. 1.5). In accordance with the usual definition of

axons and dendrites, the peripheral process (conducting toward the cell body) should be called a dendrite, whereas the central process is an axon. Both processes are, however, morphologically and functionally axons (e.g., by conducting action potentials and by being myelinated).

The dorsal root fibers form synaptic contacts—in part directly, in part indirectly through the interneurons—with neurons in the spinal cord, sending their axons to various parts of the brain. Such axons, destined for a common target in the brain, are grouped together in the spinal white matter, forming **tracts** (Latin: *tractus*). Such tracts are named after the location of the cell bodies and after the target organ. A tract leading from the spinal cord to the cerebellum, for example, is named the "spinocerebellar tract" (tractus spinocerebellaris).

Interneurons Enable Cooperation between Different Cell Groups in the Spinal Cord

The axons of the third type of spinal neuron do not leave the spinal cord. Usually, the axons ramify extensively and establish synaptic contacts with many other neurons in the cord, within the segment in which the cell body is located, and in segments above and below (Fig. 6.7). Such neurons are called **spinal interneurons**, to emphasize that they are intercalated between other neurons.[1] Many spinal interneurons are found in an intermediate zone between the dorsal and ventral horns, where they receive major synaptic inputs from sensory fibers in the dorsal roots. Many of these interneurons establish synaptic contacts with motoneurons in the ventral horn, thus mediating motor responses to sensory stimuli. Most interneurons, however, receive additional strong inputs from other spinal interneurons and from the brain.

As mentioned, spinal interneurons also send collaterals to terminate in segments of the cord other than the one in which their cell body and local ramifications are found. Such collaterals enter the white matter, run there for some distance, and reenter the cord at another segmental level, to ramify and establish synaptic contacts in the gray matter (Fig. 6.7). Axons of this kind in the white matter are called **propriospinal fibers** (i.e., fibers "belonging" to the spinal cord itself), to distinguish them from the long ascending and descending fibers that connect the cord with the brain.

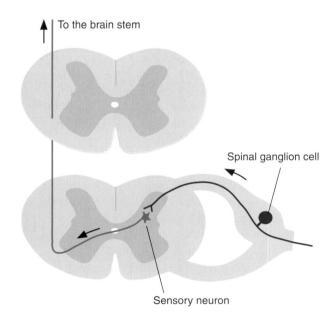

To the brain stem

Spinal ganglion cell

Sensory neuron

FIGURE 6.9 *Sensory neuron in the gray substance of the spinal cord.* The neuron, which sends its axon to the brain stem, is synaptically contacted by sensory afferents that enter the cord through the dorsal root (pseudounipolar ganglion cell). The presentation is very simplified; in reality, every sensory neuron is contacted by numerous dorsal root afferents.

1 Strictly speaking, most neurons in the CNS are interneurons according to this definition—including, for example, spinal neurons with axons ascending to the brain. In practice, the term "interneurons" is nevertheless restricted to neurons with an axon ramifying near the cell body, thus synaptically coupling neurons within one nucleus.

Propriospinal neuron is, therefore, another term used for a spinal interneuron.[2]

Propriospinal fibers provide opportunities for cooperation among the spinal segments. Most of movements necessitate close coordination of the activity in many segments, each controlling different groups of muscles. Some propriospinal connections are very long and interconnect segments in the cervical and lumbar parts of the cord that control muscles in the forelimb and hindlimb, respectively. Cooperation between the forelimbs and hind limbs is necessary, for example, during **walking**.

Spinal interneurons are discussed further in Chapter 13, under "Sensory Fibers Are Links in Reflex Arcs: Spinal Interneurons," and in Chapter 22, under "The Pyramidal Tract Can Open and Close Spinal Reflex Arcs."

The Spinal Gray Matter Can Be Divided into Zones Called Rexed's Laminae

Systematic observations with the microscope of transverse sections of the spinal cord stained to visualize cell bodies show that neurons with different sizes and shapes are also differently distributed (Fig. 6.10; see also Fig. 13.16). Essentially, neurons with common morphological features are collected into transversely oriented bands or zones. What appear as bands in the transverse plane are, three-dimensionally, longitudinal slabs or sheets. This laminar pattern is most clear-cut in the dorsal horn, whereas in the ventral horn neurons are collected into regions that form longitudinal columns rather than plates (see Fig. 21.2). Nevertheless, the columns in the ventral horn, as well as the slabs in the dorsal horn, are termed **laminae**. This pattern was first described in 1952 by the Swedish neuroanatomist Bror Rexed and has since proved to be of great help for investigations of the spinal cord. Altogether, Rexed described 10 laminae; **laminae I–VI** constitute the dorsal horn, whereas **lamina IX** is made up of columns of motoneurons in the ventral horn. **Lamina II (substantia gelatinosa**; Figs. 6.8, 6.10, and 6.11) is of particular importance for the control of signals from pain receptors, and thus how much a painful stimulus hurts. **Lamina VII** constitutes the transition between the dorsal and ventral horns and contains mainly interneurons. **Lamina VIII**, located medially in the ventral horn, contains many neurons that send axons to the other side of the cord (commissural fibers).

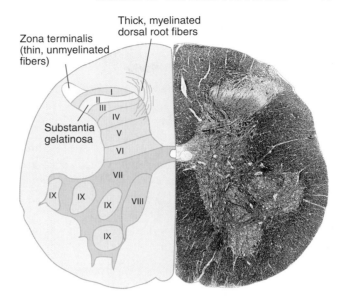

FIGURE 6.10 *Cross section of the spinal cord at the lumbar level (lumbar intumescence)*. **Left:** Photomicrograph of section stained to show myelin and neuronal cell bodies. **Right:** The borders between Rexed's laminae. The groups of motoneurons in the ventral horn (α and γ motoneurons) constitute lamina IX; the zona terminalis (tract of Lissauer) consists primarily of thin dorsal root fibers.

Even though the cell bodies are arranged in laminae, the dendrites extend much wider, as shown in Fig. 6.12. Thus, a neuron belonging to a particular lamina receives synaptic inputs from nerve terminals in neighboring laminae. Nevertheless, experimental studies of the connections of the spinal cord and of the functional properties of single spinal neurons have shown that the various laminae differ in these respects. Thus, the laminae may be regarded, at least to some extent, as the nuclei of the spinal cord. We will return to Rexed's laminae when dealing with the functional organization of the spinal cord in later chapters.

The Spinal Nerves Divide into Branches

The dorsal (sensory) and ventral (motor) roots join to form spinal nerves, as described. Each spinal nerve then divides into several **branches (rami)** just outside the intervertebral foramen (Figs. 6.5 and 6.6). The thickest one, the **ventral ramus** (ramus ventralis), passes ventrally. A thinner branch, the **dorsal ramus** (ramus dorsalis), bends in the dorsal direction. In contrast to the spinal roots, the ventral and dorsal rami contain both sensory and motor fibers. This is caused by mixing of fibers from dorsal and ventral roots as they continue into the spinal nerves.

The dorsal rami innervate muscles and skin on the back, whereas the ventral rami innervate skin and muscles on the ventral aspect of the trunk and neck and, in addition, the extremities. Thus, the ventral rami

---

2 It was formerly believed that propriospinal neurons—that is, spinal neurons with axons entering the white matter but not leaving the spinal cord—and interneurons represented two distinct cell groups. Recent studies have shown that spinal interneurons have local (intrasegmental) branches, as well as collaterals destined for other segments (intersegmental).

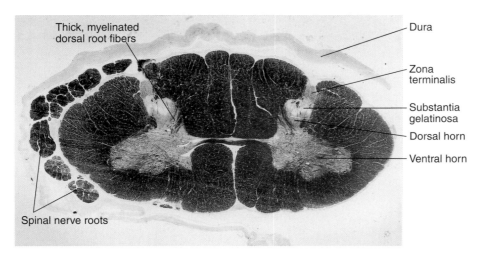

Thick, myelinated dorsal root fibers

Dura

Zona terminalis

Substantia gelatinosa

Dorsal horn

Ventral horn

Spinal nerve roots

FIGURE 6.11 *Cross section of the spinal cord at the cervical level (cervical intumescence).* The broad ventral horns contain the motoneurons that supply muscles of the arm and shoulder girdle. Compared with the lumbar cord (Fig. 6.10), the cervical cord contains more white matter in proportion to gray matter; this is because all descending and ascending fibers to and from the lower levels pass through the cervical cord.

innervate much larger parts of the body than the dorsal ones, which explains why the ventral rami contain more nerve fibers and are considerably thicker than the dorsal ones. Some of the ventral rami join each other to form **plexuses** (see Fig. 21.1).

Each spinal nerve also sends off a small branch, the **meningeal ramus**, which passes back through the intervertebral foramen to reenter the vertebral canal (Fig. 6.5). These branches supply the meninges of the spinal cord with sensory and autonomic (sympathetic) fibers.

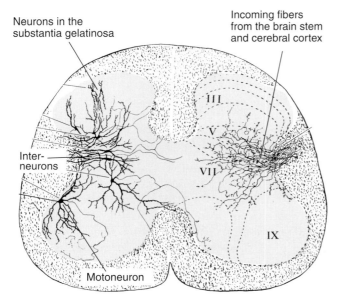

Neurons in the substantia gelatinosa

Incoming fibers from the brain stem and cerebral cortex

Interneurons

III

V

VII

IX

Motoneuron

FIGURE 6.12 *Dendritic arborizations of spinal neurons extend beyond the laminae of their cell bodies.* Composite drawing based on observations in many Golgi-impregnated transverse sections from the spinal cord of the cat. The dendrites extend far, not only in the transverse plane as shown here but also longitudinally. To the right (at **A**) are the terminal ramifications of axons descending to the cord from higher levels of the CNS. (From Scheibel and Scheibel 1966.)

The Spinal Cord Consists of Subunits that Are Controlled from the Brain

Each segment of the spinal cord is to some extent a functional unit, since, as we will see in Chapter 13, a pair of spinal nerves relates to a particular "segment" of the body (see Fig. 13.14). A spinal segment may be regarded as the "local government" of a part of the body: it receives sensory information from its own district, processes this information, and issues orders through motor nerves to muscles and glands to ensure adequate responses. However, just as local governing bodies in our society must take orders from higher ones (e.g., county versus national governments), the spinal segments have only limited independence. Many of the functional tasks of the spinal cord are under strict control and supervision from higher levels of the CNS. This control is mediated by fibers from the brain stem and cerebral cortex, which descend in the white matter of the cord and terminate in the gray matter of the spinal segments that are to be influenced. The brain also ensures that the activity of the various spinal segments is coordinated, so that it serves the body as a whole and not only a small part. To be able to carry out this coordination, the brain must continuously receive information about conditions in all the "local districts" of the body and in the spinal segments related to them. This information is mediated by long, ascending fibers (forming various tracts) in the white matter of the cord that terminates in the brain stem. The local cooperation among spinal segments is taken care of by the numerous propriospinal fibers coming from spinal interneurons.

THE BRAIN STEM

The brain stem represents the upward (rostral, cranial) continuation of the spinal cord (Fig. 6.1). It consists of several portions with, in part, clear-cut surface borders between them (Figs. 6.13 to 6.15). Whereas the lowermost (caudal) part of the brain stem is structurally similar to the spinal cord, the upper parts are more complicated. The subdivisions of the brain stem are as follows (from caudal to rostral): the **medulla oblongata** (often just called medulla), the **pons** (the bridge), the **mesencephalon** (the midbrain), and the **diencephalon**. Usually, however, often we use a more restricted definition including only the parts that extrude from the base of the brain: the medulla, pons, and mesencephalon.

The Brain Stem Contains the Third and Fourth Ventricles

A continuous, fluid-filled cavity varying in diameter stretches through the brain stem (Fig. 6.2). It is the upward continuation of the thin central canal of the spinal cord, and it continues rostrally into the cavities of the cerebrum (see Figs. 7.3 and 7.5). Together, these cavities constitute the ventricular system of the brain and spinal cord. The cavity in the brain stem has two dilated parts: one, the **fourth ventricle**, is at the level of the medulla and pons, whereas the **third ventricle** is situated in the diencephalon. We return to the ventricular system in Chapter 7.

The Cranial Nerves

Examination of the internal structure of the brain stem shows that it is more complicated than that of the spinal cord (see, e.g., Fig. 6.16). Even though gray matter is generally located centrally, surrounded by a zone of white matter in both the brain stem and the cord, the gray matter of the brain stem is subdivided into several regions separated by strands of white matter. The white matter of the brain stem consists of myelinated fibers, as in other parts of the CNS. The regions with gray matter contain various nuclei, or groups of neurons with common tasks.

Many of the nuclei belong to the **cranial nerves**. In total, there are 12 pairs of cranial nerves, which, with the exception of the first, all emerge from the brain stem (Figs. 6.13 and 6.15). They correspond to the spinal nerves but show a more complex and less regular organization. Thus, there is no clear separation of

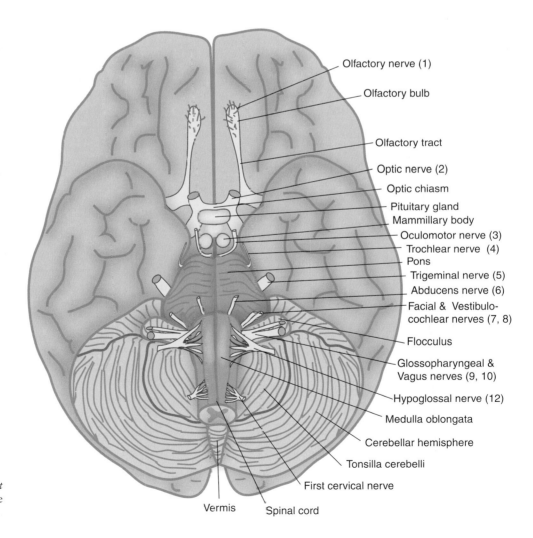

FIGURE 6.13 *The basal aspect of the brain.* Only some of the cranial nerves are shown.

Labels (clockwise): Olfactory nerve (1); Olfactory bulb; Olfactory tract; Optic nerve (2); Optic chiasm; Pituitary gland; Mammillary body; Oculomotor nerve (3); Trochlear nerve (4); Pons; Trigeminal nerve (5); Abducens nerve (6); Facial & Vestibulocochlear nerves (7, 8); Flocculus; Glossopharyngeal & Vagus nerves (9, 10); Hypoglossal nerve (12); Medulla oblongata; Cerebellar hemisphere; Tonsilla cerebelli; First cervical nerve; Spinal cord; Vermis

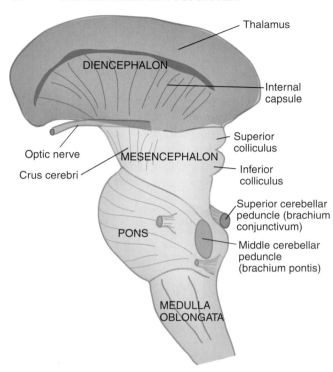

FIGURE 6.14 *The brain stem, as viewed from the left side.* The levels of sections shown in several of the following figures are indicated.

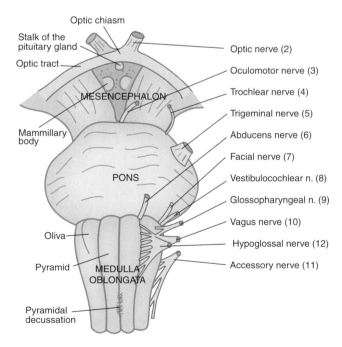

FIGURE 6.15 *The cranial nerves.* The brain stem is seen from the ventral side.

sensory (dorsal) and motor (ventral) roots. The cranial nerves are numbered from rostral to caudal, in accordance with where they emerge on the surface of the brain stem. Figure 8.9 shows the places on the base of the skull where the cranial nerves leave through small holes or fissures.

Many of the cranial nerves contain fibers that conduct impulses out of the brain stem; that is, the fibers are efferent, or motor. These fibers belong to neurons with their cell bodies in nuclei that are called **motor cranial nerve nuclei**. They correspond to the groups (columns) of neurons in the ventral and lateral horns of the spinal cord. The cranial nerves, like the spinal nerves, also contain sensory, afferent fibers that bring impulses from sense organs. The brain stem cell groups in which these afferent fibers terminate are, accordingly, called **sensory cranial nerve nuclei**; they correspond to the laminae of the spinal dorsal horn. The sensory fibers entering the brain stem have their cell bodies in ganglia just outside the brain stem, **cranial nerve ganglia**, corresponding to the spinal ganglia of the spinal nerves. Most cranial nerves are mixed—that is, they contain both motor and sensory fibers—but a few are either purely sensory or purely motor.

The only cranial nerve not emerging from the brain stem is the first cranial nerve, the **olfactory nerve** (nervus olfactorius). This consists of short axons coming from sensory cells in the roof of the nasal cavity, which, immediately after penetrating the base of the skull, terminate in the **olfactory bulb** (bulbus olfactorius) (Fig. 6.13). The other cranial nerves are briefly mentioned in the next section in connection with a description of the main structural features of the brain stem. The cranial nerves and their central connections are treated more thoroughly in later chapters, particularly Chapter 27.

The Reticular Formation Extends through Central Parts of the Brain Stem

Among the cranial nerve nuclei and other clearly delimited cell groups, there are more diffuse collections of neurons. In microscopic sections stained to visualize the neuronal processes, a network-like pattern is seen. The old anatomists therefore termed this part—present in the core of most of the brain stem—the **reticular formation** (formatio reticularis; Figs. 6.16–6.18; see also Fig. 26.1). In reality, however, the reticular formation is not one homogeneous structure but, rather, a conglomerate of cell groups with different connections and functional tasks. For example, some parts of the reticular formation are primarily concerned with control of **circulation** and **respiration**; other parts regulate **sleep** and **wakefulness**. However, the collective term, the reticular formation, is still in common use, and it may be practical to retain it to denote parts of the brain stem

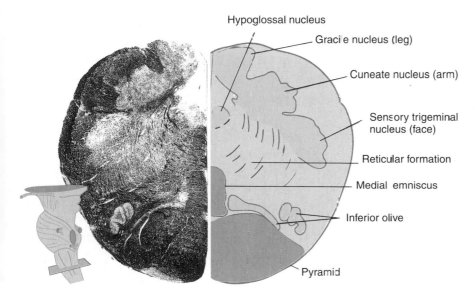

Hypoglossal nucleus
Gracile nucleus (leg)
Cuneate nucleus (arm)
Sensory trigeminal nucleus (face)
Reticular formation
Medial lemniscus
Inferior olive
Pyramid

FIGURE 6.16 *Lower part of the medulla oblongata*. Cross section. Inset shows level and plane of the section. Left half shows photomicrograph of a section with darkly stained myelinated fibers (Woelke method); that is, white matter appears dark and gray matter appears light.

with certain common anatomic features, without implying that they have common functional tasks. The reticular formation is treated more comprehensively in Chapter 26.

The Medulla Oblongata

Ventrally in the midline, the medulla has a longitudinal sulcus, which is a continuation of the ventral median fissure of the cord (Fig. 6.15). The sulcus ends abruptly at the lower end of the pons. The so-called **pyramids** protrude on each side of the longitudinal sulcus. Each pyramid is formed by a thick bundle of axons belonging to the **pyramidal tract**, which conveys signals from the cerebral cortex to the spinal cord and is essential for our control of voluntary movements (the pyramidal tract is discussed in Chapter 22). Close to the lower end of the medulla, on the transition to the cord, bundles of fibers can be seen to cross the midline, forming the **pyramidal decussation** (Fig. 6.15). Lateral to the pyramid is an oval protrusion (the olive), which is formed by a large nucleus, the **inferior olivary nucleus**

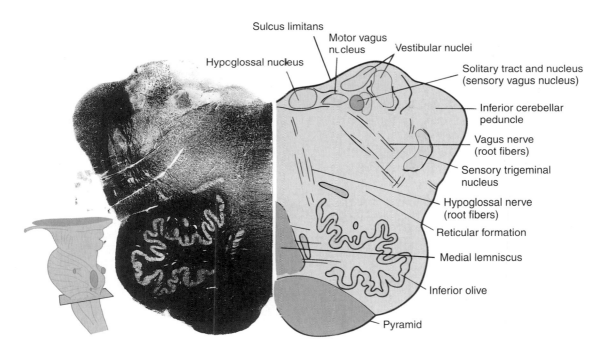

Sulcus limitans
Motor vagus nucleus
Vestibular nuclei
Hypoglossal nucleus
Solitary tract and nucleus (sensory vagus nucleus)
Inferior cerebellar peduncle
Vagus nerve (root fibers)
Sensory trigeminal nucleus
Hypoglossal nerve (root fibers)
Reticular formation
Medial lemniscus
Inferior olive
Pyramid

FIGURE 6.17 *Upper part of the medulla oblongata*. Cross section; myelin stained.

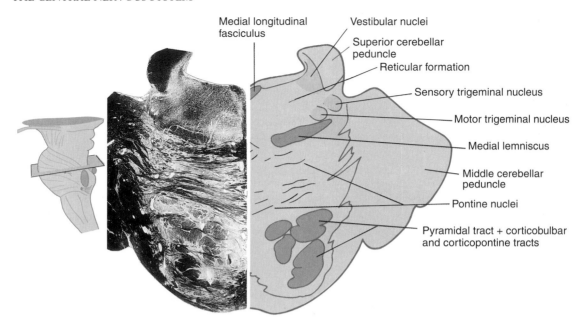

Medial longitudinal fasciculus
Vestibular nuclei
Superior cerebellar peduncle
Reticular formation
Sensory trigeminal nucleus
Motor trigeminal nucleus
Medial lemniscus
Middle cerebellar peduncle
Pontine nuclei
Pyramidal tract + corticobulbar and corticopontine tracts

FIGURE 6.18 *Upper part of the pons.* Cross section; myelin-stained.

(inferior olive), which sends its efferents to the cerebellum. Between the olive and the pyramid is a row of small bundles of nerve fibers (Fig. 6.15; see also Fig. 27.1), which are the rootlets of the **hypoglossal nerve** (the twelfth cranial nerve, nervus hypoglossus). This nerve supplies the striated muscles of the tongue with motor fibers. Lateral to the olive, the rootlets of the **glossopharyngeal** and **vagus nerves** (ninth and tenth cranial nerves, nervus glossopharyngeus and nervus vagus) leave the brain stem. These two nerves supply the pharynx, the larynx, and most of the viscera with motor and sensory fibers. The **accessory nerve** (eleventh cranial nerve, nervus accessorius) runs cranially along the lateral aspect of the medulla. Most of its fibers come from the upper cervical spinal segments but enter the cranial cavity to leave the skull together with the glossopharyngeal and vagus nerves (see Fig. 27.8). The accessory nerve supplies two muscles in the neck with motor fibers.

Figure 3.16 shows a cross section through the **lower part of the medulla**, at a level below the caudal end of the fourth ventricle. The section is stained so that regions with white matter (the myelinated fiber tracts) are dark, whereas gray matter (the nuclei) appears light. The ventrally located bundle of cross-sectioned fibers is the **pyramidal tract,** forming the pyramid (Fig. 6.15), and containing about 1 million fibers. Dorsal to the pyramid lies a highly convoluted band of gray matter, the **inferior olivary nucleus**. The **dorsal column nuclei,** the **gracile** and **cuneate** (nucleus gracilis and nucleus cuneatus), are located dorsally in the medulla. The efferent fibers from these nuclei arch ventrally and take up a position close to the midline dorsal to the

pyramids, where they form a triangular area of cross-sectioned fibers. This is an important sensory tract, the **medial lemniscus** (lemniscus medialis), that leads from neurons in the dorsal column nuclei to nuclei in the diencephalon (see Fig. 13.17). The dorsal column nuclei receive afferent fibers that ascend in the dorsal columns (or dorsal funicles) and convey impulses from sense organs in the skin and muscles and around joints. Close to the midline, just ventral to the central canal, lies the **hypoglossal nucleus,** consisting of the cell bodies of the motor fibers that form the hypoglossal nerve. The efferent fibers of the hypoglossal nucleus pass ventrally and leave the medulla at the lateral edge of the pyramid (Fig. 6.15). Lateral to the motor cranial nerve nuclei are found several sensory cranial nerve nuclei, among them the big **sensory trigeminal nucleus** that receives sensory impulses from the face, carried in the **trigeminal nerve** (the fifth cranial nerve, nervus trigeminus). Note how the nuclei that are transmitting sensory impulses from the leg, arm, and face are distributed from medial to lateral in the dorsal part of the medulla (Fig. 6.16).

A cross section through the **upper part of the medulla** (Fig. 6.17) shows partly the same fiber tracts and nuclei as the section at a lower level (Fig. 6.16). In addition, we may notice the big **vestibular nuclei** situated dorsally and laterally under the floor of the fourth ventricle (these nuclei also extend cranially into the pons; see Fig. 19.7). They receive sensory impulses from the vestibular apparatus in the inner ear via the **vestibular nerve** (the eighth cranial nerve). One of the main efferent pathways from the vestibular nuclei forms a distinct tract, the **medial longitudinal fasciculus** (fasciculus longitudinalis medialis), close to the midline under the floor of the fourth ventricle (Fig. 6.18). This tract terminates in the motor nuclei of the cranial nerves supplying the eye muscles, thus conveying influences on eye movements from the receptors for equilibrium. Further, Fig. 3.17 shows the motor and sensory **nuclei of the vagus**, and some of the fibers of the **vagus nerve**, which pass laterally and ventrally, to leave the medulla lateral to the olive (Fig. 6.15).

The Pons

The pons forms a bulbous protrusion at the ventral aspect of the brain stem, with clear-cut transversely running fiber bundles (Figs. 6.13 and 6.14). It is sharply delimited both caudally and cranially. The transverse fiber bundles are formed by fibers from large cell groups in the pons, the pontine nuclei, and terminate in the cerebellum. The fiber bundles join at the lateral aspect of the pons to form the **middle cerebellar peduncle** (brachium pontis) (Figs. 6.14 and 6.18). Several cranial nerves leave the brain stem at the ventral aspect of the pons. At the lower (caudal) edge, just lateral to the midline, a thin nerve emerges on each side. This is the **abducens nerve** (the sixth cranial nerve, nervus abducens) that carries motor fibers to one of the external eye muscles (rotates the eye laterally). Still at the lower edge of the pons, but more laterally, two other cranial nerves leave the brain stem. Most ventrally lies the **facial nerve** (seventh cranial nerve, nervus facialis), which brings motor impulses to the mimetic muscles of the face (it also contains some other kinds of fibers that are considered in Chapter 27). Closely behind the facial nerve lies the **vestibulocochlear nerve** (the eighth cranial nerve, nervus vestibulocochlearis), which carries sensory impulses from the sense organs for equilibrium and hearing in the inner ear. The **trigeminal nerve** (the fifth cranial nerve, nervus trigeminus) leaves the brain stem laterally at middle levels of the pons. The largest portion of the nerve consists of sensory fibers from the face, whereas a smaller (medial) portion contains motor fibers destined for the masticatory muscles.

In a **cross section** through the pons, the large **pontine nuclei** can be seen easily (Fig. 6.18). As mentioned, the neurons of the pontine nuclei send their axons to the cerebellum. Because their main afferent connections come from the cerebral cortex, the pontine nuclei mediate information from the cerebral cortex to the cerebellum. The **medial lemniscus** borders the pontine nuclei dorsally and has turned around and moved laterally compared with its location in the medulla (Fig. 6.16). In the lower part of the pons, the nucleus of the abducens nerve, the **abducens nucleus**, is located dorsally and medially, whereas the **facial nucleus** lies more ventrally and laterally (see Fig. 27.11; Fig. 17.11 also shows the course taken by the efferent fibers of the abducens and facial nuclei, forming the sixth and seventh cranial nerves, respectively).

Figure 6.18 also shows the **sensory trigeminal nucleus** laterally (this nucleus extends as a slender column through the medulla, pons, and mesencephalon; see also Figs. 6.16–6.18, and 27.2). Medial to the sensory nucleus lies the **motor trigeminal nucleus** (the masticatory muscles), but this nucleus is present only in the pons.

The Medulla and Pons Seen from the Dorsal Side

At the dorsal side of the medulla oblongata, at caudal levels, there are two longitudinal protrusions, the **gracile** and **cuneate tubercles** (Fig. 6.19). These are formed by the **dorsal column nuclei**, mentioned earlier (they are relay stations in pathways for sensory information from the body to the cerebral cortex). The most medial of these nuclei, the **gracile nucleus**, receives impulses from the leg and lower part of the trunk, whereas the laterally situated **cuneate nucleus** receives impulses from the arm and upper part of the trunk. Further laterally, another oblong protrusion (tuberculum cinereum) is formed by the **sensory trigeminal nucleus**, the relay station for sensory impulses from the face.

Rostral to the upper end of the dorsal column nuclei, there is a flattened, diamond-shaped area, the **rhomboid fossa**, extending rostrally onto the posterior face of the pons (Fig. 6.18). This constitutes the "floor" of the fourth ventricle (Fig. 6.19). Laterally and rostrally, the **cerebellar peduncles** delimit the rhomboid fossa (these have been cut in Fig. 6.19). Some of the cranial nerve nuclei and some fiber tracts form small protrusions medially at the floor of the fourth ventricle— notably the hypoglossal nucleus (hypoglossal trigone), the vagus nucleus (vagal trigone) and more rostrally the root fibers of the facial nerve—the latter forming the **facial colliculus**. (Figure 27.11 explains how the facial colliculus is formed.)

The Mesencephalon (Midbrain)

The part of the brain stem rostral to the pons, the **mesencephalon**, is relatively short (Figs. 6.14 and 6.15). Ventrally, an almost half-cylindrical protrusion is present on each side of the midline—the **crus cerebri**, or **cerebral peduncle** (Figs. 6.15 and 6.20).[3] Crus cerebri consists of nerve fibers descending from the cerebral cortex to the brain stem and spinal cord; among these fibers are those of the pyramidal tract. The fibers continue into the pons, where they spread out into several smaller bundles among the pontine nuclei (Fig. 6.18).

---

3 Strictly speaking, the term cerebral peduncle denotes both the crus cerebri and parts of the mesencephalon dorsal to the crus except the colliculi (the latter collectively termed the "tectum"). The region between the crus cerebri and the tectum is called the tegmentum and includes the periaqueductal gray, the red nucleus, and the substantia nigra. Previously, however, the crus cerebri and the cerebral peduncle were both applied to the ventralmost, fiber-rich part.

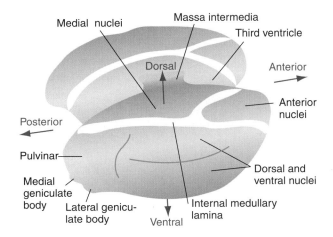

FIGURE 6.22 *The thalamus*. Drawing of the thalami of both sides, to indicate their three-dimensional form.

different parts of the cerebral cortex (see Fig. 34.7). For example, the lateral and medial geniculate bodies are relay stations for visual and auditory impulses, respectively. Thus, fibers of the optic nerve end in the lateral geniculate body while fibers from the inferior colliculus end in the medial geniculate body.

The **optic nerves** from the two eyes unite just underneath the diencephalon (Figs. 6.13 and 6.15) to form the **optic chiasm** (chiasma opticum, or just chiasma), in which there is a partial crossing of the optic nerve fibers (see Fig. 16.14). In their further course from the optic chiasm to the lateral geniculate body, the fibers form the **optic tract** (Figs. 6.15 and 6.24). The fibers from the lateral geniculate body to the visual cortex form the **optic radiation** (Fig. 16.15).

Anterior and inferior to the thalamus lies the **hypothalamus** (Fig. 6.23), which exerts central control of the autonomic nervous system—that is, with control of the visceral organs and the vessels. The hypothalamus forms the lateral wall of the anterior part of the third ventricle. The border between the thalamus and the hypothalamus is marked by the shallow **hypothalamic sulcus** (Figs. 6.23 and 6.24). The **mammillary body** (corpus mammillare), a special part of the hypothalamus, protrudes downward from its posterior part (Figs. 6.13, 6.23, and 6.29). The **fornix** is a thick, arching bundle of fibers originating in the cerebral cortex (in the so-called hippocampal region in the temporal lobe) and terminating in the mammillary bodies (see Fig. 32.2). The major efferent pathway of the mammillary body goes to the thalamus, forming a distinct fiber

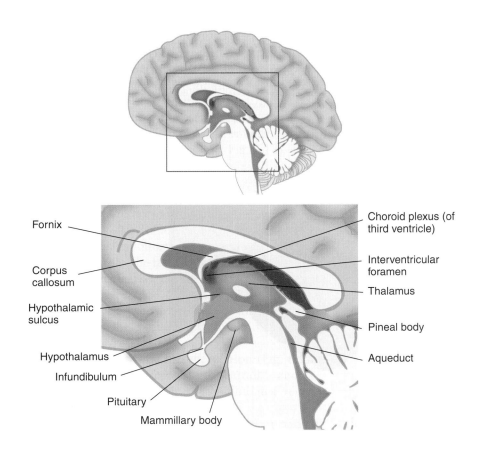

FIGURE 6.23 *The hypothalamus*. Drawing of midsagittal section showing the upper parts of the brain stem. The hypothalamus is indicated in red.

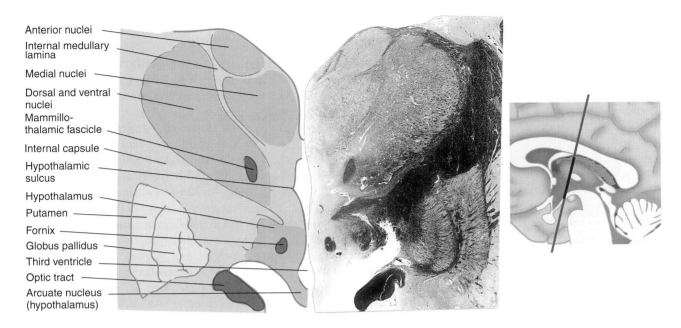

Anterior nuclei
Internal medullary lamina
Medial nuclei
Dorsal and ventral nuclei
Mammillo-thalamic fascicle
Internal capsule
Hypothalamic sulcus
Hypothalamus
Putamen
Fornix
Globus pallidus
Third ventricle
Optic tract
Arcuate nucleus (hypothalamus)

FIGURE 6.24 *The diencephalon.* Frontal section; myelin stained.

bundle, the **mammillothalamic tract** (fasciculus mammillothalamicus) (Figs. 6.24 and 30.6). In front of the mammillary bodies, the floor of the third ventricle bulges downward like a funnel and forms the stalk of the pituitary gland, the **infundibulum**. The region between the mammillary bodies and the infundibulum is called the **tuber cinereum** (see Fig 30.3). It contains neuronal groups that influence the activity of the pituitary gland.

The **pituitary** (Figs. 6.13 and 6.23) consists of a **posterior lobe**, developed from the CNS, and an **anterior lobe**, developed from the epithelium in the roof of the mouth. The anterior lobe, secreting several hormones that control important bodily functions, is itself under the control of the hypothalamus. This is discussed further in Chapter 30.

Epithalamus and the Pineal Body

The diencephalon also includes a small area called the epithalamus, located posteriorly in the roof of the third ventricle. In addition to a small nucleus, the **habenula** (Fig. 6.21), the epithalamus contains the **pineal body** or gland (corpus pineale) (Figs. 6.19, 6.23, and 6.31). This peculiar structure lies in the midline (unpaired) and is formed by an evagination of the roof of the third ventricle. It contains glandular cells, **pinealocytes**, which produce the hormone **melatonin** (and several neuropeptides). It also contains large amounts of **serotonin**, which is a precursor of melatonin. Melatonin influences several physiological parameters, especially those that show a cyclic variation. This is discussed more thoroughly in Chapter 30, under "Hypothalamus and Circadian Rhythms" and under "Melatonin."

The **habenula** (Fig. 6.21) lies just underneath the pineal body (one on each side). This small nucleus (composed of several subnuclei) receives afferents from the hypothalamus and the septal nuclei, among other sources. Its main efferents go to nuclei in the mesencephalon. The functional role of the habenula is not known, but the pathway from the hypothalamus via habenula to the mesencephalon may be engaged in the bodily expressions of strong **emotions**—for example, rage or fear. The habenula is one among several neuronal groups that are altered in severe **depression**.

THE CEREBRUM

The cerebrum has an ovoid shape and fills most of the cranial cavity. Whereas its convexity—that is, its upper and lateral surfaces—are evenly curved, the basal surface is uneven. In the center of the basal surface, the brain stem emerges (Fig. 6.13). The cerebrum is almost completely divided in two by a vertical slit, the **longitudinal cerebral fissure** (fissura longitudinalis cerebralis), so that it consists of two approximate half-spheres or **cerebral hemispheres** (Figs. 6.25 and 6.26). Each of the cerebral hemispheres contains a central cavity, the **lateral ventricle** (Figs. 6.29 and 7.3). The lateral ventricles are continuous, with the third ventricle through a small opening, the **interventricular foramen** (Fig. 6.37).

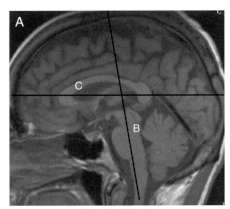

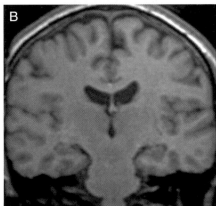

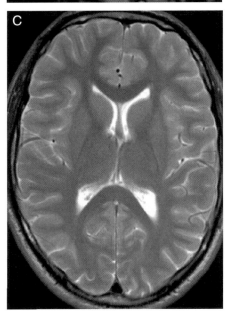

FIGURE 6.28 *Magnetic resonance images (MRI) in the three conventional planes.* **A:** Midsagittal plane. **B:** frontal (coronal) plane; corresponding to Fig. 3.27. **C:** Horizontal (transverse) plane. A and B are T1 weighted with water appearing dark. C is T2 weighted with water appearing white. (Courtesy of Dr. S. J. Bakke, Rikshospitalet University Hospital, Norway.)

is of special significance for the execution of voluntary movements. Destruction of this gyrus in one hemisphere, cause pareses in the opposite side of the body. Many of the fibers in the pyramidal tract come from the precentral gyrus, and, as mentioned, most of these fibers cross the midline on their way to the spinal cord. The **postcentral gyrus**, situated just posterior to the central sulcus, is the major receiving region for sensory impulses from the skin, the musculoskeletal system, and the viscera. This region is called the **somatosensory cortex (SI)**. The tracts that conduct impulses from the sense organs to the cortex are also crossed. Thus, destruction of the postcentral gyrus on one side leads to lowered sensibility (for example, of the skin) on the opposite side of the body. We have previously mentioned the **medial lemniscus**, which is part of the pathways from the sense organs to the postcentral gyrus. The fibers of the medial lemniscus terminate in a subdivision of the **lateral thalamic nucleus** (Fig. 6.24), and the neurons there send their axons to the postcentral gyrus.

The **visual cortex**—the main cortical region receiving information from the eyes—is located in the occipital lobe around a deep sulcus (fissure), the **calcarine sulcus** (sulcus calcarinus) (Fig. 6.26). The impulses start in the retina and are conducted in the optic nerve and the optic tract to the **lateral geniculate body** (Figs. 6.21 and 6.22), and from there to the visual cortex (see Fig. 16.14). The visual cortex can be distinguished from the surrounding parts of the cortex in sections perpendicular to the surface: it contains a thin whitish stripe running parallel to the surface (caused by a large number of myelinated fibers). Because of the stripe, this part of the cortex was named the **striate area** by the early anatomists (see Fig. 16.18).

The **auditory cortex**—the cortical region receiving impulses from the cochlea in the inner ear—is located in the superior temporal gyrus of the temporal lobe (Fig. 6.25; see also Fig. 17.11). The pathway for auditory impulses is synaptically interrupted in the **medial geniculate body** (Figs. 6.21 and 6.22).

The **olfactory cortex** is a small region on the medial aspect of the hemisphere near the tip of the temporal lobe. It is part of the so-called **uncus** (Fig. 6.26; see also Fig. 18.3) and extends somewhat onto the adjoining **parahippocampal gyrus**. The olfactory cortex receives fibers from the **olfactory bulb** (bulbus olfactorius) through the **olfactory tract** (tractus olfactorius) (Fig. 6.13). The cortex of the parahippocampal gyrus extends into the **hippocampal sulcus** (fissure), forming a longitudinal elevation, the **hippocampus** (Figs. 6.27 and 6.31; see also Fig. 32.2). The hippocampus belongs to the phylogenetically oldest parts of the cerebral cortex and has a simpler structure than the newer parts. The hippocampus and adjoining cortical regions in the medial part of the temporal lobe are of particular interest with regard to **learning** and **memory** (this is treated further in Chapter 32).

The Cerebral Cortex Consists of Six Cell Layers

Examination of a microscopic section cut perpendicular to the surface of the cerebral cortex shows that the neuronal cell bodies are not randomly distributed (see Figs. 34.1 and 34.2). They are arranged into **layers** or **laminae** parallel to the surface. Each layer is characterized by a certain shape, size, and packing density of the cell bodies (compare with the Rexed's laminae of the spinal cord). We number the layers from the surface inward to the white matter. **Layer 1** is cell poor and consists largely of dendrites from neurons with cell bodies in deeper layers and of axons with terminals making synapses on the dendrites. **Layers 2** and **4** are made up of predominantly small, rounded cells and are therefore called the **external** and **internal granular layer**, respectively. These two layers have in common that they largely have a receiving function: many of the afferent fibers to the cerebral cortex terminate and form synapses in layers 2 and 4. Fibers conveying sensory information from lower levels of the CNS end predominantly in layer 4, and consequently this layer is particularly well developed in the sensory cortical regions mentioned above. **Layers 3** and **5** contain cells that are larger than those in layers 2 and 4 are, and the cell bodies tend to be of pyramidal shape, hence the name **pyramidal cells**. Many of the pyramidal cells in layer 5 send their axons to the brain stem and spinal cord, where they influence motor neurons. Layer 5 is therefore especially well developed in the motor cortex in the precentral gyrus. The pyramidal neurons in layer 3 send their axons primarily to other parts of the cerebral cortex, either in the same hemisphere (association fibers) or to cortex in the hemisphere of the other side (commissural fibers). The cell bodies of **layer 6** are smaller and more spindle-shaped than those in layer 5 are. Many of the neurons send their axons to the thalamus, enabling the cerebral cortex to influence the impulse traffic from the thalamus to the cortex (feedback connections).

There are also numerous **interneurons** in the cerebral cortex, providing opportunity for cooperation between the various layers (interneurons with "vertically" oriented axons) and between neurons in different parts of one layer (interneurons with "horizontally" oriented axons). The layers are obviously not independent units.

The Cerebral Cortex Can Be Divided into Many Areas on a Cytoarchitectonic Basis

We mentioned that some layers are particularly well developed in certain regions of the cortex—for example, layer 4 in the sensory receiving areas and layer 5 in the motor cortex. There are many more differences when all layers all over the cortex are systematically compared. Such **cytoarchitectonic** differences (i.e., differences in size, shape, and packing density of the cell bodies) form the basis of a parcellation of the cerebral cortex of each hemisphere into approximately 50 **cortical areas** (areae). Maps of the cerebral cortex showing the positions of the various areas were published by several investigators around year 1900 and are still in use. The German anatomist Brodmann (see Fig. 20.3) published the most widely used map. Such cytoarchitectonically-defined areas have later been shown, in many cases, to differ also with regard to connections and functional properties. The numbering of the cortical areas may appear illogical. For example, the motor cortex in the precentral gyrus corresponds to area 4 of Brodmann. This borders posteriorly on area 3 but on area 6 anteriorly. Area 3 borders on area 1, which borders on area 2, and so on (see Fig. 34.3). It is not necessary to learn the position of more than a few of the cortical areas, however, and these will be dealt with in connection with the various functional systems in Parts II–VI of this volume.

The Basal Ganglia

The interior of the hemispheres contains large masses of gray substance. Largest among these are the so-called **basal ganglia**, which perform important tasks related to the control of movements.[5] Other nuclear groups (the amygdala, the septal nuclei, and the basal nucleus) are discussed in Chapter 31, and the basal ganglia are discussed in Chapter 23. Here we mention only a few main points with regard to the anatomy of the basal ganglia.

The basal ganglia receive massive afferent connections from the cerebral cortex and acts, by way of their efferent fibers, primarily back on motor regions of the cortex. Sections through the hemispheres show that the basal ganglia consist of two main parts (Figs. 6.29 and 6.30). In a horizontal section (Fig. 6.30) one large part lies lateral to the internal capsule, and a smaller part lies medial to the internal capsule and anterior to the thalamus. The largest part is called the **lentiform nucleus** (nucleus lentiformis) because of its shape. It consists of two closely apposed parts: the lateral or external part is the **putamen**, and the medial or internal part is the **globus pallidus**. The part of the basal ganglia situated medial to the internal capsule is the **caudate nucleus** (nucleus caudatus). The name describes its form: a large part of the nucleus forms a long, curved "tail" (Fig. 7.4, see also Fig. 23.1). The putamen and the caudate

5 The name basal ganglia has been retained from a time when all collections of neurons were called ganglia, regardless of whether they were located inside or outside the CNS. Today we use the term ganglion only for collections of neurons outside the CNS, as discussed in Chapter 1. However, the name basal ganglia is so well established that is not practical to exchange it.

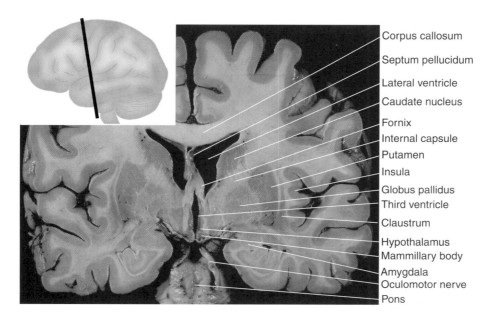

Corpus callosum
Septum pellucidum
Lateral ventricle
Caudate nucleus
Fornix
Internal capsule
Putamen
Insula
Globus pallidus
Third ventricle
Claustrum
Hypothalamus
Mammillary body
Amygdala
Oculomotor nerve
Pons

FIGURE 6.29 *The cerebral hemispheres.* Frontal section, placed more frontally than as shown in Fig. 3.27, showing the basal ganglia and amygdala.

nucleus together are called the **striatum** (or neostriatum). The caudate nucleus consists of an anterior bulky part, the **caput** (head), and a progressively thinner **cauda** (tail). The cauda extends first backward and then down and forward into the temporal lobe, located in the wall of the lateral ventricle. Figure 7.4 shows how

this peculiar form can be explained on the basis of the embryonic development of the cerebral hemispheres.

The **claustrum** forms a sheet of grey matter lateral to the putamen (Fig. 6.29). It has reciprocal connections most parts of the cerebral cortex. Little is known about its function or clinical significance, but based on its

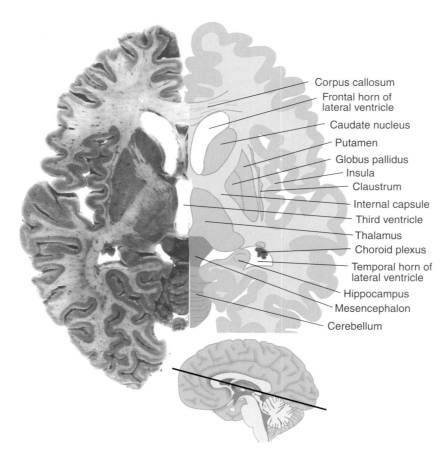

Corpus callosum
Frontal horn of lateral ventricle
Caudate nucleus
Putamen
Globus pallidus
Insula
Claustrum
Internal capsule
Third ventricle
Thalamus
Choroid plexus
Temporal horn of lateral ventricle
Hippocampus
Mesencephalon
Cerebellum

FIGURE 6.30 *The internal structure of the cerebral hemisphere.* The left half is a photograph of a horizontal section through the left hemisphere. Compare with Fig. 6.28.

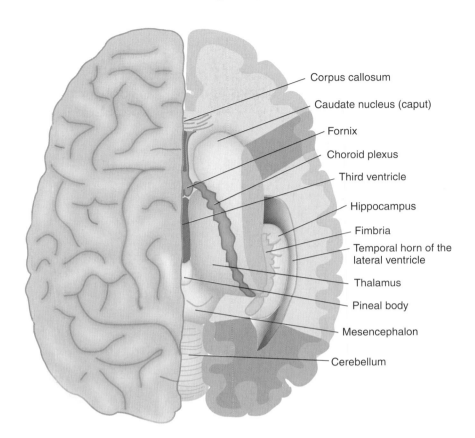

Corpus callosum

Caudate nucleus (caput)

Fornix

Choroid plexus

Third ventricle

Hippocampus

Fimbria

Temporal horn of the lateral ventricle

Thalamus

Pineal body

Mesencephalon

Cerebellum

FIGURE 6.31 *The internal structure of the cerebral hemispheres.* The upper parts of the right hemisphere has been cut away to open the lateral ventricles. In the anterior part, the caudate nucleus forms the bottom and lateral wall of the ventricle. In the temporal horn of the ventricle, the hippocampus forms the medial wall.

connections it has been suggested to deal with sensory integration. One hypothesis proposes that by virtue of its integrative potential, claustrum may be linked with the formation of conscious percepts.

THE CEREBELLUM

The cerebellum (the "little brain") is first and foremost of importance for the execution of movements; like the basal ganglia, it belongs to the motor system. The cerebellum is located in the posterior cranial fossa, dorsal to the brain stem (Figs. 6.2 and 6.32). It is connected with the brain stem anteriorly by way of three stalks of white matter on each side: the inferior, middle, and superior cerebellar peduncles (Figs. 6.14 and 3.19). In general, the **inferior cerebellar peduncle**, or **restiform body** (corpus restiforme), contains fibers that carry impulses from the spinal cord to the cerebellum, whereas the **middle cerebellar peduncle**, or the **brachium pontis**, conveys information from the cerebral cortex. The **superior cerebellar peduncle**, or the **brachium conjunctivum**, contains most of the fibers conveying impulses out of the cerebellum—that is, the cerebellar efferent fibers.

Like the cerebrum, the cerebellum is covered by a layer of gray substance, the **cerebellar cortex** (cortex cerebelli), with underlying white matter. Enclosed in the white matter are regions of gray matter, the **central (deep) cerebellar nuclei** (see Fig. 24.14). From the neurons in these nuclei come the majority of efferent fibers that convey information from the cerebellum to other parts of the CNS (the cerebral cortex, various brain stem nuclei, and the spinal cord).

The cerebellar surface is extensively folded, forming numerous narrow sheets, or **folia**, that are predominantly oriented transversely (Fig. 6.32). The fissures and sulci between the folia are partly very deep; the deepest among them divide the cerebellum into **lobes** (Fig. 6.32A; see also Fig. 24.2). In addition, the cerebellum can be subdivided macroscopically on another basis. In the posterior part of the cerebellum a narrow middle region is situated deeper than the much larger lateral parts (Fig. 6.32B). This middle part of the cerebellum is called the **vermis** (worm) and is present also in the anterior part of the cerebellum, although not as clearly distinguished from the lateral parts as posteriorly. The lateral parts are called the **cerebellar hemispheres**. A small bulbous part on each is connected medially with a thin stalk to the vermis. This part is

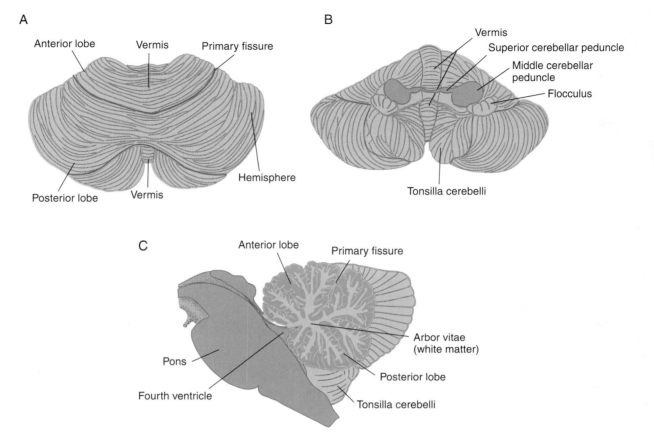

FIGURE 6.32 *The cerebellum.* A: Seen from the rostroposterior aspect. B: Seen from the ventral aspect (the side facing the brain stem). C: Midsagittal section showing the cerebellar cortex as a thin layer with white matter underneath (white matter indicated in black in the drawing).

called the **flocculus** (Fig. 6.31B) and lies close to the middle cerebellar peduncle, just posterior to the seventh and eighth cranial nerves (Fig 6.13). A midsagittal section through the cerebellum (Fig. 6.32C) shows clearly the deep sulci and fissures. The white substance forms a treelike structure called the **arbor vitae** (the tree of life, which is not very fitting since the cerebellum is not necessary for life). The fourth ventricle, extending into the cerebellum like the apex of a tent, is also evident in the midsagittal section.

7 | The Coverings of the Brain and the Ventricular System

OVERVIEW

The central nervous system (CNS) is well protected against external forces as it lies inside the skull and the vertebral canal. In addition to this bony protection, the CNS is wrapped in three membranes of connective tissue—the **meninges**—with fluid-filled spaces between the membranes. In fact, it is loosely suspended in a fluid-filled container. The innermost membrane—**pia**—is thin and adheres to the surface of the brain at all places. The outermost membrane—**dura**—is thick and fibrous and covers the inside of the skull and spinal canal. The **arachnoid** is a thin membrane attached to the inside of the dura. The **subarachnoid space** is with **cerebrospinal fluid** (CSF) and lies between the pia and the arachnoid.

The **ventricular system** consists of irregularly shaped, fluid-filled cavities inside the CNS. There are four dilatations or ventricles. The two lateral ventricles are largest and are located in the cerebral hemispheres. They communicate with the third ventricle lying between the two thalami. The third ventricle, situated between the cerebellum and the brain stem, communicates with the fourth ventricle via the narrow **cerebral aqueduct.** Vascular **choroid plexuses** in the ventricles produce about 0.5 liters of CSF per day. The CSF leaves the ventricular system through openings in the fourth ventricle and enters the subarachnoid space. Drainage of CSF occurs through small evaginations—**arachnoid villi**—of the arachnoid emptying into venous sinuses and along cranial and spinal nerve roots and then into extracranial lymphatic vessels. The CSF has a protective function, it minimizes accumulation of harmful substances in the nervous tissue, and it probably serves as a signal pathway.

THE MENINGES

The Pia Mater, the Arachnoid, and the Subarachnoid Space

The innermost one is the vascular **pia mater** (usually just called pia). It follows the surface of the brain and spinal cord closely and extends into all sulci and depressions of the surface (Figs. 7.1 and 7.2). Thin vessels pass from the pia into the substance of the brain and supply the external parts, such as the cerebral cortex, with blood (the deeper parts of the brain are supplied by vessels entering the brain at its basal surface). The next membrane, the **arachnoid**, does not follow the uneven surface of the brain but extends across depressions, fissures, and sulci. Between the pia and the arachnoid exists a narrow space, the **subarachnoid space**, which is filled with CSF (Figs. 6.1, 7.1, and 7.5). Numerous thin threads of connective tissue connect the pia with the arachnoid, thus spanning the subarachnoid space. The depth of the subarachnoid space varies from place to place because the arachnoid, as mentioned, does not follow the surface of the brain. Where it crosses larger depressions, the subarachnoid space is considerably widened, forming so-called **cisterns** filled with CSF. Several cisterns are found around the brain stem, but the largest one, the **cisterna magna**, or **cerebellomedullary cistern**, is located posterior to the medulla below the cerebellum (Figs. 6.1 and 7.5). The CSF enters the cisterna magna from the fourth ventricle (Fig. 7.5).

The subarachnoid space is continuous around the whole CNS. Substances released into the subarachnoid space at one place therefore quickly spread out. A **subarachnoid hemorrhage**, for example, most often caused by rupture of a vessel at the base of the brain, quickly leads to mixing of the CSF with blood. Thus, a sample of CSF taken from the dural sac at lumbar levels will be bloody.

The Dura Mater

The outermost membrane, the **dura mater** (usually just called the dura), is thick and strong because it consists of dense connective tissue (Figs. 7.1, 7.2, and 7.5). The dura covers closely the inside of the skull, and its outermost layers constitute the periosteum. The arachnoid follows the inside of the dura closely so that there is only a very narrow space between these two meninges, the **subdural space** (Figs. 7.1 and 7.2). The dura extends down into the vertebral canal to enclose the spinal cord. It extends further down than the cord, however, forming a sac around the roots of the lower spinal nerves (the cauda equina). This **dural sac** extends down to the

A

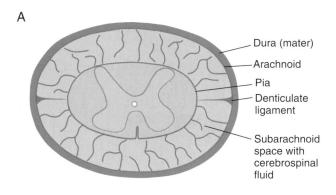

- Dura (mater)
- Arachnoid
- Pia
- Denticulate ligament
- Subarachnoid space with cerebrospinal fluid

B

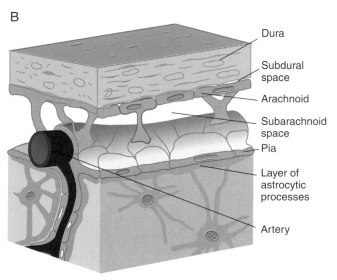

- Dura
- Subdural space
- Arachnoid
- Subarachnoid space
- Pia
- Layer of astrocytic processes
- Artery

FIGURE 7.1 *The meninges and the subarachnoidal space of the spinal cord.*

level of the second-third sacral vertebra (Fig. 6.3). Thus below the level of the first and second lumbar vertebrae (the lower end of the cord), the dural sac contains only spinal nerve roots and CSF (Fig. 6.3). This is a safe place to perform a **lumbar puncture**—that is, enter the subarachnoid space with a needle to take samples of the CSF, as there is no danger of harming the cord.

Anchoring of the Brain and Spinal Cord

In a few places, the dura forms strong infoldings, serving to restrict the movements of the brain within the skull. Large movements can stretch and damage vessels and nerves connecting the brain with the skull (one of the possible effects of head injuries). From the midline, the **falx cerebri** extends down between the two hemispheres (Figs. 7.2 and 8.7). Posteriorly, the falx divides into two parts that extend laterally over the superior face of the cerebellum and attach to the temporal pyramid. These two folds meet in the midline and form the **cerebellar tentorium** (see Fig. 8.9). In the anterior part of the tentorium, there is an elongated opening for the brain stem. If the pressure in the skull above the tentorium increases (due to bleeding, a tumor, or brain edema), part of the temporal lobe may be pressed down or **herniate** between the tentorium and the brain stem, harming the brain stem temporarily or permanently.

The **spinal cord** is anchored to the meninges partly by the spinal nerves and partly by two thin bands, the **denticulate ligaments** (Fig. 7.1A), extending laterally from the cord to the arachnoid and dura (this is not a continuous ligament but one that forms 21 lateral extensions from the cord to the dura). The spinal cord nevertheless moves considerably up and down in the dural sac with movements of the vertebral column (the length of the vertebral canal varies by almost 10 cm from maximal flexion, when it is longest, to maximal extension).

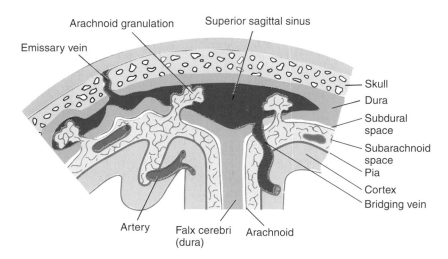

- Emissary vein
- Arachnoid granulation
- Superior sagittal sinus
- Skull
- Dura
- Subdural space
- Subarachnoid space
- Pia
- Cortex
- Bridging vein
- Artery
- Falx cerebri (dura)
- Arachnoid

FIGURE 7.2 *The meninges, the subarachnoidal space, and the superior sagittal sinus.* Schematic of a frontal section through the head, with the skull and the brain. See also Figs. 1.27 and 3.37.

The Meninges and Stiffness of the Neck

Infection of the meninges, **meningitis,** typically produces stiffness of the neck. Every attempt to bend the neck or the back forward evokes an immediate reflexive muscular resistance. When the doctor tries to lift the patient's head off the pillow, the neck is kept straight. The infection causes inflammation of the meninges, which also extends onto the vessels and the nerve roots in the subarachnoid space. Forward bending (flexion) of the vertebral column elongates the spinal canal, as mentioned, and that stretches the meninges, the vessels, and the nerve roots. Most likely, this accounts for the intense pain associated with any effort to flex the back or neck (similar to the pain felt by stretching an inflamed area of the skin or a joint capsule). Straining or coughing also causes pain in patients with meningitis. However, other means than infections by bacteria and viruses can produce such **irritation of the meninges.** For example, one strong irritant is blood in the subarachnoid space. Thus, stiffness of the neck is by itself only a sign of meningeal irritation and does not indicate a specific cause.

Meningeal irritation usually causes a strong **headache.** This occurs most dramatically with **subarachnoid hemorrhage,** in which an intense headache starts abruptly the moment the bleeding starts and blood flows into the subarachnoid space. In such instances, the cause is usually spontaneous rupture of an **aneurysm** (a sac-like dilatation) on one of the arteries at the base of the skull.

THE CEREBRAL VENTRICLES AND THE CEREBROSPINAL FLUID

We have mentioned the ventricular system several times in connection with treatment of the various parts of the brain. Here we consider the ventricular system as a whole, along with the CSF.

The Location and Form of the Ventricles

The thin central canal of the cord continues upward into the brain stem. There the canal widens to form the **fourth ventricle** at the posterior aspect of the medulla and pons (Figs. 6.1, 7.3, and 7.5). The ventricle has a tentlike form with the apex projecting into the cerebellum and two **lateral recesses** (recessus lateralis). The diamond-shaped **rhomboid fossa** at the dorsal aspect of the brain stem (Fig. 6.19) forms the "floor" of the fourth ventricle, while the cerebellar peduncles form the lateral walls.

The **third ventricle** is a thin slitlike room between the two thalami (see Figs. 6.27, 6.30, 6.31, 7.3, and 7.5). During embryonic development, the primordia of the hemispheres become closely apposed to the diencephalon (see Fig. 9.13). The loose masses of connective tissue between the hemispheres form an approximately horizontal plate that constitutes the roof of the third ventricle. The choroid plexus is attached to the inside of the roof (see Figs. 6.23 and 7.5).

The two **lateral ventricles** represent the first and second ventricles, but these terms are not used. From a central part in the parietal lobe, the lateral ventricles have processes called horns into the three other lobes: an **anterior (frontal) horn,** a **posterior (occipital) horn,** and an **inferior (temporal) horn** extending downward and anteriorly into the temporal lobe (Fig. 7.3; see also Figs. 6.29 and 6.31). The anterior horn is the largest and is bordered medially by the **septum pellucidum,**[1] whereas the head of the caudate nucleus bulges into it from the lateral side (Figs. 6.29 and 7.5). The central part of the ventricle lies just above the thalamus (Fig. 6.31). The inferior horn starts at the transition between the central part and the posterior horn and follows the temporal lobe almost to its tip (Fig. 7.3). Medially in the inferior horn there is an elongated elevation, the hippocampus (Figs. 6.27 and 6.31), formed by invagination of the ventricular wall from the medial side by the **hippocampal fissure.**

The **curved form** of the lateral ventricles can be understood on the basis of the embryonic development of the cerebrum (Fig. 7.4). Both the lateral ventricles and the nervous tissue in its walls (such as the caudate nucleus and the hippocampus) eventually obtain a curved shape.

The Cerebrospinal Fluid Is Produced by Vascular Plexuses in the Ventricles

All of the ventricles are filled with a clear, watery fluid, the **CSF.** Most of the fluid is produced by vascular tufts, the **choroid plexus.**[2] This is present in all four ventricles (Fig. 7.5), but the largest amount of choroid plexus is in the lateral ventricles (Fig. 6.31). The plexuses arise in early embryonic life by invaginations of the innermost membrane (the pia mater) at sites where the wall of the neural tube is very thin (Fig. 7.6). An elaborate structure of thin, branching protrusions, or **villi,** arises here (Fig. 7.7). The choroid plexuses attach to the wall of the ventricles with a thin stalk (**tela choroidea**). The surface of the villi is covered by **simple cuboid**

1 There is a thin slit between the septum pellucidum of the two sides that has nothing to do with the ventricles. In embryonic development, the slit is continuous with the room between the two hemispheres but is later closed when the corpus callosum grows across the two hemispheres. Downward, the fornices close the slit (Fig. 6.29).

2 Early observations in experimental animals suggested that the choroid plexus is not solely responsible for CSF production. Thus, removal of the choroid plexus did not prevent development of hydrocephalus after blocking the CSF drainage. It is now assumed that in humans 10% to 30% of the CSF is produced by brain interstitial fluid passing through the ependyma.

The CSF has an important **protective function** because the brain almost floats in it. Thus, theoretically **buoyancy** reduces the weight of the brain to about 50 g, which means less traction on vessels and nerves connected to the CNS. Further, the effect on the brain of blows to the head is dampened because water has to be pressed aside before the brain hits its hard surroundings (the skull).

Another possible functional role of the CSF can be deduced from the fact, mentioned above, that water and solutes pass freely between it and the extracellular fluid (interstitium) of the nervous tissue. This means that diffusion into the CSF may minimize **accumulation of harmful substances** in the nervous tissue (such as potassium ions during prolonged periods of intense neuronal activity). This would be of significance, however, only for neurons that are fairly close to the ventricles, as the diffusion of molecules in the labyrinth-like brain interstitium is slow (much slower than in free water). Thus, after injecting representative substances in the brain, the concentration is reduced by 90% some 1 to 3 mm away from the injection site.

Regardless of the normal functions of substances in the CSF, examination of the CSF composition gives valuable information of the extracellular fluid of the brain. This fluid compartment is difficult to examine directly, but because the ependyma is freely permeable, one can safely assume that the composition of the CSF matches fairly well the environment of the neurons.

Cerebrospinal Fluid as a Signal Pathway

The concentration of the hormone **melatonin** (which influences sexual functions and circadian rhythms by binding to receptors in the hypothalamus) is twice as high in the third ventricle as in the lateral ventricles and 100 times higher than in cerebral arteries. This suggests that melatonin is secreted into the CSF and uses this as its main transport medium, whereas the bloodstream is of minor importance.

Some studies indicate that substances in the CSF might be of importance for **sleep**. Thus, by transferring CSF from a sleep-deprived animal, the recipient becomes sleepy. The responsible substance has not been identified but **interleukin 1β** (IL-1β) is a likely candidate. Thus, its concentration in the CSF increases by sleep deprivation and has also been shown to induce sleep. The further signal pathway of IL-1β from CSF to relevant neurons is not known, but it finally influences the neurons in the reticular formation that are responsible for regulation of sleep and wakefulness.

Several **growth factors** are synthesized and secreted by the choroid plexus. While the choroid plexus epithelium expresses receptors for such growth factors—suggesting an autocrine function—they may also be expected to act on nervous tissue close to the ventricles.

Circulation and Drainage of the Cerebrospinal Fluid

About **one-half liter** of CSF is produced each day, yet the total volume of fluid in the ventricles and the subarachnoid space is only 130 to 140 mL (approximately 20 mL is in the ventricles).[3] In addition, approximately 75 mL surrounds the spinal cord. Thus, the total amount is renewed several times a day. This means that effective means of drainage must exist.

The fluid produced in the lateral ventricles flows into the third ventricle through the **interventricular foramen** (of **Monro**) (Fig. 7.5; see Fig. 6.23). From there the fluid flows through the narrow **cerebral aqueduct** to the fourth ventricle. The choroid plexuses in the third and fourth ventricles add more fluid. The fluid leaves the ventricular system and enters the subarachnoid space (more specifically, the cisterna magna) through three openings in the fourth ventricle: one in the midline posteriorly (the **foramen of Magendie**) and two laterally (the lateral recesses or **foramina of Luschka**) (Fig. 7.5). The fluid then spreads out over the entire surface of the brain and spinal cord. From the base of the brain, there is an upward stream along the lateral aspects of the hemispheres toward the midline (Fig. 7.5). The flow velocity is uneven, however, as shown by following the spread of injected substances. After injection into the lateral ventricles labeled substances are detectable after a few minutes in the subarachnoid space, but then moves very slowly over the cerebral hemispheres (several hours) and down to the lumbar cistern (one hour).

The routes of CSF **drainage** are not completely known, although emptying into venous sinuses by way of **arachnoid villi** is usually assumed to constitute the main route. The arachnoid villi are small evaginations of the arachnoid. Several villi together form macroscopically visible protrusions called **arachnoid granulations**, which are particularly prominent along the superior sagittal sinus (Figs. 7.2 and 7.5). Passage of fluid from the subarachnoid space to the venous sinuses is presumably caused by a difference in hydrostatic pressure, the pressure being higher in the subarachnoid space (about 15 cm of H_2O) than in the sinuses (7–8 cm of H_2O). Nevertheless, we do not actually know how much of the CSF that is drained in this way.[4]

3 The total volume of the ventricles has been determined mainly by use of plastic casts in fixed brains. The average total volume is probably some less than 20 cm^3. The individual variations are surprisingly large, however (the normal range is probably from 7 to 30 cm^3). Most studies have examined only the lateral ventricles, finding an average volume of about 7 cm^3 for each. The volumes of the third and fourth ventricles appear to be some less than 1 cm^3 for each. Even though the ventricular size increases somewhat with age, this can explain only a small fraction of the individual variations. In the same individual, however, the two lateral ventricles are quite similar in volume.

4 One reason for questioning the role of the arachnoid granulations in CSF drainage is that they are not present prenatally while the choroid plexuses are well developed by the end of the embryonic period (about 8 weeks after fertilization). Therefore, in the fetus and newborn other routes seem to be responsible for most or all of the CSF drainage.

Another, and perhaps quantitatively more important route of drainage, is along cranial and spinal **nerve roots** and then into **extracranial lymphatic vessels** (the nervous tissue contains no lymphatics). Animal experiments indicate that drainage through the **cribriform plate** (where the olfactory nerve fibers enter the skull, see Fig. 8.10) may be of particular significance.

Brain Edema, Herniation, and Hydrocephalus

Because the CNS and the CSF are located in a closed container with rigid walls, the pressure inside the container increases if, for some reason, the amount of substance inside it increases. The intracranial pressure is the same for the nervous tissue and the CSF, but it can be measured most conveniently in the latter. For each heartbeat, for example, the pressure inside the cerebral ventricles increases slightly because more blood is pumped into the brain. Correspondingly, the pressure increases on coughing and straining because the drainage of venous blood from the cranial cavity and the vertebral canal is reduced.

Regardless of cause, any **intracranial expansive process** leads to increased intracranial pressure. When the pressure increases, the blood pressure increases to maintain cerebral blood flow. Thus, abnormally elevated blood pressure, usually combined with slowing of the heart rate, is one of the signs of severely increased intracranial pressure. However, an increase above a certain level reduces blood flow and the functioning of the brain suffers (with signs of confusion and eventually loss of consciousness). This occurs, for example, in patients with **brain edema**. This is a dangerous complication of acute brain damage caused by, for example, head injuries. The edema is caused by extravasation of fluid from the brain capillaries. Similarly, an **intracranial hemorrhage**, which may arise from vessels inside or outside the brain substance, can also cause a dangerous increase of the intracranial pressure. If the expansion process is located in the posterior fossa (below the cerebellar tentorium; see Fig. 8.9), the **cerebellar tonsils** (see Figs. 6.13 and 6.32C) may be dislocated downward into the foramen magnum and thus compress the medulla (tonsillar herniation). If the expansive process is located above the tentorium (in the middle or anterior fossa), the **uncus** of the temporal lobe (see Fig. 6.26) can be dislocated downward beneath the edge of the tentorium and compress the brain stem at the level of the mesencephalon (see Figs. 6.29 and 8.9). Both forms of **herniation** may lead to serious brain damage or death.

A condition with increased amount of CSF and dilatation of the ventricles is called **hydrocephalus**. It is usually assumed that the condition arises because of increased intraventricular pressure due to obstruction of the drainage of the CSF—for example, by closure of the aqueduct (inflammation, tumor, bleeding) or the outlets from the fourth ventricles. Even if this may be the cause in some, it cannot explain all cases of hydrocephalus. Thus, some persons develop hydrocephalus in spite of apparently normal intraventricular pressure and no sign of obstruction (communicating or normal pressure hydrocephalus).

If obstruction of CSF flow from the ventricles occurs in an adult, in whom the sutures of the skull have grown firmly together, the intracranial pressure increases markedly, with dramatic symptoms. If the condition arises in early childhood before closure of the sutures, however, the size of the head grows abnormally, with the skull yielding to the increased intracranial pressure. This may continue for some time with surprisingly few signs of cerebral dysfunction, but the development of the brain will eventually suffer, with results such as mental retardation. Hydrocephalus in children may be treated by shunting the CSF directly into a big vein outside the skull.

Examination of the Cerebrospinal Fluid and the Ventricles

Examination of the CSF can provide valuable information about neurological diseases. A sample of the fluid is usually withdrawn with a thin needle from the subarachnoid space in the dural sac—that is, below the level of the second lumbar vertebra (lumbar cistern). This way there is no risk of damaging the spinal cord (see Fig. 6.3). When the tip of the needle is in the subarachnoid space, the intracranial pressure can also be measured. Examination of the fluid, in part under the microscope, can give information about possible bleeding into the subarachnoid space and about infections and inflammations of the brain itself (**encephalitis**) or the meninges (**meningitis**). In the latter case, there are numerous leukocytes in the CSF. The concentration of proteins, normally very low, may increase in certain diseases (e.g., in **multiple sclerosis**, in which the proteins are antibodies against components of the nervous tissue).

The **shape** and **size** of the ventricles can be determined noninvasively in living subjects by use of computer tomography (CT) and magnetic resonance imaging (MRI) (see Figs. 6.2, 6.28, 23.4, and 32.11). Atrophy of the nervous tissue of the brain—for example, atrophy of the cerebral cortex, which occurs in dementia—leads to dilatation of the ventricles, whereas expansive, space-occupying processes like hemorrhages and tumors may distort and compress the ventricles.

8 | The Blood Supply of the CNS

Of all cell types in the body, neurons are the most sensitive to interruption of their supply of oxygen (anoxia). Only a few minutes' stop in the blood flow may cause neuronal death. The oxygen consumption of the brain is high even at rest. Therefore, the blood supply of the central nervous system (CNS) is ample, and the brain receives about 15% of the cardiac output at rest. Regulatory mechanisms ensure that the brain gets what it needs—if necessary, at the expense of all other organs. The arteries of the brain lie within the cranial cavity and are mostly devoid of anastomoses (connections) with arteries outside the skull. Therefore, other arteries cannot take over if the intracranial ones are narrowed or occluded.

The cerebral blood flow is largely controlled by the local conditions in the nervous tissue, that is, there is a high degree of **autoregulation**. Local changes in the concentrations of ions, oxygen, carbon dioxide, and various signal substances determine the resistance offered by the arterioles. Brain vessels receive sensory innervation from the trigeminal nerve.

In most organs, small-molecule substances pass the capillary wall, and their concentration is therefore similar in the blood plasma and in the interstitial fluid. In contrast, the CNS exerts strict control of what is let in. The **blood–brain barrier** (a similar barrier exists between the blood and the cerebrospinal fluid [CSF]) is due mainly to special, selective properties of the brain capillaries.

In a few small regions adjoining the ventricles, the capillaries are fenestrated and hence let substances from the blood pass through easily. At such places, neurons are exposed to substances of the blood that do not enter other parts of the brain. These regions are called **the circumventricular organs**.

Broadly speaking, the **internal carotid artery** supplies most of the cerebral hemispheres, whereas the **vertebral artery** supplies the brain stem and the cerebellum. **Communicating arteries** at the base of the skull establish anastomoses between the posterior (vertebral) and the anterior (internal carotid) cerebral circulations.

CEREBRAL MICROCIRCULATION AND THE BLOOD–BRAIN BARRIER

The brain has a very high density of capillaries, and neurons are seldom more than 10 µm from the nearest capillary. The total length of all capillaries in the brain are said to be 400 miles, and their total surface area more than 20 m². To understand the normal properties and the responses to disease of brain capillaries, however, they cannot be studied in isolation. The term **neurovascular unit** serves to emphasize the close structural and functional relationship between neurons, glial cells, associated capillary-endothelial cells, basal lamina, and pericytes (Fig. 8.1).

Regulation of Cerebral Circulation

Regulation of the blood flow is one among several factors governing the composition of the brain's extracellular milieu—that is, the concentration of ions, neuroactive substances, nutrients, and water (osmolarity). Control of the properties of astrocytes and the blood–brain barrier are other important factors (see Chapter 2, under "Astroglia and the Control of Neuronal Homeostasis").

The cerebral circulation exhibits a high degree of **autoregulation**—that is, conditions in the brain itself determine the blood flow. If the blood pressure falls, the arteries dilate. This reduces vascular resistance so that the blood flow is upheld. If the blood pressure rises, the opposite happens: the arteries constrict. This is an important control mechanism, since increased capillary hydrostatic pressure may cause brain edema. The brain maintains almost constant blood flow as long as the systolic pressure is between 60 and 160 mm Hg. If the pressure falls below 60 mm, however, the flow falls steeply and the person becomes unconscious.

Among the many factors that control cerebral blood flow, local changes in the immediate surroundings of the neurons have an important role. These are changes in concentrations of ions (among them H^+ ions), CO_2 and O_2. **Hypoxia** (abnormally low concentration of O_2) and **hypercapnia** (above-normal concentration of CO_2) both cause marked vasodilatation and increased cerebral blood flow. Increased local blood flow is closely coupled to increased neuronal activity, and this phenomenon is utilized in studies of correlations between changes in brain activity and behavior (see "Regional Cerebral Blood Flow and Neuronal Activity").

Autonomic circulatory control seems to play a minor part in the brain (in contrast to in most other organs), even though **sympathetic fibers** innervate brain vessels. Such fibers release norepinephrine, neuropeptide Y (NPY) and possibly ATP, and stimulation causes vasoconstriction.

A

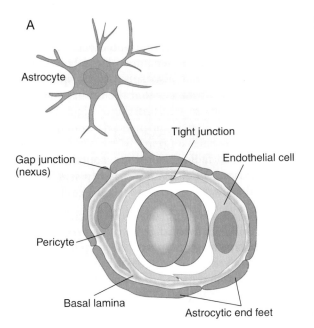

B

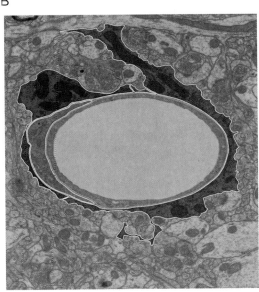

FIGURE 8.1 *The blood–brain barrier/neurovascular unit.* **A:** Schematic drawing showing the main features. Important elements are tight junctions between the endothelial cells and a continuous layer of astrocytic end feet. Gap junctions establish low-resistance connections between the astrocytes. The basal lamina also contributes to the barrier properties of the neurovascular unit. Not shown in the figure, although included in the term neurovascular unit, are neurons that are in contact with processes of the astrocyte (see Figs. 2.3 and 2.5). **B:** Electron micrograph showing a brain capillary (hippocampus) and its relationship to processes of three astrocytes (the processes are marked with different colors). The electron micrograph is one among many in a true series of ultrathin sections, used for three-dimensional reconstruction of the astrocytic processes. This makes it possible to decide that the marked processes belong to different astrocytes. (Courtesy of Drs. Thomas Misje Mathiisen and Ole Petter Ottersen, Department of Anatomy, Institute of Basic Medical Sciences, University of Oslo, Norway.)

Nevertheless, under normal conditions, activity of sympathetic fibers appears to have only marginal effects on blood flow. Thus, although sympathetic activity can constrict large brain arteries, peripheral small vessels dilate (probably because of local control). Brain arteries are also supplied by **serotonergic fibers** that arise in the raphe nuclei of the brain stem and that, on stimulation, mainly cause vasoconstriction.

Finally, brain arteries receive **sensory innervation** from the **trigeminal nerve**. These fibers contain substance P, calcitonin gene–related peptide (CGRP), and neurokinin. Electric stimulation of such sensory fibers causes vasodilatation, presumably by peripheral release of neuropeptides. The trigeminal arterial innervation, along with the vascular serotonin receptors, is an important factor in the pain of **migraine** attacks. Thus, the most effective drugs to prevent the pain of migraine are serotonin-receptor agonists. The drugs are thought to act, at least in part, by preventing release of neuropeptides from trigeminal vascular nerve endings, thereby reducing perivascular inflammation.

Regional Cerebral Blood Flow and Neuronal Activity

Neuroimaging techniques, such as positron emission tomography (PET) and functional magnetic resonance imaging (fMRI), permit the visualization of brain regions activated in conjunction with specific behaviors and mental operations (see Chapter 11, under "Methods to Study Neuronal Activity and Connectivity in the Living Brain: PET and fMRI"). This is especially valuable for the study of speech, abstract problem solving, and other functions that can be studied only in humans. PET and fMRI are based on the existence of a relationship between the **regional cerebral blood flow** (rCBF) and the neuronal activity in that region. Thus, increased

merely responses to the disease processes (which may nevertheless contribute to the disease manifestations).

Some Parts of the Brain Lack a Blood–Brain Barrier

In a few small regions adjoining the ventricles, the capillaries are fenestrated and hence let substances from the blood pass through easily. At such places, neurons are exposed to substances of the blood that do not enter other parts of the brain. These regions are called **the circumventricular organs** (Fig. 8.2). Among these, the **area postrema** is found in the lower end of the fourth ventricle, whereas the **subfornical organ** lies in the roof of the third ventricle just underneath the fornix close to the interventricular foramen. Both the area postrema and the subfornical organ contain many neurons that send their axons to other parts of the CNS and can thus mediate various specific influences on the nervous system. Neurons in the area postrema are involved in the **vomiting reflex** when this is elicited by toxic substances of the blood (see also Chapter 27, under "The Vomiting Reflex"). Neurons in the subfornical organ monitor the **salt concentration** of the blood. They send signals to the hypothalamus that can initiate responses necessary to maintain the fluid balance of the body. Further, neurons in the subfornical organ respond to circulating peptides involved in regulating **energy balance** (see Chapter 30, under "Regulation of Digestion and Feeding").The subfornical organ and other parts of the circumventricular organs are probably also targets of substances in the blood that induce **fever** and other symptoms of infections (see Chapter 30, "Hypothalamic Neurons Are Influenced by Hormones and Fever").

The **median eminence** (eminentia mediana) in the hypothalamus (see Fig. 30.6C) also lacks a blood–brain barrier. This region does not contain neuronal cell bodies but receives nerve fibers from other parts of the hypothalamus. Hormones released from nerve terminals in the median eminence are transported by the bloodstream to the anterior pituitary (see Chapter 30, under "The Influence of the Hypothalamus on the Anterior Pituitary").

The two endocrine glands that are from the brain, the **posterior pituitary** and the **pineal body**, also lack a blood–brain barrier. As with the median eminence, this is related to their release of hormones directly into the bloodstream.

ARTERIAL SYSTEM

The Brain Receives Arterial Blood from the Internal Carotid and the Vertebral Arteries

Broadly speaking, the internal carotid artery supplies most of the cerebral hemispheres, whereas the vertebral artery supplies the brain stem and the cerebellum.

The **internal carotid artery** (arteria carotis interna) enters the cranial cavity through a canal at the base of the skull (the carotid canal in the temporal bone) and then divides into three branches (Fig. 8.3):

1. The **ophthalmic artery** passes to the orbit through the optic canal and thus does not supply the brain itself (although, strictly speaking, the retina is part of the CNS). The **central retinal artery** (a. centralis retinae) enters the eye through the optic nerve and supplies the retina.

2. The **anterior cerebral artery** runs forward over the optic nerve and along the medial aspect of the hemisphere (Figs. 8.3 and 8.5). It supplies most of the cortex on the medial aspect of the hemisphere (except the most posterior parts and the inferior aspect of the temporal lobe). Its branches reach only a short distance onto the convexity of the hemispheres, supplying the leg representations of the motor and somatosensory areas. Shortly after its origin, the anterior cerebral artery gives off thin branches that penetrate the base of the hemisphere to supply anterior portions of the basal ganglia and hypothalamus.

3. The **middle cerebral artery** is the largest branch. It curves laterally into the lateral cerebral fissure and follows this backward and upward (Figs. 8.3, 8.4, and 8.5). On its way, numerous branches are given off that supply most of the cerebral cortex on the convexity of the hemispheres, notably the motor and somatosensory cortical areas, except for their most medial parts (with neuronal groups concerned with the motor and sensory functions of the legs; see Figs. 22.5 and 22.9), which are supplied by the anterior cerebral artery. The deep parts of the cerebrum, such as most of the basal ganglia and the internal capsule, receive their own branches from the middle cerebral artery, **lenticulostriate arteries** (Fig. 8.4), and by a separate branch of the internal carotid artery, the **anterior choroid artery** (Fig. 8.3).

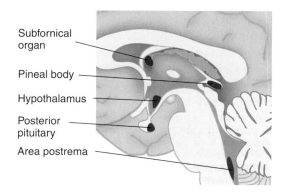

Subfornical organ

Pineal body

Hypothalamus

Posterior pituitary

Area postrema

FIGURE 8.2 *Regions of the brain devoid of blood–brain barrier.*

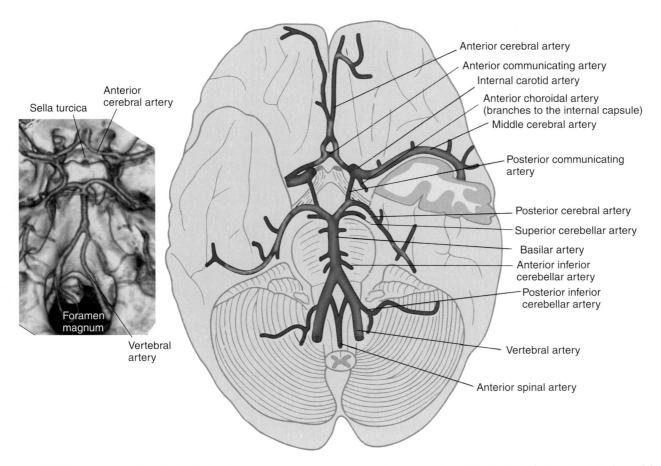

FIGURE 8.3 *The main arteries of the brain.* Anastomoses occur between the branches of the internal carotid artery and the vertebral artery and between the two anterior cerebral arteries, forming an arterial circuit at the base of the brain. **Left:** Arteries at the base of the brain as reconstructed from MRIs. (Courtesy of Dr. S.J. Bakke, Rikshospitalet University Hospital, Oslo, Norway.)

The vertebral artery (Fig. 8.3) enters the posterior fossa after ascending through the transverse foramina of the cervical vertebrae (see Fig. 27.7). When passing from the atlas through the foramen magnum, the artery is highly convoluted, enabling it to follow the large movements in the upper cervical joints without being overstretched or compressed. Nevertheless, extreme movements—particularly in elderly people with sclerotic arteries—may temporarily occlude the vertebral artery. This may lead to loss of consciousness due to lack of blood supply to the brain stem. Backward bending of the head combined with rotation is particularly apt to compress the vertebral artery. Further, the vertebral arteries supply the following branches:

1. The **basilar artery** arises when the vertebral arteries of the two sides unite at the lower level of the pons to form (Fig. 8.3).
2. The vertebral arteries and the basilar artery send off numerous branches to supply the medulla oblongata, the pons, the mesencephalon, and the cerebellum. The largest branches are the posterior inferior cerebellar, anterior inferior cerebellar, and the superior cerebellar arteries (Fig. 8.3):

a. The **posterior inferior cerebellar artery** supplies the lateral part of the medulla and inferior parts of the cerebellar hemispheres. It usually originates from the extracranial portion of the vertebral artery; more seldom from the basilar artery.

b. The **anterior inferior cerebellar artery** supplies lateral parts of the pons and parts of the cerebellum (see Chapter 27, under "Lateral Pontine Infarction").

c. The **superior cerebellar artery** supplies the dorsal aspect of the cerebellum and parts of the pons and the mesencephalon.

d. The **labyrinthine artery** is a small branch from the anterior inferior cerebellar artery (or, less frequently, from the basilar artery). It supplies the labyrinth in the inner ear (its occlusion will therefore cause deafness on the side of occlusion and vertigo).

e. Several thin branches—called **perforator arteries**—penetrate the brain stem from the basilar artery along its course. Some arise from the dorsal aspect of the basilar artery and supply midline structures in the pons and mesencephalon. Others course laterally for a variable distance before they penetrate the brain stem.

3. The **posterior cerebral arteries** are the two end branches of the basilar artery and arise at the upper end of the pons. The posterior cerebral artery curves posteriorly around the mesencephalon and continue at the medial side of the hemisphere to the occipital lobe (Figs. 8.3 and 8.5). The posterior cerebral artery supplies large parts of the occipital lobe, notably the visual cortex, and the inferior aspect of the temporal lobe containing higher visual association areas (e.g., necessary for the recognition of objects). Perforating branches leave the first part of the posterior cerebral artery to supply the cerebral peduncle (the crus cerebri with descending tracts as well as nuclei dorsal to the crus, such as the oculomotor nucleus). Some branches supply the dorsal parts of the mesencephalon and posterior parts of the diencephalon.

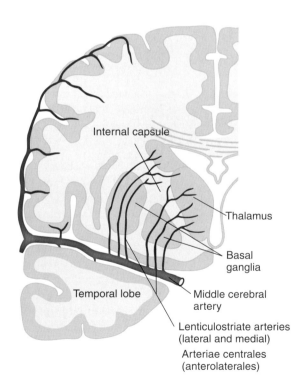

FIGURE 8.4 *Course of the middle cerebral artery.* In the depth of the lateral fissure, this artery gives off branches to the internal capsule and to the basal ganglia.

Communications between the Major Brain Arteries

At the base of the brain, there is a connection on each side between the middle and the posterior cerebral arteries, the **posterior communicating artery** (arteria communicans posterior) (Fig. 8.3). This means that, as long as the communicating artery is open, if one of the two main arterial trunks (the internal carotid or the vertebral artery) is narrowed or even occluded, the other may compensate for the loss. There is also a corresponding communicating artery between the two anterior cerebral arteries, called the **anterior communicating artery** (Fig. 8.3). In this manner a circle of anastomosing arteries is formed at the base of the skull, the **circle of Willis** (circulus arteriosus cerebri), which may be of great clinical significance. It explains, for example, how some people may have a totally occluded internal carotid artery on one side without any neurological signs. In addition, the communicating arteries can most likely become wider when the occlusion of the internal carotid artery develops slowly over the years.

The Spinal Cord Receives Arteries at Many Levels

In general, the arteries of the cord are arranged with one artery running in the midline anteriorly, the **anterior spinal artery**, and one on each side running along the rows of posterior roots, the **posterior spinal arteries** (Fig. 8.6). All three arteries begin cranially as branches of the vertebral arteries but receive contributions from the small arteries that enter the vertebral canal along with the spinal nerves.

Individual Variations in Size and Distribution of Cerebral Arteries Have Clinical Significance

The **symptoms** produced by occlusion of one arterial branch are variable because of individual differences in the size and exact distribution of the various arterial branches. Thus, if one artery is small, another supplying a neighboring territory is usually large. The anterior and posterior inferior cerebellar arteries are examples of this phenomenon: sometimes one of them supply the total territory normally supplied by both. Even the two vertebral arteries often differ markedly in size in one person, explaining why symptoms caused by occlusion of the artery may vary from minimal to life threatening.

Less than 50% of the population appears to have a "typical" **circle of Willis**, that is, the communicating arteries are symmetrical and with a certain cross-sectional diameter. In some persons the anterior communicating artery is very thin or missing; in others this may concern the posterior communicating artery on one or both sides. Therefore, the ability of the carotid artery of one side to compensate for the loss of the corresponding artery of the other side would be expected to vary

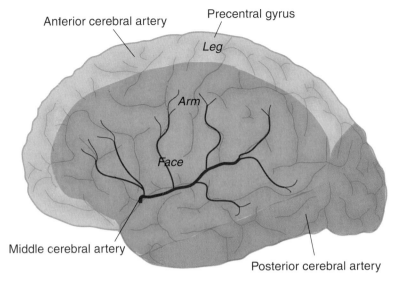

Anterior cerebral artery

Precentral gyrus

Leg

Arm

Face

Middle cerebral artery

Posterior cerebral artery

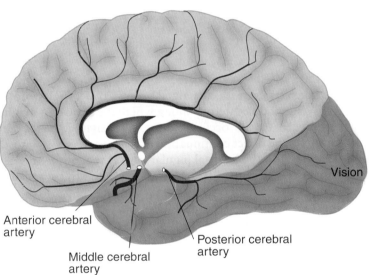

Vision

Anterior cerebral artery

Middle cerebral artery

Posterior cerebral artery

FIGURE 8.5 *The parts of the brain supplied with blood from the main arterial branches.*

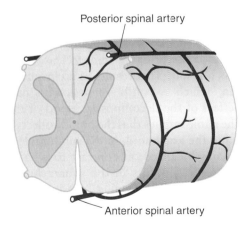

Posterior spinal artery

Anterior spinal artery

FIGURE 8.6 *The arterial supply of the spinal cord.*

considerably among individuals. Similar individual variations exist with regard to the ability of the anterior (carotid) and posterior (vertebral) circulations to compensate each other.

VENOUS SYSTEM

The Venous Blood Is Collected in Sinuses

The cerebral veins can be divided into deep and superficial types. The latter partly accompany the arteries on the surface of the brain. All of the veins empty into large **venous sinuses** that are formed by folds of the dura (Figs. 8.7–8.9).

The **superficial veins** at the dorsal parts of the hemispheres run upward and medially and empty into the large **superior sagittal sinus** in the upper margin of the falx cerebri. Where the falx cerebri meets the tentorium

II | DEVELOPMENT, AGING, AND PLASTICITY

THE fully developed nervous system consists of incredibly complex networks of connections. There are billions of neurons in the human brain, and each one is probably, on average, connected with several thousand others. The number of possible combinations of synaptic contacts is therefore astronomic. Indeed, a section of nervous tissue stained to reveal all neuronal processes might appear as a chaotic jungle. Nevertheless, we have ample evidence that this is very far from the case: order exists everywhere, and the mutual connections between neuronal groups are far from random. This leads to a number of questions, such as: How do the thousands of individual cell groups find their highly specific positions in the brain? How do the complicated and precisely organized networks arise during development of the individual? What roles do genetic and environmental factors play in the final structure and performance of the brain? Such questions are dealt with in **Chapter 9**. In **Chapter 10**, we discuss the changes taking place in the aging brain and their consequences for function. A common theme in Chapters 9 and 10 is nervous system plasticity—that is, its ability to adapt structurally and functionally to altered demands. In **Chapter 11**, we discuss plastic changes in the nervous system as the basis for recovery of function after damage to the central nervous system. We will argue that a common theme in all rehabilitative efforts is to facilitate learning.

week, the embryo resembles an elongated disc. In the second week the disc is covered on the upper or dorsal side and along the edges by primitive epithelium, the ectoderm, whereas the under or ventral side is covered by an epithelium—the endoderm—which later forms the intestinal tract and its glands. Between these two epithelial layers develops the mesoderm that later differentiates into the musculoskeletal system. In the third week (after 18 days) the development of the nervous system starts, with formation of a thickening, the neural plate, in the prospective cranial end of the disc (Figs. 9.1 and 9.2). The thickening is due to growth of the ectodermal cells so that they form a tall, simple, columnar neuroepithelium. Diffusible substances— called morphogens[1]—from the underlying mesodermal cells induce formation of the neural plate (see also "Neuromeres and Hox Genes" later). The differentiation of ectodermal cells to neuroepithelium proceeds in a cranial-to-caudal direction. A longitudinal infolding of the ectoderm occurs by the end of the third week (Fig. 9.1). This neural groove is subsequently closed in the fourth week; the closing starts in the middle part (Fig. 9.2) and forms the neural tube, which is soon covered by the ectoderm dorsally (Figs. 9.1 and 9.2) The wall of the tube is formed by primitive neuroepithelial cells, which proliferate enormously and develop into neurons and glial cells. The lateral edge of the neural plate forms a distinct cell group, the neural crest, which later forms a longitudinal column on each side of the neural tube (Fig. 9.1). The neural crest produces the neurons of the peripheral nervous system, among them spinal ganglion cells and autonomic ganglion cells. The neural crest also produces Schwann cells and satellite cells (a kind of glia) in the ganglia.

The Neural Crest Produces More Than Neurons and Glia

Experiments with labeling of neural crest cells before they migrate (Fig. 9.1) show that some differentiate into non-nervous structures. These include the smooth muscles of the eye (intrinsic eye muscles) and, most likely, the **pia** and the **arachnoid** (the dura mater is believed to originate from the mesoderm). Migrated neural crest cells also form the dermis and subcutis of the **face** and the cartilaginous skeleton of the **visceral arches**. Finally, neural crest cells produce endocrine

1 **Morphogens** are substances that spread by diffusion from a localized source and govern the embryological development and patterning of organs and body parts. Their effects depend on their concentrations—often so that high and low concentrations exert opposite effects. Among several morphogens involved in patterning of the human nervous system, the protein **sonic hedgehog** plays an important role at very early stages. For example, sonic hedgehog is expressed by the notochord when the dorsal–ventral differentiation of the neural tube begins. It also acts at later stages to guide axonal growth, attracting outgrowing axons in low concentrations, and repelling them in high concentrations (as shown for retinal ganglion cell axons growing from the eye toward the brain).

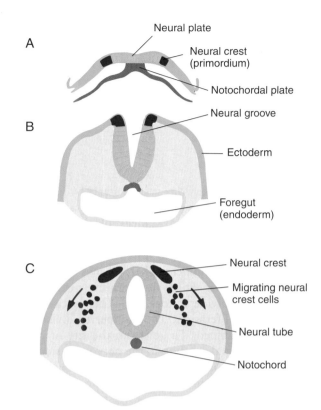

FIGURE 9.1 *Formation of the neural tube and the neural crest.* Schematic cross sections through embryos at different stages of development. **A:** The formation of the neural tube is induced by substances diffusing from the underlying mesoderm (notochordal plate). Approximately 17 days. **B:** The neural tube is formed by growth and folding of the neural plate. Approximately 21 days **C:** The neural crest gives origin to spinal ganglion cells and autonomic ganglion cells (and some other cell types). The neural crest cells migrate into the body to form ganglia. Approximately 24 days.

cells of the **adrenal medulla, melanocytes** of the skin, and parts of the **septum** that divides the pulmonal artery and the aorta.

Early Development of the Cranial End of the Neural Tube

Whereas the caudal end of the neural tube—which develops into the spinal cord—retains its simple tubular form, the expanded cranial end undergoes marked changes. This occurs because different parts grow at different rates, and because the tube bends, forming **flexures** (Fig. 9.3). In the fourth week three swellings or **primary vesicles** take shape (Figs. 9.3 and 9.4). The cavities inside the primary vesicles are continuous and develop into the ventricular system of the brain (see Fig. 7.3). The most cranial vesicle is called the **prosencephalon** (forebrain), the middle one the **mesencephalon** (the midbrain), and the caudal-most one the **rhombencephalon** (hindbrain). A ventrally directed bend—the **cervical flexure**—arises at the junction between the rhombencephalon and the spinal cord (Fig. 9.3). Later, a **mesencephalic flexure**

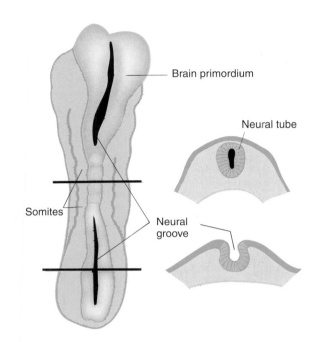

FIGURE 9.2 *The neural plate and closure of the neural groove.* Drawing of a 22-day-old human embryo, approximately 1 mm long. The central nervous system is shown in pink. (Based on Hamilton, Boyd, and Mossman 1972.)

arises between the rhombencephalon and the mesencephalon. A dorsally directed bend—the **pontine flexure**—later divides the rhombencephalon into two parts (Fig. 9.5).

Early in the fourth week, the ventral aspect of the prospective brain exhibits shallow, transverse grooves. These are external signs of segmentation of the cranial end of the neural tube, and each segment is called a **neuromere**. The segmentation is most obvious in the rhombencephalon, and we use the term **rhombomere** in this region. Although their external signs disappear by the sixth week, the neuromeres are important because they represent the first segregation of neurons that later differentiate into the various nuclei of the brain stem. Thus, several cranial nerves and their nuclei are first laid down according to a segmental pattern, like the spinal nerves, although later development makes the cranial nerve pattern less regular.

The mesencephalon changes little during further development, in contrast to the two other primary vesicles. The **prosencephalon** develops into the diencephalon and the cerebral hemispheres, whereas the **rhombencephalon** differentiates into the medulla oblongata, the pons, and the cerebellum (Figs. 9.4 and 9.5). The rostral end of the prosencephalon produces two more vesicles (one on each side), called the **telencephalon** (Figs. 9.4 and 9.5), which later forms the cerebral cortex and basal ganglia. In addition, the **olfactory bulbs** (see Fig. 3.13) arise as evaginations from the ventral aspect of the telencephalon. The remaining caudal part of the prosencephalon forms the diencephalon, which includes the thalamus and hypothalamus. At an early stage (Fig. 9.3), cuplike evaginations—the **eye vesicles**—are formed from the prosencephalon (the part later to become the diencephalon). The eye vesicles develop into the retina and the optic nerve. The rhombencephalon develops two parts: the **myelencephalon** forming the medulla oblongata, and the **metencephalon** forming the pons and most of the cerebellum (the cerebellum also develops from the mesencephalon, as discussed next).

FIGURE 9.3 *Early stages of brain development.* **Left:** Drawing of a 28-day-old human embryo, approximately 3.5 mm long. **Right:** Drawings of the cranial part of the neural tube (the brain primordium) isolated and magnified compared with the drawing of the embryo. Arrows indicate the flexures of the neural tube. The lower left is cut through (seen from the dorsal aspect) to show the primary vesicles and the ventricular space. (Based on Hamilton, Boyd, and Mossman 1972.)

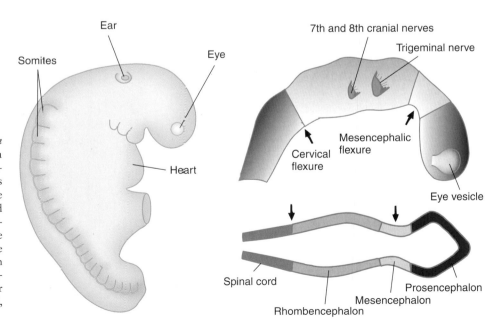

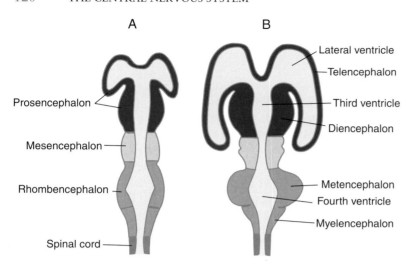

FIGURE 9.4 *Different divisions of the brain primordium.* Schematic of the cranial part of the neural tube (straightened out and cut open horizontally). **A:** Approximately the same stage as in Fig. 4.3. **B:** The same stage as in Fig. 4.13A. Note the development of the telencephalon (the hemispheres) that gradually covers the diencephalon.

Early Phases in the Development of the Neuroepithelium

Initially, the wall of the neural tube consists of only one layer of cylindrical neuroepithelial cells (Figs. 9.1 and 9.2), bounded externally by the **external limiting membrane** (covered by the pia) and internally toward the cavity by the **internal limiting membrane**. These are basal membranes built of extracellular material, which always develop with surface epithelia. Intense **proliferation** of neuroepithelial cells soon leads to several layers of nuclei. The epithelium does not become truly stratified, however, because all cells retain a thin process reaching the internal limiting membrane (pseudostratified epithelium; Fig. 9.6). The outermost cells move toward the cavity of the neural tube (the future ventricles

and central canal). The innermost layer, the **ventricular zone**, borders the cavity. In the ventricular zone, the cells divide mitotically (Figs. 9.6 and 9.13A). The future neurons, the **neuroblasts**, afterward migrate outward to form the **mantle zone** that later becomes the gray matter. A layer without neurons, the **marginal zone**, forms external to the mantle zone and becomes the white matter. The neurons of the mantle zone send axons into the marginal zone. These axons loop back to the mantle zone, however, to synapse on neurons there (these are the first association connections to arise). Other axons leave the neural tube as motor fibers growing peripherally to contact muscle cells and glands (Fig. 9.7). After neuroblast production ends, various types of glial cells are produced by mitosis of neuroepithelial cells that remain in the ventricular zone. The last to be produced

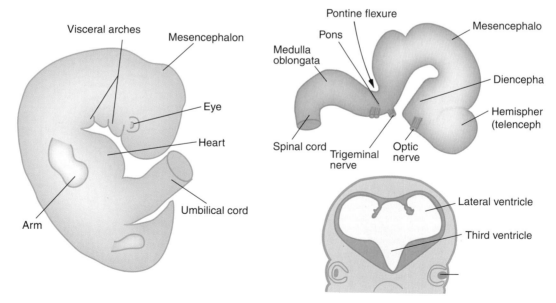

FIGURE 9.5 *Early development of the brain.* **Left:** Drawing of a 36-day-old human embryo, approximately 11 mm long. **Right:** The cranial part of the neural tube at the same stage. (Based on Hamilton, Boyd, and Mossman 1972.)

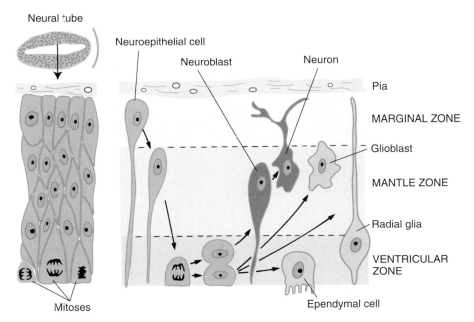

Neural tube

Neuroepithelial cell

Neuroblast

Neuron

Pia

MARGINAL ZONE

Glioblast

MANTLE ZONE

Radial glia

VENTRICULAR ZONE

Ependymal cell

Mitoses

FIGURE 9.6 *Differentiation of the neuroepithelium.* **Left:** Drawing of a section through the wall of the neural tube at an early stage (cf. Fig. 9.7A). **Right:** Arrows show how the neuroepithelial cells move while they differentiate into different cell types.

are the **ependymal cells**. These retain their internal position and cover the ventricular face of the neural tube (Fig. 9.6). The cavity is filled with cerebrospinal fluid produced by tufts invaginated from the wall into the cavity (see Fig. 7.6). These tufts—the future **choroid plexus**—are covered by ependymal cells.

The simple layering of the neural tube, with the mantle zone (gray matter) inside and the marginal zone (white matter) outside, is retained with minor changes in the spinal cord. In the cranial part of the neural tube (the future brain), however, major alterations in the mutual positions of gray and white matter occur. In the developing cerebellar and cerebral cortices, for example, neurons migrate from the mantle zone through the marginal zone and form a layered sheet of gray matter externally, just under the pia.

Neuromeres

We mentioned that the rostral part of the neural tube shows transient, external signs of segmentation—each segment constituting a **neuromere**. Although this phenomenon was observed in the nineteenth century, modern cell biological methods were necessary for closer study of their role in the development of the nervous system. Neuromeres are most convincingly shown in the rhombencephalon, where they are called **rhombomeres**. It is assumed that the mesencephalon consists of two neuromeres, whereas the prosencephalon probably consists of six. The great interest in neuromeres and other external signs of segmentation arose because they provide information about the mechanisms that control the early development from the undifferentiated neural.

Each rhombomere represents a unit of neurons that do not mix with neurons of other rhombomeres during subsequent development. This neuronal specification takes place just when the rhombomere boundaries arise. The rhombomeres arise when adjoining groups of neurons begin to express different surface markers. The neurons of one rhombomere, among other things, have a specified future peripheral target (the neurons of the neural crest in the head region are also specified with regard to their peripheral target before they start to migrate peripherally). The motor trigeminal nucleus,

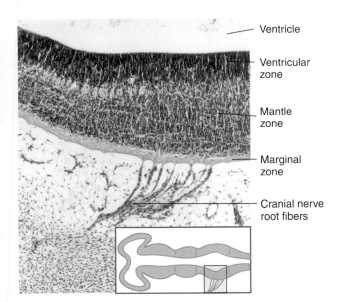

Ventricle

Ventricular zone

Mantle zone

Marginal zone

Cranial nerve root fibers

FIGURE 9.7 *Outgrowth of cranial nerves from the rhombencephalon.* Photomicrograph of a horizontal section through a chicken embryo at about the same stage as in Figure 4.3. Thin bundles of axons leave the marginal zone and penetrate the connective tissue that surrounds the brain primordium.

for example, is formed in rhombomeres r2 and r3, whereas the motor facial nucleus develops in r4 and r5. The motor and sensory cranial nerve axons already have a specified target when they start growing out from the neural tube (Fig. 9.7). Thus, when a rhombomere is transplanted to another place in the chicken embryonic brain, it develops as if it were still in its original place and not corresponding to its new location. Such specification must be caused by the switching on of certain genes—which start to express themselves by production of mRNA—while probably other genes are switched off.

Hox *Genes*

Many so-called **Hox** genes have been identified that are expressed in a pattern corresponding to neuromeric boundaries in vertebrates. Most of these genes code for proteins that act as **transcription factors**. These bind to DNA of other genes and regulate their transcription. Typically, transcription factors are expressed temporarily during specific phases of development. (*Hox* genes not only control regional development of the nervous system but also act in pattern formation in other parts of the body.) When a certain *Hox* gene is switched on, a cascade of changes in the expression of other genes is initiated, producing signal molecules that give the neuronal groups their identity—for example, regarding location and connections. A crucial question is, of course, what controls the regionalized expression of *Hox* genes giving rise to the rhombomeres? One important factor is **retinoic acid (vitamin A)**, which normally occurs with an anteroposterior (rostrocaudal) concentration gradient in the embryo (highest concentration posteriorly or caudally). The retinoic acid seems to stem from the mesoderm adjacent to the neural tube. In low concentrations, retinoic acid acts on *Hox* genes that specify anterior parts of the neural tube, while in high concentrations it induces differentiation of posterior parts. This explains why adequate dietary levels of vitamin A are necessary for the normal development of the CNS, but also why too much also may cause malformations (as may occur in women treated for acne with retinoic acid in early pregnancy).

Neuromeric borders, identified with genetic markers, are more reliable indicators of future borders between anatomically and functionally different areas than are borders between brain vesicles. For example, the cerebellum, traditionally regarded as arising only from the metencephalon, is also formed by neurons in the adjoining part of the mesencephalon. The rostral border of neurons forming the cerebellum coincides with a border for the expression of the ***engrailed 2*** gene.

Further Development of the Spinal Cord and the Brain Stem

In the fourth week, the proliferation of neuroblasts in the mantle zone produces a large ventral thickening and a smaller dorsal one on each side of the neural tube. These thickenings are called the **basal plates** and the **alar plates**, respectively (Figs. 9.8, 9.9, and 9.10). A shallow furrow, the **sulcus limitans**, marks the border between them. This remains visible in the lower part of the brain stem in the adult (see Fig. 3.17), while it disappears early in the spinal cord. The basal plate contains neuroblasts that later become motor neurons, whereas many alar plate neuroblasts become sensory neurons. This corresponds to the functional division between the ventral and dorsal horns of the cord. In the adult brain stem, the sulcus limitans marks the border between the motor and the sensory cranial nerve nuclei (Fig. 9.11). In the open part of the rhombencephalon—later to become parts of the medulla and the pons—the motor nuclei lie medially and the sensory nuclei laterally (see Figs. 27.2 and 27.3). This is caused by lateral

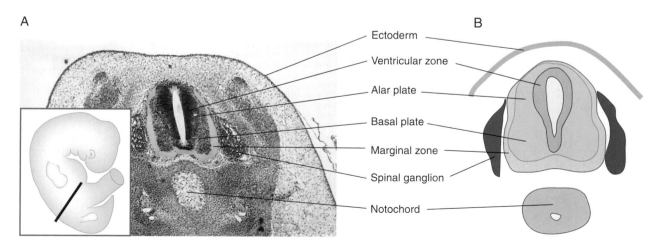

A

B

Ectoderm

Ventricular zone

Alar plate

Basal plate

Marginal zone

Spinal ganglion

Notochord

FIGURE 9.8 *Early development of the spinal cord.* **A:** Photomicrograph of a cross section of a chicken embryo (corresponding approximately to a 6-week-old human embryo; cf. Fig. 9.5). **B:** Drawing based on a photomicrograph of the human spinal cord at about 7 weeks' gestation.

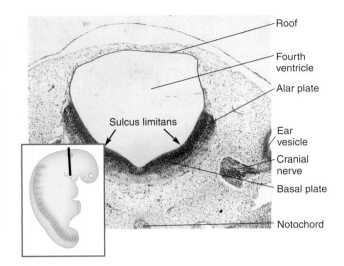

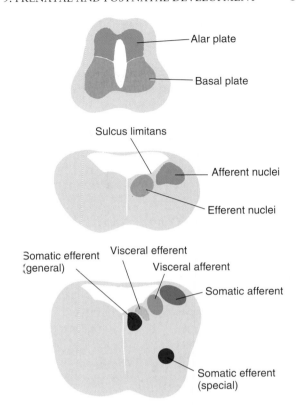

FIGURE 9.9 *The rhombencephalon.* Early stage of development, approximately as in Fig. 9.3. Photomicrograph of a cross section of a chicken embryo. **Inset:** A human embryo at a corresponding stage of development. Note the thin rhombencephalic roof attached to the edge of the alar plate.

bending of the alar plates—away from each other—so that the roof of the rhombencephalon becomes only a thin membrane (Figs. 9.9 and 9.10). At a later stage, the **cerebellum** develops from the margins of the alar plates (the **rhombic lip**).

At an early stage, several neuronal groups in the brain stem **migrate** from their "birthplace" in the alar or basal plates. In the pons, neuroblasts move from the rhombic lip in a ventral direction and form the pontine nuclei (see Fig. 3.18). Similarly, in the medulla the inferior olive (another nucleus projecting to the cerebellum; see Fig. 3.17) is formed by neuroblasts moving ventrally from the rhombic lip. Another example is the **motor**

FIGURE 9.10 *Development of the cranial nerve nuclei.* Schematic. Three stages are shown to explain the mutual positions of the nuclei. After their formation, the special somatic efferent nuclei move ventrolaterally. See also Figs. 17.2 and 17.3.

cranial nerve nuclei that innervate visceral (branchial) arch muscles (see Fig. 9.10). These neurons move in a ventral direction during early development after they have started to send out axons. The course of the root fibers in the brain stem therefore shows the path followed by the migrating neurons (see Fig. 27.11).

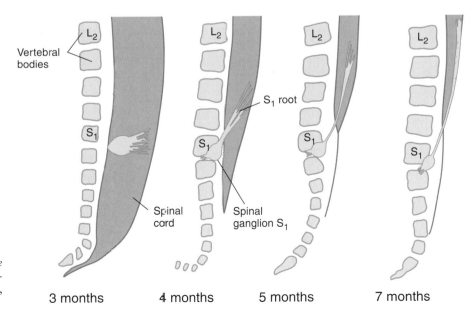

FIGURE 9.11 *Relationship between the lengths of the spinal cord and the vertebral column.* (Based on Hamilton, Boyd, and Mossman 1972.)

Until the eighth to ninth week, the spinal cord extends the full length of the spinal canal of the embryo. After that, however, the vertebral column and the coverings of the cord grow more rapidly than the spinal cord itself, producing a gradually increasing length difference (Fig. 9.11). This explains the oblique course of the **spinal nerves** in the vertebral canal before they leave through the intervertebral foramina. The lower end of the cord is at the level of the third lumbar vertebra at birth, in contrast to the first lumbar vertebra in adults. The dural sac, containing spinal nerve roots (the cauda equina), continues down to the second sacral vertebra (see Fig. 3.3).

Cranial Nerves and Visceral Arches

Cranial nerves 5, 7, 9, and 10 (trigeminal, facial, glossopharyngeal, and vagal; see Figs. 6.15 and 6.19) innervate structures developed from visceral arches (or branchial arches). In fish, the two upper visceral arches are parts of the viscerocranium surrounding the oral cavity. They are not equipped with gills, in contrast to the lower (3–6) arches that are true respiratory organs. In mammals, none of the visceral arches has respiratory functions. Parts of them are used for new tasks, whereas other parts have regressed. There are no signs of gill development at any stage of human embryogenesis. The term "branchial arch" (from Greek *brankhion*, gill) is therefore not quite appropriate.

A visceral arch consists of a skeletal part (cartilage, later replaced by bone in some arches), muscles, skin, mucous membranes, and a nerve of its own. As mentioned, neural crest cells give rise to the skeletal part. In human embryos, some visceral arches appear as ventral bulges in the head and cervical region (Figs. 9.3 and 9.5). The **first visceral arch**—producing the upper and lower jaw with attached masticatory muscles, along with the hammer and the anvil of the middle ear—is innervated by the **fifth cranial nerve** (the trigeminal). The second visceral arch—forming, among other things, the upper part of the hyoid bone, the stirrup of the middle ear, and the facial muscles—is innervated by the **seventh cranial nerve** (the facial). The **third visceral arch**—forming most of the hyoid bone and the posterior part of the tongue—is innervated by the **ninth cranial nerve** (the glossopharyngeal). The **fourth, fifth, and sixth visceral arches** form the cartilaginous skeleton of the larynx and the muscles of the larynx and the pharynx. These structures are innervated for the most part by the **tenth cranial nerve** (the vagus).

Cranial nerves 3, 4, 6, and 12 (the oculomotor, trochlear, abducens, and hypoglossal; see Fig. 3.14) innervate structures that most likely develop from segmentally arranged **somites** (somites are paired cubical masses giving rise to muscles, the axial skeleton, and the dermis of the skin). These nerves are homologous to spinal ventral roots. As for the **eleventh cranial nerve** (the accessory), it is not settled whether the two muscles it innervates (the sternocleidomastoid and trapezius) develop from somites or from visceral arches. The latter hypothesis is supported by the fact that the accessory nerve root fibers, coming from the upper cervical segments, exit the cord more dorsally than the spinal ventral roots (corresponding to the level where visceral arch nerves leave the brain stem; see Fig. 27.8).

Further Development of the Diencephalon

The diencephalon represents the caudal part of the original prosencephalic vesicle (Figs. 9.4 and 9.5). The lateral wall in this part becomes thicker at an early stage and develops into the **thalamus** (Fig. 9.12A). The floor plate forms the **hypothalamus** and the **posterior pituitary** (see Figs. 6.22 and 6.24). The latter arise as an evagination of the floor plate. The furrow (hypothalamic sulcus; see Fig. 6.23) marking the border between the thalamus and the hypothalamus might be a continuation of the sulcus limitans (Fig. 9.10) It is not settled, however, whether the arrangement with basal and alar plates continues rostrally into the diencephalon. The thin roof plate of the diencephalon forms by invagination the **choroid plexus** of the third ventricle (see Fig. 7.5). Further, the roof plate produces the **pineal body** by evagination (see Fig. 6.23). The **eye vesicles** occur at an earlier stage (before the further differentiation of the prosencephalon; Fig. 9.3) but retain connection with the diencephalon by the future optic nerve (Fig. 9.5).

Further Development of the Telencephalon

In the fifth week, development of the **cerebral hemispheres** starts with the appearance of one vesicle on each side of the prosencephalon (Figs. 9.4 and 9.5). These are called the **telencephalic (cerebral) vesicles**. Their cavities form the lateral ventricles, which initially have wide openings to the third ventricle (interventricular foramen, Fig. 9.12A). The mantle zone of the basal part of the telencephalic vesicle thickens rapidly to form the corpus striatum of the **basal ganglia** (Fig. 9.12A). The thinner overlying part, called the **pallium**, becomes the cerebral cortex. The pallium grows dorsally, rostrally, and caudally in relation to the diencephalon (Fig. 9.4). The caudal and ventral parts of the hemispheres later fuse with the diencephalon (Fig. 9.12B).

The basal ganglia primordium is later divided into two parts—the lateral and medial **corpus striatum**—by descending axons from the cerebral cortex. These descending axons form the **internal capsule** (Fig. 9.12B). As development proceeds, the caudate nucleus and the thalamus come to lie medial to the internal capsule whereas the lentiform nucleus (the putamen and the globus pallidus) lies laterally (see Fig. 13.2).

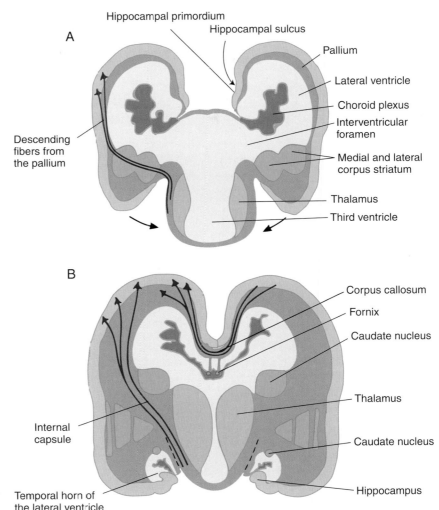

Hippocampal primordium

Hippocampal sulcus

A

Pallium

Lateral ventricle

Choroid plexus

Interventricular foramen

Descending fibers from the pallium

Medial and lateral corpus striatum

Thalamus

Third ventricle

B

Corpus callosum

Fornix

Caudate nucleus

Thalamus

Internal capsule

Caudate nucleus

Temporal horn of the lateral ventricle

Hippocampus

FIGURE 9.12 *Development of the telencephalon.* **A:** Early stage, in which the telencephalon is still separated from the diencephalon. Descending fibers have started their growth from the pallium (primordium of the cerebral cortex) to the brain stem and the spinal cord. **B:** The telencephalon is now attached to the diencephalon laterally, and the medial and lateral striatum have been separated by the internal capsule. The hippocampus has changed its position, due to the growth of the hemispheres (cf. Fig. 3.36). (Based on Hamilton, Boyd, and Mossman 1972.)

In the medial wall of the pallium, just above the attachment of the choroid plexus, a thickening arises that bulges into the lateral ventricle (Fig. 9.13A). This is the beginning of the **hippocampus**, which is partly separated from the rest of the pallium by the hippocampal sulcus. As the hemispheres grow, their shape changes so that the temporal lobes come to lie ventrally. This produces the characteristic curved shape of the lateral ventricles and the structures in their wall, such as the hippocampus and the caudate nucleus (see Figs. 7.4 and 31.2). The hippocampus thus moves from the position in Fig. 4.12A to that in Fig. 4.12B.

The **choroid plexus** of the lateral ventricles is formed by invagination of the thin part of the pallium (together with the pia) close to the dorsal aspect of the diencephalon (Fig. 9.12B; see also Fig. 7.6).

Development of the Cerebral Cortex

At first, the telencephalic vesicle consists of only one layer of neuroepithelial cells. These proliferate, however, producing rapid growth of the prospective cerebral hemisphere. At a later stage, we can differentiate a ventricular zone, mantle zone, and marginal zone, just as in other parts of the neural tube (Fig. 9.13A). At the beginning of the **eighth week**, neuroblasts from the mantle zone **migrate** into the marginal zone and start establishing the **cortical plate** (Fig. 9.13B), which in due course will develop into the mature cerebral cortex by waves of cells migrating toward the cortical surface. The peak of migratory activity probably occurs between the third and fifth months, while migration ends in the third trimester. By the end of the seventh month the cortex has developed six layers, as in the mature cortex (see Figs. 33.1 and 33.2). Synapses begin to occur in the fourth month (earliest in the prospective somatosensory cortex).

The deepest cortical layers are established first; thus, neurons destined for superficial layers have to pass through the deep layers. Neuroepithelial cells in the ventricular zone that have ceased dividing are termed **postmitotic**. The exact time a neuron becomes postmitotic—its **birth date**—appears to decide which cortical layer it will join. Radially oriented glial cells, **radial glia** (Fig. 9.6), with processes extending from the ependyma to the pia,

A   B

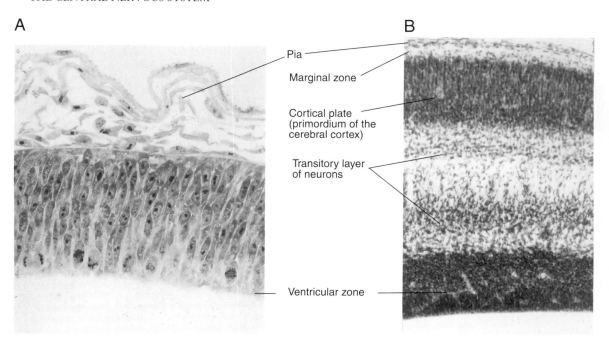

Pia

Marginal zone

Cortical plate
(primordium of the
cerebral cortex)

Transitory layer
of neurons

Ventricular zone

FIGURE 9.13 *Differentiation of the prosencephalic neuroepithelium to the cerebral cortex.* **A:** Photomicrograph of a cross section through the neural tube (prosencephalic part) at an early stage (chicken embryo, corresponding to early fourth week gestation in humans). Mitotic activity occurs in the ventricular zone. **B:** Photomicrograph of a section through the telencephalon (rat) at a much later stage than in A, corresponding approximately to the fourth to fifth month in human development. The ventricular zone is densely packed with neuroblasts that will soon migrate toward the cortical plate. In further development, the cortical plate develops into the adult six-layered cortex.

guide the migration of postmitotic neurons toward the cortex. The phenotype of postmitotic neurons, for example, whether they will develop into interneurons or projection neurons, appears to be specified at the time they start migrating toward their final destination.

Shortly after the establishment of the cortical plate, thalamocortical fibers start to invade the telencephalic wall, although they must "wait" several weeks below the cortical plate before they find their final destination in the developing cortex. The earliest afferent fibers to arrive, however, are **monoaminergic** (at about 7 weeks).

While probably all progenitors of projection neurons arise in the ventricular zone and migrate radially to their final destination, many prospective cortical **interneurons** arise from subcortical sites in the ventral forebrain. They then migrate tangentially along the cortical plate for varying distances before they change course and migrate perpendicularly into the cortex.[2]

Specification of Cortical Cytoarchitectonic Areas

The adult cerebral cortex consists of many areas that differ structurally and functionally (see Fig. 33.4).

The differentiation of the cortical plate into distinct areas (see Fig. 33.4)—a process called **arealization**—depends on both genetic factors intrinsic to the developing cortical progenitor cells and extrinsic influences. In the beginning, local patterning centers in the periphery of the ventricular zone produces gradients of **morphogens** that define four main, overlapping domains in the cortical plate.[3] The morphogens in turn initiate more discrete expressions of transcription factors in cortical progenitor cells. These transcription factors are involved in the further differentiation of the cortical plate into areas with sharp borders (as well as in other aspects of cortical development).

Among **extrinsic influences**, thalamocortical afferents appear to be of particular importance for the mature **cytoarchitectonic** characteristics of an area. For example, the characteristic cytoarchitectonic differences between the primary sensory areas (compare Figs. 33.2 and 33.4) depend on from which specific thalamic nucleus the areas receive their afferents. For example, transplanting a piece of visual cortex to the somatosensory cortex makes the transplanted tissue acquire the cytoarchitectonic features that are typical of the somatosensory cortex. Further, immature projection neurons transplanted from one area to another develop axonal

2 All cortical interneurons are **GABAergic** but fall into different groups structurally and with regard to whether they co-express the neuropeptide **somatostatin** (SST), **parvalbumin** (PVA), or **calretinin** (CR). The three main groups of GABAergic interneurons seem to be specified at the time they migrate from the so-called ventricular (ganglionic) eminences.

3 For example, the arealization of the frontal cortex seems to be initiated by two **fibroblast growth factors** (Fgf8 and Fgf17).

ramifications appropriate for the area to which they are transplanted. Thus, the local environment contributes significantly to the neuronal phenotype.

In addition to the genetically determined development described here, proper use of cortical areas is critical for the realization of their functional specialization. This involves **use-dependent** plastic processes, stabilizing useful synaptic connections, and eliminating those that prove to be superfluous or maladaptive.

Migration and Migration Disorders

We know some of the factors governing neuronal migration, such as recognition molecules, adhesion molecules, cytoskeletal components, and others. There is a complex interplay among them, and the different factors must be present in the proper concentration at the proper time and place. For example, the early presence of certain neurotransmitters influences neuronal motility by acting on ion channels that increase the intracellular Ca^{2+} concentration. The glycoprotein **reelin** (among other factors) governs the final positioning of migrating neurons in the cortex. Because reelin is produced by **Cajal-Retzius cells** in the marginal zone (Fig. 9.6), it would seem logical that a concentration gradient of reelin between the marginal and ventricular layers is critical for normal development. The mechanisms behind the effects of reelin appear to be more complex, however. Nevertheless, mice with a mutated gene for reelin exhibit characteristic malformations of layered structures; in the cerebral cortex, the late-arriving neurons do not migrate past those that arrived first to occupy the outer layers. Although the neurons survive and establish apparently normal connections, the brain does not function normally. Another mutation, shown in some humans, affects the migration *before* the neurons enter the cortical plate and is associated with a smooth cortex lacking the normal six-layered structure (**Miller-Dieker lissencephaly**). This is just one example of a large and varied group of malformations in humans—**migration disorders**—caused by delayed or deficient migration of postmitotic neurons.

Migration disorders affect primarily the cerebral cortex and the cerebellum. Many are inherited recessively, although ischemia, radiation, and other influences can cause migration disorders (as shown in animal experiments). In the cerebral cortex, migration disorders typically are associated with defective development of the gyri (Fig. 9.14), which may be lacking (**lissencephaly**), too small (**polymicrogyria**), or show other abnormalities. Usually, such a cortex is called **dysplastic**, and some use the term "dysplastic cortex" as synonymous with migration disorders.

Migration disorders cause a number of syndromes characterized by **cognitive** and behavioral defects (mental retardation is common). Typical of many such syndromes

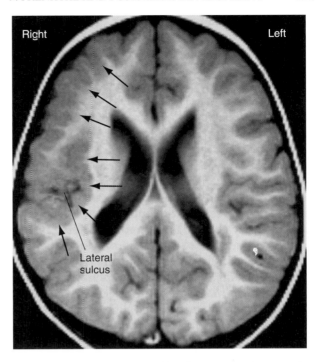

FIGURE 9.14 *Neuronal migration disorder.* Horizontal T1-weighted MRI. The right frontal cortex is dysplastic: it is thicker than normal with obliteration of normal sulci (polymicrogyria). Similar alterations occur around the lateral sulcus. (Courtesy of Dr. S.J. Bakke, Rikshospitalet University Hospital, Norway.)

is **epilepsy** (which is often difficult to treat pharmacologically). This is compatible with the fact that migration disorders also are associated with molecular abnormalities of cortical neurons. Thus, animal experiments suggest that epilepsy can arise in dysplastic cortex because of an imbalance between the expression of excitatory and inhibitory receptors (up-regulation of amino-methylisoxazole propionic acid [AMPA] receptors and down-regulation of $GABA_A$ receptors).

Programmed Cell Death and Competition for Trophic Factors

As previously mentioned, many more neurons are formed during the proliferation phase than are found in the mature nervous system. Cell death usually coincides in time with the period during which the neurons establish synaptic contacts. For the most intensively studied neuronal groups, such as spinal motoneurons and retinal ganglion cells, the amount of elimination depends on **target size**. If the target (e.g., striated muscle cells) is experimentally expanded, more motoneurons survive, whereas reducing the target size increases elimination. This can be explained by the neurons needing a sufficient supply of a growth-promoting substance—a **trophic factor**—to survive. The target cells produce limited amounts of this trophic factor; that is, there is not enough to keep all neurons alive. The neurons

die shortly after. A defective closure of the spinal cord (most often in the lumbosacral part) is termed **spina bifida** because the vertebral arch and soft tissue dorsal to the cord do not develop normally. This condition may vary in severity. In the most serious cases the vertebral arches, muscles, and skin are absent and there is herniation of the coverings of the cord that contain degenerated nervous tissue (**meningomyelocele**). Less severe cases may involve herniation of the coverings but keep the spinal cord intact, whereas the least affected have only partial lack of the vertebral arch (**spina bifida occulta**). In the most serious cases, the cord does not develop normally, leading to pareses and sensory disturbances of the legs. When the nervous supply is deficient, the muscles do not develop to their normal size and strength.

Reduced drainage of the cerebrospinal fluid caused by, for example, abnormal narrowing or obliteration of the cerebral aqueduct (see Fig. 7.5) leads to **hydrocephalus**. If left untreated, this will cause death or seriously impair brain development (see also Chapter 7, under "Brain Edema, Herniation, and Hydrocephalus").

MECHANISMS FOR ESTABLISHMENT OF SPECIFIC CONNECTIONS

The main morphologic features of the nervous system—such as its macroscopic form, the positions of major nuclei and their interconnections—arise before birth and shortly after. In a sense, this represents the **hard wiring** of the brain. In this section, we discuss mechanisms important for forming the brain's "wiring diagrams." The growth of axons is often surprisingly goal-directed, indicating the existence of guiding mechanisms. We will discuss some mechanisms that can aid axons in selecting their target. The number of known interacting players at the cellular and molecular levels is enormous, and many more are probably yet to be identified. It should therefore not come as a surprise that we cannot fully explain how the amazing connectional specificity of the mature nervous system arises.

Trial and Error

Although trial and error cannot explain the overall development of orderly connections in the nervous system, it nevertheless plays a role at the local level. Indeed, modern imagining methods permitting in vivo observation of growing neurons show that growth and retraction of neuronal processes are highly dynamic processes. Thus, at the same time as growth cones randomly explore their immediate environment and new spines bud from dendrites, errors are corrected continuously by retraction of unsuccessful growth cones and spines. The development of neuronal networks is therefore a

very complex interplay of simultaneous building up and tearing down, resembling the work of a sculptor who adds excess of clay to be able to carve out the fine details.

Distances Are Small in the Early Embryo

Knowing the complexity of the mature nervous system, one might think that most of the human genome must be devoted to specification of neuronal connections. This is not the case of course. We should bear in mind that the whole embryo is only a few millimeters to a couple of centimeters during the stages of most intense axonal outgrowths. Thus, the distances that axons have to grow to reach their targets are usually very short. Further, the topography of the nervous system at these early stages is also much simpler than later, as not all nuclear groups develop simultaneously. Our present knowledge suggests that combined actions of several mechanisms, each of them relatively simple, can explain how the specificity of the nervous system arises.

Time of Neuronal "Birth"

The genetically programmed time of neuronal birth can explain the development of specific connections in many cases (Fig. 9.15). If, at the time of axonal outgrowth from one neuronal group, only certain neurons are present in the direction of growth, the axons will hit their correct target without specific recognition molecules. In addition, programming of neurons for maximal synapse formation during a limited period ensures that synapses are established upon arrival of the proper axons. The time during which neurons readily produce synapses is usually limited. Axons encountering a particular neuronal group at a later stage cannot establish synapses, and therefore they either retract or grow past to other targets.

Trophic Factors

Timing of neuronal birth and maturation cannot explain all aspects of specificity, however. For example, what decides the direction of **axonal outgrowths**? For some neurons, such as pyramidal cells in the cerebral cortex, the initial growth direction is genetically determined. After that, however, signals in the environment of the axons determine the growth direction. Thus, cortical pyramidal cells are occasionally "inverted" with their apical dendrite pointing toward the white matter instead of toward the cortical surface. In such cases, the axons start growing toward the pial surface but soon reverse direction and grow toward the white matter, as do normal pyramidal cells (see Fig. 33.5). Such findings are best explained by the target organs producing growth-promoting substances—**trophic factors**—that

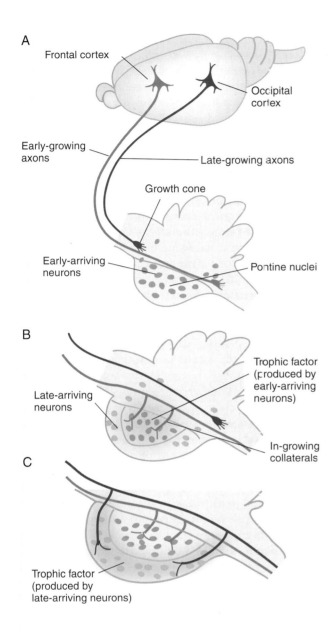

A

Frontal cortex

Occipital cortex

Early-growing axons

Late-growing axons

Growth cone

Early-arriving neurons

Pontine nuclei

B

Late-arriving neurons

Trophic factor (produced by early-arriving neurons)

In-growing collaterals

C

Trophic factor (produced by late-arriving neurons)

FIGURE **9.15** *Development of topographically organized connections: example from the corticopontine projection (cf. Fig. 14. 7).* **A:** Because the axons from the frontal lobe start growing earlier than axons from the occipital lobe, they have reached further down in the brain stem. At this stage, neurons migrate into the ventral pons to form the pontine nuclei. **B:** At a later stage, the early-arriving pontine neurons produce a trophic substance that attracts collaterals from the descending axons. However, only the axons from the frontal lobe are sufficiently mature to emit collaterals at this stage (2 days elapse from the time the axons arrive in the pons until they can form collaterals). Immature neurons continue to invade the ventral pons and form a shell around the early-arriving neurons. **C:** Late-arriving pontine neurons are now sufficiently mature to produce the trophic factor, whereas the early-arriving ones have stopped their production. At this later stage, only the axons from the occipital lobe can emit collaterals. Thus, axons from different parts of the cerebral cortex end in different parts of the pontine nuclei, forming the orderly topographic arrangement seen in the adult (see Fig. 24.8). In this example, the topographic arrangement can be explained by genetically programmed differences in the time of birth for neurons in various parts of the cerebral cortex and the pontine nuclei. Other mechanisms may operate as well. (Based on experimental studies in the rat by Leergaard, Lakke, and Bjaalie 1995.)

diffuse in the tissue. Axons then grow in the direction of increasing concentration of the factor, which binds to specific receptors, so that only axons expressing the receptor are attracted. This may explain why axons from a neuronal group in some cases grow toward their correct target even if the neuronal group has been moved to another site before axonal outgrowth.

Cell-Adhesion Molecules and Fasciculation

In other instances, neurons or glia along the route apparently express specific molecules that function as "**signposts.**" When the first **pioneer axons** have reached their target, the rest of the axons can get there simply by following the pioneers. (The pioneers may have a relatively simple task because, as mentioned, the distances they grow are very short and the "landscape" is simple.) Axons with a common target can express at their surface **neuronal-cell adhesion molecules** (N-CAMs) that make them sticky (N-CAMs are proteins related to the immunoglobulins). Axons expressing a particular kind of N-CAM are then kept together, whereas others are repelled or inhibited in their growth. In this way axons with common targets form bundles, or fascicles, and the phenomenon is termed **fasciculation.** The well-defined tracts of the nervous system arise in this way.

Growth Cones and Their Interactions with N-CAMs and Other Molecules

The many trophic factors, "signpost" molecules, recognition molecules, and N-CAMs governing the establishment of specific connections mostly act on the axonal **growth cone.** The growth cone is an expanded part of the tip of a growing axon (Figs. 9.15). It continuously sends out small extensions, or **filopodia,** as if exploring its immediate surroundings (Fig. 9.16). Filopodia encountering the proper molecules in the tissue are stabilized, and this determines the direction of further growth, while other filopodia retract. The stabilization depends on increased number of **actin** molecules in the filopodia and of **microtubules** in the axon. Several N-CAMS influence the growth of the axon when they are present near the growth cone. These N-CAMs can be expressed at the surface of both the growth cone and the nearby cells. Binding of the N-CAM molecules to each other causes stickiness. In other instances, N-CAMs bind to specific receptors in the growth cone membrane and thus activate intracellular second messengers (by influx of Ca^{2+} ions). There are also **extracellular molecules** with actions on the growth cone, such as **laminin,** which is bound to the basal lamina. Laminin binds to receptors in the growth cone membrane. Laminin can occur transiently along the path of growing axons in the peripheral nervous system, guiding the growth

ability to form and receive synapses, as discussed above.) Figure 9.15 illustrates how topographic maps in the **pontine nuclei** may arise. In the adult, axons from the cerebral cortex end in a precise topographic pattern in the pontine nuclei. Functionally different parts of the cerebral cortex connect with different parts of the nuclei (Fig. 24.9). This pattern appears to arise because axons from different parts of the cortex start growing at different times and because subgroups of pontine neurons are born at different times.

Although the basic pattern of topography is genetically determined, proper use of the system is necessary to obtain maximum precision of spatial arrangements. We return to this next in considering the environmental effects of experience on the development of the nervous system.

Prenatal Development of a Neuronal Network

We use as an example the development of the **spinal network** that controls **locomotion**. This network arises long before locomotor movements are of any use. In human fetuses, rhythmic movements of the extremities (although uncoordinated) occur as early as 10 weeks after fertilization. At first, the spinal network initiates movements without any sensory information or commands from higher levels of the CNS. Gradually the coordination improves to complete locomotor patterns (improvement continues after birth when the system is used in a goal-directed manner). The prenatal improvement is probably due to several factors: altered electric properties of the neurons, expression of novel transmitters and receptors, and development of the connections among the network neurons. These alterations depend on the development of descending connections from the brain stem (especially important might be those that contain serotonin). Maturation of the locomotor function starts with the forelimb and proceeds caudally to the hind limb, in parallel with the growth of descending axons.

Postnatal Growth of the Brain

The weight of the human brain triples during the first year of life (from 300 to 900 g), and at the same time major changes of synaptic density take place, as discussed in the preceding text. After the first year, the weight increases more slowly to reach adult values around the age of 5 to 7 (1400 g for men and 1250 g for women). This weight gain is caused by the growth of existing neurons and their processes, the myelination of axons, and the proliferation of glial cells. The neuronal growth mainly involves expansion of the dendritic trees and formation of axon collaterals with nerve terminals. The growth of dendritic arbors is especially marked in the human cerebral cortex during the first 2 years of life (Fig. 9.17). There is good evidence that increased dendritic ramifications relate to an increased number of synapses. Myelination of corticocortical connections takes place during the same period and is a sign of functional maturation. Increased conduction velocity enhances both the precision and the capacity of the neural networks; that is, their potential for information processing increases.

Human Brain Weights

Typical values of average adult brain weight from large autopsy studies are about 1400 g in men and 1250 g in women. Usually, such studies are based on brains of

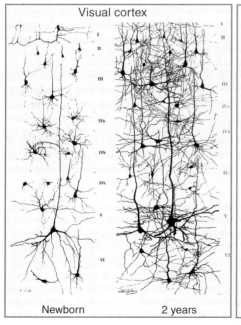
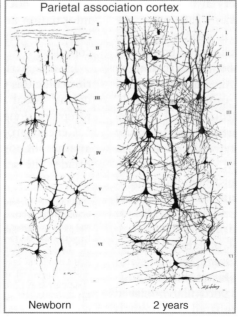

FIGURE 9.17 *Postnatal development of the human cerebral cortex.* Drawings based on Golgi sections from the visual cortex showing the increase in dendritic arborizations from birth and until the age of 2 years. The increase in dendritic arborization is most likely related to the increase in the number of synapses per neuron. (From Conel 1939.)

adults between the ages of 20 and 40 years. More interesting than average weight is the range of variation among normal individuals. An investigation of brains from 200 persons 17 to 40 years of age reported variations from 1120 to 1780 g in men and from 1070 to 1550 g in women. Older autopsy studies indicate that adult brain weight (volume) is reached between ages 5 and 10. An MRI study of 85 normal children, aged 5 to 17, did not find any volume increase after the age of 5. MRI studies show a weak correlation between brain volume and IQ, both among children and adults.

THE ROLE OF THE ENVIRONMENT IN DEVELOPMENT OF THE NERVOUS SYSTEM

Growth and Use-Dependent Plasticity

Although the brain's postnatal weight gain is largely genetically determined, the final functional state of the various neural systems and networks depends critically on their proper use during a certain period: they must be used at the proper time and in a meaningful way. The ensuing **use-dependent** structural changes occur mainly at the synaptic level, determining the final number of synapses, their precise distribution, and postsynaptic effects. Both establishment and elimination of synapses occur at high rates during the development toward a fully functioning system. As we have discussed, an enormous surplus of synapses arises in infancy, with subsequent synaptic elimination as the neuronal networks mature. Nevertheless, networks that are properly used appear to end up with a higher number of synapses than networks not subjected to normal challenges.[8]

"Enriched Environments" and Synaptic Plasticity

Numerous animal experiments have shown robust effects of environmental conditions on brain structure and biochemistry, as well as on behavior. Early experiments showed, for example, that dendritic arborizations were more extensive in the cerebral cortex of rats raised in an **enriched environment** (a simulated natural environment with ample space and access to toys) than in rats raised in standard laboratory cages.[9] Brains of wild and tame animals represent a naturally occurring analog of experiments with enriched environments. Indeed, wild animals have somewhat larger brains than tame animals of the same species. The responsible influence must occur quite early, because animals born in the wild and later tamed have the same brain size as wild animals. The difference is not genetic, however, because individuals of the first generation born in captivity have smaller brains than their wild relatives have. Experimental enrichment in the early postnatal period of rats induced increased synaptic density in the **hippocampus** and improved performance in certain learning and memory tasks. Results from experiments on the **motor system** further support the association between synaptic plasticity and learning: Among young adult rats doing different motor tasks, some developed more synapses per neuron in the cerebellar cortex than others did. The decisive factor was not the amount of motor activity but that the activity implied learning of new motor behaviors. Other experiments show that learning of specific skills is associated with synaptic changes in cortical areas involved in the task. For example, as monkeys gradually improved their performance in distinguishing tones of different frequencies, the part of the **auditory cortex** representing the particular frequencies increased in size. Similar changes occur in the motor cortex during learning of motor skills.

The preceding examples strongly suggest that formation and modification of synapses are closely linked with **learning**. It is plausible, for example, that life in the wild (or in an artificially enriched environment) requires the acquisition of a broader repertoire of adaptive behaviors than life in the cage or the bin. In general, there is good reason to assert that task-specific networks become operational during childhood because of learning processes driven by active interactions between the individual and his or her environment.

Information Must Be Meaningful

Nerve impulses are not by themselves sufficient for normal development, as shown in many animal experiments. For example, in goldfish exposed only to diffuse light (devoid of information) at the time retinal axons form synapses in the optic tectum, the normal ordered map of the visual environment does not develop properly. Another example concerns the development of connections from the retina to the visual cortex. At first, neurons in the visual cortex are influenced with equal strength from each eye. Soon after birth, however, neurons in the cortex segregate into groups, with a dominant input from one eye and a weaker input from the other. This phenomenon is called **eye dominance**. When all impulse traffic from the retina is blocked in kittens, eye dominance does not develop: each neuron continues to respond equally well to signals from either eye. Artificial electric stimulation of the

8 Kittens that do not use their vision during the phase of maximal synapse production (sensitive period), end up with about two-third of the normal number of synapses in the visual cortex. Generalizing from this observation, one-third of synapses in the cerebral cortex may depend on proper use of the functional system in which they participate.
9 It should be emphasized that so-called enriched environments are enriched only as compared with standard laboratory conditions. The latter is a situation of **deprivation** rather than of normality. Both the standard and the enriched-conditions are therefore highly artificial. Nevertheless, when interpreted with caution, experiments with enriched environments give robust evidence of the role of environmental factors in brain development and function.

system "waits" for the right signals. However, if time passes without proper use, the networks seem to be taken over by other systems. In this way, they become less and less accessible for their proper inputs. One example concerns children that are born blind: as adults, their visual areas are activated by somatosensory stimuli (e.g., during Braille reading).

Examples of Sensitive Periods in Humans

Infants born with opaque lenses in their eyes—cataracts—can develop normal vision if the lens is removed at a very early stage. The longer the time before operation, the smaller the chances are that the child will attain normal vision. Persons attaining their sight after puberty (for example, by removal of an opaque lens) have grave difficulties using their sight. The "new" sense may cause trouble rather than being the expected blessing. Some choose to return to life as a blind person. A boy operated on at the age of 8 illustrates this problem. Several months of patient training were needed before he could recognize objects by sight (objects he was familiar with from the use of other senses). The surgeon who treated the boy concluded afterward: "To give back his sight to a congenitally blind patient is more the work of an educationalist than of a surgeon" (cited by Zeki, 1993 , 216). The main reason for the problems encountered by this boy (and others in his situation) is most likely that he had not established the cortical networks needed for integrating visual information with other sensory modalities. Thus, his brain was not capable of using the wealth of information provided by his eyes. In contrast, if the visual system has been used normally during the sensitive period in infancy and early childhood, even many years of temporary blindness have no serious effects on visual capacities.

Another example concerns children who are born deaf and later receive a cochlear implant that supplies the brain with information about sounds of different frequencies. Experience shows that such children can develop useful language and hearing behavior if the implant is provided early—that is, during the first 2 to 3 years of life. As with vision, access to auditory information during the sensitive period is necessary for proper development of the hearing system. To use sounds as basis for development of language, for example, numerous specific connections must be formed in the brain between the auditory cortex and other areas of the cerebral cortex. Such connections cannot be properly formed after the sensitive period. At least in part, this is due to other systems taking over the parts of the cerebral cortex that are normally engaged in auditory functions. Thus, deaf children activate the auditory cortex when using sign language (this is called cross-modal plasticity). Cochlear implants in such children do not restore sound-activation of the auditory cortex.

10 | The Nervous System and Aging

OVERVIEW

Many presumably harmful changes occur in the brain as we grow older. There are, for example, reductions of average brain **weight, synaptic numbers,** and **neurotransmitters.** There is also a loss of myelinated nerve fibers, and together all these changes would be expected to cause less efficient communication in neuronal networks. Age-related changes appear to affect especially networks of the **prefrontal cortex** and the **medial temporal lobe**—regions critically involved in memory and other cognitive functions. Nevertheless, most healthy elderly persons function remarkably well in spite of biologic alterations—with only a minor reduction of recent memory and some slowing of movements and mental processes. This is believed to result from compensatory, use-dependent plasticity initiated in response to the biologic changes. Thus, elderly individuals seem to activate larger parts of the brain when solving mental tasks (often both hemispheres are activated in contrast to strictly unilateral activation in younger people). Aging also entails a fairly marked loss of **peripheral receptors,** which may compromise vision, hearing, and balance. Such loss of peripheral receptors is often more bothersome than the changes occurring in the brain.

In **neurodegenerative diseases,** loss of neurons and their processes usually proceeds for many years before symptoms occur. This is at least partly due to compensatory processes going on in parallel with neuronal loss. The emerging symptoms depend mainly on which parts of the brain are subject to the neuronal loss. In spite of being caused by different mutations, **misfolding** of intracellular proteins occurs in many neurodegenerative diseases. Misfolding appears to initiate cytotoxicity. Neurodegenerative diseases with massive loss of neurons in the cerebral cortex lead to **dementia,** with Alzheimer's disease as the most common. This disease is characterized by—in addition to cortical neuronal loss—degeneration of the cholinergic **basal nucleus** (of Meynert) and marked loss of acetylcholine in the cortex.

AGE-RELATED CHANGES IN THE NORMAL BRAIN AND THEIR CONSEQUENCES

Biologic Changes and Their Interpretations

Comparisons of the brains of young and old persons have revealed several biologic differences. These include a reduction of average brain **weight**, enlargement of ventricles (indicative of tissue atrophy), the appearance of **degenerative patches**, and **neuronal shrinkage** (that occurs primarily in very old people). **Dendritic trees** and **synaptic numbers** appear to be reduced in the cerebral cortex. Reduced **blood flow** of the whole brain or certain regions has been found in several studies. Several other changes, particularly in **neurotransmitters** and their **receptors**, have been reported. With imaging techniques, several alterations have been reported, notably changes of both **gray** and **white matter**. The relationship between biologic changes and impairments of brain performance is still debated, however. This is partly because of conflicting evidence on several important points and uncertain interpretations of findings. Interpretations are hampered, for example, because the biologic differences usually represent small group averages, while the individual differences within each age group may be much larger. Because detailed information of a person's behavioral and cognitive performance is seldom available when examining the brain after death, correlations must be tentative. In animal experiments, formal testing can be performed before examining the brain, enabling more affirmative conclusions regarding the correlation between behavior and age-related brain alterations. Unfortunately, some biologic alterations that are well documented in aged rats and monkeys are controversial in humans.

Nonuniform Distribution of Changes

In spite of the uncertainties just mentioned, one important point seems clear: Alterations of brain structures with advancing age are not uniformly distributed but, rather, are concentrated in specific parts of the brain. Thus, changes in a small part of the cortex may cause functional deficits without significantly affecting overall numbers of neuronal elements. Most consistently, changes have been observed in the **hippocampal formation** and the **prefrontal cortex**. In general, psychological tests show that functions of the brain that are served by these altered parts of the brain also show the most marked reductions by normal aging.

Elderly People Differ Widely with Regard to Brain Functions

It should be emphasized that individual differences with regard to brain functions are as marked among the

Loss of Peripheral Sensory Receptors with Age

For everyday problems of the elderly, changes in the CNS may be less important than loss of sensory cells and neurons of the peripheral sensory organs. These losses are of sight and hearing in particular, but joint sense and sense of equilibrium also deteriorate with advancing age. For example, animal experiments show that muscle stretch receptors (muscle spindles) lose dynamic sensitivity. This might result in slower reflex responses to unexpected, sudden movements of the limbs. In general, thick myelinated, fast conducting fibers are more vulnerable during aging than thin fibers. Especially, impaired proprioception and cutaneous sensation in the lower extremities may contribute to increased risk of falling among the elderly.

Transmission of sensory signals at lower levels of the CNS is serial—that is, the different links in the chain are coupled one after another (see Fig. 14.1). If one link is completely broken, all transmission stops, and the brain cannot compensate for the loss of sensory information. This contrasts with the high degree of parallel processing taking place at higher levels, particularly in the cerebral cortex.

Dizziness and Loss of Vestibular Receptors

Studies of eye movements show that the **vestibuloocular reflex (VOR)** is less accurate in persons older than the age 75 than in younger persons. This reflex ensures that the gaze is kept fixed at one point in the environment when the head rotates (to keep the retinal image stable). Further, **optokinetic eye movements** become more sluggish in old age. Such eye movements are elicited when the environment moves—for example, when looking out of a car—so that the gaze is kept fixed. Suppression of the VOR, which is necessary when the head rotates in the same direction as the visual scene, is also impaired in many elderly persons. All these changes may cause difficulties with vision and orientation while moving, especially if the movement is rapid. This may be an important factor in the dizziness bothering many elderly people. At the cellular level, a major cause of impaired equilibrium and eye movements may be loss of sensory cells in the vestibular apparatus. A 40% loss has been reported in persons 75 years of age.

Plasticity May Compensate for Age-Dependent Losses

As we grow older, potentially harmful changes occur in the brain, as discussed in the preceding text. Yet, most elderly people manage remarkably well and show only minor functional deficits, which often become apparent only in situations with high demands. As said by Denise Park and Patricia Reuter-Lorenz (2008, p. 183): "The puzzle for cognitive neuroscientists is not so much in explaining age-related decline, but rather in understanding the high level of cognitive success that can be maintained by older adults in the face of such significant neurobiological changes." There is now much evidence that this seeming paradox arises because the nervous system remains plastic throughout life (even though the plasticity decreases with advancing age). Thus, even in old age we can learn and thereby upheld functions that are threatened by loss of neuronal elements. Probably, this process is not principally different from what takes place at any age when the brain is challenged—be it by damage or disease, need for new skills, or novel environments.

Interestingly, brain-imaging studies show that elderly and young people have different patterns of **cortical activation** during cognitive tasks, even when performance is equal. In particular, processes that are strongly lateralized in the young are more evenly divided between the two hemispheres in the elderly (Fig. 10.1). Much evidence supports that this activation pattern in the elderly is a sign of functional compensation rather than of faulty processing. For example, the tendency to use both hemispheres is associated with higher performance compared with other elderly persons using mainly one hemisphere. Elderly persons show less hippocampal activation than young people on certain **memory** tests, presumably because of age-related alterations in the hippocampal region. Among the elderly, those showing increased prefrontal activation (compared with young persons and age-matched controls) performed better on memory tests than those with less prefrontal activation. This suggests that increased prefrontal activation in the

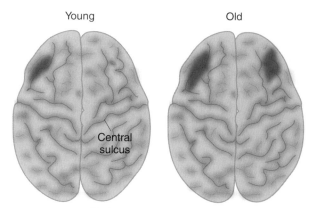

Prefrontal activation during a demanding cognitive task

FIGURE 10.1 *Altered brain activation patterns in the elderly.* Comparisons with functional MRI of young and elderly people (older than 65 years) during execution of various cognitive tasks shows clear differences. This figure shows (in a very simplified form) that during a demanding verb-generation task, elderly persons activate the prefrontal cortex on both sides, whereas young people activate only one side (differences are apparent also in other parts of the brain). This extra activation most likely is due to compensatory (plastic) processes. It would mean that elderly people, while solving the task as well as young people, must allocate more resources to the task.

elderly compensates for reduced performance of the hippocampal region. Disrupting cortical processing by transcranial magnetic stimulation (TMS) supports that the bilateral frontal activation in the elderly is of functional significance. Thus, in the young, TMS of the left prefrontal region influenced memory performance most severely, while in older adults application to either the left or the right hemisphere reduced their performance equally. Also for successful **motor performance**, larger parts of the cortex and the cerebellum are recruited in elderly than in young persons.

Together, these and other observations strongly suggest that plastic changes occur in the aging brain, and that they counteract the detrimental effects of age-related loss of neural elements.

The Benefit of Experience

Normal aging does not affect everyday activities significantly. Indeed, it appears that all activities (motor or intellectual) that have become highly automated by long practice are quite resistant to age-dependent decline. Both speed and precision can then be maintained into advancing age. We need only think of musicians, such as Rubinstein and Horowitz, performing with excellence after 80. Preserved superior spatial memory in old taxi drivers provides another example of the effect of experience. Further, a study comparing young and old bridge and chess players concluded that there was no clear age-related decline in performance, with prior experience being more important than the player's age. A generally reduced short-term memory in the older players is presumably compensated by superior card recognition and specific memory for cards. Thus, old experienced players remembered more cards after a 1-second exposure than young untrained ones did, and this difference persisted even if the younger players were given more time. Another example of the beneficial effect of experience comes from a study comparing old and young bank employees. Although the older employees scored on average less on reasoning tests than the younger ones did, this did not correlate with poorer job performance. In conclusion, specific experience and continuous training appears to be more important for performance than normal age-related reductions in cognitive functions.

Presumably, continuous use of neural systems makes them more resistant to age-related impairment. One reason may be that more neurons are included in task-specific networks.[2] This might make the networks more robust and less vulnerable to a loss of synapses and

other elements. Further, age-related changes may be slowed by use-dependent production of growth factors and neurotrophins. Finally, by continuously challenging the systems, compensation by recruiting additional neuronal groups would counteract the inevitable negative effects of aging on the brain.

Physical Exercise May Protect the Aging Brain

There is evidence from both experimental animals and humans that physical training (especially cardiovascular conditioning) can improve cognition. This has also been examined specifically with regard to the aging population. For example, a study including more than 5000 women older than 65 years showed that those with the highest level of physical activity were less likely to develop cognitive decline during the next 6 to 8 years. Other studies indicate that **aerobic capacity**—as expressed in maximal oxygen uptake—is the factor most clearly linked with beneficial effects on cognitive functions. Especially executive cognitive processes—such as planning, task coordination, and working memory—seem to benefit from aerobic training. Increased production of **BDNF** (brain derived neurotrophic factor)—known to enhance neuronal plasticity—may mediate some of the effects of physical training on the brain.

NEURODEGENERATIVE DISEASES AND DEMENTIA

Dementia

Dementia can be defined as an acquired, global impairment of intellect, reason, and personality, but without impairment of consciousness. It is uncommon before the age of 60 but occurs with increasing frequency, especially after the age of 75. One-third of people older than 85 years of age may exhibit signs of dementia; although with varying severity. Dementia can have different causes, but all cases share extensive damage to neurons and connections of the cerebral cortex. One cause of dementia is loss of brain tissue due to ischemic brain lesions. Usually, the patient has suffered from repeated small infarctions of the white matter, causing **vascular cognitive impairment** (VCI).[3] Dementia can also be caused by **intoxications** (alcohol, solvents, and carbon monoxide), large **tumors**, or **infections** (for example, HIV).

Neurodegenerative diseases leading to progressive neuronal loss, however, cause most cases of dementia. Most people in the latter group have **Alzheimer's disease** (AD). This disease was described just after 1900 as

---

2 London taxi drivers were found to have larger hippocampi than controls, and the difference increased with increasing experience (Maguire et al. 2000). Presumably, this represents a learning effect caused by their long-term engagement in spatial navigation.

3 Vascular cognitive impairment was formerly termed vascular dementia, and that term is still widely used. Cerebrovascular lesions may be the main cause in as many as 15% of all patients with dementia.

a distinct kind of dementia, which characteristically developed before the age of 60 (**presenile dementia**). Around 1970 it was realized, however, that the majority of cases of dementia beginning after age 60 also are of the Alzheimer kind. Despite all the research since then, so far, no one theory can explain the complex biochemical and pathological aspects of this devastating disease. **Frontotemporal dementia** (FTD) is less common than Alzheimer's disease and affects different parts of the cerebral cortex. This explains why the symptoms differ in these two forms of dementia. In many patients, multiple cerebrovascular lesions may coexist with Alzheimer pathology, aggravating the cognitive deficits (mixed type dementia).

Common Molecular Mechanisms in Neurodegenerative Diseases

Alzheimer's disease, Parkinson's disease, Huntington's disease, amyotrophic lateral sclerosis (ALS), and other neurodegenerative diseases have in common that neurons slowly die in a long period preceding the debut of neurologic symptoms. These diseases affect different parts of the nervous system, occur in different age groups, and show different heritability. They therefore present as separate disease entities. They may nevertheless share basic cellular malfunctions that eventually cause neuronal death. One common finding is that neurons accumulate large amounts of **misfolded** proteins, which thereby induce cytotoxicity. Various factors, such as gene mutations, environmental influences, and aging may induce misfolding of proteins. Most likely, a modest amount of misfolded proteins occurs normally, and cellular processes are disturbed only when the amount of misfolded proteins exceeds the cell's capacity to remove them. Disturbed cellular processes comprise transcription, energy handling, axonal transport, synaptic function, and apoptosis. Apparently, different mutations can produce similar clinical pictures, the crucial point being which neuronal populations are affected. Thus, dementia will ensue if sufficient numbers of neurons in certain parts of the cerebral cortex die, regardless of the cause of cellular death. Neurodegenerative diseases are characterized by clumps of misfolded proteins—**inclusion bodies**—in the neuronal cytoplasm. Most likely, damaging effects of the misfolded proteins is exerted before they are collected in clumps, with the latter representing just the end stage in a cascade of molecular events.

Alzheimer's Disease

There is now little doubt that Alzheimer's disease (AD) represents a distinct disease entity, not just an exaggerated form of normal aging. The disease manifests itself by gradual decline of mental functions. Impaired recent memory is an early sign: the person forgets appointments and names, repeats questions, and may appear confused and helpless. There is typically a loss of interest and initiative, and a neglect of daily activities. Initial symptoms are usually vague and hard to distinguish from normal aging. In some patients, the early signs of dementia may be misdiagnosed as depression. If such patients receive antidepressant drugs, their condition can deteriorate dramatically with confusion, loss of bladder control, and other symptoms. This may probably be explained, at least in part, by the anticholinergic effect of such drugs.

Microscopically, **senile plaques** and **neurofibrillary tangles** in the cerebral cortex characterize AD. The latter consist of thickened, intraneuronal fibrils. The senile plaques are patchy, degenerative changes with extracellular deposits of amyloid and other proteins, in which **amyloid β-protein** (Aβ) is a major component. The plaques also contain many abnormal axon terminals. Aβ is formed from a large membrane protein called **amyloid precursor protein** (APP). We do not know the function of APP, but it is present normally in most neurons and is transported anterogradely in the axons to the terminals. Aβ is normally secreted from neurons, and we do not know why it precipitates in AD. The **neurofibrillary tangles** consist of a specific kind of filament (**paired helical filaments**; PHF). A major component of PHF is an abnormal kind of the microtubule-associated protein **tau**. The protein lacks its normal ability to attach to microtubules, however, and this may explain why tau aggregates as abnormal filaments.

There is a marked loss of **synapses** in AD, as shown via electron microscopic observations. Most notable are losses in the layers two and three of the cerebral cortex (see Fig. 33.1) that send out and receive association connections. Figure 10.2 shows the typical distribution of early changes in the form of cortical atrophy. The pathologic changes are more severe in the **association areas** of the frontal and temporal lobes than in the primary sensory and motor areas. The earliest changes appear to occur regularly in the **entorhinal cortex** (part of the hippocampal region in the medial temporal lobe). It appears that severity of dementia shows a closer correlation with the degree of synaptic loss than with the density of senile plaques and neurofibrillary tangles. What causes the cell loss (and loss of synapses) is not quite clear, although both Aβ and tau are involved in the process. Neither is the relationship between these two actors clear. The so-called **amyloid-cascade hypothesis** implies that overproduction of Aβ leads to amyloid precipitation that induces formation of neurofibrillary tangles, which then cause neuronal death.

Alzheimer patients have a severe neuronal loss in a diffusely distributed cell group at the base of the cerebral hemispheres, called the **basal nucleus** (of Meynert) (Fig. 10.3). Many neurons in this nucleus are cholinergic and send

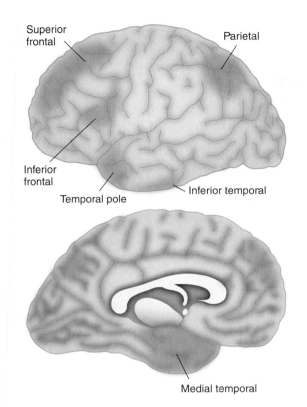

Superior frontal

Parietal

Inferior frontal

Temporal pole

Inferior temporal

Medial temporal

FIGURE 10.2 *The distribution of cortical atrophy in early stages of Alzheimer's disease.* The blue patches show approximate locations of regions with the most marked thinning of the cortex, based on quantitative analysis of MRI data. More extensive parts of the cortex become atrophic as the disease progresses. (Based on data of Dickerson et al. 2009.)

their axons to the cerebral cortex (see Chapter 31, under "Cholinergic Neurons Projecting to the Cerebral Cortex"). Loss of neurons in the basal nucleus may therefore explain why Alzheimer patients have severely reduced amounts of **acetylcholine** in the cortex. Acetylcholine raises the

excitability and improves the signal-to-noise ratio of cortical neurons, enhancing their ability to handle information rapidly and accurately. These facts form the basis of the first pharmacological treatment of AD, which aimed at increasing the amount of acetylcholine available in the cerebral cortex.

The relationship between the loss of basal nucleus neurons and the pathological changes in the cerebral cortex is not clear, however. Thus, not all aspects of the functional impairment in AD can be induced by destruction of the basal nucleus in experimental animals. Further, transmitters other than acetylcholine are also affected by AD. Many monoaminergic neurons die in the locus coeruleus and the raphe nuclei, which may explain why the levels of **norepinephrine** and **serotonin** in the cortex are markedly reduced. Depleting the cerebral cortex of acetylcholine, norepinephrine, or serotonin (rats) triggers a rapid rise of APP synthesis. Such transmitter depletion can be produced by destroying the basal nucleus, the raphe nuclei, or the locus coeruleus. These findings suggest, first, that APP synthesis is normally controlled by synaptic actions and, second, that precipitation of amyloid might be caused by loss of transmitter actions.

Even though patients with AD are quite similar with regard to brain pathology and clinical manifestations, they differ in terms of causal factors. **Heritability** plays a variable role but is especially important in patients with an early onset of symptoms (before 60 years). Many in the latter group inherit the disease dominantly. These patients have mutations of three genes: two genes coding for **presenilins** (1 and 2) and the *APP gene*. All three mutations increase Aβ synthesis. The much more common late-onset AD shows less obvious familial accumulation of cases. A large number of genes have been implicated as possible risk factors, however.

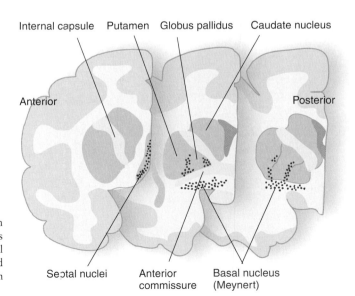

Internal capsule   Putamen   Globus pallidus   Caudate nucleus

Anterior

Posterior

Septal nuclei   Anterior commissure   Basal nucleus (Meynert)

FIGURE 10.3 *The basal nucleus (of Meynert).* Frontal section through the left hemisphere (monkey). The cholinergic neurons of the basal nucleus are indicated with red dots. The basal nucleus is continuous anteriorly with the septal nuclei and other cholinergic cell groups of the forebrain. (Redrawn from Richardson and DeLong 1988.)

For example, persons with the *ApoE4* gene (coding for a apolipoprotein) run a much higher risk of AD than do persons with genes for another variety of apolipoprotein. Apolipoproteins normally transport cholesterol in the blood. ApoE4, however, also binds to amyloid β-protein and is present in senile plaques and neurofibrillary tangles. Therefore, it may facilitate the precipitation of amyloid.

Frontotemporal Dementia

Perhaps as many of 15% of all patients with dementia have **frontotemporal dementia** (FTD), formerly called **Pick's disease.** It can be distinguished from AD by the distribution of degenerative changes, which affect primarily frontal and temporal parts of the cerebral cortex. Further, the initial symptoms are behavioral aberrations, typical for lesions of the affected regions, rather than loss of memory (patients with FTD are often misdiagnosed as suffering from a psychiatric disease). Both FTD and AD, however, are associated with abnormal phosphorylation of the microtubule-associated protein **tau.**

11 | Restitution of Function after Brain Damage

OVERVIEW

Whatever the nature of the insult, brain damage ultimately leads to loss of neurons and their interconnections. Although new neurons are produced in limited parts of the adult brain, there is no effective replacement of lost neurons after brain damage. Reduced or abolished blood supply—ischemia—initiates a cascade of cellular events ending in cell death. Excessive release of **glutamate** and ensuing **excitation** appear to be crucial steps in a vicious cycle. In a region with focal ischemia (e.g., caused by occlusion of an artery) there is central zone where all cells will die and a peripheral zone—the **penumbra**—with diminished supply, in which neurons may silenced but do not die. They may be rescued if circulation is restored within a certain time (e.g., by thrombolytic drugs or reduction in edema).

The nervous system retains its **plasticity** throughout life, and this property is a prerequisite for recovery of function after damage of nervous tissue. Yet what changes do occur in the brain when a patient recovers functions after a stroke or other acute brain insults? Judging from animal experiments and brain imaging studies of human stroke patients, recovery is due to a learning process in which remaining parts of the brain are modified. We call this process **substitution**. The modification is driven by continuous efforts to perform tasks that were made difficult or impossible by the brain damage. Crucial factors determining the degree of progress are **motivation, focused attention, and amount of training**. Stroke patients who have recovered activate much larger parts of the cortex than normal persons when performing simple movements. In addition, plastic changes may be **compensatory**, in the sense that they do not restore the lost function but reduces disturbing symptoms or enable goal attainment by other means than those enabled by the damaged parts of the brain.

Infants with **early brain damage** may in some cases recover remarkably well, especially if lesions (even very large ones) are confined to one hemisphere. In other instances, with bilateral or lesions affecting deeper parts of the brain (basal ganglia, brain stem), complex functional impairments become stable and may even worsen during the first years of life. This may at least partly be due to a disturbance of ongoing developmental processes.

BRAIN INJURIES AND POSSIBLE REPARATIVE PROCESSES

Ischemic Cell Damage

Abolished or reduced blood supply to an organ is called **ischemia**. Regardless of cause, even a few minutes of severe brain ischemia can produce massive neuronal death, but, surprisingly, the neurons often do not die until several hours after the ischemic episode. This is so because the lack of oxygen (hypoxia) and glucose triggers a cascade of events, in which each step takes some time but results eventually in neuronal death. Although many factors are implied, **glutamate** and glutamate receptors are under particularly strong suspicion as the main villains of this drama. Thus, ischemia leads to excessive release of glutamate (see later, "The Glutamate Hypothesis," and Chapter 5, under "NMDA Receptors: Mediators of Both Learning and Neuronal Damage"). In an ischemic region, whether it is due to edema, bleeding (e.g., after head injuries), or vascular occlusion, there is usually a central zone where the ischemia is so severe that all neurons die.[1] Outside this region, however, there is a zone—the **penumbra** (from Latin *paere* = almost, and *umbra* = shadow)—characterized by neurons that are nonfunctional (unexcitable) but still viable.

The discovery of the delay between an ischemic episode and irreversible cell damage initiated an enormous research activity to find drugs that prevent or reduce the brain damage. In clinical situations, **focal ischemia** due to occlusion of a brain artery by thrombosis or embolus is more common than **global ischemia** (shutting down the blood supply to the whole brain, as can occur in cardiac arrest). In cases of focal ischemia hopes were raised to reduce the size of the brain infarct by

---

1 Cell death in the central region completely devoid of blood supply is due to necrosis, as judged from the electron microscopic appearance. There is some evidence that apoptosis may cause cell death in the penumbra.

keeping neurons in the penumbra alive until the circulation improves (improvement may occur spontaneously or by use of thrombolytic drugs that dissolve the vascular obstruction). So far, however, the results with **glutamate-receptor blockers** (especially of the N-methyl-D-aspartate [NMDA] receptor) have been disappointing in humans in spite of convincing results in animal experiments. One problem has been intolerable side effects with the doses that are necessary to obtain protection. This might not be surprising considering that glutamatergic transmission participates in virtually every neuronal network. Another reason for the failure of numerous attempts to achieve neuroprotection after stroke may be that although the activation of NMDA receptors undoubtedly is harmful in the early stages of a stroke, it may be necessary for recovery in the delayed phase. Further, it appears that the cellular events evolving in the penumbra are much more complex than assumed—with regard to both the number of substances involved and the temporal profile of cellular changes.

Excessive release of glutamate cannot readily explain *all* aspects of ischemic cell death, however. For example, after global ischemia, the cell death is not diffusely distributed. Especially **vulnerable** are the neurons in the CA1 field of the hippocampus (see Fig. 32.10). Regional differences in glutamate release or glutamate receptors are probably not the reason. More likely explanations concern differences among regions regarding the presence and regulation of neurotrophic factors.

The Glutamate Hypothesis of Ischemic Cell Damage

According to the glutamate hypothesis, the sequence of events after a temporary stop of blood flow may be as follows (Fig. 11.1):

1. The loss of energy supply rapidly reduces the activity of the sodium–potassium pump, leading to (among other things)
2. Increased extracellular K^+ concentration that depolarizes the neurons so they fire bursts of action potentials, which leads to
3. Steadily worsening imbalances of ion concentrations across the cell membrane that make the neuron incapable of firing action potentials (electrically silent), while at the same time
4. The extracellular glutamate concentration rises steeply (because, among other things, the ionic imbalances reverse the pumping of glutamate by high-affinity transporters), leading to
5. Enormous activation of glutamate receptors, among them NMDA receptors; this in turn is believed to induce
6. Cell damage, probably because of an uncontrolled rise in intracellular Ca^{2+} concentration. This may harm the cell in various ways, for example, by activating

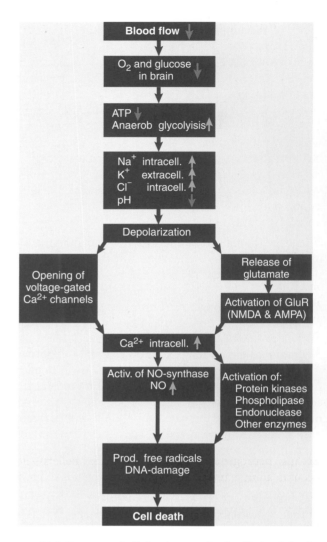

FIGURE 11.1 *Sequence of cellular changes after focal ischemia leading to cell death (hypothetical).* (Based on Samdani et al. 1997.)

enzymes that degrade proteins and nucleic acids and by activating nitric oxide (NO) synthases that leads to production of free radicals. In turn this destroys other vital enzymes.

7. Before the strong inflow of calcium there is an inflow of Na^+ accompanied by Cl^- and water, which causes neurons and glia to swell.

That **NMDA receptors** are involved in ischemic cell death is indirectly supported by animal experiments involving NMDA-receptor blockers. If such drugs are given even a few hours after an ischemic episode, they reduce or prevent the cell damage. Also, blockers of AMPA receptors provide protection against ischemic cell death in such experiments.

Neurogenesis: Production of New Neurons in the Adult Brain

In adult mammals, new neurons are produced continuously in parts of the subventricular zone and the dentate gyrus of the hippocampal formation (see Fig. 32.10). The neurons produced in the subventricular zone migrate into the olfactory bulb (claims that some also populate the cerebral cortex have not been substantiated). Although only a minority of the newly formed neurons appears to survive, some are incorporated into existing networks. The finding that the number of surviving neurons is use-dependent further strengthens the assumption that the new neurons are of functional significance. Neurogenesis thus seems to represent an additional but spatially restricted form of plasticity, supplementing the ubiquitous synaptic plasticity discussed earlier in this book. It remains to be determined, however, how much and in what way neurogenesis contributes to the role of hippocampus in memory formation.

Nevertheless, adult neurogenesis has attracted much interest and raised hopes that it may be induced in regions with neuronal loss due to injury or disease. Indeed, increased neurogenesis occurred in the subventricular zone after ischemic brain injury in rats, and some neurons were incorporated in adjacent parts of the striatum. The clinical relevance of such observations is not yet known, however.

Why Is Neurogenesis and Regeneration So Restricted in the Human Brain?

Because neurogenesis—contrary to earlier beliefs—*does* occur in adult mammals, one may ask why it is so limited in distribution. Thus, in reptiles and birds neurogenesis occurs in large parts of the nervous system. One reason may be that new neurons might be disturbing rather than beneficial if not properly integrated with existing networks, and that the increasing complexity of the mammalian brain has rendered successful integration of new neurons less likely. Mutations that diminished neurogenesis may therefore have given an evolutionary advantage. The situation in the dentate gyrus may be special because of its specific role in memory acquisition—perhaps "ordinary" synaptic changes are insufficient or less efficacious than addition of new neurons.

Further, it is probably not coincidental that the mature CNS produces substances that **inhibit axonal growth** (such substances are not present during early development). An uncontrolled axonal growth in the mature brain might cause harm rather than help restitution. Correspondingly, although supply of growth promoting factors after brain damage might rescue sick neurons and promote axonal growth, it might also be expected to disturb the connections and functions of the healthy neurons.

Axonal Regeneration in the CNS—Hope for Spinal Cord Repair?

Why do severed axons regenerate in the peripheral nervous system but not in the CNS? This question, puzzling neuroscientists for a century, has recently been answered at least partly. Thus, in the adult brain, the **growth cone** of an axon trying to regenerate quickly collapses due to the presence of inhibitory substances. Among several such substances, **myelin-associated proteins** produced by oligodendroglia have been most thoroughly studied. The proteins bind to receptors in the membrane of the growth cone and activate intracellular pathways that quickly down-regulate protein synthesis. In addition, scar formation at the site of injury also inhibits axonal regeneration.

Central axons may regenerate under certain conditions, however. Thus, the proximal stump of a cut central axon can grow into a piece of peripheral nerve if it contains viable **Schwann cells**. Indeed, growth of central axons for several centimeters has been demonstrated in nerve transplants in experimental animals. Another special kind of glial cell—**olfactory ensheathing cells (OECs)**—can also induce growth of central axons and has been subject to clinical trials. These cells cover the olfactory-receptor cell axons that extend from the nasal mucosa to the olfactory bulb. Interestingly, the olfactory receptor cells are renewed throughout life, and the OECs provide a permissive environment enabling the axons to grow into the CNS. Local supply of substances that block the growth-inhibiting proteins combined with transplantation of OECs is now used experimentally in patients with transverse lesions of the cord in the hope of inducing axonal regeneration across the lesion. So far, however—in spite of positive results in experimental animals—such procedures have not provided convincing functional improvement in patients. Animal studies (rodents) suggest that a combination of regeneration-promoting local measures and active rehabilitation might give the best results.

Collateral Sprouting Can Aid Restitution

Neurons that have lost their afferents may be supplied with new ones from normal axons in the vicinity. This is called **collateral sprouting**. After cutting afferent axons to a neuronal group (deafferentation), the axons degenerate and glial cells remove their nerve terminals. In a relatively short time, however, new nerve terminals fill the vacant synaptic sites. This probably occurs because a trophic substance becomes available from the deafferented neurons. The trophic substance stimulates nearby normal axons to send out sprouts. Obviously, collateral sprouting can only act locally in restoration of neuronal activity. There is no evidence that it can restore connections between more distant cell groups. Nor do all systems seem to exhibit collateral sprouting. Neither can collateral sprouting restore the original pattern of innervation because the neurons responsible for that pattern are gone. Thus, there will always be a loss of specificity of connections, compared with the normal situation. Indeed, restitution of function seen after brain damage usually entails a loss of precision; for example, recovery of movement force is usually better than recovery of the ability to carry out delicate movements.

Although collateral sprouting probably aids recovery in many situations, it may not always be beneficial. For example, after a stroke that damages the motor pathways descending from the cerebral cortex, axon collaterals from sensory neurons may fill the vacant synaptic sites on motor neurons in the cord. This would not help to improve the voluntary control of the muscles but might, rather, contribute to the abnormally increased reactivity of the muscles to sensory stimuli that is characteristic of such cases (as in **spasticity**).

Can We Help Restitution by Neurotrophic Factors, Drugs, or Transplantation?

The well-established effects of **neurotrophins** and **growth factors** on plasticity and neuronal survival raise the question of whether they can be used therapeutically. Thus, one might expect that raising the level of such substances in the damaged brain might rescue neurons and stimulate the plastic changes necessary for restitution. The application in the CNS of such substances meets difficulties, however. Because they are proteins, the substances do not pass the blood–brain barrier readily, and even if they are delivered directly into the cerebrospinal fluid, their tissue penetration is restricted. Also, long-term supply of proteins to the brain may have uncontrollable actions and perhaps dangerous side effects. Therefore, the hope is to develop drugs that can stimulate the synthesis of specific neurotrophic factors in the brain itself or to improve their penetration of the blood–brain barrier.

Drugs that increase brain levels of **monoamines** (e.g., amphetamine) help recovery after brain lesions in experimental animals, apparently by increasing plasticity. From a theoretical point of view, it seems likely that the same would apply to humans. Indeed, some studies suggest that amphetamine speeds up recovery in stroke patients. Presumably, the effect would be best when combined with function-specific training.

Another means of helping restitution might be to replace lost neurons by **transplantation** of neural precursor cells—**neuroblasts**—into damaged regions. Embryonic neurons can still send out axons, provided the embryo is so young that the neuroblasts have not yet sent out axons. Besides numerous animal experiments, this approach has been tried in a limited number of patients with Parkinson's disease, giving promising results. Animal experiments show convincingly that neuroblasts can survive and send out axons after transplantation to an adult brain. If they are transplanted to a site where the adult neurons have been destroyed, the axons may even reach the normal targets of the destroyed neurons. Functional restoration has also been demonstrated in some studies. Embryonic neuroblasts are obviously not affected by the myelin-associated factors that normally inhibit axonal growth in the mature CNS.

Many problems complicate the transplantations of embryonic tissue, however. One is the ethical issue of using brains of early abortions for therapy. Neuroblasts grown in culture may replace embryonic cells, however. Such cells may also be genetically modified to, for example, improve survival in the host. Other problems with neural transplantations are technical, such as the necessity for growth over long distances in the human brain (as compared with the rat) and survival of a sufficient number of neuroblasts. The chances of success are best with restoring diffusely organized, fairly short connections, whereas chances are presumably remote with precisely organized, long-ranging connections in the human brain.

BRAIN PROCESSES UNDERLYING RECOVERY OF FUNCTION

Substitution and Compensation

Differentiated neurons are unable to divide mitotically, and the brain does not possess a store of undifferentiated neurons that can multiply and replace lost ones (with some possible exceptions, as discussed earlier). Thus, as a rule, dead neurons are not replaced. We also know that cut axons do not regenerate in the CNS (the latter in contrast to the peripheral nervous system). Therefore, a reparative process in which the damaged structures regenerate or are replaced by new ones cannot explain the recovery of function after brain damage. Rather, recovery must be due to changes among the remaining undamaged neurons and glial cells. Indeed, there is much evidence to suggest that neural circuits **reorganize** to adapt to a novel situation. We discuss two kinds of adaptation next, both of which can probably best be regarded as **learning processes**.

In one type of adaptation—which we call **substitution**—intact neuronal groups take over and substitute for the damaged parts. The neuronal groups responsible for the substitution normally carry out tasks similar to those of the damaged ones. Thus, after a stroke destroys the cell groups that are responsible for initiating certain kinds of movement, the cells responsible for other kinds of movements may take over to some extent. For example, other cortical areas may partially substitute for functions lost when a lesion destroys the **primary motor cortex**, and neuronal groups that normally control only one side of the body may expand their activity to the other side as well. Substitution can seldom restore a system to its premorbid functional level, however. After all, an amateur, who still has to take care of his former duties, has replaced a specialist!

The other kind of adaptation, called **compensation**, implies that any remaining structures change their normal activity to diminish disturbing symptoms produced by the injury. This is relevant when the brain damage not only leads to loss of functions, such as muscular weakness or sensory loss, but also produces disturbing phenomena such as involuntary movements or sensory confusion. For example, unilateral destruction of the **vestibular apparatus** in the inner ear initially causes severe dizziness and disturbances of posture and eye movements. This is due to a mismatch between the vestibular information reaching the brain from the two sides of the body. The symptoms usually subside quickly, because the vestibular system compensates by altering its sensitivity and information handling. Although this does not normalize the sense of equilibrium, it reduces disturbing symptoms. By substitution, the brain can learn to rely on other sources of information to control posture and movements. Thus, the postural adjustments necessary for the upright position gradually improve because visual information substitutes for vestibular. When denied the use of vision (as in the dark), the person becomes very unsteady.

Some patients do not recover useful function of a body part after brain injury. To some extent goals can still be achieved by using other movement strategies, for example, using the (normal) left arm instead of the paralyzed right, using a stick to keep balance, using both hands instead of one, and so forth. Also in such cases, the degree of success depends on a learning process, even though the level of performance as a rule will be severely reduced compared with the normal situation. This may also be regarded as a form of compensation, and should be distinguished from substitution.

Restitution after a Stroke Can Be Divided into Two Phases

After a person has a stroke, there is usually a **first phase** of rapid improvement lasting from days to weeks, followed by a **second phase** of slower progress lasting from months to years. Acute damage to neural tissue is usually caused by head injuries with crushing of neural tissue and bleeding or by vascular occlusion caused by thrombosis or an embolus. Secondary changes occur in the penumbra (the tissue surrounding the damaged area) such as edema (tissue swelling) and disturbed local circulation. If the edema subsides quickly and the circulation improves in the penumbra, neurons will regain their normal activity (compare with the transient weakness and loss of cutaneous sensation produced by pressure on a peripheral nerve). This is probably why there is often a marked improvement of the patient's condition during the first week or two after the accident.

For example, an arm that was totally paralyzed the day after a stroke may in a matter of days be only slightly weaker and clumsier than before the stroke. However, when the condition deteriorates rapidly after the initial insult, the reason is usually that the edema worsens and compromises the blood supply to more and more of the brain.

Certainly, plastic changes occur shortly after an injury (hours, days), as witnessed by animal experiments. Thus, there is probably no sharp distinction between the rapid and the slow phases of recovery—the nervous system starts its adaptation to the new circumstances immediately.

Methods to Study Neuronal Activity and Connectivity in the Living Brain

Throughout this book, references are made to studies using brain imaging techniques, particularly those that enable determination of regional cerebral blood flow (see Chapter 8, under "Regional Cerebral Blood Flow and Neuronal Activity"). Because of the link between a change of neuronal activity and local cerebral blood flow, the flow of blood through specific parts of the brain can be correlated with certain stimuli or specific sensory, motor, or mental activities. Computer tomography (CT) can be used to visualize the distribution of a radioactive substance in the living brain. This method, called **positron emission tomography** (PET), is based on the use of isotopes that emit positrons. Positrons fuse immediately with electrons, producing two gamma rays going in opposite directions, thus permitting the identification of their origin in the brain with the aid of a powerful computer. PET produces images that show the distribution of an inhaled or injected radioactively labeled substance at a given time. By labeling substances of biological interest, one can determine their distribution in the body. In the case of **blood flow** measurement, radioactively labeled water is injected into the bloodstream. **Functional MRI (fMRI)** is the other main method to visualize dynamic changes in the brain. This method is based on the fact that the magnetic properties of hemoglobin depend on whether or not it is oxygenated, and small differences in blood oxyhemoglobin concentration can be detected with MRI. For unknown reasons, the oxygen uptake of nerve cells does not increase simultaneously with increased activity. Thus, it appears that neurons work anaerobically during a brief period of increased activity, despite a sufficient oxygen supply. The glucose uptake increases, however, and so does the blood flow. When the blood flow increases without increased oxygen uptake, more oxygen remains in the blood after passing the capillaries—that is, the arteriovenous O_2 difference is reduced. MRI can detect this change, and in this way the regions of increased or reduced blood flow can be visualized. An advantage over PET is that the picture of blood flow changes can be compared with the precise MRI picture of the same person's brain. This permits localization of blood flow changes to anatomic structures with a spatial resolution down to less than 2 mm.

A drawback of blood flow measurement as an indicator of neuronal activity is its low time resolution compared with the time scale for signal transmission in the brain. In this respect, recording the electrical activity of the brain is superior. This is usually done by placing many electrodes on the head and is called **electroencephalography** (**EEG**, see Chapter 26, under "Electroencephalography"). EEG has been developed to enable study of topographic patterns of cerebral activation in relation to the performance of specific tasks, and coherence of EEG activity in different cortical areas suggests that the areas are functionally interconnected.

A drawback with EEG is its low spatial resolution, which means that only a crude correlation is possible between electrical activity and its origin in the brain. A more recent technique, **magnetic encephalography** (**MEG**), records the magnetic fields produced by the electric activity of the brain. The spatial resolution is much better than with EEG—at best, down to a few millimeters. (For both methods, however, the spatial resolution becomes poorer the deeper in the brain the source of activity is located.) A further advantage with the MEG technique is that it can be combined with MRI. This enables precise localization of the brain areas participating in a task, at the same time as the temporal aspects are analyzed (such as the sequence in which various cell groups are activated).

Electric stimulation of the brain through the skull (transcranially) requires an intensity that causes pain, and is therefore seldom used. With **transcranial magnetic stimulation** (**TMS**; also termed magnetic brain stimulation), however, neurons in the cerebral cortex can be activated painlessly with a short, intense magnetic pulse applied to the head. The magnetic field penetrates the skull and creates an electric current in the brain, primarily in the outer parts of the cerebral cortex. Magnetic brain stimulation also enables study of how disruption of normal activity in a specific part of the cortex affects behavior and cognitive functions.

Connectivity in the living brain can be studied with **TMS** and with **diffusion-weighted imaging** (**DWI**). TMS has been used to study the connections between the motor cortex and the spinal cord in healthy persons and in persons with motor dysfunction (e.g., multiple sclerosis). It can also be used to study whether parts of the brain are interconnected, and in particular, whether connectivity changes in the course of therapeutic interventions (such as rehabilitative training programs for stroke patients). DWI (and further developments of this method) enables visualization of major pathways in the brain, such as connections among various cortical areas, and between the cerebral cortex and subcortical nuclei. The method cannot determine the polarity of connections and the spatial resolution is limited. Provided the results are critically evaluated in conjunction with experimental tracing data from primates, the method gives important information.

Studies of Recovery after a Stroke in Humans

Many stroke patients have muscular weakness (pareses) in the opposite side of the body as a dominating symptom. This is called **hemiplegia** (*hemi*, half; *plegia*, from Greek *plegé*, stroke). The symptoms are caused by destruction (due to occlusion of an artery or a bleeding) of motor pathways from the cerebral cortex to the brain stem and the cord (see Fig. 22.3). Usually, the injury occurs in the internal capsule (see Fig. 22.13) where the descending fibers from the cerebral cortex are collected. When such injuries cause hemiplegia, we use the term **capsular hemiplegia**. Because patients with this clinical condition are so common, and because the site of their injury is usually well localized, they have been the subjects for many studies of restitution. Some examples elucidating mechanisms behind restitution in humans are presented here.

Regional cerebral blood flow is closely linked with neuronal activity. Thus, when we find altered blood flow—using **PET** or **fMRI** brain imaging—in a specific part of the brain after a stroke, it is taken as evidence of altered activity caused by the stroke. One group of patients with capsular hemiplegia was tested 3 months after the stroke. They were then completely or substantially recovered; for example, they could all perform opposition movements with the fingers. The test was to touch the thumb sequentially with the fingers, in a rhythm determined by a metronome. In normal control persons, this task is associated with increased blood flow primarily in the opposite **motor cortex** (and in subcortical motor regions like the cerebellum and the basal ganglia). This fits with the fact that the pyramidal tract, which is necessary for precise finger movements, originates in the motor cortex and is crossed. The patients differed from the controls by showing increased activity in cortical areas that are not normally activated in this kind of simple, routine movement, notably in parts of the, **insula, posterior parietal cortex,** and **cingulate gyrus.** In controls, these areas show increased activity with complex movements and problem-solving tasks that require extra attention. The regions have in common that they send association connections to the **premotor area** (PMA; see Fig. 22.10) and by this route can influence voluntary movements. Indeed, increased activity is also present in the premotor area. In addition, some of the patients differed from the controls by showing increased activity in motor cortical areas on the same (ipsilateral) side as the affected hand. Such findings suggest that functional recovery after hemiplegia is related to the patients learning to use larger parts of the cerebral cortex for control of simple finger movements than before the damage, and their using motor areas on the same side as the pareses. A large number of studies confirm the above findings, although the exact distribution of activation may vary somewhat among studies. Use of **transcranial magnetic stimulation** (TMS) in restituted stroke patients has furthermore showed that not only are cortical activation differently distributed but there is also evidence of altered connectivity, as assessed in a resting situation. Further support for **structural changes** during recovery comes from use of MRI-based morphometry, suggesting that an intense rehabilitative training program is associated with increased cortical gray matter in the regions most activated by movements.

The involvement of larger parts of the cerebral cortex may explain why simple, previously effortless movements require so much more **attention** and **mental energy** than before the stroke. There is evidence that descending fibers from various cortical motor areas, such as the primary motor cortex (MI), the supplementary motor area (SMA), and premotor area (PMA) occupy different parts of the internal capsule. Thus, when a capsular stroke damages the most powerful and direct pathway from the cortex to the motor neurons—arising in MI—other, parallel, descending pathways may be "trained" to activate motor neurons more powerfully than before the stroke.

The Contribution of the Undamaged Hemisphere to Recovery

Although many observations suggest that the undamaged hemisphere participates in recovery, the responsible mechanism is not clear. In particular, results are conflicting as to whether or not descending motor pathways from the undamaged hemisphere contribute—the other possibility being actions via the lesioned hemisphere and its remaining descending connections. One should note that most studies involve a small number of patients with somewhat differently placed lesions, making it difficult to draw general conclusions. The weight of evidence suggests that different mechanisms may operate during recovery in patients with a similar functional and clinical picture.

Some observations support that use of **uncrossed motor pathways** contribute to recovery. For example, a group of patients with strokes affecting the pyramidal tract in the posterior part of the internal capsule (as verified with MRI) had initially severe paresis of the hand contralateral to the stroke, but they gradually recovered the ability to perform fractionate finger movements. In these patients, transcranial magnetic stimulation of the motor cortex of the undamaged hemisphere evoked movements of both hands—not just

of the contralateral hand, as in normal persons. Further, in some recovered stroke patients, involuntary movements of the unaffected fingers—**mirror movements**—accompany voluntary movements of the paretic fingers. Finally, a peculiar experiment of nature strongly suggests that the undamaged hemisphere participates in recovery in some patients. Thus, two patients with purely motor symptoms who were in good recovery from capsular hemiplegia suffered a second stroke in the internal capsule of the other hemisphere. As expected, their previously normal side now became paretic, but so did also the recovered side. This phenomenon is difficult to explain if we do not assume that the restitution had involved the use of motor pathways from the normal hemisphere to ipsilateral muscles.

Most patients do not exhibit mirror movements, however, and several studies found no evidence of contribution of descending pathways from the undamaged hemisphere (e.g., with the use TMS).

Examples of Substitution from Animal Experiments

Substitution implies that neuronal groups and pathways that normally participate only marginally gradually take over the responsibility for the execution of a task. Clinical recovery after brain damage resembles a long-term learning process, involving strengthening of specific synaptic connections by repeated use.

Some redirecting of impulse traffic can occur even immediately after the damage, however. When the arm region of the **motor cortex** in monkeys doing specific wrist movements is cooled, the movements immediately become slower and weaker. This is expected because the cooling inactivates many pyramidal tract neurons. Activity in the somatosensory cortex increases simultaneously, however, as if this region were prepared to take over immediately. If the somatosensory cortex is then also cooled, the monkey becomes paralytic and is unable to do the movements at all. Cooling of the somatosensory cortex alone has almost no effect on the movements and is not accompanied by increased activity in the motor cortex. These data suggest that the impulse traffic can be switched very rapidly from one path to another, so that command signals for movements are redirected to the somatosensory cortex. If the motor cortex were permanently inactivated, we might expect that establishment of new synapses would gradually strengthen the new impulse routes. Further experiments indicate that this is indeed what happens. After the first link of the disynaptic pathway from the **cerebellum** to the motor cortex is severed in monkeys (Fig. 11.2A), voluntary movements become jerky and uncoordinated. In 2 to 3 weeks, however, most symptoms disappear, and movements are carried out almost as before (Fig. 11.2B). Thus, considerable restitution has occurred, despite permanent damage to the connections.

also innervate other cell groups than they normally do. This may be due to a lack of normal competition among outgrowing fiber tracts.

Finally, we will mention one other possible factor—although speculative—that may help to explain unsuccessful restitution after early brain damage. Prenatal brain damage occurs in a brain that is not yet geared to motivated, goal-directed behavior; establishment of functional networks is still mainly under genetic control. Thus, when emerging neuronal networks are disturbed there is presumably little pressure on functional restitution, in contrast to what is usually the case when damage occurs postnatally. This may allow haphazard plastic changes that are not tempered by a pressure to re-establish connectivity that is necessary for certain behaviors.

Early Damage of the Corticospinal (Pyramidal) Tract

Direct connections from the cerebral cortex to the spinal cord are necessary for the acquisition and performance of most skilled movements. Although corticospinal fibers reach the cord at the seventh gestational month, the development of synaptic connections in the cord and myelination of the corticospinal fibers go on at least until the child is 2 to 3 years old. Some connections are strengthened and others are removed during this period. Presumably, this represents a sensitive period for establishment of specific corticospinal connections. Initially, connections from each hemisphere are bilateral, but at the age of 2 the hand is controlled exclusively from the contralateral hemisphere; that is, the relevant corticospinal fibers do all cross (in the medulla). This development is at least partly use-dependent and governed by the child's efforts to learn new skills.

A frequent kind of cerebral palsy is **hemiplegia** caused by a perinatal stroke. Typically, disturbed movement control and posture in these children appear not immediately but during the first 3 years of life, and often skills acquired early are later lost. This is probably due to plastic processes that are detrimental to normal motor development. Thus, it appears that any remaining corticospinal fibers from the damaged hemisphere are prevented from establishing synaptic connections in the cord by competition from the much stronger connections of the undamaged hemisphere. Indeed, the undamaged hemisphere retains and strengthens its ipsilateral connections to the cord, rather than being weakened as would normally occur (this is shown in animal experiments and indirectly by use of TMS in human infants). Children with cerebral palsy doing **mirror movements** express this: that is, voluntary movements with one hand are always accompanied by the same movement with the other hand. Why this abnormal innervation pattern is associated with poor function is not so obvious, however. In any case, animal experiments show that stimulation of the damaged hemisphere can rescue the remaining fibers and prevent the poor functional outcome. Further, it appears that in infants with cerebral palsy early specific training (constraint-induced movement therapy) of the impaired arm can improve the functional outcome. Probably, in such cases use-dependent plasticity serves to prevent the gradual loss of connections from the damaged hemisphere.

III | SENSORY SYSTEMS

THE first chapter in this part covers the basic features that are common to all sensory receptors, or sense organs. Such knowledge will make reading the following chapters easier. The next three chapters treat various aspects of the **somatosensory system**, which is primarily concerned with sensory information from the skin, joints, and muscles. Chapter 13 deals with the peripheral parts of the somatosensory system; that is, the sense organs and their connections into the central nervous system. Chapter 14 deals with the central pathways and neuronal groups concerned with processing of somatosensory information, while Chapter 15 discusses pain in some more depth. (Sensory information from the internal organs—visceral sensation—is dealt with mainly in Chapter 29.) In Chapter 16, we describe the **visual system**, from the peripheral receptors in the eye to the higher association areas of the cerebral cortex. Chapter 17 deals with the **auditory system** (hearing); Chapter 18 with the **vestibular system** (sense of equilibrium); and finally Chapter 19 discusses **olfaction** and **taste**.

We use the term **system** to indicate that each of these senses is mediated, at least in part, in different regions of the nervous system. In neurobiology, a system usually means a set of interconnected neuronal groups that share either one specific task, or several closely related tasks. Sensory systems are designed to capture, transmit, and process information about events in the body and in the environment, such as light hitting the eye or the fullness of the bladder. We also use the term "system" for the parts of the nervous system that deal with tasks other than sensory ones. The motor system, for example, initiates appropriate movements and maintains bodily postures.

We use the term "system" rather loosely here: we do not imply that each system can be understood independently of the rest of the nervous system. Further, it is often arbitrary as to which system a particular neuronal group is said to belong. Thus, usually a cell group is used in the operations of several systems. Especially at higher levels of the brain, information from various systems converges. Cortical neuronal groups, for example, may be devoted to both sensory processing and motor preparation. **Convergence** of information from several sensory systems seems necessary for us to perceive that the different kinds of information actually concern the same phenomenon, whether it is in our own body or in the environment. How do we know, for example, that the round object with a rough surface we hold in the hand is the same as the orange we see with our eyes?

Sometimes the term system is misused, so that it confuses rather than clarifies; this happens when we lump structures about which we know too little, or cell groups that have such widespread connections that they do not belong to a particular system. The wish to simplify a complex reality—and the nervous system is indeed overwhelmingly complex—can sometimes become too strong.

12 | Sensory Receptors in General

OVERVIEW

Sensory signals from nearly all parts of the body are transmitted to the central nervous system (CNS), bringing information about conditions in the various tissues and organs and in our surroundings. The structures where sensory signals originate are called **sense organs**, or **receptors**. The receptors are formed either by the terminal branches of an axon (the skin, joints, muscles, and internal organs) or by specialized sensory cells (the retina, taste buds, and inner ear) that transmit the message to nerve terminals. We are using the word "receptor" differently here than in earlier chapters where we applied it to molecules with specific binding properties. A **sensory unit** is a sensory neuron with all its ramifications in the periphery and in the CNS. The **receptive field** of the sensory neuron is the part of the body or the environment from which it samples information. These terms are applied to neurons at all levels of the sensory pathways, from the spinal ganglia to the cerebral cortex. Because of **convergence**, the receptive fields are larger at higher than at lower levels of the CNS.

Sensory receptors are built to respond preferentially to certain kinds of stimulus energy, which is called their **adequate stimulus** (mechanical, chemical, electromagnetic, and so forth). Regardless of the nature of the stimulus, it is translated into electric discharges conducted in axons; that is, the language of the nervous system. This process is called **transduction** and involves direct or indirect activation of specific cation channels. Activation produces a **receptor potential**, which is a graded depolarization of the receptor membrane (similar to a synaptic potential). We **classify** receptors by their adequate stimulus (e.g., mechanoreceptor, photoreceptor, and so forth), by their degree of adaptation, and by the site from which they collect information. For example, many receptors are rapidly adapting, meaning that the respond mainly to start and stop of a stimulus. Others are slowly adapting, and continue to signal a stationary stimulus. Receptors in the muscles and connective tissue are termed **proprioceptors**, while **exteroceptors** capture information from our surroundings (e.g., light, something touching the skin, and so on). **Enteroceptors** (interoceptors) inform about stimuli arising in the visceral organs. In general, contrasts and brief, unexpected stimuli and are perceived much more easily than steady and familiar ones. This is partly because the majority of receptors **adapt** rapidly, and partly because sensory information is heavily **censored** on its way to the cerebral cortex.

SENSORY UNITS AND THEIR RECEPTIVE FIELDS

Regardless of the structure of the receptor, a sensory neuron transmits the signal to the CNS. We use the term **sensory unit** for a sensory neuron with all its ramifications in the periphery and in the CNS (Figs. 12.1 and 12.2). Such primary sensory neurons have their cell bodies in ganglia close to the cord or the brain stem (similar neurons are found in the retina). The **receptive field** of the sensory neuron is the part of the body or the environment from which it samples information. The receptive field of a cutaneous sensory unit is a spot on the skin (Fig. 12.1; see also Fig. 13.10). For a sensory neuron in the retina, the receptive field is a particular spot on the retina, receiving light from a corresponding part of the visual field. We can determine the receptive field of a sensory unit by recording with a thin electrode the action potentials produced in an axon or a cell body, and then we can systematically explore the area from which it can be activated.

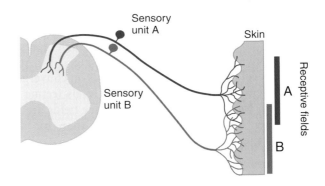

FIGURE 12.1 *Sensory units and receptive fields.* Simplified representation of two sensory units (A and B), which in this case are spinal ganglion cells. The peripheral process of each unit (fibers) ramifies in an area of the skin, which is the receptive field of this particular unit, and the receptive fields of the two units overlap. The density of terminal nerve fiber branches—endowed with receptor properties—is highest in the central part of the receptive field. Therefore, the threshold for eliciting action potentials is lower centrally than peripherally in the receptive field.

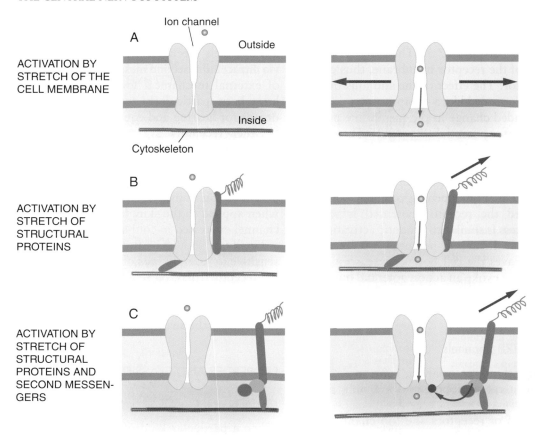

FIGURE 12.3 *Possible means for mechanical stimuli to evoke receptor potentials via TRP ion channels.* (Based on Christensen and Corey 2007.)

modality as when the receptor is stimulated by its adequate stimulus.

Adequate Stimulus

Most receptors are built to respond only or preferably to one kind of stimulus energy: mechanical, chemical, thermal, and so forth. The kind of stimulus to which the receptor responds most easily—that is, with the lowest threshold—is called the **adequate stimulus** for the receptor. We also say that the receptor is **specific** for this type of stimulus, whether it is mechanical, chemical, electromagnetic (light), or thermal (warmth, cold). As we shall see, each of these broad groups of stimuli is registered by receptors with different properties.

Receptors are classified according to the nature of their adequate stimulus, that is, their stimulus specificity. A large group of receptors, the **mechanoreceptors**, responds primarily to distortion of the tissue in which they lie and thus inform the CNS about mechanical stimuli. Such receptors are numerous in the skin, in deep tissues such as muscles and joint capsules, and in internal organs. Another large group of receptors,

chemoreceptors, responds primarily to certain chemical substances in the interstitial fluid surrounding the receptor. Many chemoreceptors respond to substances produced by or released from cells as a result of tissue damage and inflammation, regardless of the cause—mechanical trauma, burns, infection, and so forth. Other kinds of chemoreceptors are the receptors for taste and smell. Receptors in the retina responding to visible light are called **photoreceptors**. **Thermoreceptors** respond most easily to warming or cooling of the tissue in which they lie.

Threshold

Even when stimulated by their adequate stimulus, receptors vary enormously with regard to the strength of the stimulus needed to activate them; that is, they have different **thresholds** for activation. For example, in the retina, the rods are much more sensitive (have lower threshold) to light than the cones. Another example concerns mechanoreceptors, many of which have a **low threshold** and send signals even on the slightest touch of the skin or a just barely perceptible movement of a joint. Other mechanoreceptors have a **high threshold** and require very strong stimulation to respond: we usually perceive such stimuli as painful.

Adaptation

Receptors differ in other ways, too. Many receptors send action potentials only when a stimulus starts (or stops). If the stimulus is continuous, this kind of receptor ceases to respond and thus provides information about changes in stimulation only. Such receptors are called **rapidly adapting**. When after a short time we cease noticing that something touches the skin, this is partly because so many of the receptors in the skin are rapidly adapting. Other receptors, however, continue responding (and thus sending action potentials) as long as the stimulus continues. Such receptors are called **slowly adapting** (or nonadapting). Receptors responsible for the sensation of pain exemplify slowly adapting receptors. It would not be appropriate if the body were to adapt to painful stimuli because these usually signal danger and threat of tissue damage. Receptors that signal the position of the body in space and the position of our bodily parts in relation to each other must also be slowly adapting; if not, we would lose this kind of information after a few seconds if no movement took place. That adaptation is a property of the receptors themselves can be verified by recording the action potentials from the sensory fibers supplying various kinds of receptors. For example, afferent fibers from receptors excited by warming of the skin stop sending signals if the same stimulus is maintained for some time, whereas afferent nerve fibers from sense organs in a muscle continue to send signals as long as the muscle is held in a stretched position.

Dynamic and Static Sensitivity

Many receptors respond more vigorously to rapid changes in the stimulus than to slow ones (they adapt rapidly). For example, rapid stretch of a muscle produces much higher firing frequency in the sensory nerve fibers leading from the muscle than when the same stretch is applied slowly (see Fig. 13.8). Such a receptor can therefore inform about the velocity of stretching, not just its magnitude. This property of a receptor is called **dynamic sensitivity**. A receptor that continues to produce action potentials with a constant frequency as long as the stimulus is constant (slowly adapting or nonadapting) is said to have **static sensitivity**. Often, one receptor has both kinds of sensitivity (see Figs. 13.8 and 16.8). The majority of receptors, however, have dynamic sensitivity and are rapidly adapting. This helps to explain the everyday experience that we are much more aware of changing stimuli than those that are constant—such as an insect moving on the skin or a moving light, as opposed to stationary ones.

Origin of Stimulus

Receptor classification can be based on the origin of the stimuli the receptors capture. For example, mechanoreceptors may—depending on their location—give information of very different events (even though all are mechanical). A low-threshold mechanoreceptor in the wall of the urinary bladder provides information about its degree of distension, mechanoreceptors in the inner ear inform us about sound (movement of air molecules), whereas mechanoreceptors around the root of a hair respond to the slightest bending of the hair.

We usually distinguish between **exteroceptors, proprioceptors**, and **enteroceptors. Exteroceptive** signals reach the body from the outside, from our environment. Most exteroceptors are located in the skin, whereas the receptors in the eye and the internal ear represent important special kinds of exteroceptors that respond to teleceptive signals. **Proprioceptive** signals originate in the body itself. The term is, however, restricted mostly to signals arising in the musculoskeletal system, including the joints. **Enteroceptive** signals arise from the internal (visceral) organs, such as the intestinal tract, lungs, and the heart.

Comprehensive Classification of a Receptor

By the descriptions discussed in the preceding text, we can classify receptors by the characteristics we want to emphasize. We can also give a complete description of the receptor by mentioning all the characteristic properties: for example, a proprioceptive, fast-adapting, low-threshold mechanoreceptor (informing about joint rotation), or an enteroceptive, slowly adapting chemoreceptor (in the wall of an artery informing about the oxygen tension of the blood).

RECEPTORS AND SUBJECTIVE SENSORY EXPERIENCE

Receptor Type and Quality of Sensation: An Uncertain Connection

The kind of conscious sensory experience it evokes is perhaps the most interesting among a receptor's many characteristics. How do I describe what I feel when a particular kind of receptor sends signals to the brain? We use the term pain receptor or **nociceptor** to describe receptors that, when stimulated, produce pain. Stimulation of **cold receptors** causes a feeling of coldness, stimulation of **warm receptors** gives a feeling of warmth, and so on. Only exceptionally is it possible, however, to know whether a sensory experience is evoked by stimulation of one receptor type only, or by the simultaneous activation of several kinds. The connection between the conscious sensory experience and the responsible receptors is therefore often uncertain. Because only human beings can inform the observer directly of what they feel, animal experiments alone cannot resolve the question of the relationship between receptors and conscious sensations. Moreover, the very same receptors that can be examined physiologically cannot be examined anatomically in human beings. Important insight has nevertheless emerged from correlation of observations obtained in animals with psychophysical observation in humans (see Chapter 13, under "Microneurographic Studies of Human Skin Receptors").

In most cases, our conscious sensory experiences are due to signals from several kinds of receptor. The brain interprets a barrage of signals and the context in which they arise, and provides us with a unitary sensation. The sensation of taste is an example: it depends not only on signals from taste receptors (on the tongue) but also on signals from olfactory receptors (with some contribution from mechanoreceptors and thermoreceptors in the mouth).

The Brain Does Not Receive "True" Information

Not all signals reaching the CNS from the receptors are consciously perceived. In particular, enteroceptive signals are mostly processed only at a subconscious level. For signals from all kinds of receptors, however, a considerable selection and suppression of signals take place at all levels of the sensory pathways in the spinal cord and the brain, to leave out "irrelevant" information. At the same time, "relevant" signals are usually enhanced in the CNS (see also Chapter 13, under "Inhibitory Interneurons Improve the Discriminative Sensation"). We mentioned that receptive fields of sensory cells expand or shrink in a context-dependent manner, and that most receptors respond more strongly to changing than to constant stimuli. Therefore, sensory information is censored and does not provide the brain with an objective representation of the physical world (see Fig. 16.9). Usually, such weighting of sensory signals is advantageous because it ensures that the most behaviorally relevant information is prioritized while irrelevant or less important signals are suppressed. An example concerns our need to be able to distinguish sensory signals that we produce ourselves by voluntary movements from signals that arise from external perturbations. As rule, our self-produced sensory signals are inhibited while the unforeseen external ones are enhanced.

Central Analysis

We cannot explain how it happens that action potentials, which are of the same kind in all nerve fibers, evoke entirely different conscious sensations, depending on where the stimulus arises. One prerequisite is that different kinds of sensory information are analyzed by different neurons (i.e., neurons located in anatomically distinct parts of the CNS). A complete mixing of information from different receptor types would not be compatible with our discriminative abilities. It is equally, clear, however, that there must be ways in which the brain can bring the different kinds of information together, making meaning and unity out of the innumerable bits and pieces of sensory information. Such a synthesis may not necessarily be due to convergence of all relevant information onto a single cell group. Rather, we now believe the final processing to depend on extensive interconnections among cortical areas dealing with different aspects of sensory information (these aspects are treated further in Chapter 16, under "How Are Data from Different Visual Areas Integrated?" and Chapter 34, under "Parietal Association Areas").

In an elegant study, de Lafuente and Romo (2005) trained monkeys to respond to cutaneous stimuli that were barely detectable, while at the same time recording neuronal activity in the cerebral cortex. In turned out that whenever the monkey responded to the stimulus (as a sign of perception), there was activity among neurons in the premotor cortex of frontal lobe as well as in the somatosensory cortex. Activity in the somatosensory cortex alone was apparently not sufficient for perception. On the other hand, there was frontal activation in instances when the monkey (erroneously) responded without the stimulus being strong enough to evoke activity in the somatosensory cortex. This example serves further to emphasize that our conscious sensations are not hard-wired to the signals from sensory receptors, but depends critically on central analysis.

13 | Peripheral Parts of the Somatosensory System

OVERVIEW

The term **somatosensory** includes, strictly speaking, all sensations pertaining to the body (*soma*). It is therefore more comprehensive than the significance commonly assigned to it—namely, sensory information specifically from **skin, joints**, and **muscles** only. In this chapter, we discuss receptors (sense organs) located in the skin and in the musculoskeletal system and the neurons leading from them into the central nervous system (CNS). Receptors in the skin and in deep tissues are either **free** or **encapsulated**. The terminal ramifications in encapsulated receptors are surrounded by connective tissue cells, serving as a filter ensuring that only certain kinds of stimuli reach the axon terminal. We distinguish between **exteroceptors**, located in the skin, and **proprioceptors** in muscles and connective tissue around the joints. Regardless of their location, somatosensory receptors can be classified by their adequate stimulus as **mechanoreceptors, thermoreceptors**, and **chemoreceptors**.

High-threshold receptors usually signal impending tissue damage, and are termed **nociceptors**. They are all free nerve endings, but differ with regard to stimulus specificity. Some respond only to intense mechanical stimuli, others to chemical (inflammatory) substances, while others detect extreme heat or coldness. Many nociceptors respond to several kinds of stimuli (**polymodal nociceptors**), while others do not respond to "normal" pain-provoking stimuli but require prolonged stimulation to become active (**silent nociceptors**). In addition to signaling impending acute tissue damage, nociceptors probably play an important role in monitoring the composition of the tissue fluid and thus contribute to bodily **homeostasis**.

Thermoreceptors respond to even very small changes of the temperature of their surroundings (especially in the skin). They are much less sensitive to steady-state temperature. Cold receptors detect cooling below the normal skin temperature, while warm receptors detect a rise in temperature.

Low-threshold mechanoreceptors in the skin and in the deep tissues share many physiological properties. In general, they signal deformation of the tissue in which they reside. Their capsular elements and relation to surrounding tissue components—such as collagen fibrils or muscle fibers—determine the kind of stimulus they respond to with the lowest threshold. Further, capsular elements and membrane receptor proteins determine whether the receptor is **rapidly** or **slowly adapting**.

Cutaneous low-threshold mechanoreceptors are of four types: **Meissner corpuscles** reside in the dermal papillae of glabrous skin (e.g., on fingertips) and respond to the slightest impression on the skin. They are rapidly adapting, thus signaling only when something touches (or leaves) the skin—not when the skin remains impressed. Like Meissner corpuscles, **Merkel disks** respond to small impressions of the skin but are slowly adapting. **Ruffini corpuscles** are located in the dermis and respond to stretching of the skin. They are slowly adapting, and probably signal the steady tension (important, e.g., when holding objects). **Pacinian corpuscles** are large, lamellate structures located on the transition between the dermis and the subcutaneous tissue. They are extremely rapidly adapting and are well suited to signal vibration (>100 Hz). The receptive fields of Meissner corpuscles and Merkel disks are small (especially on distal parts of the extremities), making these receptors of crucial importance for **discriminative sensation**.

Among **proprioceptive** low-threshold mechanoreceptors, the **muscle spindles** are the most elaborate. They consist of a small bundle of thin, so-called **intrafusal** muscle fibers encircled by sensory nerve endings. Although each muscle spindle is much shorter than the muscle in which it lies, it is connected with connective tissue strands to both tendons of the muscle. Thus, when the muscle elongates, the muscle spindle is stretched and the sensory endings are depolarized. The muscle-spindle sensory endings have both dynamic and static sensitivity, making them suited to record the actual muscle length at any time, length change, and direction and velocity of change. Signals from muscle spindles contribute to reflex control of movements and to **kinesthesia**—that is, our conscious perception of joint positions and movements. **Tendon organs** are located at the musculotendinous junction, and measure the force of muscle contraction. **Joint receptors** are located in the fibrous joint capsule and in ligaments around the joints. They can signal movements and steady positions but their contributions to movement control and kinesthesia are not well understood.

Dorsal root fibers conducting from somatosensory receptors are classified according to **conduction velocity** into myelinated A fibers and unmyelinated C fibers. The thickest A fibers conduct from low-threshold mechano-receptors, whereas thin A fibers (Aδ) and C fibers conduct from nociceptors and thermoreceptors. The thin (Aδ and C) and thick dorsal root fibers end almost completely separated in the cord. Probably all primary sensory neurons release a classical transmitter with fast synaptic actions in the spinal cord. Probably all primary sensory neurons release a classical **neurotransmitter** with fast synaptic actions in the spinal cord. In addition, many contain several **neuropeptides**, such as substance P and others. Apparently, release of neuropeptides from the peripheral branches of sensory neurons contributes to local inflammation in several diseases (e.g., arthritis, asthma, and migraine).

The ventral branches of the spinal nerves form **plexuses** supplying the arms and the legs. Each nerve emerging from these plexuses contains sensory and motor fibers arising from several segments of the spinal cord. In the peripheral distribution of the fibers, however, the **segmental** origin of the fibers is retained. Thus, sensory fibers of one dorsal root supply a distinct part of the skin. The area of the skin supplied with sensory fibers from one spinal segment is called a **dermatome**.

EXTEROCEPTORS: CUTANEOUS SENSATION

The skin and the subcutaneous tissue contain receptors that respond to stimuli from our surroundings. Among the almost indefinitely varied sensory experiences that can be evoked from the skin, we usually distinguish only a few, regarded as the basic modalities: **touch, pressure, heat, cold,** and **pain**. There is indirect evidence that each of these sensations can be evoked by stimulation of one receptor type. Yet it is important to realize that terms such as "pain," "cold," and "touch" refer to the quality of our subjective sensory experience evoked by certain kinds of stimuli. Thus, a classification of sensations on this basis does not enable us to conclude that for each subjective quality of sensation there exists one particular kind of receptor.

Sensations—such as itch, tickle, dampness, or dryness; the texture of surfaces; and the firmness or softness of objects—are thought to arise from the simultaneous stimulation of several kinds of receptors in the skin and also in deeper tissues. As discussed in Chapter 12, our conscious sensory experience is the result of an interpretation in the brain of information from a multitude of receptors.

Functionally, skin receptors—like receptors in other parts of the body—can be classified by their adequate stimulus as **mechanoreceptors, thermoreceptors,** and **chemoreceptors**.

Free and Encapsulated Receptors

We conveniently subdivide receptors in the skin (and in deep tissues) on a structural basis into **free** and **encapsulated**, although there are numerous transitional forms. In encapsulated receptors, the terminal ramifications of the sensory axon are surrounded by a specialized capsule-like structure of connective tissue cells (Fig. 13.1A, C, and D), whereas such a structure is lacking around the free receptors or endings (Fig. 13.1E). The encapsulation serves as a **filter**, so that only certain kinds of stimuli reach the axon terminal inside. **Schwann cells** cover the axonal ramifications of the free receptors, except at their tips (Fig. 13.1E), where their receptor properties presumably reside. Free receptors are the most numerous and widespread, being present in virtually all parts of the body. In the skin, free receptors are particularly numerous in the upper parts of the dermis, and they even extend for a short distance between the cells of the deeper layers of the epidermis.

Free receptors that are structurally indistinguishable can nevertheless have different adequate stimuli. The **cornea** of the eye, for example, contains only free nerve endings but functionally there are at least four different receptors. Thus, anatomically identical receptors can differ functionally as a result of their expression of different repertoires of membrane channels and receptor molecules.

Nociceptors

Receptors that on activation evoke a sensation of pain are termed nociceptors. A more precise, **physiological definition** would be: a receptor that is activated by stimuli that produce tissue damage, or would do so if the stimulus continued. In Chapter 15, we discuss the relationship between nociceptor stimulation and the experience of pain. In the skin and, as far as we know, in all other tissues from which painful sensations can be evoked, nociceptors are **free nerve endings**. It is characteristic that most stimuli we experience as painful are so intense that they produce tissue damage or will do so if the stimulus is continued. Functionally, skin nociceptors are of three main types. One type responds to intense mechanical stimulation only (such as pinching, cutting, and stretching), and is therefore termed a **high-threshold mechanoreceptor**. The other is also activated by intense mechanical stimuli but in addition, by intense **warming** of the skin (above 45°C)[1] and by **chemical**

---

1 Heat activates nociceptors by opening the nonselective cation channel **TRPV1** (and apparently also other varieties of the TRPV channel). Interestingly, **capsaicin**, responsible for the pungency of hot peppers, activates the heat-sensitive channel. On continued presence, however, capsaicin desensitizes the receptor thus alleviating ongoing pain. Drugs that selectively block the TRPV1 channel have been tested in animals and found effective in alleviating inflammatory pain but also causing a rise in body temperature. Thus, the TRPV1 channel apparently contributes not only to thermal and chemical nociception but also to control of body temperature.

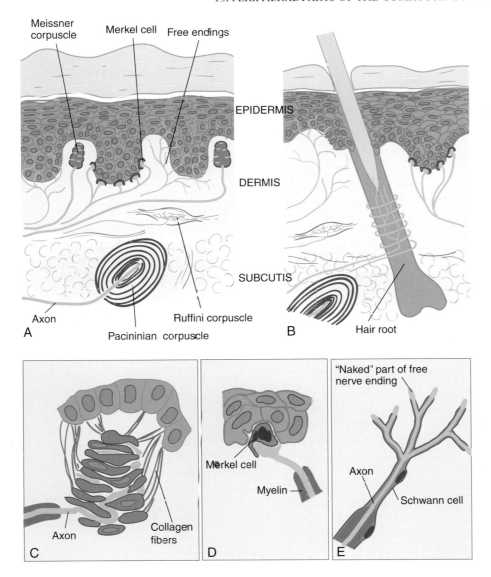

FIGURE 13.1 *Cutaneous receptors.* Schematic of receptors as they appear in sections through the skin. Sensory nerve fibers and receptors in (**A**) glabrous skin (palms of the hands and soles of the feet) and (**B**) hairy skin. Nerve endings in hairy skin wind around the hair follicles and are activated by the slightest bending of the hair. **C:** Meissner corpuscle (from glabrous skin). The axon (red) follows a tortuous course between flat, specialized connective tissue cells. The whole sense organ is anchored to the epidermis with thin collagen fibers. **D:** A disk of Merkel (present in both glabrous and hairy skin). The axonal terminal is closely apposed to a Merkel cell in the epidermal cell layer. **E:** Free nerve endings are covered by Schwann cells except at their tips, where the receptor properties reside.

substances that are liberated by tissue damage and inflammation. Because such receptors can be activated by different sensory modalities, they are termed **polymodal nociceptors**. In addition, recent studies indicate that many nociceptors are purely sensitive to chemical substances released in inflamed tissue. Since such receptors are unresponsive to most nociceptive stimuli used in animal experiments, they are termed **silent nociceptors**. Silent nociceptors typically require stimulation for 10 to 20 minutes to become active; thereafter, however, they may continue firing for hours. They are present in skin, muscles, and visceral organs and may constitute about one-third of all nociceptors. They appear particularly suited to communicate about disease processes in the tissues, and are probably important for communication between the immune system and the brain.

Many substances can excite nociceptors, and specific membrane receptors and ion channels have been identified for some. **ATP**, for example, excites nociceptors by binding to purinoceptors (Fig. 13.2). Because ATP is normally present only intracellularly, its extracellular occurrence is an unequivocal sign of cellular damage. The peptide **bradykinin**, which is produced by the release of proteolytic enzymes from damaged cells, acts on specific membrane receptors in nociceptors. Several other mediators of **inflammation**—such as prostaglandins,

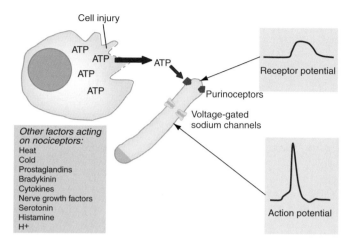

FIGURE 13.2 *Nociceptor activation.* ATP is one among many substances that activate nociceptors. Because the extracellular ATP concentration is extremely low normally, ATP is a very sensitive signal of impending cell damage. Binding of ATP to specific receptors depolarizes the nerve terminal (receptor potential). If the receptor potential reaches threshold an action potential arises due to opening of voltage-gated sodium channels. The action potential is conducted to the CNS. Some other means of activating nociceptors are listed.

histamine, serotonin, substance P, and adenosine—may contribute to nociceptor activation and sensitization. **H$^+$ions** (pH < 6) activate nociceptors effectively and, in addition, seem to increase their responses to inflammatory substances.

A characteristic feature of nociceptors is their tendency to be **sensitized** by prolonged stimulation (this is the opposite phenomenon of adaptation). Sensitization is due to accumulation of inflammatory products that up-regulate voltage-gated Na$^+$ channels and transient receptor potential (TRP) channels expressed in sensory neurons. Sensitization partly explains why even normally non-noxious stimuli (such as touching the skin) may be felt as painful when the skin is inflamed. A condition of abnormal intensity of pain compared to the strength of the stimulus is called **hyperalgesia**. As discussed later in this chapter, hyperalgesia may also be caused by altered properties of neurons in the CNS, especially in the spinal dorsal horn. The term **allodynia** is used when innocuous stimuli, such as light touch, evoke intense pain.

Signals from nociceptors are conducted in thin myelinated (Aδ) and unmyelinated (C) fibers. This is further discussed later in this chapter, under "Classification of Dorsal Root Fibers in Accordance with Their Thickness."

Nociceptors, Voltage-Gated Sodium Channels, and Inherited Channelopathies

Sensory neurons express a multitude of ion channels and receptors, among them several kinds of voltage-gated sodium (Na$^+$) channels. Such channels are expressed in all neurons and are necessary for excitability and impulse conduction. Ten voltage-gated sodium channels have been identified, sharing a basic structure but with somewhat different properties and distribution. Sensory neurons express several kinds, and some of these occur primarily in small nociceptive spinal ganglion cells. Nerve injury as well as inflammation cause rapid changes in the expression of several voltage-gated sodium channels, thus rendering the ganglion cells hyperexcitable (as mentioned earlier in relation to hyperalgesia).

One channel—**Na$_V$1.7**—appears to be particularly important for the generation of action potentials in axons leading from nociceptors. Rare inherited diseases caused by mutations of the gene (*SCN9A*) coding for Na$_V$1.7 shed light on the function of this channel. Two gain-of-function mutations cause attacks of intense pain but with different mechanisms. Patients with **paroxysmal extreme pain disorder** suffer from attacks of pain in the eyes, jaw, and rectum, apparently caused by incomplete inactivation of the Na$_V$1.7 channel. Patients with **erythromelalgia** (primary erythermalgia) experience burning pain and redness in the hands and feet. The mutation in the latter patients cause the channel to open to easily (lowered threshold). A third variety of inherited Na$_V$1.7 channelopathy was quite recently found among members of a Pakistani family. Those afflicted show complete absence of pain sensitivity and suffer serious injuries as they grow up. The mutation in these patients appears to cause a loss of function of the Na$_V$1.7 channel, resulting in abolished impulse traffic from nociceptors.

Other voltage-gated sodium channels, expressed in nociceptive ganglion cells, also appear to be involved in clinical pain conditions. Great efforts are now being made to develop drugs that can block specific voltage-gated sodium channels. Nonspecific blockers, such as **lidocaine**, have long been used for local anesthesia.

Silent Nociceptors, the Immune System, Homeostasis, and Sickness Behavior

Since mediators released in inflamed tissues activate them, silent nociceptors most likely contribute to the pain that follows tissue damage. Nevertheless, in contrast to other nociceptors they may not function primarily as a warning system for impending tissue damage but, rather, play a long-term role in evaluating the status of the tissue microenvironment. Thus, they would play a role in bodily **homeostasis**. Signals from silent nociceptors may be particularly important to modulate the activity of the **immune system**. Thus, we know that the nervous system can influence the properties of the cells of the immune system, as we shall return to in Chapter 30. To do this, the nervous system needs information from the "battlefield" of the immune system. Silent nociceptors seem well suited to carry out this task, as substances released from leukocytes activate them. We know, for example, that cytokines released in the gastric mucosa stimulate nerve fibers in the **vagus nerve**. This produces **sickness behavior** in rats: they move less around, lose appetite, are uninterested in their surroundings, and so forth. In addition, cytokines in the bloodstream can reach neurons in certain parts of the brain, either by passing the blood–brain barrier or by acting on places devoid of a blood–brain barrier. It seems likely that signals from silent nociceptors—not only in the skin but also in deep tissues and visceral organs—contribute to "how we feel," or the subjective feeling of the physiological state of the body.

Thermoreceptors

Free endings of thin sensory nerve fibers are responsible for the perception of heat and cold. Although warm and cold receptors look the same, they express different kinds of TRP channels. **Cold receptors** respond with an increase of firing frequency to cooling of the skin below the normal temperature (about 32°C). They stop responding, however, at very low skin temperatures. Surprisingly, cold receptors can also be excited by skin temperatures above 45°C. This explains why a hot shower may feel cold at the beginning (until we feel pain, as mentioned previously, temperatures above 45°C excite polymodal nociceptors). This phenomenon is called **paradoxical cold** (sensation). Signals from cold receptors are conducted in thin myelinated (Aδ) fibers. **Warm receptors** respond to warming of the skin above the normal temperature up to about 45°C. The signals are conducted in unmyelinated (C) fibers.

The **adequate stimulus** for thermoreceptors is the temperature of the tissue surrounding them or, rather, changes in the temperature. The receptors send action potentials with a relatively low frequency at a steady temperature, whereas a small change in the temperature elicits a marked change in the firing frequency. A heat receptor, for example, fires at constant room temperature with a low frequency, but warming the skin even slightly increases in the firing rate. The response is particularly brisk if the warming happens rapidly (thus, we perceive lukewarm water as hot if the hand is cold when put into it). A change in skin temperature of 0.2°C is sufficient to cause a marked change in firing rate from a thermoreceptor. Thus, the thermoreceptors do not give an objective measure of the actual skin temperature but, rather, signal **changes** that may be significant in our adjustment to the environment (to keep the body temperature constant). Thus, they are important for the maintenance of bodily **homeostasis**.

Mechanoreceptors of the Skin

The study of receptors for pain and temperature sensation is more difficult than the study of mechanoreceptors. These are particularly well studied, therefore, and among them, we know most about the low-threshold mechanoreceptors. The following account mainly deals with low-threshold mechanoreceptors of the skin. High-threshold mechanoreceptors in the skin are nociceptors and do not differ significantly from such receptors in muscles and around joints. As far as we know, they are always free nerve endings (Fig. 13.1E).

There are several kinds of **low-threshold mechanoreceptors** in the skin, ranging from free receptors to those with an elaborate capsule. Some adapt slowly or not at all; others adapt very rapidly. For example, receptors found close to the roots of **hairs** (Fig. 13.1B) are rapidly adapting. They are activated by even the slightest bending of a hair, as can easily be verified by touching the hairs on the back of one's own hand. If the hair is held in the new position, however, the sensation disappears immediately. Unmyelinated afferent fibers from hairy skin that signal light touch may be of special importance for mediating **emotional** aspects of touch (rather than precise, discriminative information).[2]

Although the thick, **glabrous skin** on the palm of the hand and on the sole of the foot lacks hair, the elaborate encapsulated receptors are particularly abundant at these locations and are obviously related to the superior sensory abilities of these parts—the fingers, in particular (Table 13.1). One such receptor is the **Meissner corpuscle**, which mediates information about touch. Meissner corpuscles are small oval bodies located in the dermal papillae just beneath the epidermis—in fact, as close to the surface of the skin as possible without being directly exposed (Fig. 13.1A and C). Several axons approach the corpuscle and follow a tortuous course inside the capsule between the lamellae formed by connective tissue cells.[3] Meissner corpuscles respond by sending action potentials even when indenting only a few micrometers the skin overlying the receptor. If the skin is kept indented, however, the receptor stops sending action potentials. On release of the pressure, a few action potentials are again elicited. Meissner corpuscles are thus **rapidly adapting** and obviously have a low threshold for their adequate stimulus. These corpuscles are presumably well suited to, among other things, signal **direction** and **velocity** of objects moving on the skin.

2 A woman with selective loss of large-diameter myelinated sensory fibers provided an opportunity to study the properties of **low-threshold C-fibers** (Olausson et al. 2002). Light touch (stroking with a soft brush) applied to the back of the hand was felt as a very faint and diffuse but pleasant pressure (no sensation was evoked by brushing the palm of the hand, corresponding to the lack of unmyelinated low-threshold afferents from glabrous skin). Interestingly, functional magnetic resonance imaging (fMRI) showed activation of the insula—known to be related to affective aspects of sensation—but not in SI that is responsible for the discriminative aspects.

3 In addition to a thick myelinated axon, the Meissner corpuscle receives thin unmyelinated axons. The latter contain neuropeptides and express receptors typical of nociceptors. So far, however, there is no direct evidence of a contribution from Meissner corpuscles in nociceptive signaling.

TABLE 13.1

RECEPTIVE FIELDS	ADAPTATION	
	Rapid	Slow
Small	Meissner corpuscles: Glabrous skin, in dermal papillae Touch: moving stimuli Vibration < 100 Hz	Merkel disks: Close to the epithelium Touch (judging form & surface of objects)
Large	Pacinian corpuscles: Border dermis-subcutis; Vibration > 100 Hz	Ruffini corpuscles: Dermis, parallel to the skin surface; stretch of the skin (friction)

Ruffini corpuscles are also low-threshold mechano-receptors and are **slowly adapting**. They consist of a bundle of collagen fibrils with a sensory axon branching between the fibrils (Fig. 13.1A). The collagen fibrils connect with those in the dermis, and stretching of the skin in the direction of the fibrils is the adequate stimulus for the receptor. Stretching the skin tightens the fibrils, which, in turn, leads to deformation and depolarization of the axonal ramifications, thus producing action potentials in the afferent fiber. It is therefore assumed that Ruffini corpuscles function as low-threshold **stretch receptors** of the skin, informing us about the magnitude and direction of stretch.

Another kind of **slowly adapting**, low-threshold mechanoreceptor in the skin is the **Merkel disk** (Fig. 13.1A and D), present particularly on the distal parts of the extremities, the lips, and the external genitals. An axon ends in close contact with a large epithelial cell in the basal layer of the epidermis. Even after several minutes of constant pressure on the skin overlying the Merkel disks, the receptor continue to send action potentials at about the same rate.

A final type of low-threshold mechanoreceptor, **Pacinian corpuscles** (Fig. 13.1A), are found at the junction between the dermis and the subcutaneous layer; they are also present at other locations, such as in the mesenteries, vessel walls, joint capsules, and in the periosteum. Pacinian corpuscles are large (up to 4 mm long) ovoid bodies, which can be seen macroscopically at dissection. A thick axon is surrounded by numerous lamellae, which are formed by a special kind of connective tissue cell. Between the cellular lamellae there are fluid-filled spaces. Pacinian corpuscles are very **rapidly adapting**, eliciting only one or two action potentials in the afferent fiber at the onset of indentation of the skin. The adequate stimulus is therefore extremely rapid indentation of the skin. In practice, this is achieved by **vibration** with a frequency of 100 to 400 Hz. If a vibrating probe

is put in contact with the skin, the frequency of action potentials in the afferent fiber follows closely the frequency of vibration. Vibration with a frequency below 100 Hz appears to be signaled by Meissner corpuscles.

Itch and Tickle

Itching is a peculiar, unpleasant sensation evoked by stimulation of free nerve endings in superficial parts of the skin and mucous membranes. The signals are conducted in unmyelinated sensory fibers to the spinal cord. From the cord to higher levels, the signals follow the pathways for pain, because cutting these also abolishes the sensation of itching. (In fact, we know that weakly painful stimuli, such as scratching the skin, suppress the sensation of itching.) Further, liberation of **histamine** in the skin, for example, from mast cells in allergic reactions, evokes itching. The leaves of stinging nettle (*Urtica dioica*) provoke intense itching because they contain histamine. Microneurographic studies in humans have identified a subgroup of peripheral sensory units (with unmyelinated fibers) that react vigorously to histamine and produce itching when stimulated. These units have been regarded as itch-specific (even though capsaicin and inflammatory substances such as prostaglandin E and bradykinin also activate them). Further, some units in the dorsal horn (lamina 1) respond primarily when histamine is applied in their receptive fields. Histamine appears to evoke activity in the same parts of the cerebral cortex as painful stimuli do, as shown via functional magnetic resonance imaging (fMRI). Nevertheless, animal experiments suggest that itch involves neuronal groups—from the cord to the cortex—that are at least partly separate from those treating noxious stimuli. Thus, the sensation of itch may be served by a specific subdivision of the neural system for pain. Itching is a symptom in several diseases (cancer, metabolic disorders, skin diseases, and others). Histamine does not seem to be involved in such cases, however.

Tickling is another peculiar sensory phenomenon. It is evoked by stimulation of low-threshold mechanoreceptors, but we do not know which subgroup is involved. The sensation of tickling is strongly influenced by the **context** in which it is evoked: the same stimulus may be experienced as tickling in one situation and merely as light touch in another. For example, we know that we are unable to tickle ourselves, probably because the brain can easily distinguish sensory signals produced by our own actions and those coming from other sources. We also know that our emotional state influences whether or not a stimulus is felt as tickling. This example may serve to emphasize a point we will return to repeatedly: the sensory messages sent from the receptors are subject to extensive processing before a conscious sensation is produced.

What Information Is Signaled by Low-Threshold Cutaneous Mechanoreceptors?

Together, the four types of low-threshold mechanoreceptors described in the preceding text are thought to mediate the different qualities of our sense of touch and pressure, which are so well developed in glabrous skin (fingers, toes, and lips). One important aspect is the ability to judge the speed and direction of a moving object in contact with the skin, as well as the friction between them. Thus, we may perceive quickly that an object is slipping from our grip and judge from the friction the force needed to stop the movement. Two of the receptor types, Merkel disks and Ruffini corpuscles, are slowly adapting and, as long as the stimulus lasts, continue to provide information about slight pressure and stretching of the skin, respectively (Table 13.1). The other two, Meissner and Pacinian corpuscles, are rapidly adapting and signal only the start and stop of stimuli. It seems likely that Meissner corpuscles would be particularly well suited to signal the direction and speed of a moving stimulus. It should be noted that low-threshold mechanoreceptors in the skin also contribute to joint sense (see later), and control of posture and movements (see Chapter 18, under "Receptors of Importance for Upright Posture," and Chapter 21, under "Cutaneous Receptors and the Precision Grip").

Microneurographic Studies of Human Skin Receptors

Studies with techniques that enable **recording** from and **stimulation** of peripheral nerves in conscious human beings have provided important information with regard to the functional properties of receptors (Fig. 13.3). The Swedish neurophysiologists Hagbarth and Vallbo pioneered this technique around 1970. With the use of very thin needle electrodes, one records the activity of single sensory axons within a nerve, such as the median nerve at the forearm. Thus, it is possible to determine the receptive field of this particular sensory unit, along with its adequate stimulus. In glabrous skin of the fingers and palms, four types of low-threshold mechanoreceptors have been so characterized. Most likely, they correspond to the four encapsulated types described earlier (Table 13.1). Thus, there are two types of rapidly adapting sensory units: one with a small receptive field (most likely the Meissner corpuscle), and the other with a large and indistinct receptive field (Pacinian corpuscle). The two other types of sensory units are slowly adapting; again, one has a small receptive field (Merkel disk) and the other a large but direction-specific receptive field (most likely the Ruffini corpuscle).

Stimulation of the axons of the sensory units that have just been recorded enables correlations to be made between the conscious sensory experiences evoked by stimulation of only one sensory unit. Stimulation of single sensory units that most likely end in Meissner corpuscles produces a feeling of light touch, like a tap on the skin with the point of a pencil. As a rule, the person localizes the feeling to exactly the point on the skin previously found to be the receptive field of the sensory unit. Activating a sensory unit that presumably leads off from Merkel disks evokes a sensation of light, steady pressure (as long as the stimulus lasts). Stimulating axons that appear to end in Pacinian corpuscles gives a feeling of vibration.

Receptive Fields of Cutaneous Sensory Units

It has been known for a long time that cutaneous sensation is punctate; that is, there are distinct tiny spots on the skin that are sensitive to different sensory modalities. We therefore use the terms "cold," "warm," "touch," and "pain" spots. Cold spots are most easily demonstrated. Between the spots sensitive to cooling of the skin, there are others where contact with a cold object is felt only as pressure. This is so because each sensory unit distributes all its peripheral ramifications within a limited area of the skin. Thus, the sensory unit can be activated only from this part of the skin, which constitutes its **receptive field** (Fig. 13.3; see Fig. 12.1). Certain parts of the skin lack ramifications belonging to "cold" sensory units; consequently, sensations of cold cannot be evoked from such areas. Correspondingly, many small spots on proximal parts of the body—for example, on the abdomen and the upper arm—lack nociceptors; therefore, insertion of a sharp needle at such places is felt only as touch. The receptive fields of nociceptive sensory units are so closely spaced, however, that one has to make a thorough search to find painless spots.

The **size** of the receptive field depends on the area of the skin receiving axonal branches from the sensory neuron. In general, the **density** of sensory units—that is, the number of units innervating; for example, 1 cm^2 of the skin—is highest in distal parts of the body (fingers, toes, and lips), and the receptive fields are smaller distally than proximally (Fig. 13.3). This explains why the stimulus threshold is lower and the ability to localize a stimulus is more precise in the palm of the hand than at, for example, the upper arm.

Discriminative Sensation

The punctate arrangement of the cutaneous sensation is important for our ability to **localize** stimuli. Being able to determine that *two* pointed objects (such as the legs of a compass) touch the skin rather than one must mean that separate units innervate the two spots. Not surprisingly, the distance between two points on the skin that, when touched, can be identified as two is shortest where the density of sensory units is highest, and the receptive fields are smallest—that is, on the fingertips (Fig. 13.3A and B). Determining this distance gives a measure of what

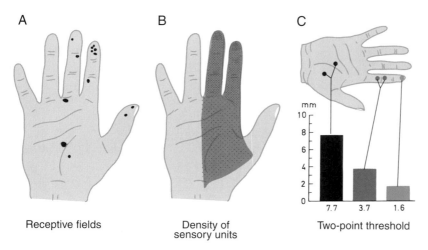

A   Receptive fields

B   Density of
sensory units

C   Two-point threshold

FIGURE 13.3 *Receptive fields.* **A:** Size and location of the receptive fields of 15 sensory units, determined by recording from the median nerve. All of these sensory units were rapidly adapting and were most likely conducting from Meissner corpuscles. Within each receptive field there are many Meissner corpuscles, all supplied by the same axon. **B:** Relative density of sensory units conducting from Meissner corpuscles (i.e., number of sensory units supplying 1 cm²). The density increases distally and is highest at the volar aspect of the fingertips. **C:** Two-point discrimination. The numbers give the shortest distance between two points touching the skin that can be identified by the experimental subject as two (reducing the distance further makes the person experience only one point touching the skin). Average of 10 subjects. (Based on microneurographic studies by Vallbo and Johansson 1978.)

we call **two-point discrimination** and is often used clinically. The smallest distance at which two stimuli can be discriminated is the **two-point threshold** (Fig. 13.3C). A useful test for this kind of discriminative sensation is the writing of letters or figures on the skin (with the subject's eyes closed). The figures that can be interpreted are quite small on the fingertips, somewhat larger on the palms, much larger on the upper arm, and even larger on the trunk. As one might expect, the pathways conducting the sensory signals from the spots on the skin are arranged topographically so that signals from different parts of the skin are kept separate at all levels up to the cerebral cortex.

Lateral Inhibition: Inhibitory Interneurons Improve the Discriminative Sensation

The two-point threshold (Fig. 13.3C) does not depend solely on the size and density of the cutaneous receptive fields. Inhibitory interneurons in the cord (and at higher levels) restrict the signal traffic from the periphery of a stimulated spot, thereby improving the discriminative ability compared with what might be expected from the anatomic arrangement of receptive fields (Fig. 13.4). The cutaneous sensory units (neurons) send off collaterals in the CNS that activate inhibitory interneurons that, in turn, inhibit sensory neurons in the vicinity. This phenomenon is called **lateral inhibition,** and occurs at all levels of the sensory pathways and in all sensory systems. Figure 13.4 shows an example with a pencil pressed lightly onto the skin. The sensory units with receptive fields in the center of the stimulated spot receive the most intense stimulation. Therefore, they excite the inhibitory interneurons strongly, with consequent strong inhibition of sensory units leading from the periphery of the spot. Sensory units with receptive fields in the periphery are less strongly stimulated but receive strong inhibition. Thus, they cannot inhibit the transmission of signals from the center of the spot. Together, the impulse traffic from the periphery of the

stimulated area is reduced, and we perceive the stimulated area as smaller as and more sharply delimited than it really is. In this way, the CNS receives distorted sensory information.

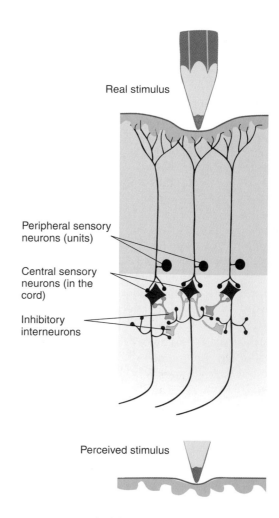

Real stimulus

Peripheral sensory neurons (units)

Central sensory neurons (in the cord)

Inhibitory interneurons

Perceived stimulus

FIGURE 13.4 *Lateral inhibition.* Simplified presentation of how inhibitory interneurons in the CNS can improve the precision of the sensory information reaching consciousness.

PROPRIOCEPTORS: DEEP SENSATION

As mentioned, the term "proprioceptive" is used for sensations pertaining to the **musculoskeletal system**—the muscles, tendons, joint capsules, and ligaments. There are many similarities between proprioceptors and cutaneous receptors. For example, numerous free receptors (belonging to thin myelinated and unmyelinated axons) occur in the muscles, the muscle fascia, and the dense connective tissue of joint capsules and ligaments. Many of these are nociceptors as in the skin.

Here we are dealing primarily with specialized sense organs in muscles and around joints, which are of crucial importance for control of posture and goal-directed movements. These are low-threshold mechanoreceptors, and the signals from them are conducted centrally in thick, myelinated axons. The adequate stimulus of these receptors is stretching of the tissue in which they lie. Whether the receptors are located in a muscle or in a joint capsule, joint movement is the natural stimulus that leads to their activation.

We first discuss specialized sense organs in muscles—muscle spindles and tendon organs—and then discuss receptors in joint capsules and ligaments. In Chapters 18 and 21, we treat the role of proprioceptors in control of movements.

Classification of Muscle Sensory Fibers

Muscle afferents, that is, sensory fibers leading from muscles, are classified according to size into groups I to IV (size or thickness is closely related to conduction velocity). **Group I** muscle afferents contain fast conducting, thick myelinated fibers, while **group II** contain medium-sized myelinated fibers, and **group III** comprises the thinnest myelinated fibers. **Group IV** contains the slowly conducting unmyelinated fibers. Group I is further divided into **Ia** and **Ib** fibers, with Ib fibers conducting slightly more slowly than Ia fibers. Signals from low-threshold mechanoreceptors in muscles—that is, from muscle spindles—are conducted in group I and II fibers, while the tendon organs are supplied with Ib fibers. Unfortunately, other terms are used for classification of cutaneous sensory fibers and efferent (motor) fibers. Broadly, group I and II fibers correspond with regard to conduction velocity to Aα and Aβ fibers, while group III and IV correspond to Aδ and C fibers, respectively (see later in this chapter under "Classification of Dorsal Root Fibers in Accordance with Their Thickness").

Nociceptors in Muscle and Tendon

As mentioned, muscles are supplied with numerous free nerve endings of thin myelinated and unmyelinated axons (i.e., the most slowly conducting fibers). Microscopic examination of muscle nerves in experimental animals shows that almost 40% of all the axons are either thin myelinated or unmyelinated sensory fibers, terminating in free endings (Fig. 13.5). Many—probably the majority—of the unmyelinated and thin myelinated axons lead from nociceptors in the muscle. This has been shown by recording the activity of single sensory units that innervate a muscle while systematically exploring their adequate stimuli. Such units were excited by both strong mechanical stimuli and substances liberated in inflamed tissue (such as bradykinin, known to provoke pain in humans). Inflammation also **sensitizes** the nociceptive sensory units; making them respond to normal movements (this may partly explain the muscle soreness after heavy exercise). Like cutaneous nociceptors, those in muscle are also sensitized by prolonged stimulation, and some sensory units are activated by **ischemia**. For example, muscle ischemia caused by a thrombotic artery, produces pain in humans.[4]

Microneurographic studies have identified sensory units in human muscle nerves that have nociceptor-like properties similar to those described in the preceding text in experimental animals. Thus, human units are slowly adapting, have a high threshold for mechanical stimuli, and can be activated by inflammatory substances. Electrical stimulation of small nerve fascicles in human muscle nerves produces pain as the only sensory experience. The pain is felt to be deep (not in the skin) and has a cramp-like quality. The subject localizes the pain to the muscle supplied by the nerve, not to the site of nerve stimulation that is at a distance from the muscle (recording and stimulation of single sensory fibers have confirmed these findings). If the stimulation continues, or its intensity is increased, the pain radiates to other regions than the muscle itself (this phenomenon is called **referred pain**; see later, "Spinothalamic Cells Receive Signals from Both Somatic and Visceral Structures: Referred Pain").

A small number of axons from nociceptors in a muscle **tendon** have been investigated with microneurography. Stimulation of such a sensory unit produced a sharp pain, different from the muscle pain described above. The subject localized the pain to the tendon.

Ergoreceptors and Other Kinds of Free Receptors in Muscles

Not all of the thin, slowly conducting sensory fibers in a muscle nerve are nociceptors. Thus, in experimental animals, some of these fibers have a low mechanical threshold; that is, ordinary muscle contraction or gentle

---

4 Animal experiments using cultured dorsal root ganglion cells indicate that the adequate stimulus for many muscle nociceptors is a combination of protons, ATP, and lactate, acting on ASICs (acid sensing ion channels), P2X (purinergic type 2), and TRPV receptors, respectively. Increased levels of these metabolites would presumably mediate the pain provoked by heavy muscular exercise (causing ischemia).

the dynamic sensitivity of the primary sensory ending, since there is no extra increase in firing rate of the Ia fiber during the stretch phase. Under the influence of γ_s, the primary sensory ending behaves more like a secondary one.)[7]

Even though this description of the properties of muscle spindles is based on experiments in animals, there is evidence that it applies to the human muscle spindle. Certainly, however, results from anesthetized animals, often with the spinal cord isolated from the rest of the brain, do not enable us to draw conclusions as to the functions of the muscle spindle in intact organisms, for example, in human voluntary movements and in proprioception. It may seem paradoxical that the muscle spindle is among the most studied sense organs, yet its functional roles remain only partially understood.

Muscle Spindles in Humans and α–γ Coactivation

The activity of group Ia afferent fibers in the nerves of the arm and the leg has been recorded in conscious human subjects via **microneurographic** techniques. It appears (unexpectedly, based on animal experiments) that in a resting muscle there is little or no impulse traffic from the muscle spindle. Indirectly, this shows that there is no fusimotor (γ) activity, either. But if the muscle contracts isometrically (i.e., without change of length), there is a sharp increase of the firing frequency of Ia fibers, which must be caused by increased fusimotor activity that occurs simultaneously with the increase in α-motoneuron activity (which evokes the contraction of the extrafusal fibers). This phenomenon of simultaneous activation of α and γ motoneurons is called **α–γ coactivation**. This ensures that the sensitivity of the muscle spindle is increased whenever the muscle is being used. In fact, the firing rate of the Ia fiber is maintained or increased even if the muscle is shortened during active contraction. This must mean that the fusimotor activity (firing rate of the γ motoneurons) increases during active shortening of the muscle.

The preceding example of α–γ coactivation does not mean that the γ motoneurons are activated only in conjunction with the α motoneurons, even though direct proof of separate activation is scarce. There are situations in which it would be desirable to have increased sensitivity of the muscle spindle without simultaneous muscle contraction. One piece of indirect evidence comes from studies of stretch reflexes during **mental imagery**. In such a situation—when the subject imagines the performance of a movement—the stretch reflex response of the relevant muscles is increased without concomitant increase of α-motoneuron excitability, so

it appears that the sensitivity of the muscle spindle has been increased by **selective activation** of γ motoneurons. It is also difficult to understand why the elaborate γ system has developed if its activity were always to reflect that of the α system. In fact, there are collaterals of α axons, so-called β **axons**, that innervate some intrafusal muscle fibers, and in submammalian species (e.g., in the frog) there are only β fibers. During evolution, the β system appeared first.

Signals from Muscle Spindles Reach Consciousness

There is good evidence that signals from muscle spindles contribute to our conscious awareness of joint angle and movement (discussed further later in this chapter). Signals from a single muscle spindle are not sufficient to produce a conscious sensation, however (in contrast to some cutaneous and joint low-threshold mechanoreceptors), so that microneurographic stimulation of single spindle afferents from human intrinsic hand muscles does not evoke any sensation. Many muscle spindles must obviously be activated simultaneously for the signals to be consciously perceived, and presumably this always happens when a muscle is stretched. Therefore, it seems unnecessary and perhaps also disturbing ("noise") to the brain if every muscle spindle were to evoke a sensation on its own.

Especially in weak contractions, different parts of a muscle undergo different length changes; consequently, the muscle spindles would fire with different frequencies. In this way the signals from single muscle spindles may provide useful feedback to the motor control machinery in the cord about smaller parts of the muscle. The cerebral cortex is presumably concerned only with the muscle as a whole and extracts necessary information by integrating the signals from the numerous muscle spindles.

The Tendon Organ

The other kind of proprioceptive receptor we describe here is the tendon organ, also called the **Golgi tendon organ**. It is built more simply than the muscle spindle and consists of a sensory nerve fiber that follows a convoluted course among collagen fibrils of the tendon, close to the musculotendinous junction (Fig. 13.5). The number of tendon organs in a muscle appears to be only slightly lower than the number of muscle spindles. The thick, myelinated fiber leading from the tendon organ belongs to group I and is called a **group Ib** fiber. There is no efferent innervation of the tendon organ (in contrast to the muscle spindle): its sensitivity cannot be controlled from the CNS.

The **adequate stimulus** of the tendon organ is stretching the part of the tendon in which it lies. Stretching tightens the collagen fibers, and thus the axonal branches

---

7 Because the bag fibers appear to be solely responsible for the dynamic sensitivity of the muscle spindle, it has been assumed that dynamic γ fibers end on bag fibers and static γ fibers end on chain fibers. This is not fully clarified, however.

between them are deformed (probably stretched, similar to the group Ia afferents). This depolarizes the receptor and, if the stimulus is of sufficient intensity, evokes action potentials in the afferent Ib fiber. Recording the activity of Ib fibers shows that the receptor is **slowly adapting**. It is important to realize that the tendon organ, in contrast to the muscle spindle, is coupled in **series** with the extrafusal muscle fibers. Both passive stretch and active contraction of the muscle increase the tension of the tendon and thus activate the tendon organ receptor. The tendon organ, consequently, can inform the CNS about the **muscle tension**. In contrast, the activity of the muscle spindle depends on the muscle length and not on the tension.

Recording from single group Ib fibers in the dorsal root of anesthetized cats (Fig. 13.10) confirms what was expected on the basis of the structure of the tendon organ. In addition, however, such experiments have shown that the tendon organ is much more sensitive to tension produced by **active contraction** than to that produced by passive stretch. The tendon organ therefore appears to be primarily concerned with signaling how hard the muscle is contracting rather than with how hard it is passively stretched.

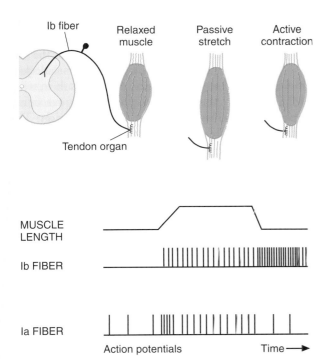

FIGURE 13.10 *Functional properties of the tendon organ.* The experimental setup is as in Fig. 13.8. Action potentials are recorded from isolated Ib fibers in the dorsal roots. Vertical lines on the lower rows indicate the firing frequency. Both passive stretching and active contraction of the muscle increase the firing frequency of the Ib fiber, but active contraction produces the greatest increase. The firing frequency of a Ia fiber during the same experiment is shown for comparison.

Why Tendon Organs Are More Sensitive to Contraction than to Passive Stretch

Structural details may explain why the tendon organ is more sensitive to active contraction than to passive stretch. Each tendon organ is directly attached to a small bundle of extrafusal muscle fibers. If one or a few of these contract, the tension set up in this particular small part of the tendon is much higher than the tension measured for the whole muscle. To obtain the same tension in this particular tendon organ by passive stretch, higher overall tension of the muscle would have to be produced. The muscle fibers attached to one tendon organ appear to belong to several motor units (see Chapter 21, under "Motor Units"). Because each tendon organ probably monitors the tension produced by only a few motor units, the CNS is informed not only of the overall tension produced by the muscle but also of how the workload is distributed among the different motor units.

The Actions of Ib Afferents on Spinal Motoneurons

Activation of the group Ib afferents from tendon organs was shown a long time ago to inhibit (via interneurons) motoneurons of the muscle in which the tendon organs lie (homonymous inhibition). Although these experiments were performed on anesthetized animals, and therefore should be interpreted with caution, the task of the tendon organ was said to be to prevent contractions from being too strong. More recent studies have shown that the effects of the Ib afferents in the cord are not limited to homonymous inhibition. In awake animals, the effect on the motoneurons depends on the locomotor phase, and the effect is reversed from inhibition to excitation when moving from the swing phase to the standing phase. Thus, tendon organs in hind limb extensors excite extensor motoneurons when the leg is in the standing phase (via excitatory interneurons). In this case the signals from the tendon organ serve to amplify the contraction of the extensor muscles that keep the upright position. This is an example of how higher motor centers (in the brain stem and cerebral cortex) can switch the impulse traffic from one route to another in the cord, depending on the motor task. Further examples of this phenomenon are provided in Chapter 21.

Perception of Muscle Force

Our conscious perception of how hard the muscles contract may depend on two sources of information. One is the total activity of neurons in the motor cortex that send commands to the muscles that contract. This requires that other parts of the brain—for example, the somatosensory cortex—receive a copy of the motor commands sent to the muscles. This is called **efference copy**, or **corollary discharge**. Based on previous experience, the

them rapidly adapting. Receptors with such properties, which are influenced by joint movements, are found in muscles, around the joints, and in the skin. The accumulated evidence today indicates that **muscle spindles, joint receptors**, and **skin receptors** all contribute to kinesthesia. Muscle spindles appear to contribute most importantly to kinesthesia with regard to large joints, such as the **hip** and knee joints, whereas joint receptors and skin receptors may have more significant contributions with regard to **finger** and toe joints.

Significance of Various Receptors for Kinesthesia

The views on which receptor types are responsible for kinesthesia have undergone considerable changes. At the beginning of the past century, the newly discovered muscle spindle was held solely responsible but during the 1950s and early 1960s investigations indicated that joint receptors had the necessary properties to signal all the information needed for kinesthesia. It was also argued that the muscle spindle cannot give the necessary information, since the firing rate of its afferent nerve fibers depends not only on the actual position and movements of a joint but also on whether the γ motoneurons are active. While it was held that signals from the muscle spindles do not reach consciousness, it has now been convincingly demonstrated that signals from the muscle spindles can reach consciousness and that they contribute to our kinesthetic sense. A simple demonstration to this effect was performed by vibrating the biceps muscle in a normal subject. **Vibration** is known to stimulate the primary sensory endings of muscle spindles (the stimulus consists of brief stretches of the muscle). The subject, who is blindfolded, feels that the forearm is moving downward even though no such movement is occurring—that is, there is an illusory extension movement at the elbow joint. This corresponds to a lengthening of the biceps muscle, and under normal circumstances would be the normal cause of an increased firing rate in muscle spindle afferents.

Reexamination of the properties of joint receptors showed a striking paucity of slowly adapting joint receptors (type 1) that are active in midrange positions of the joint, the range in which the precision of kinesthesia is best. Because most type 1 receptors appear to reach their maximal firing rate only toward extreme joint positions, it seems unlikely that joint receptors alone can provide all the necessary information. Further, examination of patients with **artificial joints** who lack joint capsules (and thus, presumably, most of their joint receptors) show that their kinesthesia is only slightly reduced, at least with regard to the hip joint and the metacarpophalangeal joints. Presumably, muscle spindles (not tendon organs) are responsible for the remaining kinesthesia in such cases, even though skin receptors may contribute as well (particularly for the metacarpophalangeal joints). For the knee joint, however, elimination of

presumably all afferent signals from the joint capsule and the overlying skin by local anesthesia does not impair kinesthesia appreciably. Local anesthesia of finger joint capsules and the skin of the fingers provides more marked reduction of kinesthesia, but even in such cases the loss of kinesthesia is not complete.

Proprioceptors, Balance, and Voluntary Movements

Patients with neuropathies causing loss of thick myelinated fibers in their peripheral nerves have problems with voluntary movements, especially when they cannot see the moving parts. They also depend on visual information to keep upright and perceiving the position of their body parts. Their problems must be caused by the loss of information from low-threshold mechanoreceptors, presumably mainly proprioceptors. Most disturbed are movements requiring **coordination** of several joints, such as slicing bread, hitting a nail with a hammer, unlocking a door, and so forth. The regulation of muscular force is inaccurate, and they have particular problems with maintaining a **constant force** for some time. Presumably, information from proprioceptors is necessary for a continuous upgrading of the central motor program, so that the commands issued to the muscles are adapted to the actual position of the body parts. Thus, the influence of gravity changes continuously during a movement, and so do the mutual forces exerted by the parts (e.g., between the arm and the forearm). The movements become inaccurate and insecure if the force of muscle contraction is not adapted to these changes, which may differ slightly every time we, for example, raise a glass of water. Such **proprioceptive feedback** is particularly important for small, precise movements, when unforeseen disturbances occur during the movement, and when we learn new movements. Vision can only partially compensate for the loss of proprioceptive information.

As mentioned, **kinesthesia** does not depend solely on information from proprioceptors; cutaneous receptors also contribute. Patients with peripheral **neuropathies** and loss of proprioceptive information usually also have reduced cutaneous sensation that may contribute to their disturbances of posture. Thus, specifying the individual contribution of muscle spindles, tendon organs, joint receptors, and cutaneous receptors to the control of voluntary movements is difficult. Further, when information of one kind is reduced, the patient will learn to rely more on information from other kinds of receptors. In addition, the analysis is complicated by the fact that the various proprioceptors differ regarding their contribution to kinesthesia in different joints, and this probably is true for control of voluntary movements as well. The brain extracts what it needs for motor control from the collective information provided by all these receptors. Nevertheless, it is striking that loss of proprioceptive information is poorly compensated: the person becomes permanently dependent upon the cumbersome use of visual information to control posture and voluntary movements.

We return to proprioceptors and their central actions in Chapter 14, and discuss their relation to motor control in Chapters 18 and 21.

Clinical Examples of Loss of Somatosensory Information

In his book *The Man Who Mistook His Wife for a Hat*, the neurologist Oliver Sacks gives a vivid description of a young woman, Christina, who completely lost kinesthetic sensation. A sensory neuropathy of unknown origin deprived her suddenly of virtually all kinds of proprioceptive information. Her cutaneous sensation was only slightly reduced, and motor axons were essentially spared. Nevertheless, at first she could not stand without continuously watching her feet. She could not hold anything in her hands, and they wandered around without her awareness. When stretching out to grasp an object she usually missed it—the movement stopped too soon or too late. "Something awful's happened, I can't feel my body. I feel weird—disembodied," she said, and "I may 'lose' my arms. I think they're one place and I find they're another." After having proprioception explained, she said: "This 'proprioception' is like the eyes of the body, the way the body sees itself. And if it goes, as it's gone with me, it's like the body is blind . . . so I have to watch it—be its eyes. Right?"

Another example concerns a 36-year-old man who gradually lost both cutaneous and kinesthetic sensation of the extremities due to a sensory neuropathy (described by Rothwell and coworkers 1982). His muscle power was hardly reduced, and he did surprisingly well on several routine tests of motor function. He performed, for example, various finger movements that require cooperation between muscles in the forearm and the hand. He could move his thumb with fair precision over three different distances and with three different velocities, and he could judge reasonably well the resistance to a movement. In spite of this, his hands were almost useless in daily life. He could not hold a cup with one hand, hold a pen and write, or button his shirt. Most likely, this can be explained by lack of automatic adjustment of ongoing movements and by an inability to maintain constant muscle force for more than a few seconds (without seeing the part). The problems seemed to arise also because he was unable to do longer sequences of simple movements without constantly watching what he was doing.

THE SENSORY FIBERS AND THE DORSAL ROOTS

Afferent (sensory) fibers from the receptors follow the peripheral nerves toward the CNS. Close to the spinal cord, the sensory fibers are collected in the **dorsal roots** and enter the cord through these (see Fig. 6.5 and 13.12).

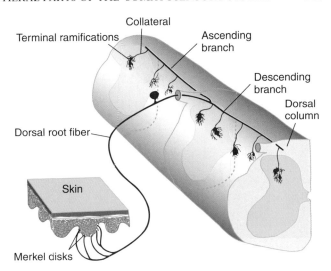

FIGURE 13.12 *Terminal pattern of a dorsal root fiber.* A dorsal root fiber (in this case conducting from Merkel disks) divides into an ascending and a descending branch after entering the cord. These branches give off several collaterals that end in the dorsal horn. The piece of the cord shown is about 1 cm long, but the axon continues beyond this in both directions. Corresponding reconstructions have been made for sensory units leading from several other kinds of receptors, and each sensory unit has a characteristic terminal pattern in the dorsal horn. (Based on Brown 1981.)

The sensory fibers of the spinal nerves have their cell bodies in the dorsal root **ganglia** (see Figs. 6.5 and 6.9). Likewise, the sensory fibers in the cranial nerves have their cell bodies in ganglia close to the brain stem (see Fig. 27.5).

As mentioned, the spinal ganglion cells are pseudounipolar (see Figs. 1.5 and 12.2) and send one long process peripherally, ending freely or in encapsulated sense organs. Functionally and structurally, both the peripheral and the central processes are axons. The **central process** enters the cord and then divides into an ascending and a descending branch (Fig. 13.12). These branches give off several collaterals ventrally to the gray matter of the cord. One sensory neuron, entering the cord through one dorsal root, can therefore influence spinal neurons at several segmental levels of the cord.

Classification of Dorsal Root Fibers in Accordance with Their Thickness

The dorsal root fibers vary in thickness, from the thickest myelinated ones, with a diameter of 20 μm and conduction velocity of 120 m/sec, to the thinnest unmyelinated fibers, with a diameter of less than 1 μm and conduction velocity of less than 1 m/sec. The thick fibers belong to the ganglion cells with large cell bodies, and the thin fibers belong to those with small cell bodies (Fig. 13.13). We have previously in this chapter described classification of sensory axons from muscle by their thickness (conduction velocity) into groups I to IV (see under "Classification of Muscle Sensory Fibers").

and from nociceptors (and thermoreceptors) follow different routes from the dorsal horn to the cerebral cortex, as we will discuss in Chapter 14.

Thin Sensory Fibers from Muscles, Joints, and Viscera: Nociception and Homeostasis

Whereas the thin afferent fibers (the majority coming from nociceptors and thermoreceptors) from the **skin** end mainly in **laminae I and II**, corresponding fibers from the **viscera** appear to end almost exclusively in **lamina I** (and, to some extent, lamina V), thus avoiding the substantia gelatinosa. Thin **muscle** and **joint** afferents appear to terminate in the same parts of the dorsal horn as the fibers from viscera (although there are some conflicting data). Another feature of afferents from muscles and joints is their extensive rostrocaudal distribution in the cord. For example, afferent fibers from a single **facet joint** of the back terminate in seven to eight segments of the cord (cat). It is a common experience that pain of visceral origin has different qualities than pain evoked from the skin; visceral pain is much more diffuse and difficult to localize. In addition, pain that arises in muscles and joints is less precisely localized than cutaneous pain and radiates out from the site of the noxious stimulus. We also mentioned that muscle pain has a cramp-like quality. Presumably, the anatomic arrangements in the dorsal horn may contribute to such differences.

Lamina I of the dorsal horn has attracted interest because of its possible role in **homeostasis**. Due to the unique convergence of thin sensory fibers (especially C fibers) from virtually all tissues of the body—many of them chemoreceptors—lamina I neurons may monitor the metabolic status of the organism (such as the concentration of lactic acid and other metabolites produced in working muscles). At higher levels of the CNS, information from lamina I neurons most likely elicits appropriate autonomic and endocrine adjustments, while increasing afferent activity is perceived as discomfort and pain. The latter feelings are, of course, strong "recommendations" to the brain to change behavior (so that homeostasis is reestablished).

Primary Sensory Fibers and Neurotransmitters

Probably all primary sensory neurons release a classical transmitter with fast synaptic actions in the spinal cord. Among other evidence, this is based on the observation that boutons originating from dorsal root afferents contain small, clear vesicles, which have been shown in other parts of the nervous system to contain this kind of neurotransmitter. It has been estimated that at least 70% of all dorsal root fibers release an excitatory amino acid transmitter. Both ionotropic and metabotropic **glutamate receptors** are present in the dorsal horn, with the highest concentration in the dorsalmost laminae (I and especially II). **NMDA** receptors have attracted much interest because of their possible role in development of central sensitization in chronic pain. There is also evidence that some primary sensory fibers release **ATP** (probably together with glutamate), exerting fast, excitatory synaptic actions.

Several **neuropeptides** are present in the central and peripheral terminals and in the cell bodies of spinal ganglion cells, as shown with immunocytochemical techniques. These include **substance P** (SP), **vasoactive intestinal polypeptide** (VIP), **cholecystokinin** (CCK), **somatostatin, calcitonin gene-related peptide** (CGRP), **galanin,** and others. Many ganglion cells contain more than one neuropeptide; for example, 80% of all SP-containing cells contain CGRP as well. The neuropeptides probably always colocalize with a classical transmitter with a fast, excitatory action. The peptides appear to mediate slow, modulatory synaptic actions in the dorsal horn, probably largely by acting on **extrasynaptic receptors** (see Fig. 5.1). When applied locally in the dorsal horn, SP and CGRP increase the release of glutamate. Further, SP receptors (neurokinin receptors) and N-methyl-D-aspartate (NMDA) receptors (glutamate) interact, making the NMDA receptors more sensitive to glutamate. Release of SP in the dorsal horn might therefore enhance and prolong the excitation produced by incoming signals from sensory receptors. We return in Chapter 15 to how this phenomenon may relate to increased pain sensitivity.

A relationship seems to exist between the kind of **tissue** a neuron innervates and its neuropeptide content. For example, many more of the ganglion cells innervating viscera contain SP and CGRP than do those cells innervating the skin. About two-thirds of the ganglion cells supplying joints contain SP and CGRP. The evidence so far is too limited, however, to draw conclusions regarding relations between neuropeptides, sensory modalities, and tissue or organ specificity.

Neuropeptides in Spinal Ganglion Cells and Nociceptors

Most of the neuropeptides are found only in **small ganglion cells** (Fig. 13.13) which have thin axons; these are probably mainly C fibers but also some Aδ fibers. Substance P, for example, is present in most of the small ganglion cells (in about 20% of all, large and small together). The **neuropeptide receptors** are concentrated in **laminae I and II** (with the exception of CGRP receptors). These data suggest that the neuropeptides are particularly involved in transmission from **nociceptors** and **thermoreceptors.** Correspondingly, several neuropeptides and their receptors in the dorsal horn are up- or down-regulated in conjunction with **inflammation, nerve injury,** and **enduring pain.** Especially SP and its receptors (**neurokinin 1**, or **NK-1**) are likely to be involved in processing of signals from nociceptors. Thus, SP is released from dorsal root fibers in the dorsal horn on nociceptor activation, and microinjection of SP in the dorsal horn make neurons more susceptible to sensory stimulation. Blocking NK-1 receptors prevents this effect.[11]

Inflammatory Diseases and Release of Neuropeptides from Peripheral Branches of Sensory Neurons

The function of neuropeptides present in the peripheral ramifications of primary sensory neurons is less understood than their functions in the central terminals. We do not know, for example, whether these peptides are released under normal circumstances and take part in the normal homeostatic control. We know, however, that the peptides can be released in the peripheral tissue by **noxious stimuli** and by **antidromic activation** of the axon (see Chapter 29, under "Antidrome Signals and the Axonal Reflex"). Several of these peptides, when released in the tissues, have profound effects on vessels, as shown in the skin and mucous membranes. **SP** and **VIP** both produce vasodilation, and thereby increased blood flow and extravasation of fluid from the capillaries leading to edema. Furthermore, SP can activate cells of the immune system, resulting in phagocytosis and release of inflammatory mediators. Inhalation of irritating gases may provoke release of SP from peripheral sensory fibers in the **airways**, and the same takes place in the **skin** upon strong mechanical stimulation, such as scratching. The liberation of SP in such cases is probably due to an axonal reflex because afferent signals from the receptors are transmitted not only toward the spinal cord but also distally in branches of the sensory fibers (that is, distally in the branches that were not stimulated).

Injury to the nerve or the innervated tissue changes the neuropeptide content of the ganglion cells. For example, **experimental arthritis** leads to a marked increase of SP and CGRP in the cell bodies of the ganglion cells that innervate the affected joint (the arthritis is produced in animals by injecting the joint with a local irritant). SP enters the synovial fluid, and induces release of such substances as prostaglandins and collagenase

from leukocytes. Such substances may contribute to the damage of the joint cartilage in arthritis. Blocking the SP receptors (NK-1) or depleting the nerves of SP with **capsaicin** reduces the inflammatory reaction. Therefore, peripheral release of neuropeptides is now believed to play a role in several human diseases, including **rheumatoid arthritis, asthma, inflammatory bowel disease,** and **migraine.**

Sensory Fibers Are Links in Reflex Arcs: Spinal Interneurons

Sensory information reaching the spinal cord through the dorsal roots is further conveyed to higher levels of the CNS. In addition, many of the spinal neurons that are contacted by dorsal root fibers are not links in ascending sensory pathways but have axons that ramify within the cord—that is, they are **spinal interneurons**. The axons of these interneurons establish synaptic contacts with other spinal neurons, among them **motoneurons** (see Fig. 6.6) and **sympathetic neurons** in the intermediolateral cell column (see Fig. 3.8), giving origin to efferent fibers to smooth muscles and glands. In this manner, **reflex arcs** (see Fig. 21.9) for several important somatic (skeletal muscle) and autonomic (visceral) reflexes are established. Most, if not all, spinal interneurons also establish connections between neurons at different segmental levels (propriospinal fibers). Each spinal interneuron thus establishes synaptic contacts with a large number of other neurons in the spinal cord. Signals entering the cord through one dorsal root may influence neurons at several segmental levels, by both their own ascending and descending collaterals and their influence on interneurons with propriospinal collaterals (Fig. 13.12; see also Fig. 21.10).

How far the signals from one dorsal root fiber spread from interneuron to interneuron depends on the other synaptic influences these interneurons receive. For example, **descending connections** from the brain can selectively facilitate or inhibit spinal interneurons. This enables the impulse traffic from dorsal root fibers to be directed so that certain reflex arcs are used, whereas others are "switched off," in accordance with the need of the organism as a whole. **Presynaptic inhibition** is an important mechanism in this respect (see Fig. 4.7). For example, separate groups of interneurons mediate presynaptic inhibition of group I muscle afferents, group II muscle afferents, and group Ib tendon organ afferents. Spinal reflexes are treated in more detail in Chapter 21.

---

11 Although SP is clearly associated with nociception, the correlation is not absolute (as judged from studies combining physiological and immunocytochemical characterization of single spinal ganglion cells). Thus, an SP-containing ganglion cell is not necessarily nociceptive, and many nociceptive neurons do not contain SP.

this chapter under "Transmission of Sensory Signals Is Controlled from the Brain").

Thalamocortical Pathway to SI and SII

The neurons of the VPL and the VPM send their axons into the internal capsule (Fig. 14.2) and further through this to the **postcentral gyrus**. This part of the cortex, made up of cytoarchitectonic fields 3, 1, and 2 (after Brodmann; see Fig. 34.3), constitutes the **primary somatosensory area, SI** (Figs. 14.2 and 14.6). In addition, some fibers from the VPL and the VPM end in the **secondary somatosensory area, SII**, situated in the upper wall of the lateral cerebral fissure (Fig. 14.6). On **electrical stimulation** of SI or SII, conscious human subjects report sensory phenomena such as tingling, itching, numbness, and so forth. Just as the somatosensory pathways are **somatotopically** organized, this is also the case within SI and SII (Figs. 14.2 and 14.7). Fibers conducting signals from the leg end most medially within the postcentral gyrus, then follow fibers conveying signals from the trunk, arm, and face successively in the lateral direction.

Epileptic Seizures Demonstrate the Cortical Somatotopic Pattern

On irritation of the cortex within the postcentral gyrus—for example, by a chip of bone from a skull fracture—the patient may experience fits of abnormal sensations. In the same person, the fits have the same characteristic pattern each time: The sensations are felt in one particular part of the body and then spread gradually to other parts. The spreading follows the known somatotopic pattern within SI (see Fig. 14.8). For example, the patient may first experience a tingling sensation in the thumb; then it moves to the index finger and the other fingers; then to the forearm, upper arm, shoulder, and even further. Such epileptic seizures are called **Jacksonian fits** (after the famous British neurologist, Hughlings Jackson). They signify the presence of a local disease process of the brain, and the starting point of the abnormal sensations indicates the focus of the disease. Often the sensory phenomena are followed by muscle spasms (convulsions) due to spreading of the abnormal cortical electrical activity to the motor cortex of the precentral gyrus.

Single-Unit Properties in the Dorsal Column–Medial Lemniscus System

As mentioned, the dorsal columns contain primarily fibers coming from **low-threshold mechanoreceptors** in the skin, muscles, and joints. Recording the activity of single units in the dorsal columns has confirmed this and has shown that there is a predominance of **rapidly adapting** sensory units; relatively few are slowly adapting. They have small **receptive fields**, mostly at the **distal**

parts of the extremities. Recordings from neurons in the cluster regions of the dorsal column nuclei show that many neurons are activated by only one kind of receptor. Some are activated only by joint movements, others only by light touch of the skin, others only by vibration, and so forth. These neurons are called **modality specific** (because they only react to one kind of stimulus) and **place specific** (because they are activated only from one restricted part of the body).

Neurons in the **VPL** and **SI** also have the same characteristic response properties as those described for the neurons of the dorsal column nuclei, even though an increasing number of neurons are activated by more than one kind of receptor. In addition, the receptive field tends to be somewhat larger for neurons in SI than, for example, in the dorsal column nuclei.

Some of the axons that end in the dorsal column nuclei do not belong to primary sensory units but to neurons with their cell bodies in the dorsal horn (**postsynaptic dorsal column neurons**). Unexpectedly, these postsynaptic neurons are activated not only from cutaneous low-threshold receptors but also from **visceral nociceptors**. We return later in this Chapter to these special dorsal-column sensory units and their possible role in nociception (see under "Additional Pathways from Nociceptors").

Functions of the Dorsal Column–Medial Lemniscus System

Most of the axons at all levels of the dorsal column–medial lemniscus system are thick and rapidly conducting. This, together with the data from single-unit recordings mentioned above, enable us to conclude that the dorsal column–medial lemniscus system is particularly well suited to bring fast and precise information from the skin and musculoskeletal system about the type of stimulus, the exact site of the stimulus, and when the stimulus starts and stops. Thus, it provides information about the **sensory quality** and the **spatial and temporal characteristics** of any stimulus of low intensity ("what," "where," and "when"). The next question is then: how is this information used by the CNS? Unfortunately, on this point conclusions are largely based on the deficits observed when the system is not working. Further, because of the adaptive changes taking place after an injury, we have to distinguish between the acute and long-term functional deficits. Other problems of interpretation arise because with incomplete lesions, functional deficits may be revealed only by tests that require full use of the system.[3]

---

3 For example, experiments in cats show that sparing as little as 10% of the fibers of the dorsal columns—as compared with a lesion comprising all fibers—markedly reduces the sensory deficits with regard to, for example, the discrimination of surfaces with different roughness.

Most studies (with some exceptions) indicate that in monkeys, as in humans, **acute damage** to the dorsal columns produces severe **ataxia** (insecure and incoordinate movements), which recedes partly or completely within weeks to months after the damage. In some patients, the ataxia may be so severe that they cannot walk without support. Observations some time after the damage indicate, however, that the dorsal column–medial lemniscus system is not necessary for all aspects of cutaneous sensation and kinesthesia. First, temperature and pain perception are unaltered by lesioning the dorsal columns; second, light touch of the skin can easily be felt, as can passive joint movements. Two-point discrimination may not be appreciably reduced, and some reports even indicate that the ability to recognize objects by manipulation may be retained (clinical observations do not support the latter point, however). What appears to be consistently impaired is the ability to solve tasks that require spatially and, in particular, temporally very accurate sensory information. Thus, a coin pressed into the palm of the hand may perhaps be recognized, but the patient is unable to decide which is the larger of two coins. The patient may also correctly identify that something is moving on the skin, but not the direction of the movement. To ask the patient to identify figures written on the skin, for example, is one sensitive test of the function of the dorsal column–medial lemniscus system. Further, some careful clinical observations indicate that the perception of joint position and movement is abnormal after lesions of the dorsal columns.

The above-described sensory deficits occurring after lesions of the dorsal columns have in common that they concern spatial and temporal comparisons of stimuli, or what we call **discriminative sensation**. Such sensory information is crucially important for the performance of many **voluntary movements**; indeed, disturbances of voluntary movements are characteristic of the lesions that affect the dorsal column–medial lemniscus system. After the acute phase, the movement deficits first concern movements that require fast and reliable feedback information from the moving parts. For example, the ability to adjust the grip when an object is slipping is clearly reduced. Delicate movements, such as writing and buttoning, are performed only with difficulty after lesions of the dorsal columns. It is not possible to throw an object accurately or to perform a precise jump, presumably because such activities require feedback information from skin receptors to judge the pressure exerted on the hand by the object or by the ground against the sole of the foot.

In conclusion, the dorsal column–medial lemniscus system is of primary importance for complex sensory tasks, such as determination (comparison) of direction and speed of moving stimuli. Further, many precise voluntary movements—especially of the hand—depend on the fast sensory feedback provided only by this system.

In fact, after damage to the system, the motor deficits may be more disturbing than the purely sensory ones.

The Dorsal Columns and Kinesthesia

Observations in humans have provided conflicting results as to whether lesions of the dorsal column–medial lemniscus system give impaired kinesthesia. A thorough clinical study by Nathan and coworkers (1986, p. 1032), however, concluded that complete lesions of the dorsal columns do produce clear-cut and enduring kinesthetic deficits. But they emphasize that: "routine examination of tactile sensibility does not show up these defects as well as everyday activities of living. The further one gets away from this testing situation, the easier it is to see the effects of these disturbances of sensibility." One example may illustrate this point: a patient with damage to the dorsal columns was aware of a toe being passively moved by the examiner; nevertheless, his shoe would easily slip off his foot without his noticing, and he was unable to roll over in bed because he did not realize that one leg was hanging off the bed.

In monkeys, Vierck and Cooper (1998) described deficient kinesthetic sensation of the hands after cutting the cuneate fasciculus, although only specific and detailed testing revealed the problems. Thus, the perception of passive finger movements was impaired only if the movements were small or slow. This is indeed what you would expect when eliminating a system devoted to very precise sensory information. It is furthermore worth noticing that the monkeys had more obvious problems with precise hand movements than with kinesthesia.[4]

Clinical Examination of the Dorsal Column–Medial Lemniscus System

Many of the deficits that occur after damage to the dorsal column–medial lemniscus system may not be revealed by a routine neurological examination. Nevertheless, they may render the patient severely handicapped in daily life. We described earlier in this chapter similar symptoms occurring after loss of thick myelinated nerve fibers in the peripheral nerves. This is not surprising because many of these fibers continue into the dorsal columns. The deficits may be more severe with peripheral loss, however, because reflex effects from low-threshold

---

4 In the legs, however, no defect of joint sense occurred in monkeys after lesions of the dorsal columns at thoracic or cervical levels. This can perhaps be explained by less rigorous testing of the legs than of the hands. Another explanation is possible however. Thus, primary afferent fibers conveying signals from slowly adapting low-threshold mechanoreceptors in leg muscles and joints leave the gracile fasciculus at the low thoracic level (in monkeys). Then they enter the dorsal horn, where they synapse on second-order sensory neurons. The axons of the latter continue in the dorsal part of the lateral funiculus, not in the dorsal columns. Thus, a lesion of the dorsal columns at cervical levels would not interrupt signals from leg proprioceptors. We do not know, however, whether this arrangement pertains also to humans.

Terminations of the Spinothalamic Tract and Further Projections to the Cortex

The **thalamic** termination site of the spinothalamic tract is more extensive than that of the medial lemniscus, and the same holds for the further signal transmission to the cerebral cortex. Many of the spinothalamic fibers end in the **VPL** with a **somatotopic** pattern (Fig. 14.4), but not in exactly the same parts as the fibers of the medial lemniscus (corresponding fibers from the spinal trigeminal nucleus end in the VPM). The terminal ramifications are also different for the two pathways, and nociceptor-activation of VPL neurons requires more summation than activation from low-threshold mechanoreceptors. In addition, many of the spinothalamic fibers arising in lamina I end more posteriorly in the **ventromedial nucleus** (VM). Spinothalamic fibers also end in parts of the **intralaminar nuclei** (e.g., the central lateral nucleus, CL), in the **mediodorsal nucleus** (MD), and some other nuclei.

The multiple terminations of spinothalamic fibers probably explain how signals from nociceptors, by way of thalamocortical fibers, can reach several regions of the cortex in addition to SI and SII. Recordings of single-unit activity in monkey **SI** indicate that neurons activated by high-intensity (presumably noxious) cutaneous stimuli are concentrated in a narrow zone at the transition between Brodmann's **areas 3** and **1** (Fig. 14.6). This may primarily concern signals relayed through the VPL, whereas signals from other parts of the thalamus receiving spinothalamic fibers may directly and indirectly influence other cortical areas, such as the **anterior cingulate gyrus** and the **insula** (this is further treated later in this chapter,

under "Which Parts of the Cerebral Cortex Process Nociceptive Information?").

Does the Spinothalamic Tract Consist of Distinct Discriminative and Affective Parts?

The spinothalamic tract has been proposed to consist of two anatomically and functionally different components. One part—ending in the lateral thalamus (mainly in VPL and VPM) with further transmission to SI—would be responsible for the discriminative aspects of pain perception; that is, our ability to localize a painful stimulus and to judge its quality (sticking, burning, cramp-like, and so forth). The other part—consisting of fibers ending in the medial thalamus (especially in the intralaminar nuclei) and projecting on to the **insula**—would be responsible for the affective, emotional aspects of pain. There is much evidence, however, that this division is at least an oversimplification. For example, many spinothalamic fibers send collaterals to both lateral and medial thalamic nuclei (and to parts of the reticular formation in the brain stem). Furthermore, microstimulation of the lateral thalamus in humans (presumably in the ventromedial nucleus) evoked pain that could be precisely localized *and* at the same time evoked strong emotions (anxiety, discomfort).

Spinothalamic Cells Receive Signals from Both Somatic and Visceral Structures

Recording from spinothalamic cells in the spinal cord has shown that many can be activated by nociceptive stimuli applied to **visceral organs** and to the **skin**. Signals from

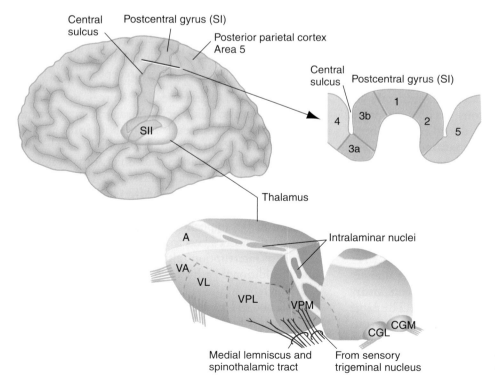

FIGURE 14.6 *The somatosensory cortex (SI) and its thalamic afferent nucleus.* **Upper left:** The location of the SI and SII and parts of the posterior parietal cortex in the left hemisphere. **Upper right:** The extension of the various cytoarchitectonic areas of the central region. **Below:** The VPL—supplying the SI and SII with somatosensory signals—is marked on a schematic drawing of the left thalamus. The main afferent pathways to the VPL are also indicated. A, anterior thalamic nucleus; LG, lateral geniculate body; MG, medial geniculate body; VA, ventral anterior nucleus; VL, ventral lateral nucleus; VPM, ventral posteromedial nucleus; VPL, ventral posterolateral nucleus.

the skin and viscera converge onto the same neuron, which then conveys the information to the thalamus. Nociceptive signals from **muscles** and skin can also converge onto the same spinothalamic neuron. Sensory convergence of this kind pertains to regions of the skin and deep tissues and to visceral organs that receive sensory innervation from the same segments of the cord. The primary sensory fibers can activate the spinothalamic cells monosynaptically or through one or more interneurons (polysynaptically). In addition, in some spinal ganglion cells the peripheral process divides, with one branch innervating the skin and the other a visceral organ or a muscle.

The observations of convergence on spinothalamic cells and branching of sensory fibers may help explain why pain arising from a visceral organ is often felt as if it comes from the skin. This phenomenon is called **referred pain** and is discussed further in Chapter 29.

What Tracts in the Anterolateral Funiculus Can Mediate Alone: A Case History

A woman with a knife-stab partly severing the cord at the Th$_3$ level illustrates what the anterolateral funiculus alone can mediate of somatic sensations (Danzinger and coworkers 1996). The lesion, which was verified during open surgery, severed the cord completely except for the anterolateral fascicle and adjoining parts of the lateral funicle on the left side. Shortly after the accident, with some difficulty, she was able to perceive and localize light touch on both sides of the body below the lesion. She was able to perceive passive joint movements on the left side, but not vibration. Eighteen years after the lesion her sensibility was virtually unchanged. The lesion did not abolish control of the bladder and the rectum, and she retained some voluntary control of movements of the left leg (whereas the right leg was paralytic, she was, for example, able to lift the left leg 30° in the supine position).

Additional Pathways from Nociceptors

Other pathways than the spinothalamic tract may transmit signals from nociceptors to consciousness, even if their contribution may be minor under normal conditions. It should be emphasized that nociceptive signals reach numerous subcortical nuclei (in the rat apparently more than 20), many of which have ascending projections. Concerning transmission from **visceral nociceptors**, postsynaptic fibers in the **dorsal columns** seem to contribute in addition to the spinothalamic tract. There is also evidence that signals in the dorsal columns may contribute to chronic pain in some instances (this is further discussed in Chapter 29, under "Visceral Pain"). Further, many nociceptor-activated spinal neurons send their axons to brain stem nuclei that mediate automatic responses to noxious stimuli, such as changes of blood pressure, heart rate, sweating, breathing, muscle tone, bladder and bowel function, and so forth. Parts of the **reticular formation**, the **PAG** (periaqueductal gray), and the **parabrachial nucleus** all receive signals from nociceptors and participate in automatic behavioral responses to nociceptor activation. Among these, the parabrachial nucleus is special since it receives spinal afferents mainly from **lamina I**, which contains many neurons specifically activated from nociceptors.[6] In addition, these brain stem nuclei send fibers rostrally to end in the **amygdala, hypothalamus**, and **thalamus**. Such connections are probably involved in the varied affective, autonomic, endocrine, and behavioral responses to noxious stimuli but may also gain access to the cortical network responsible for pain perception. Whereas the spinothalamic tract is mainly crossed, these other pathways are bilateral. Thus, unilateral stimuli would reach the thalamus (and cerebral cortex) of both sides.

We know that nociceptive neurons are easily **sensitized** by prolonged stimulation. For example, recordings during brain surgery in humans with **chronic pain syndromes** revealed neurons in the reticular formation and thalamus that responded to noxious stimuli; while such responses were not found in the same regions in pain-free controls (the patients were undergoing brain surgery for movement disorders). These and other data strongly suggest that various cell groups and pathways—in addition to the spinothalamic tract—are recruited under special, poorly understood circumstances.

After interruption of the spinothalamic tract by **cordotomy**, pain usually returns in some months to a year. This probably depends, at least partly, on transmission of nociceptive signals in pathways other than the spinothalamic tract (nociceptor-activated postsynaptic units in the dorsal columns, spino–parabrachial–amygdala connections, and others). Presumably, after severance of the dominant spinothalamic pathway, other minor pathways, which normally do not contribute significantly to our pain perception, take over.

Homeostatic Surveillance: A Task of Ascending Tracts from Lamina I?

As mentioned, perception of pain and temperature are particularly dependent on the spinothalamic tract, although, as witnessed by clinical observations, this tract can also mediate a relatively crude sense of touch and pressure. In a broad perspective, pathways leading from nociceptors constitute an **alarm** system: they report that something is wrong in the body and a change

---

6 In the cat, the majority of lamina I neurons with an ascending axon terminate in the parabrachial nucleus and the PAG (twice as many in the parabrachial nucleus as in PAG). Only about one sixth appears to terminate in the thalamus. If this is so also in humans, it would underscore the role of lamina I in homeostatic control.

of behavior is required to avoid damage. Especially many neurons in **lamina I**—responding to a variety of potentially harmful tissue substances and to heat and cold—seem suited for this task. The system notifies impending cell damage regardless of cause (metabolites, inflammatory mediators, extreme temperatures, or mechanical forces), and is an integral part of the defense systems of the body. Pain elicits a **stress response** consisting of autonomic, somatic, and endocrine components aiming at restoring homeostasis. Activation of brain stem nuclei (parabrachial nucleus, PAG), the hypothalamus, and the amygdala elicits the stress response, either by ascending tracts carrying signals from nociceptors or by descending signals from the cortical pain network (or both). In daily life, most of the signals conveyed through Aδ and C fibers do not reach consciousness: small adjustments prevent the sum of stimulation to reach a level sufficient to cause pain. We alter position, change clothing, or protect ourselves in other ways without needing to pay attention. Persons born without the ability to feel pain illustrate the importance of the alarm system: they incur frequent and serious injuries of various kinds such as burns, wounds, infections, overstretched joints, and fractures.

The Brain Controls the Transmission of Sensory Signals

Descending fibers from the cerebral cortex and the brain stem end in the relay nuclei of the somatosensory pathways. One important group of such connections arises in **SI** (the primary somatosensory area) and terminates in the **thalamus** (VPL and other nuclei), the **dorsal column nuclei**, the **sensory trigeminal nucleus**, and the **dorsal horn** of the cord (see Fig. 22.8). These connections are somatotopically organized and enable selective control of sensory signal transmission from particular parts of the body and from particular receptor types. Physiological studies indicate that descending connections from the SI sometimes can **facilitate** signal transmission through the sensory relay nuclei, but **inhibitory** effects appear to be most common. The latter effects are mediated via inhibitory interneurons. Generally, it appears that signals from somatosensory receptors are continuously regulated to adapt to changing needs—for example, whether sensory information is received passively or actively sought, whether it is needed for movement control, or just arise as a trivial result of self-initiated movements (see later, "Why We Cannot Tickle Ourselves").

Recordings from single units of the medial lemniscus in conscious monkeys have shown reduced impulse traffic from cutaneous receptors immediately before a voluntary movement. There is indirect evidence of the same phenomenon in humans: the threshold for perceiving a vibratory stimulus is elevated immediately before a voluntary movement. Perhaps this happens because proprioceptive signals are of greater importance than cutaneous ones in this particular situation. During walking, signals from mechanoreceptors in the sole of the foot are let through to the motor cortex immediately before heel strike, while the traffic is inhibited during most of the stance phase.

We know from daily life that we have the ability to leave out sensory signals that are irrelevant at the moment. Without such filtering mechanisms, we would be flooded by sensory information. The sensory information finally reaching the cerebral cortex is therefore "censored" and distorted compared with the stimuli received by the receptors.

Later in this chapter we deal specifically with descending control of transmission in the "pain pathways."

Why We Cannot Tickle Ourselves

The fact that we are unable to tickle ourselves is an interesting special case of sensory-information control. Identical signals from cutaneous low-threshold mechanoreceptors can be perceived as tickling if they are caused by another person stroking our skin but as mere touch if a self-initiated movement causes them. In the latter situation, the activation of SI is reduced. Apparently, only signals that are unexpected or unpredictable are let through to SI without suppression. Presumably, experience has provided us with (subconscious) knowledge of the sensory signals that a certain motor command will produce. The cerebellum may have a role in such situations by informing the cerebral cortex about which somatosensory signals might be expected. Probably, the cerebellum receives a copy of the motor command issued from the motor cortex (**efference copy**).

THE SOMATOSENSORY CORTICAL REGIONS

As mentioned, the sensory signals conducted in the medial lemniscus finally reach the two somatosensory areas, SI and SII. In addition, the spinothalamic tract sends signals to several other parts of the cerebral cortex. Both SI and SII receive somatotopically-organized projections from the VPL and VPM (Figs. 14.7 and 14.8), transmitting signals primarily from low-threshold mechanoreceptors and, to a lesser extent, from nociceptors. Somatosensory signals also reach other cortical regions, however, such as the **motor cortex** (MI) in the precentral gyrus. Not unexpectedly, primarily signals from **proprioceptors** are conveyed to the motor cortex.

The parts of SI receiving sensory signals from the feet, hands, and face are much larger than those receiving signals from other parts of the body (Fig. 14.8). Further, the region devoted to the thumb is larger than that devoted to the palm of the hand, which, in turn, is larger than that devoted to the forearm, and so on. This is mainly a reflection of the much higher **density of sensory units** that supply the skin at distal parts of the extremities

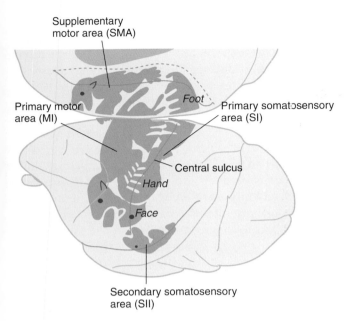

FIGURE 14.7 *The somatosensory regions SI and SII and their somatotopic organization (monkey).* Motor areas (MI and SMA) are also shown. (After Woolsey 1958.)

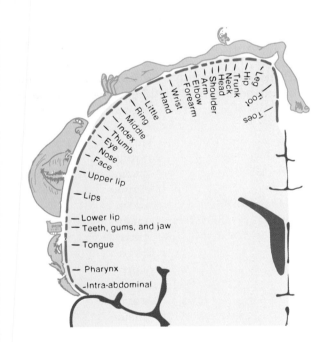

FIGURE 14.8 *Relative size of the cortical regions representing various body parts.* Schematic section through the postcentral gyrus (SI) of the human brain. Based on electrical stimulation during brain surgery under local anesthesia. (After Penfield and Rasmussen 1950.)

(and parts of the face) than more proximal parts of the trunk. To use this very detailed information from the most densely innervated parts of the body, a large volume of cortical gray matter—that is, many neurons—has to be available for information processing. A **magnification factor** gives a numerical representation

of the cortical representation of certain body parts. Similar overrepresentations exist within the visual and auditory systems.

Various **brain-imagining techniques**, such as fMRI and PET, have brought a wealth of information on the contribution of specific cortical areas in motor, sensory, and cognitive processes. We refer to results from such studies throughout this book. A brief description of these and other methods for study of the living human brain are found in Chapter 11 (see under "Methods to Study Neuronal Activity and Connectivity in the Living Brain").

The Primary Somatosensory Area (SI)

The primary somatosensory area, in particular, has been the subject of intense anatomic and physiologic investigations. The subdivision of SI into different **cytoarchitectonic areas**—3, 1, and 2 of Brodmann (see Figs. 22.4 and 33.2)—corresponds to functional differences. These areas extend as narrow strips from the midline laterally along the postcentral gyrus: that is, perpendicular to the somatotopic arrangement (Fig. 14.6; see also Fig. 33.3). Animal experiments, particularly by the American neurophysiologist Mountcastle, show that the cytoarchitectonic subdivisions differ with regard to the kinds of receptor from which they receive information. **Area 3a**, on the transition to the MI (see Fig. 22.4), receives sensory signals from **muscle spindles** in particular.[7] Neurons in **area 3b** are mainly activated by stimulation of **cutaneous receptors** (predominantly by low-threshold mechanoreceptors). Neurons receiving information from rapidly adapting receptors appear to be separated from those receiving from slowly adapting receptors. **Area 2** is influenced by **proprioceptors** to a larger extent than area 3b is; for example, many neurons are most easily activated by bending of a joint. Within each of the cytoarchitectonic subdivisions it appears that the whole body has its representation; thus there are probably three **body maps** within SI. The map in Fig. 14.7 therefore gives a somewhat misleadingly simplified presentation.

Figure 14.8 shows the representation of body parts based on electric stimulation of the cortical surface in conscious patients (during neurosurgery for therapeutic reasons). The patient tells where she feels something when a certain cortical site is stimulated. Although later studies overall agree with the findings of Penfield and Rasmussen (Fig. 14.8), an exception seems to concern the representation of the **genitals**, that most likely are represented on the convexity near the lower part of the

---

7 Some have argued that area 3a should be considered a part of the MI rather than of SI. In certain respects, anatomically and physiologically, area 3a represents at least a transitional zone. Like the other subdivision of SI, area 3a receives thalamic afferents from VPL, whereas MI (area 4) receives them from VL. The afferents from other parts of the cortex are more like those of MI than of the other parts of SI, however.

abdomen (and not on the medial aspect of the hemisphere close to the foot, as originally indicated by Penfield and Rasmussen).[8]

Even though many neurons in SI are activated only or most easily from one receptor type—that is, they are **modality-specific**—there are other neurons in SI with more **complex properties**. For example, many neurons have large receptive fields, indicating that they receive convergent inputs from many primary sensory neurons. Further, movement of just one joint in one direction activates some neurons, while other neurons are activated by several joints. Still other neurons in SI require specific combinations of receptor inputs to be activated. Thus, processing of the "raw" sensory information already begins at the first cortical stage; SI is not merely a simple receiver of sensory information.

Efferent **association connections** from SI pass posteriorly to the **posterior parietal cortex**, which processes the sensory information (see below), and anteriorly to the **motor cortex (MI)**. The latter connections appear to be of particular importance while **learning** new movements, whereas they are not crucial for the performance of well-rehearsed movements (as judging from lesion experiments in monkeys). This may be explained by an extra need for fast and precise feedback from the moving parts during learning. The connections from SI to MI, furthermore, are necessary for motor **recovery** after cutting the connections from the cerebellum to MI, as discussed in Chapter 11 (see under "Examples of Substitution from Animal Experiments"). This may also be regarded as a learning situation.

Further Processing of Sensory Information Outside SI

Although processing somatic sensory information starts in SI, clinical and experimental observations show that the cortex posterior to SI is necessary for comprehensive utilization. The posterior parietal cortex comprises **area 5** and **area 7** (Fig. 14.6; see also Fig. 33.7) and belongs to the association areas of the cerebral cortex (these will be further discussed in Chapters 33 and 34). Areas 5 and 7 do not receive direct sensory information from the large somatosensory pathways but via numerous association fibers from SI and SII. They also receive numerous connections from other parts of the cortex. Broadly speaking, in areas 5 and 7 the bits of information reaching SI are put together and compared with other inputs, such as visual information and information about the salience of a stimulus and about intentions. Neurons in area 5 often have large receptive fields and

respond to complex combinations of stimuli, as shown in monkeys. Their activity depends not only on what is occurring in the periphery but also on whether the **attention** of the monkey is directed toward the stimulus. The posterior parietal cortex sends **efferent** connections to motor areas in the frontal lobe, thereby linking sensory information with **goal-directed movements**. Accordingly, some neurons are active in conjunction with the monkey stretching its arm toward something it wants.

In addition to the posterior parietal cortex, SII (Fig. 14.6) and adjoining areas in the **insula** (Fig. 14.9; see also Fig. 6.29) also process information from SI. The anterior part of insula integrates somatosensory information with other sensory modalities (taste and smell, and signals from vestibular receptors). Sensory units in these areas typically have large receptive fields and are activated from both sides of the body. Insula is, however, more strongly linked with processing of visceral sensory information and pain (see below, and Chapter 34, under "Insula").

Symptoms after Lesions of the Somatosensory Areas

Lesions of **SI** in humans entail reduced sensation in the opposite half of the body. A localized destruction of the SI, or of the fibers reaching it from the thalamus, may produce loss of sensation in a restricted area (corresponding to the somatotopic localization within SI). Not all sensory qualities are affected equally, however. **Discriminative** cutaneous sensation and **kinesthesia** are particularly disturbed; much less reduced (if at all) is pain sensation. As is the case with lesions of the dorsal columns, the sensory deficits gradually diminish after the time of the lesion. The least improvement with time is seen in the discriminative aspects of sensation, whereas pain sensation improves considerably. This can perhaps be explained by the fact that the pathways for signals from nociceptors are to a larger extent bilateral than are the pathways from low-threshold mechanoreceptors.

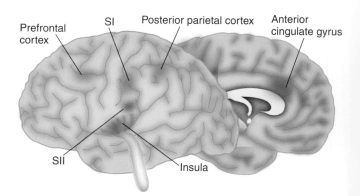

FIGURE 14.9 *Regions of the cerebral cortex showing increased activity during pain perception. (Based on data from a meta-analysis published by Peyron et al. 2000.)*

---

8 Representation of the genitals on the medial aspect of the hemisphere would be in conflict with the principle of continuous representation of body parts (Fig. 14.7). Indeed, a recent study using natural peripheral stimulation and fMRI (rather than stimulation of the cortical surface) concluded that the penis is represented on the convexity in the transition zone between the lower abdomen and the thighs (Kell et al. 2005).

It might also be explained by signals from nociceptors being distributed to areas outside the SI.

Whereas lesions of the **posterior parietal cortex** produce difficulties with the use of objects (**apraxia**), lesions of **SII** and neighboring regions in the **insula** impair the ability to recognize objects by touch (**tactile agnosia**). Similar problems with the visual recognition of objects occur after lesions of dorsal and ventral divisions of the extrastriatal visual areas, respectively.

Which Parts of the Cerebral Cortex Process Nociceptive Information?

Animal experiments show that noxious stimuli activate neuronal groups in many parts of the brain, both subcortically (in the amygdala, hypothalamus, PAG, basal ganglia, and cerebellum) and in the cerebral cortex. SI does not appear to play a central role in pain perception, however, in contrast to its crucial role in other aspects of somatosensory sensation. Although they have been elicited by electrical stimulation of SI in humans, pain sensations are an infrequent effect of such stimulation. Curiously, stimulation of other parts of the cortex did not evoke pain, either. Ablations of SI do not necessarily reduce pain perception, and only occasionally has it been reported to relieve chronic pain. Some even questioned the importance of the cerebral cortex for pain perception. However, recent studies in humans, using PET and fMRI, have demonstrated robust activation of the cerebral cortex on stimulation of nociceptors and, further, that this activation is associated with the subjective experience of pain.[9] The most consistently activated

regions are the **insula, SII,** and the **anterior cingulate gyrus** (Fig. 14.9). In addition, most studies show activation in **SI,** the **premotor area,** and the **thalamus.** Often the **prefrontal cortex** and the **posterior parietal cortex** (area 7b) are activated as well.

Most experimental studies evoked activation of the anterior cingulate gyrus (and other areas) via stimulation of skin nociceptors (injecting irritating substances or radiation heat). In fact, surgical ablation of the anterior cingulate gyrus has been used to alleviate chronic pain. Afterward, some patients report that the pain is still there, but it is less bothersome: it seems as if the affective component of the pain has been reduced (this is similar to pain perception after large lesions of the frontal lobe). This may perhaps be explained by other mental processes that involve the cingulate gyrus. For example, activation of the anterior cingulate gyrus is associated with the person directing his attention toward a stimulus. Further, activation of the anterior cingulate gyrus is associated with monitoring of cognitive and bodily processes: there is a change of activity in relation to errors. Indeed, signals from nociceptors are strong warnings that something is wrong in the body, and they forcefully direct our attention to the painful site.

The cortical pattern of activation upon nociceptor stimulation, as revealed by PET and fMRI, depends less on the mode of stimulation than on the **context** and the subject's **state of mind** (anxiety, expectations, feeling of control, and so forth). Many of the areas activated by painful stimuli may be activated in conjunction with other kinds of sensory processing and mental activities. Therefore, most likely no cortical regions are *specific* to pain processing. It seems, rather, that we experience pain when a distributed **network** of cortical and subcortical regions reaches a certain level and pattern of activity. This "pain network" (pain matrix) overlaps other cortical networks, such as networks for attention, emotional processing, and body image.

9 The interpretation of such data is not straightforward, however. For example, it is not always clear whether a change of cortical activity is an expression of altered sensory, affective, or cognitive processing. Furthermore, change of activity may be due to facilitation or inhibition of movements in response to a painful stimulus rather than to the experience of pain as such.

central mechanisms.[2] The former is clearly related to nociceptor activation; it ends when (or shortly after) the stimulus ends. The threshold for eliciting acute pain is high (see the preceding definition of a nociceptor). There is good correspondence between the intensity of nociceptor stimulation and the experience of pain. In such instances, pain is a homeostatic factor, serving as a signal to change behavior to avoid tissue damage. Chronic pain, in contrast, is characterized by a weak or absent correlation between stimulus and experience of pain. For example, **hyperalgesia**—the experience of pain on nociceptor stimulation—is more intense than normal—is often present.[3] Thus, the somatosensory system is abnormally sensitive. We all experience this altered state of the somatosensory system with, for example, a sprained ankle or a local infection, that is, in situations with inflammation. Even slight movement or touching of the injured part evokes intense pain, or it may be painful also at rest. In this situation the pain can be seen as biologically meaningful, as it ensures that the injured part gets the necessary rest; moreover, the pain subsides in parallel with the inflammation as the tissue heals. Hyperalgesia is due to **sensitization** of both the nociceptors (primary hyperalgesia) and of neurons in the dorsal horn and at higher levels (secondary hyperalgesia). Experimentally, dorsal horn neurons can be made hyperexcitable by inducing inflammation in a joint or in the skin.

Some, but not all, chronic pain patients have a lowered threshold, so that normal innoxious stimuli (such as touching the skin) can elicit intense and long-lasting pain. This phenomenon is called **allodynia** and appears to be caused by (abnormal) activation of nociceptive neurons in the cord by dorsal root fibers (Aβ) leading from low-threshold mechanoreceptors. Change of presynaptic inhibition is probably instrumental in causing such a switch in the signal traffic. (The normal situation is that activity in thick myelinated dorsal root fibers *inhibits* nociceptive neurons, as discussed later under "Analgesia Can Be Produced by Nerve Stimulation and Acupuncture".)

Another characteristic of long-lasting pain is the tendency to **radiate**—the pain spreads out from the original painful site. This is most likely due to sensitization of

(among others) spinothalamic neurons in the segments above and below the dorsal roots leading from the inflamed region (as mentioned, the dorsal root fibers divide in an ascending and a descending branch that may pass for several segments).

Glial cells seem to be implicated in development and maintenance of chronic pain. Thus, in the cord astrocytes and activated microglia release neuroactive substances (interleukins, tumor necrosis factor, nitric oxide [NO], ATP, and others). These substances may increase transmitter release from central terminals of nociceptive dorsal root fibers. Further, activated glial cells can sensitize dorsal horn neurons, among them spinothalamic ones. Activation of glial cells occurs with infections in the CNS, but also in response to release of substance P and amino acid transmitters from nociceptive dorsal root fibers.

Plastic Changes and Altered Brain Networks

Hyperalgesia, allodynia, and radiating pain are at least partly due to altered synaptic transmission in the CNS: chronic pain is associated with **plastic changes** that make neurons in many parts of the somatosensory system hyperexcitable. This is best documented in the dorsal horn but occurs also at higher levels. As with plastic changes in other systems, N-methyl-D-aspartate (**NMDA**) **receptors** have a crucial role. **Substance P** increases the sensitivity of NMDA receptors to glutamate, so that wide-dynamic range spinothalamic neurons might react more vigorously to inputs from low-threshold mechanoreceptors.

Intense pain of some duration may leave "memory traces" in the brain, so that later, minimal provocation may suffice to revive the pain. For example, a man who had a painful spine fracture reexperienced the pain when, many years later, he suffered a myocardial infarction. Electric stimulation during brain surgery indicates that part of the somatosensory **thalamus** becomes hyperexcitable in patients with chronic pain syndromes. For example, patients with panic attacks accompanied by chest pain and patients with deafferentation pain reported their usual pain on thalamic stimulation. In contrast, patients undergoing surgery for movement disorders reported no pain on stimulation at the same thalamic sites.

It appears from morphometric studies that chronic pain conditions may cause **gray and white matter alterations** in pain-related networks. Although findings differ somewhat among studies, most report gray-matter reductions in the anterior **cingulate cortex**, the **insula**, and the **orbitofrontal cortex** (the specific cellular changes that underlie these findings are unknown, however). Further, fMRI studies show altered activation of networks related to attention in chronic pain patients. Finally, in patients with complex regional pain syndrome (CRPS), the

---

2 The indiscriminate use of the term "chronic pain" has been criticized because it lacks precision and encompasses a variety of conditions with different causes, courses, and prognoses. Indeed, definitions of chronic pain differ widely. Some define it as pain that persists longer than the course of natural healing, others that it lasts longer than three, alternatively six months. Some even use as a criterion that the pain has not responded to available (drug) treatment. The International Association for the Study of Pain defines chronic pain as: "... pain which persists past the normal time of healing ... With non-malignant pain, three months is the most convenient point of division between acute and chronic pain, but for research purposes six months will often be preferred."

3 The International Association for the Study of Pain has proposed that **hyperalgesia** be used as an umbrella term for all conditions of increased pain sensitivity (Loeser and Treede 2008). Allodynia would then be a special case of hyperalgesia.

somatosensory-cortex representation of the painful part seems to shrink but normalizes during successful therapy. Curiously, in chronic back pain patients, an *enlarged* back representation appears to occur. It seems, therefore, fair to say that while cortical reorganization in chronic pain states is well documented, its functional significance is less than clear.

Pathologic Pain

Chronic pain can occur not only on increased nociceptor activity but also after loss of sensory information, either from nociceptors or from low-threshold mechanoreceptors. We use the term **pathologic pain** here rather loosely to describe conditions in which pain occurs without any nociceptor activation (or peripheral tissue pathology)—that is, pain that has no obvious biologic function (in contrast to "normal" or "physiological" pain). Pathologic pain may have quite different causes, such as partial damage to peripheral nerves or destruction of central somatosensory pathways, for example, in the cord or in the thalamus (usually termed **neuropathic pain**). **Deafferentation pain** is pain that, paradoxically, occurs after loss of sensory information from a body part. A striking example of the latter is patients with **avulsion** of dorsal roots (this occurs sometimes with the roots of the brachial plexus upon a violent pull of the arm). In spite of no sensory nerves entering the cord, such patients often develop excruciating pain in the denervated arm. Pathologic pain also occurs in some patients below a **transverse lesion of the cord**, even though all ascending sensory pathways are interrupted. Pathologic pain may also be felt in an area of the skin with reduced sensibility in patients who have had shingles (**postherpetic neuralgia**). A stroke destroying parts of the thalamus leading to reduced sensibility in a body part is sometimes associated with chronic pain (**thalamic pain**). **Phantom pain**, often occurring for shorter or longer periods after amputations, refers to pain felt in the missing body part. Clinical evidence indicates that this peculiar phenomenon is associated with plastic changes in the brain (especially in the somatosensory cortex). It is not due to abnormal activity in peripheral nerves or ascending sensory pathways. Often, the pain occurs together with a vivid experience of abnormal movements or postures of the missing limb. Probably, the brain misinterprets the lack of sensory information from the missing body, drawing the conclusion that something is seriously "wrong" out there.

It is fair to say that our understanding of pathologic pain syndromes is far from satisfactory. It is particularly enigmatic why apparently identical injuries cause chronic pain in some patients but not in others (the majority). An association between pathologic pain syndromes and certain personality traits has not been convincingly demonstrated.

Complex Regional Pain Syndromes (CRPS): A Special Type of Pathologic Pain

In some patients, pain continues in spite of complete healing of an injury (most often in the extremities). What started as a "normal," nociceptor-driven pain continues for unknown reasons as a pathologic pain. For example, an apparently trivial fracture of the radius is sometimes followed by pain for years after the fracture has healed. Similar persistence of pain can occur after partial lesions of peripheral nerves (neuropathic pain).Usually, such patients also suffer from hyperalgesia and allodynia, and even light touch may provoke excruciating pain. Often they also show signs of **autonomic dysfunction**, such as abnormal sweating and circulatory disturbances. This condition used to be called reflex sympathetic dystrophy (RSD), reflex dystrophy, or sympathetically mediated pain. It is especially unfortunate, however, that names of poorly understood diseases implicate an etiology, like "reflex" and "sympathetic." In some cases, especially after nerve injury, the pain has a peculiar burning quality, and the name **causalgia** refers to this condition (Greek: *kausos*, heat; *algos*, pain).

The term **complex regional pain syndrome** (CRPS) was introduced in an attempt to avoid the many confusing terms for these kinds of pathologic pain conditions. CRPS is a purely descriptive term, reflecting that we do not know the pathophysiological mechanisms leading to the various symptoms. It has two subgroups, with reasonably precise definitions, corresponding largely to reflex dystrophy (CRPS type I) and causalgia (CRPS type II), respectively.

CRPS and the Sympathetic System

As mentioned, patients with complex regional pain syndromes often show evidence of autonomic dysfunction in the painful part—mainly hyperactivity of the sympathetic system. The often-used term "reflex sympathetic dystrophy" (RSD) implies that sympathetic dysfunction *causes* the syndrome. The pain relief achieved in some patients by a sympathetic block (e.g., of the stellate ganglion in case of pain in the hand) would seem to support this assumption. Nevertheless, **microneurographic** and other kinds of studies have not confirmed abnormally increased activity of sympathetic postganglionic fibers in such patients, even in those with obvious signs of sympathetic hyperactivity such as profuse sweating and extreme cutaneous vasoconstriction. This seeming paradox may perhaps be explained by **adrenergic receptors** starting to be expressed by **spinal ganglion cells** (Fig. 15.1). Thus, normal levels circulating catecholamines may activate sensory neurons. There is furthermore evidence that in some CRPS patients neuropeptides (substance P and cholecystokinin [CCK] in particular) are released from sensory nerve endings in the skin of the painful parts.

evoked by painful stimuli.[4] In pain-induced analgesia, pain in one part of the body seems to be "rewarded" by analgesia in other parts.

Opiates, Opioids, and Endorphins

Some of the dorsal horn interneurons contain opioid peptides. These neuropeptides, found in many parts of the brain, got their name because they have actions that resemble closely those of the opiate-type drugs, such as morphine. The naturally occurring (endogenous) peptides of this kind are also called **endorphins**, that is, endogenous morphine. Opioids, when injected locally in the dorsal horn, have inhibitory effects on spinothalamic cells, but it is not known whether the inhibition is caused by a direct action or is mediated by interneurons (or both). Three main groups of endorphins have so far been discovered, each with its characteristic distribution in the brain and spinal cord. Best characterized are β **endorphin**, two varieties of **enkephalin**, and **dynorphin**. Whereas β endorphin is restricted to one neuronal group in the hypothalamus (the arcuate nucleus), the enkephalins and dynorphin are present in interneurons in many parts of the CNS (among them, parts that are not concerned with aspects of pain sensation).

That **morphine** and other **opiates** can alleviate severe pain has been known for hundreds of years. Today we know that there are receptors in the brain to which opiates can bind and exert their effects. These receptors are actually receptors for the endorphins, and at least five different receptors, each with affinity for a certain subgroup of endorphins, have so far been identified. **Opiate receptors** (binding morphine) are present in, among other places, the PAG, the NRM, and parts of the spinal dorsal horn (especially laminae I, II, and V). Microinjection of morphine in the PAG can produce analgesia in experimental animals that depend at least in part on connections from the NRM to the spinal cord. The actions of morphine appear thus to be exerted both in the spinal cord and in the PAG. In the cord, binding of morphine to opiate receptors on inhibitory interneurons in the substantia gelatinosa and, presumably, on primary afferent terminals, leads to inhibition of spinothalamic cells. The action in the PAG occurs most likely by activation of the descending pathway from NRM and probably also by activation of ascending connections from the PAG acting on higher levels of the CNS. Binding of morphine in other parts of the brain, such as the amygdala and other limbic structures, is probably also important in explaining the actions of morphine.

Analgesia Can Be Produced by Nerve Stimulation and Acupuncture

Analgesia may also be produced therapeutically by stimulation of peripheral nerves. When done with surface electrodes, the procedure is called **transcutaneous nerve stimulation** (**TNS**). One kind of analgesia occurs immediately and is mediated by activity of **thick myelinated fibers** in the stimulated nerves (i.e., fibers leading from low-threshold mechanoreceptors). Selective stimulation of such fibers is elicited by electrical stimulation with **high frequency** and low intensity or by natural stimuli such as vibration, light touch, or pressure. The analgesia is restricted to parts of the body innervated by the peripheral nerves, and it usually disappears when the stimulation stops. It is mediated by activity in collaterals of the thick dorsal root fibers that inhibit impulse transmission from the thin (Aδ and C) fibers in the dorsal horn, via inhibitory interneurons and presynaptic inhibition. Melzack and Wall (1965) proposed such interaction between thick and thin dorsal root fibers in their gate-control theory. It is presumably the basis of the everyday observation that it helps to blow at a finger that hurts, that it may help to move the part that has received an acute injury, that labor pains may be alleviated by rubbing over the lower back, and so forth.

Another kind of stimulation-induced analgesia requires that **thin sensory fibers** be activated. This can be achieved by electrical stimulation of **low frequency** with relative high intensity. Classical **acupuncture** probably obtains the same effect by rotation of thin needles in the tissue. The analgesia produced by this kind of stimulation occurs with latency but may last for hours after termination of the stimulation. Analgesia is not limited to the parts of the body that were stimulated. This kind of stimulation-induced analgesia is most likely due, at least in part, to activation of the descending connections from the brain stem. The activation may happen by way of collaterals from spinothalamic and spinoreticular cells to the PAG and adjacent parts of the reticular formation. The analgesia can be reversed or prevented by intravenous injection of **naloxone**. Further, in animal experiments it has been blocked by sectioning the dorsolateral fascicle. The results of such control experiments are in part contradictory, however, and indicate that not all aspects of stimulation-induced analgesia can be explained by liberation of endorphins.

Functional Role of Pain-Modulating Systems

A dominating view today is that modulation of pain is just one among several bodily adjustments—controlled by the nervous system—to physical and mental challenges. The mental "set" and the individual's interpretation of the situation determine the choice of responses. In other words, **expectation** of what a stimulus will

---

4 Both dopamine and opioid peptides in the nucleus accumbens appear to be necessary for pain-induced analgesia. The nucleus accumbens probably exerts its effects by indirect connections to NRM or nearby regions. The PAG and the hypothalamus may be intercalated in the pathway.

cause is more decisive for the response than the stimulus itself. Nevertheless, we do not fully understand the functional role of the pain-modulating systems, nor under which conditions they are activated. It is reasonable to assume, however, that **inhibiting** systems are active in situations with severe injuries and no experience of pain (as, e.g., in war and major civil accidents). In such situations, suppression of pain may enable continuation of intense physical activity, which may be of vital importance. Markedly reduced pain sensitivity may also occur in more peaceful situations, such as sport competitions. Further, pain-suppressing systems (at several levels) appear to be active in expectation-dependent analgesia, although expectation may also increase pain perception (see next section, "Placebo and Nocebo"). Animal experiments indicate that analgesia can occur in stressful situations characterized by the inability to escape (**stress-induced analgesia**). However, the mental state of the animal seems to decide whether analgesia occurs. Thus, in one study analgesia occurred only if the animal was calm at the start of the period of stress, whereas anxious animals became hyperalgesic. This resembles the well-known effect of anxiety on the experience of pain in humans.

PLACEBO AND NOCEBO

The **placebo** effect is probably best understood as one part of a repertoire of responses to challenges that threaten our mental or physical stability (see also Chapter 30, under "Psychosomatic Relations," and Chapter 31, under "Amygdala and Conditioned Fear"). Although it has attracted most attention in connection with the treatment of pain, we now know that placebo effects concern several physiological processes. The beneficial placebo effect depends on the patient's positive expectations, but negative expectations may evoke increased pain and harmful physiological alterations. This is called the **nocebo** effect. However, placebo (and nocebo) effects may in addition involve **conditioned responses**, for example elicited by the taste of a drug that previously was experienced as effective (e.g., a painkiller).[5] In this respect, the placebo response is **learned**, depending on prior experience. Even the observation of another person receiving a beneficial treatment induces a placebo response in the observer.

As discussed, descending connections from the brain stem can inhibit or enhance nociceptive signal

transmission, depending on the situation (Fig. 15.2). Such mechanisms are most likely involved in the placebo and nocebo effects on pain. One likely pathway goes from the amygdala to the PAG. At the cortical level, expectation of pain relief reduces the activity of the pain network (Fig. 15.4A). Further, during the expectation phase cortical regions usually involved in cognitive and evaluative processes show enhanced activity (Figure 15.4B).

A common misconception is that the placebo effect works only with moderate pains and only in comparison with "weak" drugs. However, if the patient believes that the drug she gets is morphine, the placebo effect is much greater than if the patient believes it to be aspirin. Indeed, postoperative, intravenous administration of placebo (saline) in full view of the patient had the same analgesic effect as 6 to 8 mg of morphine given covertly.

The question remains, however, how **expectancy** controls the "pain network" and pain-suppressing systems. Put more broadly: how do thoughts and feelings express themselves through the body? We discuss this theme further in Chapters 31 and 32 although, admittedly, we are far from a full understanding of the **mind–body problem**.

Placebo

The word placebo (literally: "I shall please") has been used for a long time about mock medicine—that is, drugs and procedures that the doctor knows have no effect. In clinical trials, for example, inert tablets are given as a placebo to decide whether a drug has a specific effect on a disease. Thus, it is well known that a treatment without any specific effect may influence the disease and the experience of pain. We know that the effect is only present if the patient expects the treatment to work. Further, surgery produces a larger placebo effect than drugs, and injection of a drug is more efficient than oral administration.

An operation introduced in the 1950s to cure **angina pectoris** exemplifies the placebo effect of surgery. On a dubious theoretical basis, the internal mammary arteries were ligated to improve the blood supply to the ailing heart. Many patients noted improvement in their condition after the surgery. Later pathological examinations showed, however, that no improvement of the blood supply had occurred. Therefore, a study was initiated to compare two groups of patients with angina pectoris: one group underwent ligation of the artery, the other group underwent the same procedure but without ligation (a sham operation). Many of the patients in both groups noted improvement, and the improvement lasted for the observation period of 6 months. Remarkably, the improvement concerned not only reduction of pain but also objectively measurable variables, such as walking distance, drug consumption, and (in some) even the electrocardiogram. Several later studies have shown

---

5 In one study, patients received the immunosuppressant cyclosporine in association with a flavored drink. After a number of repetitions of the association, the flavored drink alone induced immunosuppression. Several other studies in experimental animals and in humans have shown similar conditioning of immune responses. The endocrine system is also subject to placebo conditioning. The conditioned immune and endocrine responses do not require conscious expectations.

pains are forgotten very quickly. Plastic changes may produce chronic pain in some persons, while in others they may enable reactivation of a long-forgotten pain in a certain body part.

Advances in basic pain research have influenced **clinical practice**; for example, new drugs are designed to attack the central synaptic changes in chronic pain directly. Further, an important aim for modern pain therapy is to prevent the occurrence of the plastic changes in the dorsal horn and elsewhere. Thus, analgesic drugs are often administered before surgery, and afterward the dosage is individualized according to the need of the patient rather than to a fixed scheme. In addition, the importance of early and efficient pain relief in patients with injuries that are apt to produce persisting pain is being realized.

16 | The Visual System

Humans are "visual animals." Like in other primates, our visual system is highly developed, and accordingly large parts of the cerebral cortex are devoted to processing of visual information. There are approximately 1 million axons in the optic nerve, constituting almost 40% of the total number of axons in the cranial nerves. The receptors for sight, **photoreceptors**, are the rods and cones of the retina. Their adequate stimulus is electromagnetic waves with a wavelength between 400 and 700 nm. The photoreceptors do not react to light with shorter (ultraviolet light) or longer (infrared light) wavelengths. The photoreceptors transform light energy to graded changes of the membrane potential with ensuing release of **glutamate**. From the photoreceptors, the signals pass to **bipolar cells** and from these to **retinal ganglion cells**. Several kinds of **interneurons** enable considerable information processing in the retina. The **rods** are responsible for vision in dim light, whereas the **cones** require daylight and are necessary for perception of visual details and colors.

The **visual pathways** start with the retinal ganglion cells sending their axons to the **lateral geniculate body** of the thalamus. The ganglion cell axons leave the eye in the **optic nerve** and pass through the **optic chiasm**, where axons from nasal half of the retina cross while axons from the temporal half pass through uncrossed. The axons continue in the **optic tract** to the lateral geniculate body. Axons from neurons in the lateral geniculate form the **optic radiation**, and end in the primary visual cortex—the **striate area**—in the occipital lobe of the same side. In this way, stimuli from the left visual field reach the right occipital lobe. The visual pathways show a precise, **retinotopical** organization at all levels. The area striata performs the first analysis of the visual information, while further processing takes place in **extrastriate** visual areas in the occipital, temporal, and parietal lobes. The processing is largely **segregated**, so that, for example, different areas deal with color and motion. Visual information from the extrastriate areas is integrated with other sensory modalities, and finally reaches the frontal lobe where visual information contributes to the control of behavior.

To understand the visual system, it is not sufficient to know the conscious use of visual information; the many reflex effects elicited by visual stimuli must also be taken into account. Among the reflex effects are those ensuring **fixation of our gaze** on the object we want to examine and follows it if it moves, and those ensuring that the visual images formed at the retina are always in focus. Such **visual reflexes**, however, are only briefly mentioned in this chapter. They are discussed more thoroughly in Chapter 25, under "Central Control of Eye Movements," and in Chapter 27, under "The Light Reflex and the Accommodation Reflex."

THE EYEBALL AND THE REFRACTING MEDIA

The Eye and a Camera Have Certain Features in Common

The **eyeball** (bulbus oculi) (Figs. 16.1 and 16.2) has a firm outer wall of dense connective tissue covered on the inside by the light-sensitive retina. Between these two layers is a vascular layer, the **choroid**, that is highly pigmented, thus ensuring that light enters the eye only through the pupil and preventing reflection of light (compare with the dull black inside a camera). The diameter of the **pupil** (the shutter) controls the amount of light allowed into the eye. Refraction of the light takes place on its way through the cornea and the lens. The curvature of the lens can be varied by the use of the **ciliary muscles**, so that the retinal image is always sharply focused (in a camera, the focusing is brought about by varying the distance between the lens and the light-sensitive film). **Extraocular muscles** (external eye muscles) attach to the eyeballs and can move them to coordinate their positions, so that the visual images hit corresponding points of the two retinas (Fig. 16.3). This is a prerequisite for our perception of one image, and not two (two slightly different images are formed in the eyes, however). We discuss the extraocular muscles more comprehensively in Chapter 25.

Structural Features of the Eye

The wall of the eye consists of three layers. Outermost is the **sclera**; then follows the **choroid**, and the **retina** is the innermost layer. The eye keeps its spherical shape because the sclera has some stiffness, but mainly because the **pressure** inside the eye is higher than outside (approximately 15 cm H_2O).

Anteriorly, the sclera has a circular opening, in which the transparent **cornea** is positioned like a glass of

the ciliary muscle reduces the diameter of the ring formed by the ciliary body. This slackens the zonular fibers and enables the lens to become rounder; that is, its curvature (convexity) and thus also the refraction of the light increase. Contraction of the ciliary muscle is required sharply to see objects that are closer to the eye than approximately 6 m. This distance is called the **far point of the eye**. In a normal—**emmetropic**—eye, the length of the eyeball is accurately adjusted to the refraction of the cornea and the lens in the relaxed state. When viewing objects at distances greater than about 6 m, the lens maintains the same convexity, and yet the image is always focused on the retina. This is because the light rays entering the eye from points at such distances are all virtually parallel and are therefore collected in the plane of the retina (like a camera focused at infinite distance). If the length of the eyeball differs from the normal (even by only a few hundred microns), the light rays are not collected in the plane of the eye and the sight is blurred. If the eyeball is too long, the light rays are collected in front of the retina. This condition is called **myopia** and is corrected by concave (−) glasses.[1] If the eyeball is too short, the light rays meet behind the retina. Convex (+) glasses correct this **hypermetropia** (in children, because of their elastic lenses, the error is easily corrected by constant accommodation).

The closer an object comes within the far point of the eye, the more the convexity of the lens must be increased by contraction of the ciliary muscle. Such adjustment of the lens for near sight is called **accommodation**. The closest distance from the eye at which we can see an object sharply is called the **near point of the eye**. One's own near point can be easily determined by fixing the eyes on an object (e.g., a finger) that is gradually moved closer to the eye, until it no longer can be viewed sharply.

The far point of the eye depends on the curvature of the lens in its "relaxed" state—that is, with no contraction of the ciliary muscle—and remains stable throughout life. The near point, however, depends on the ability of the lens to increase its curvature and moves gradually away from the eye from birth until about the age of 60. This happens because the lens becomes gradually stiffer and less elastic, so that the ability to increase its convexity declines steadily. At about the age of 45 so much accommodation is lost—or, in other words, the near point is so far away—that it is difficult to read fine print. This condition, called **presbyopia**, is corrected by the use of convex (+) glasses of appropriate strength.

---

1 A correlation exists between much reading (i.e., accommodating for long periods) and development of myopia in adolescents. Animal experiments confirm that how the eye is used influences the growth of the eyeball. Thus, when 3-month-old monkeys were equipped with +3 glasses, the length of the eye changed to compensate for the refraction error.

THE RETINA

The retina forms the innermost layer of the eye (Fig. 16.2). The outer part of the retina, which adjoins the choroid, is the **pigmented epithelium** consisting of one layer of cuboid cells with large amounts of pigmented granules in their cytoplasm. Internal to the pigmented epithelium follows a layer with **photoreceptors**, and then two further layers with neurons (Fig. 16.4). The processes of the photoreceptors contact the **bipolar cells**, which, in turn, transmit signals to the **retinal ganglion cells**. The axons of the ganglion cells leave the eye in the **optic nerve** to end in nuclei in the diencephalon and the mesencephalon. The pigmented epithelium extends forward to the edge of the pupil (Fig. 16.2), whereas the photoreceptors, bipolars, and ganglion cells are present only in the parts of the retina situated posterior to the ciliary body (pars nervosa retinae).

Unlike many other receptors, the photoreceptors are not of peripheral origin but belong to the central nervous system (CNS). The retina develops in embryonic life as an evagination of the diencephalon (see Fig. 9.3).

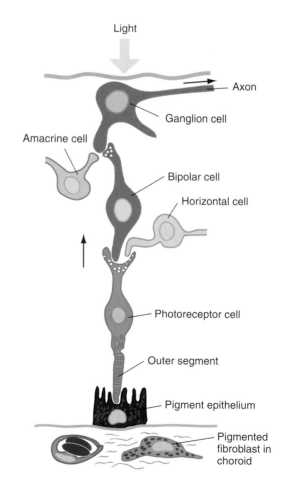

FIGURE 16.4 *The retina*. The main cell types and their interconnections (highly simplified).

Strictly speaking, the term "retinal ganglion cell" is therefore not correct, but it is nevertheless maintained.

Because the photoreceptors are located external to the two other neuronal layers, the light has to pass through the latter to reach the photoreceptors. Because there are no myelinated axons in the retina, however, the layers internal to the photoreceptors are sufficiently translucent.

In addition to the aforementioned neuronal types, the retina also contains many **interneurons**, the **amacrine cells**, and the **horizontal cells** (Fig. 16.4; these neurons are treated in more detail later in this chapter, under "Interneurons in the Retina"). The horizontal cells are responsible for **lateral inhibition** (see Fig. 13.4), among other things. More processing of sensory information takes place in the retina than in any other sense organ. Thus, the visual information transmitted to higher centers of the brain from the retina is already "distorted" by enhancement of the contrast between light and darkness and by preference for signals caused by light from moving objects.

The Retina Has a Layered Structure

Under the microscope, several distinct layers of the retina can be identified in sections cut perpendicular to its surface (Figs. 16.5 and 16.12). Externally, toward the pigmented epithelium, lie the light-sensitive parts of the photoreceptors—their **external segments**. The two types of photoreceptors, the **rods** and the **cones**, can be distinguished because the external segments of the cones are thicker and usually somewhat shorter than those of the rods. Internal to the layer of the external segments, there are three distinct layers with cell nuclei. The **outer nuclear layer** consists of the nuclei of the photoreceptors. The nuclei of the bipolar cells (and many of the interneurons) form the **inner nuclear layer**. The innermost layer of nuclei belongs to the ganglion cells—**the ganglion cell layer**. Between the nuclear layers lie processes of the neurons and their synapses, consequently termed the **outer** and **inner synaptic layers** (or plexiform layers). In the outer synaptic layer, the processes of the bipolar cells end in depressions in the processes of the photoreceptors (Fig. 16.4). The photoreceptor processes contain synaptic vesicles close to the presynaptic membrane.

A special kind of glial cell—the **Müller cells**—extends through the retina from the pigmented epithelium to the vitreous body. They are most likely a form of astrocyte.

Photoreceptors and the Photopigment

Electron microscopy reveals that the outer segments of the rods and cones are packed with folded membrane, forming a large surface containing the light-sensitive photopigment. In the rods, the folds of membrane lie mostly intracellularly, whereas in the cones they are partly invaginations of the surface membrane. The photoreceptors constantly remove and resynthesize the membrane folds.

The rods and the cones contain different kinds of photopigment. The **rods** contain **rhodopsin**, which has been the most studied. It consists of a protein part, **opsin**, and **retinal**, which is an aldehyde of the **vitamin A** molecule. Retinal is light absorbing and is changed by light (absorption of photons). Simultaneously, the opsin part is changed, and this leads to alteration of the membrane potential of the photoreceptor (hyperpolarization by closure of Na$^+$ channels). The **transduction** mechanism involves activation of G proteins and intracellular signal molecules, and structurally the photopigments resemble closely other G protein–coupled receptors (e.g., muscarinic receptors, and receptors for smell). The hyperpolarization of the photoreceptors by light stimuli affects the bipolar cells (and retinal interneurons), which then act on the ganglion cells to alter the frequency of action potentials conducted in the optic nerve to the visual centers of the brain.

The photopigment of the **cones** differs slightly from rhodopsin in the structure of the opsin molecules. Further, there are three varieties of **cone opsin** molecules, which explain why we have three kinds of cones absorbing light of different wavelengths (Fig. 16.6). The opsin of the cones is also bound to retinal, but the opsin molecule determines the wavelength sensitivity of retinal.

Dark Adaptation and Light Adaptation

When looking into the eye (e.g., through an ophthalmoscope), the color of the retina is a deep purple because of the content of rhodopsin. The reflection of light from the retina produces the red eyes of flash photography. The color bleaches quickly on illumination of the retina, but it returns slowly in the dark. The light has broken down the rhodopsin, and it takes some time to resynthesize it. We experience the time needed for this process of **dark adaptation** when entering a dark room from strong sunlight. In the beginning, we can hardly see anything, but gradually the ability to see returns. This happens in two stages; first, there is a rapid stage of improvement of about 10 minutes, and thereafter a slower stage of almost 1 hour until full light sensitivity has been restored (if the initial illumination was very intense). Because the rods are responsible for vision in dim light (scotopic vision), the dark adaptation depends on resynthesis of rhodopsin in the rods.

We experience the opposite phenomenon of dark adaptation, **light adaptation**, when moving from darkness into strong light. Also then, after first seeing nothing, vision gradually returns. The strong light bleaches the photopigment massively—that is, there is an intense,

release is reduced by light (as if darkness were the adequate stimulus). Recording from **bipolar cells** has shown that they are of two kinds: one is depolarized by light, and the other is hyperpolarized. **Glutamate**—which is the transmitter released from the photoreceptors—has a depolarizing (and therefore excitatory) effect on neurons in other parts of the CNS. With regard to the bipolars, however, one kind is hyperpolarized by glutamate, whereas another is depolarized. This is presumably due to the existence of two different kinds of postsynaptic glutamate receptor.

We can **summarize** the events as follows. When light hyperpolarizes the photoreceptors, the release of glutamate is reduced, as mentioned. This leads to less hyperpolarization, which is the same as depolarization, of one kind of bipolar; thus, some of the bipolars are depolarized and therefore increase their own transmitter release. This is an example of **disinhibition**. The opposite happens with the other kind of bipolar cell, which is hyperpolarized (receives less depolarization) and therefore reduces its transmitter release. Thus, one kind of bipolar reacts with increased transmitter release when light is turned on, the other kind when the light is turned off (Fig. 16.7).

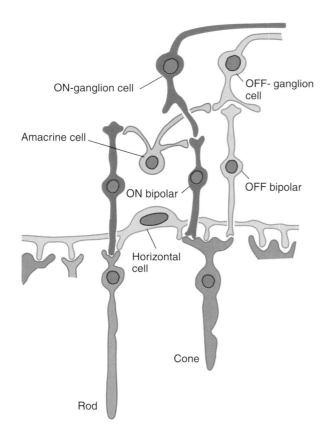

FIGURE 16.7 *ON and OFF bipolar and ganglion cells in the retina.* Simplified diagram showing the coupling of a cone to two different bipolar cells, and further coupling of the bipolars to ganglion cells that increase or decrease their activity, respectively, when light falls on their receptive fields. Amacrine cells are intercalated in the coupling of rods to ganglion cells.

The bipolar cells have depolarizing (excitatory) effects on the **retinal ganglion cells** (and on amacrine cells), and we can then understand why there are also two kinds of ganglion cells: one that is excited, and one that is inhibited by light hitting the photoreceptors to which they are coupled. We therefore use the terms ON and OFF **bipolars** and **ganglion cells**. In contrast to the photoreceptors and the bipolars, the ganglion cells produce action potentials (conducted in the optic nerve to the higher visual centers).

Couplings from Rods and Cones Are Different

Figure 16.7 shows that there are two **parallel signal pathways** from the **cones**. The ON ganglion cells increase their firing frequency with increasing intensity of light hitting the cones with which they are connected, whereas the OFF ganglion cells increase their firing frequency with increasing darkness. These two channels enable the ganglion cells to inform of a much wider range of light intensities than if there were only one channel. However, the bipolars and the ganglion cells do not inform about the absolute light intensity but the intensity in a small spot on the retina in comparison to the surroundings. This is caused by **lateral inhibition** produced by **horizontal cells** (Fig. 16.7), which are electrically coupled.

The coupling from the **rods** to the ganglion cells is more complicated than from the cones. Thus, bipolars excited by rods do not influence ganglion cells directly but via a special kind of **amacrine cells** (Fig. 16.7). These amacrines excite ON bipolars and inhibit OFF bipolars. It should be noticed that the rods and cones are coupled to the same ganglion cells. Consequently, a ganglion cell transmitting signals from cones in daylight transmits from rods in the dusk.

Interneurons in the Retina

As mentioned, the retina contains interneurons in addition to the photoreceptors, bipolars, and ganglion cells (Fig. 16.4). The **horizontal cells** send their processes in the plane of the retina—that is, perpendicular to the orientation of the photoreceptors and the bipolars (Fig. 16.7). The horizontal cell processes establish contact with the inner segments of the photoreceptors and with the dendrites of the bipolars. They therefore regulate the transmission from the photoreceptors to the bipolars. There is good evidence that the horizontal cells are responsible for the typical receptive fields of the bipolars and ganglion cells with central excitation and peripheral inhibition (or vice versa). This involves complex and unusual synaptic mechanisms that are not fully understood. The horizontal cells are interconnected with **electric synapses**, probably enabling transmission for several millimeters in the plane of the retina.

They release γ-aminobutyric acid (**GABA**) in their efferent synapses onto the inner segments of the photoreceptors. Each horizontal cell is depolarized by **glutamate** released from many photoreceptors. Thus, light hitting the photoreceptors leads to hyperpolarization of the horizontal cells; that is, they release less GABA so that the photoreceptors are disinhibited. Conversely, the horizontal cells hyperpolarize the photoreceptors in darkness.

The other kind of retinal interneuron, the **amacrine cell**, is located with its cell body in the inner nuclear layer and establishes contact with both the axons of the bipolar cells and the dendrites of the ganglion cells (Fig. 16.7). Amacrine cells are thus intercalated between bipolar cells and ganglion cells, and many bipolar cells exert their effect on ganglion cells only or mainly via amacrine cells. As mentioned, this is the rule for **rod bipolars** (bipolars connected with rods). Such amacrines (**AII**) form **electric synapses** with ON (depolarizing) bipolars and chemical **glycinergic** synapses with OFF (hyperpolarizing) bipolars. Some of the processes of the amacrine cells also extend horizontally for considerable distances. The actions of the amacrine cells are varied and complex, and there are numerous morphological varieties. They are also heterogeneous with regard to their transmitter content, and, as mentioned, some establish both chemical and electric synapses. One subgroup of amacrines contains **GABA**, for example; others contain **acetylcholine** or **dopamine**. At least seven different **neuropeptides** have been associated with amacrine cells. Twenty different kinds of amacrine cells have so far been identified, considering differences in both synaptic connectivity and transmitter content. The amacrines play an important role in influencing the activity of many ganglion cells with properties that cannot be explained by transmission directly from bipolars to ganglion cells. For example, amacrine cells appear to be partly responsible for making certain ganglion cells sensitive to light stimuli (contrasts) with a specific orientation.

Receptive Fields of Retinal Ganglion Cells

Most retinal ganglion cells have in common that they are excited most effectively by shining light on small circular spots on the retina. These are the **receptive fields** of the ganglion cells and can be defined as the **area** of the retina from which a ganglion cell can be influenced. The receptive field can of course be determined not only for ganglion cells but also for neurons at all levels of the visual pathways. The ganglion cells are typically excited from a small central circle and inhibited from a peripheral circular zone, or vice versa (Fig. 16.8A). The American neurophysiologist Stephen Kuffler first demonstrated this in the early 1950s. He introduced the terms **on-center** and **off-center** for ganglion cells that are activated and inhibited, respectively, by light hitting the central zone of the receptive field. These correspond to ON and OFF ganglion cells, described above with reference to the center of their receptive fields (Fig. 16.7). Thus, as mentioned, illumination of a small spot on the retina can lead to increased activity in one chain of neurons—forming, as it were, a channel for signal transmission to the higher visual centers—and reduced activity in another. (The arrangement of a central excitatory field and a peripheral inhibitory zone is also found in the somatosensory system.) For receptive fields of the retinal ganglion cells, the central excitatory or inhibitory part of the receptive field can be explained by direct coupling from photoreceptors to bipolars and further to ganglion cells, whereas the peripheral zone with opposite effects must involve **horizontal cells** producing lateral inhibition (Fig. 16.7). As expected, illumination of the complete receptive field—the central and peripheral zones simultaneously—gives a much weaker response from the ganglion cells than illumination of the central zone only (Fig. 16.8).

In conclusion, each ganglion cell brings information to higher visual centers about a particular small, round area in a definite position on the retina, and thus in the visual field. Together, the receptive fields of all ganglion cells cover the whole visual field with the same type of concentrically arranged receptive fields. Ganglion cells that lie side by side in the retina have overlapping, but not identical, receptive fields.

Retinal Ganglion Cells Exaggerate Contours

Recording of ganglion cell activity under different lighting conditions show that the retinal ganglion cells do not give information about absolute light intensity. Rather, their activity depends on the **contrast** of intensity between the light falling on the central and the peripheral parts of the receptive field. For example, for an on-center cell, a narrow beam of strong light hitting precisely the center of the receptive field while the peripheral zone is in darkness evokes maximal firing frequency.

This preference of the visual system for contrast in light intensity can be demonstrated, for example, by looking at a gray circular spot surrounded by black (Fig. 16.9A). Exchanging the black surrounding with a light gray makes the gray spot appear darker (even though the amount of light the eye receives from the central gray area is unchanged). This property of the visual system makes it particularly suited to detect **contours**, which are especially important for analysis of form. Our ability to judge contrasts of light intensities does not just depend on retinal mechanisms, however. For example, the brightness of an area compared with its neighbors depends on our (subconscious) judgment of how the light falls—that is, whether we assume that

CENTRAL RETINA

PERIPHERAL RETINA

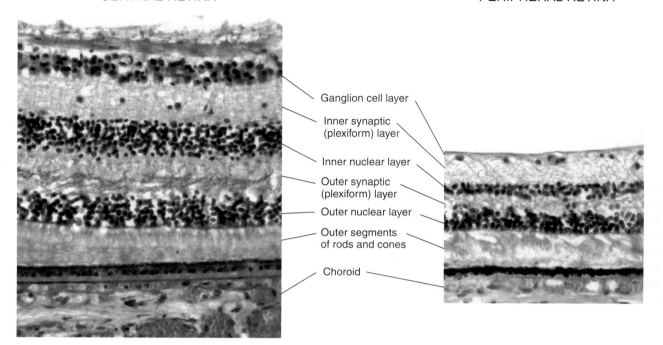

- Ganglion cell layer
- Inner synaptic (plexiform) layer
- Inner nuclear layer
- Outer synaptic (plexiform) layer
- Outer nuclear layer
- Outer segments of rods and cones
- Choroid

FIGURE 16.12 *Central and peripheral parts of the retina.* Photomicrographs illustrating how the various retinal layers differ in thickness when moving from the central to the peripheral parts of the retina. The density of ganglion cells is quite different in the two areas.

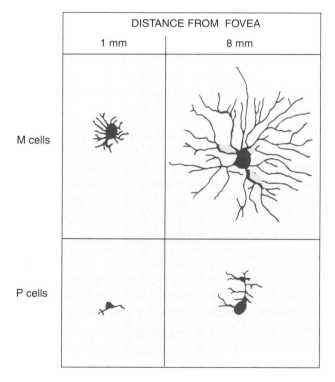

DISTANCE FROM FOVEA	
1 mm	8 mm
M cells	
P cells	

FIGURE 16.13 *Two main kinds of retinal ganglion cells (monkey).* Both types increase in size in the peripheral direction (distance from the fovea). The extension of the dendritic tree is related to the size of the receptive fields of the ganglion cells. The cells have been visualized by intracellular injection of HRP. (Based on Shapley and Perry 1986.)

There Are Two Main Kinds of Retinal Ganglion Cell

We described two kinds of retinal ganglion cell that differ according to whether they signal light or darkness (ON and OFF ganglion cells). There are, however, further specializations among ganglion cells that we should know to understand the information sent from the retina to higher visual centers.

Anatomic studies showed many years ago that the retinal ganglion cells differ greatly in size. One tendency, mentioned above, is that the **dendrites** of the ganglion cells are longer peripherally than centrally (Fig. 16.13). This relates to differences in the size of their receptive fields. However, ganglion cells with the same placement with regard to eccentricity on the retina also vary in size. It is now customary to recognize two main kinds of retinal ganglion cell, together constituting about 90% of all cells: the **M cells** and the **P cells**. As seen in Fig. 16.13, the P cells are tiny compared with the M cells, but both types are much smaller centrally than peripherally. Physiological studies of their properties indicate that the M cells primarily signal movement and contrasts of illumination, whereas the P cells are responsible for providing information about fine features (high visual acuity) and color. Both kinds can have either ON or OFF properties and can be activated under both scotopic and photopic light conditions. This is what one would expect, because signals from rods and cones converge on the same ganglion cells (Fig. 16.7). It is nevertheless possible that the M cells play a more important role than P cells in scotopic vision.

Next, we discuss the organization of the pathways followed by the signals from the retina, and we will see that information from the two main types of ganglion cells is kept separate—at least to some extent—up to the cortical level.

More about Retinal Ganglion Cells

The functional properties of the two main morphological types of ganglion cells have been clarified by intracellular staining of cells that first have been characterized by their response to various kinds of light stimuli. Particularly the cat's and the monkey's retinal ganglion cells have been studied in depth. Even though cat and monkey (and presumably human) ganglion cells have several features in common—for example, with regard to the organization of their receptive fields—there are also important differences (notably that cats lack ability to differentiate colors, and their visual acuity is much lower than in monkeys and man). What follows here is based on findings in the monkey. The **M cells** (called A cells by some authors) have a large cell body and a fairly extensive dendritic tree (Fig. 16.13). The axon is relatively thick. The **P cells** (or B cells) have smaller cell bodies, a less extensive dendritic tree, and a thinner axon than the M cells. The P cells are most numerous and probably constitute about 80% of all of the ganglion cells. A major difference is that many of the P cells respond preferentially to light with a particular wavelength—that is, they are **color-specific**—whereas M cells do not have such specificity. The M cells are more sensitive than the P cells to **contrasts** in **intensity** of illumination, however.

A further difference is that the M cells appear to respond better than the P cells to **moving stimuli**. In general, the M cells tend to respond especially when a stimulus starts and stops, whereas the P cells tend to give a signal as long as the stimulus lasts. In spite of anatomic differences between M and P cells, however, each group contains a wide variety of properties. For most properties, the two groups overlap, so that some M cells are more like typical P cells with regard to certain functional properties, and vice versa.

A **third kind** of retinal ganglion cell does not fit into the M and P groups described so far. In the monkey, they constitute about 10% of all ganglion cells. Both anatomically and physiologically, this group is heterogeneous, but the cells are usually smaller than the P cells and have thinner axons. The common feature of this group is that the cells send their axons to the **mesencephalon** rather than to the thalamus, like the M and P cells. A small fraction of the M cells sends an axon (most likely a collateral of the axon going to the thalamus) to the mesencephalon. It gives some insight into the development of the visual system to compare the proportion of retinal ganglion cells that sends axons to the mesencephalon in various species. Thus, in the cat, about 50% of the axons in the optic nerve pass to the mesencephalon, and the proportion is most likely even higher in lower mammals like the rat. In humans, it is probable that even less than 10% pass to the mesencephalon. With increasing development of the cerebral cortex, more and more of the analysis of visual information takes place at the cortical level rather than in the brain stem visual centers.

ORGANIZATION OF THE VISUAL PATHWAYS

The Visual Pathways

The axons of the retinal ganglion cells constitute the first link in the central visual pathways. All ganglion cell axons run toward the posterior pole of the eye, where they pass through the wall of the eyeball at the **optic papilla** (Figs. 16.1 and 16.11). They then form the **optic nerve**, which passes through the orbit and enters the cranial cavity. Here the two optic nerves unite to form the **optic chiasm** (Fig. 16.14; see also Fig. 6.13). In the optic chiasm some of the axons cross, and crossed and uncrossed fibers continue in the **optic tract**, which curves around the crus cerebri to end in the **lateral geniculate body** (corpus geniculatum laterale) of the thalamus (Fig. 16.15; see also Figs. 6.21 and 6.27). Here the axon terminals of the retinal ganglion cells establish synaptic contact with neurons that send their axons posteriorly into the occipital lobe. These efferent fibers of the lateral geniculate body form the **optic radiation** (radiatio optica) (Fig. 16.16). The optic radiation curves anteriorly and laterally to the posterior horn of the lateral ventricle and ends in the **primary visual cortical area**, which is situated around the **calcarine sulcus** (see Fig. 6.26). Some of the fibers of the optic radiation lie in the posterior part of the internal capsule, where they can be damaged together with the fibers of the pyramidal tract—for example, by bleeding or infarction—thus producing a combination of weakness (paresis) of the muscles of the opposite side of the body and blind areas in the opposite visual hemifield. The primary visual area is **area 17** of Brodmann, which is also called the **striate area**. The latter name (which we will use here) refers to a white stripe in the cortex, running parallel to the cortical surface. The stripe consists of myelinated fibers and is therefore whitish in a cut brain (Fig. 16.17).

Not all fibers of the optic nerve terminate in the lateral geniculate body. Some (about 10% in the monkey) terminate in the **mesencephalon**, especially in the **superior colliculus** and the **pretectal nuclei**. These fibers are of importance primarily for reflex adjustments of the

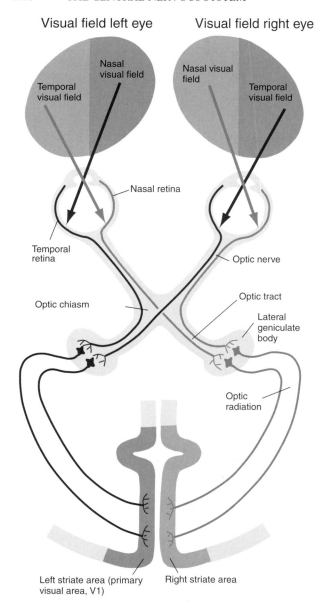

FIGURE 16.14 *The visual pathways.* For didactic reasons, the visual field of each eye is shown separately (cf. Fig. 16.3).

position of the head and the eyes. Some fibers of the optic nerve pass to the **hypothalamus** where they contribute to regulation of circadian rhythms (see Chapter 30, under "Hypothalamus and Circadian Rhythms").

Axons from the M and P Cells Terminate in Different Layers of the Lateral Geniculate Body

The human lateral geniculate body (and that of other primates, like monkeys) consists of six cell layers (Figs. 16.18 and 16.19). The two ventral-most laminas (1 and 2) are composed of large cells and are therefore called the **magnocellular layers**, whereas the dorsal four are composed of small cells and are called the **parvocellular layers** (Fig. 16.16). Anatomic and physiological studies have shown that the large retinal ganglion cells, the **M cells**, send their axons to the magnocellular layers of the lateral geniculate body, whereas the small ganglion cells, the **P cells**, send their axons (at least preferentially) to the parvocellular layers (Fig. 16.18). There is thus a division of the lateral geniculate body that largely corresponds to the functional division among retinal ganglion cells. It is now usual to speak of the two **parallel pathways**—M and P—from the retina to the lateral geniculate and further to the visual cortex. The significance of this will be discussed in connection with the visual cortex.

Signal Processing in the Lateral Geniculate Body: Corticothalamic Connections

Although the receptive fields of neurons in the lateral geniculate body are closely similar to those of retinal ganglion cells, the lateral geniculate is not merely a simple relay station. Signals from the retina are subject to modification before being forwarded to the striate area. Of special importance are strong, retinotopically organized **corticothalamic projections** from the visual cortex to the lateral geniculate. These connections most likely can control the signal traffic from the retina through the lateral geniculate and have been shown physiologically to influence the properties of the neurons. This modulation probably relates to mental states

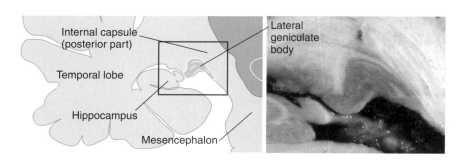

FIGURE 16.15 *The lateral geniculate body.* Drawing and photograph of frontal section through the right hemisphere. The whitish bands separating the lamellae are partly visible.

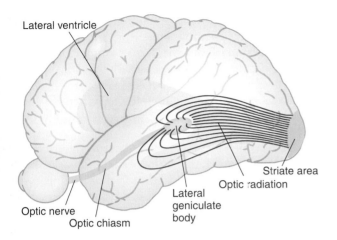

FIGURE 16.16 *The optic radiation*. The course of the fibers from the lateral geniculate body to the striate area shows how the fibers bend around the lateral ventricle and extend partly into the temporal lobe.

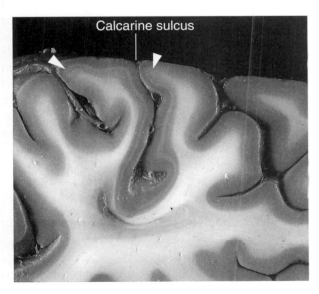

FIGURE 16.17 *The striate area*. Photograph of a section through the human occipital lobe showing the characteristic whitish stripe in layer 4 (the line of Gennari) of the striate area. Arrows mark the border between the striate area and neighboring extrastriate areas. See Fig. 33.5 for photomicrographs of a thionine-stained and myelin-stained sections from the striate area.

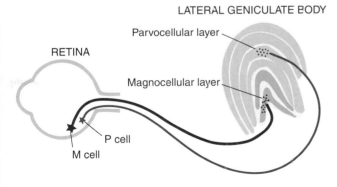

FIGURE 16.18 *The lateral geniculate body*. The two main kinds of retinal ganglion cells end in different layers of the lateral geniculate. (Based on Shapley and Perry 1986.)

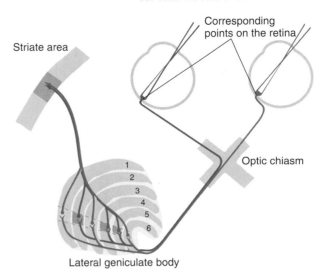

FIGURE 16.19 *Fusion of the visual images*. The signals from corresponding points on the two retinae end in different layers of the geniculate—that is, signals from the two eyes are kept separate at this level. The convergence of signals takes place in the striate area.

such as **motivation, alertness, expectation**, and stimulus **context**. Corticothalamic fibers may contribute to the suppression of vision of one eye in patients with **strabismus** (squint, cross-eyed); this has the obvious advantage of avoiding double vision. In addition, the lateral geniculate receives fibers from other sources, notably from **cholinergic** cell groups of the pontine reticular formation; these connections probably regulate the signal transmission through the lateral geniculate to the striate area, in accordance with the level of consciousness and attention.

Finally, a large number of GABAergic **interneurons** and numerous **dendrodendritic synapses** in the lateral geniculate presumably enable neurons with somewhat different receptive fields to influence each other.

Visual Signals from One Side of the Visual Field Reach the Hemisphere of the Other Side

Figure 16.14 shows how the fibers are arranged in the **optic chiasm**. The fibers coming from the nasal halves of the two retinas cross, whereas the fibers from the temporal halves pass through without crossing. In this way, the left lateral geniculate body receives fibers from the temporal retina of the left eye and from the nasal retina of the right eye. The **lateral geniculate body** thus receives light from the contralateral half of the visual field. In functional terms, the crossing of signals corresponds to that taking place in the somatosensory system.

Optic nerve fibers from the two eyes are kept separate at the level of the lateral geniculate body, since three of the six layers receive fibers from the ipsilateral eye, and the three others receive fibers from the contralateral eye (Fig. 16.19). After cutting one optic nerve, almost all cells in three of the layers degenerate (transneuronal degeneration), whereas the other three layers remain normal. Physiological experiments also show that neurons within each layer of the lateral geniculate body are influenced from one eye only: these cells are **monocular**. We first encounter cells that are influenced from both eyes—**binocular cells**—at the level of the striate area.

Fusion of Visual Images

Normally, we perceive one image of the objects we look at, even though two (slightly different) images are formed on the retina. The two images are perceived as one, and the phenomenon is called **fusion**. Fusion requires that the visual axes of the two eyes be properly aligned, so that the images fall on corresponding points on the retina (Fig. 16.3). The two maculae are obviously corresponding points, and the images fall on them when we fix the gaze on a point to see it as sharply as possible. As mentioned, the signals from the two eyes are kept separate in the lateral geniculate body, but at the cortical level many cells are influenced from both eyes—that is, they are binocular (Fig. 16.19). Convergence in the cortex of signals from corresponding points in the two eyes is a prerequisite for fusion. Fusion is not present from birth but develops gradually from about the age of 3 to 7 months. During this period, the movements of the eyes become coordinated, so that all movements are conjugated and the images fall on corresponding points when the gaze is fixed.

Strabismus (Squint)

Strabismus (squint, cross-eyed) means that the visual axes of the eyes are not properly aligned, and, accordingly, the images do not fall on corresponding points. This may be due to problems with the extraocular muscles or their nervous control, or the "pressure" on the brain to produce fusion may be too weak. The reason for weak pressure may be reduced vision on one or both eyes (e.g., due to retinal disease or a cataract). The lack of fusion in children with a squint leads to underdevelopment or suppression of vision for the eye not used for fixation. In this manner, bothersome double vision is avoided, but even a relatively brief period of strabismus in early childhood may lead to permanently reduced visual acuity. It has been shown in monkeys that strabismus (produced experimentally) leads to a reduced number of cells in the striate area that is influenced by both eyes. In one kind of squint, the child uses the two eyes alternatively for fixation, and in such patients, the visual acuity is usually conserved for both eyes.

The Visual Pathways Are Retinotopically Organized

The arrangement of the visual pathways just described concerns merely retinal halves—that is, a crude retinotopic

localization ensuring that signals from different parts of the visual field are kept separate (compare with somatotopic localization within the somatosensory pathways). But the **retinotopic localization** is much more fine-grained than what appears in Fig. 16.20. Although many fiber systems of the brain are topographically organized, no one is as sharply localized as the visual pathways, which show a true point-to-point localization.

In the **lateral geniculate body**, fibers from differently placed tiny parts of the retina end differently. Each small spot in the retina—and thus in the visual field—is "represented" in its own part of the lateral geniculate (Fig. 16.19). The retinotopic localization in the lateral geniculate is such that neurons influenced from the same part of the visual field (that is, from corresponding points on the retina) lie stacked in a column perpendicular to the layers. This has been demonstrated with various anatomic techniques, and physiologically by inserting microelectrodes perpendicular to the layers and determining the receptive fields of the cells that are encountered. The receptive fields of neurons in the lateral geniculate are quite similar to those of retinal ganglion cells (Fig. 16.8A).

The **thalamocortical** connections from the lateral geniculate body to the **striate area** are also organized with a precise retinotopic arrangement. This has been demonstrated, for example, by injection of a small amount of horseradish peroxidase in the striate area: retrogradely labeled cells are then confined to a narrow column that extends through all six layers of the lateral geniculate.

That all links of the visual pathways are retinotopically organized can be verified by shining light on a small spot on the retina. This evokes increased neuronal activity in a small region of the striate area, and when the light is shone on other parts of the retina, the evoked cortical activity changes position systematically. This kind of experiment has clarified how the **visual field** is represented in the cerebral cortex of animals. Careful examination of patients with circumscribed cortical lesions (often gunshot wounds) provides the basis for maps of the human visual cortex, as shown in Fig. 16.20. Electrical stimulation of the human occipital lobe confirms the retinotopic arrangement within the striate area. Stimulation with a needle electrode usually evokes the sensation of a flash of light in a certain part of the visual field. When the electrode is placed close to the occipital pole of the cerebral hemisphere, the person reports that the flash is located straight ahead, in agreement with the fact that fibers carrying signals from the macula end near the occipital pole. As the electrode is moved forward along the calcarine sulcus, the light flash is perceived as occurring progressively more peripherally in the visual field (at the opposite side of the stimulated hemisphere). If the electrode is placed above (dorsal to) the calcarine sulcus, the light occurs in the lower visual field, whereas stimulation below the calcarine sulcus elicits a sensation of light

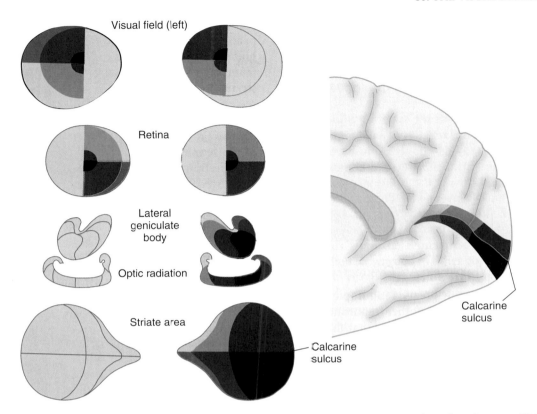

FIGURE 16.20 *Retinotopic localization of the visual pathways.* **Left:** The striate area has been unfolded. Note that information from the upper half of the visual field reaches the part of the striate area below the calcarine sulcus, whereas the lower visual field projects above. Central parts of the visual field are represented most posteriorly and peripheral parts most anteriorly in the striate area. **Right:** The extension of the striate area on the surface of the occipital lobe; most of it is buried in the calcarine sulcus. The striate area is similarly oriented in the left and the right figures.

in the upper visual field. Studies in healthy humans with positron emission tomography (PET) and functional magnetic resonance imaging (fMRI) have confirmed the main features of the retinotopic organization of the striate area.

Disease processes (e.g., a tumor) involving the visual cortex may also at times elicit sensations of light because the neurons are abnormally irritated. **Epileptic** seizures originating in the visual cortex often start with a **visual aura**—that is, the muscular convulsions are preceded by bizarre patterns of light in the visual field opposite the diseased hemisphere.

Visual Information Can Reach the Cortex via the Superior Colliculus and the Pulvinar

Not all fibers in the optic nerve end in the lateral geniculate body, as mentioned. About 10% (in the monkey) leave the optic tract to terminate in the **pretectal nuclei** and in the **superior colliculus** (see Fig. 27.19). Some fibers end in the **pulvinar** (see Figs. 6.21 and 6.22), and this nucleus (together with another thalamic nucleus, the lateral posterior nucleus, LP; see Fig. 33.7) also receives afferents from the superior colliculus. Like other thalamic nuclei, these send their efferents to the cortex, notably to the **extrastriate visual areas** (cortical areas processing information from the striate area). Thus visual information may reach the cortex even when the optic radiation or the striate area is damaged. Even though these visual pathways—which circumvent the lateral geniculate body—are retinotopically organized, they are apparently capable only of giving crude information about **movement** in the visual field. Thus, after bilateral damage of the striate area in monkeys, the animals react easily to moving stimuli, even though in other respects they behave as if they were blind. Studies of patients with damage at various levels of the visual pathways and of the visual cortex (localized with the use of MRI) indicate that, as long as parts of the extrastriate visual areas on the convexity are intact, the patients retain some capacity to recognize movements in the visual field. When sitting in front of a large screen with a random pattern of moving dots, patients with damage of the striate area (and surrounding areas on the medial aspect of the hemisphere) reacted with movements of the eyes, apparently following the moving objects. They reported that they felt something moving in front of them, and they had some ability to identify the movement direction. They had no

subtypes according to details of their properties. Why the properties of the complex cells are more complex than those of the simple ones may not be obvious, but presumably the terms were used because Hubel and Wiesel assumed that the properties of the complex cells could be explained by several simple cells acting on one complex cell. The properties of the simple cells, Hubel and Wiesel suggested, could be explained if several neurons in the lateral geniculate with round receptive fields in a row (together forming a stripe) converge on one cortical cell. It is, however, not yet entirely clear which neuronal interconnections underlie the properties of cells in the striate cortex.

Hubel and Wiesel also discovered other fundamental properties of cells in the striate area. Among other things, cells generally respond much better to a **moving** than to a stationary stimulus. Many cells respond preferentially to a line or contour that is moving in a specific direction. Such **direction-selective** cells thus can detect not only the orientation of a contour but also in which direction it is moving. Other kinds of specificities have also been described for cells in the striate area. For example, many **binocular cells** (cells that require input from both eyes) are sensitive to **disparity** of the images: that is, they require that the images from the two eyes are slightly different (disparate). This is always the case for images falling on corresponding points of the retina because the angle of view is different for the two eyes (except in the center of the macula) and also for images of objects that are nearer or farther from the fixation point. The ability to detect **binocular disparity** is important for perception of **depth** and for **stereoscopic** vision.

In addition to single cells being specific or selective with regard to their adequate stimulus, there is also a strong tendency for cells with similar properties in this respect to be located together, more or less clearly separated from cells with other properties. This is called **modular organization** (Figs. 16.23 and 16.24) and concerns properties such as orientation selectivity, wavelength (color) selectivity, and ocular dominance (i.e., which eye has the strongest influence). Such segregation of neurons in the striate area requires that fibers carrying different aspects of visual information from the lateral geniculate end at least to some extent differentially in the cortex. In agreement with this, fibers from the parvocellular layers of the lateral geniculate (Fig. 16.18) terminate deeper in lamina 4 than fibers from the magnocellular layers.

Modular Organization of the Visual Cortex

The first example of modular organization discovered by Hubel and Wiesel was the tendency for cells with similar **orientation selectivity** to be grouped together in **columns** perpendicular to the cortical surface. If we imagine that the striate area is unfolded and we are

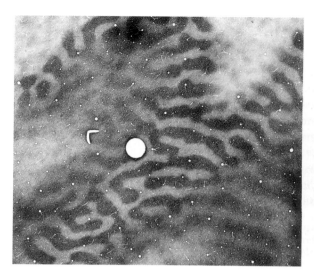

FIGURE 16.23 *Ocular dominance columns.* Photomicrograph of a section cut tangentially to the cortical surface of the striate area and stained to reveal differences in cytochrome oxidase activity. The section is from a monkey that was blind in one eye, causing reduced cytochrome oxidase activity in the regions (light stripes) of the striate area connected mainly with the blind eye. The dark stripes receive their main input from the normal eye. Magnification, ×25. (Courtesy of Dr. J.G. Bjaalie, Department of Anatomy, Institute of Basic Medical Sciences, University of Oslo.)

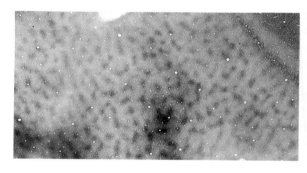

FIGURE 16.24 *Color-specific "blobs" in the striate area.* Photomicrograph of a section cut tangentially to the surface of the striate area of a normal monkey and stained to show differences in cytochrome oxidase activity. The section passes through laminas 2 to 3 and shows numerous small, darkly stained patches or blobs, which correspond to regions with color-specific neurons. Magnification, ×25. (Courtesy of Dr. J. G. Bjaalie, Department of Anatomy, Institute of Basic Medical Sciences, University of Oslo.)

viewing it from above, the groups of cells with similar orientation selectivity are located in an irregular pattern of curving bands. This has been demonstrated with the deoxyglucose method, which demonstrates the neurons that are most active at a certain time. When an experimental animal is exposed for some time to parallel stripes of light, increased glucose uptake takes place in cells distributed in bands in the striate area. Another modular organization concerns **ocular dominance**. As mentioned, many cells in the striate area respond to light from corresponding points in the two retinas, but for most cells the influence is strongest from one of the eyes. The use of various tracer techniques and the deoxyglucose method has shown that neurons sharing ocular dominance are also distributed in bands within the striate area. Such ocular dominance columns can also be demonstrated in animals with monocular blindness (Fig. 16.23). A final example of modular organization concerns **color-specific** cells (strictly speaking: wavelength specific). They are not aggregated in bands but in clumps or **blobs** in laminas 2 to 3 of the striate area of monkeys. For some unknown reason, these blobs have a higher cytochrome oxidase activity than the surrounding tissue and can thus be easily identified in sections with a simple histochemical procedure (Fig. 16.24).

Extrastriate Visual Areas

As mentioned, several areas around the striate area take part in visual processing. These are collectively called the **extrastriate visual areas** and consist mainly of Brodmann's areas 18 and 19, which in the monkey each consist of several subdivisions. Whereas V1 is often used for area 17 (the striate area), parts of the extrastriate areas are termed V2 to V5. Other parts have specific names. In total, about 30 visual areas have been characterized so far in the monkey, and each is in some way involved in the processing of visual information. Many have a more or less complete representation of the visual field and are retinotopically organized, although with different degrees of precision. Together, the visual areas occupy more than half of all of the cerebral cortex in the monkey. The interconnections between the striate area and the extrastriate areas, and among the extrastriate areas, are numerous and as a rule **reciprocal**. The complete scheme of visual association connections is therefore extremely complex and explains why it is difficult to determine the contribution of each individual area to the processing of visual information.[4]

Further Processing of Visual Information: Segregation and Integration

The properties of single neurons in the striate area suggest that these neurons together are the basis for the cortical analysis of **form, depth, movement,** and **color.** Their properties, for example, fit predictions made on the basis of psychophysical experiments in humans, such as the preference for contours and for moving

stimuli. Nevertheless, what is taking place in the striate area appears to be mainly a first analysis and sorting of raw data, which must be further processed elsewhere to form the basis for our conscious visual experiences. There is now much evidence of separate, or **segregated,** treatment of the various features of visual images (such as form, color, movement, and location in the visual field) outside the striate area, and we discuss a few examples in the next section. At some stage in the processing, however, different features of the visual image must be brought together and **integrated.** We return to this later in this chapter.

Segregation: Dorsal and Ventral Pathways (Streams) Out of the Striate Area

It has been proposed that a **ventral** stream of information concerning **object identification** ("what") passes downward from the occipital lobe to the temporal lobe, whereas another, **dorsal** stream concerned with **spatial features** and **movement** ("where") passes upward to the parietal lobe (see Fig. 16.25). This concept is partly based on results from experiments in monkeys with lesions that have been restricted to "visual" parts of either the temporal lobe or the posterior parietal cortex. Monkeys with bilateral lesions of temporal visual areas have reduced ability to identify objects; for example, they can no longer distinguish between a pyramid and a cube. In contrast, lesions of visual parts of the posterior parietal cortex reduce the ability to localize an object in space and in relation to other objects; among other symptoms, such monkeys have difficulties with performing **goal-directed movements.** It suffices with a unilateral lesion of the parietal lobe to produce deficits in the contralateral half of the visual field. This resembles

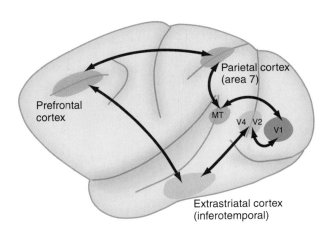

FIGURE 16.25 *Dorsal and ventral pathways out of striate area (V1).* Monkey. The ventral pathway is especially important for conscious object identification, whereas the dorsal pathway is crucial for perception of movement and space. Note convergence of information from the two pathways in the prefrontal cortex. (Based on data published by Deco and Rolls 2005.)

---

4 It is not immediately clear why the cerebral cortex is organized so that the visual field is represented repeatedly in different parts. It may be a result of the adoption of novel functions by the visual cortex during evolution, and because this probably occurs more easily by adding new areas (or duplicating an old one) than by already existing areas taking up new functions. It is presumably also a simpler solution to have several separate areas than one large area with regard to arrangement of the necessary fiber connections.

the symptoms occurring in humans after damage to the posterior parietal cortex, such as reduced ability to judge movements in the visual field and disturbed eye movements (see Chapter 34, under "More about Symptoms after Lesions of the Posterior Parietal Cortex"). The pathways taken by the signals from the striate area to the temporal and posterior parietal visual regions are not known in detail, but several visual areas are intercalated in the pathways (Fig. 16.25).

It is often stated without reservation that the ventral (temporal) and dorsal (parietal) streams out of the striate area segregate information from **P** and **M cells**, respectively. This is an oversimplification, however. For example, some convergence of information from M and P cells takes place already in the striate area (besides the more prominent segregation). The sum of evidence suggests that the subcortical pathways from the retina to the striate area are specialized for signaling simple stimulus features, whereas the further pathways do more advanced processing using as, a rule, information from both M and P cells.[5]

More about Segregated Information Processing in the Extrastriate Visual Areas

While there is no doubt that different aspects of visual information are to some degree segregated in the striate area and in the extrastriate areas, how far the segregation goes is a contentious issue. One striking example of anatomic segregation is the termination in **patches** and **bands** of projections from the striate area to other visual areas. Closer examination of such patterns and correlation with the physiological properties of cells within the patches and bands indicate the existence functionally different information channels out of the striate area, as described in the preceding text with regard to a dorsal and a ventral pathway or stream. More detailed analysis revealed a pathway from cells in the striate area that are predominantly influenced by the **magnocellular layers** of the lateral geniculate. The properties of these striate cells indicate that they signal **movement** and **depth** cues. Another pathway comes from cells that appear to be influenced by the **parvocellular layers** of the lateral geniculate. Accordingly, these striate cells have small receptive fields and are orientation-selective.

This pathway presumably signals **forms** and **patterns** and would seem particularly important for our ability to discern visual details. A third "parvocellular" pathway originates in striate neurons that are, at least to a large extent, **wavelength-specific**, signaling information about color.

These three pathways from the striate area appear to be kept separate, at least partly, also at the next station—that is, in **area V2**, which is adjacent to the striate area. From V2, information about **movement** is channeled to **area V5** (also called **MT**, the **middle temporal visual area**), whereas information about **color** is channeled primarily to **area V4**. The major outflow from V5 has been traced to the **posterior parietal cortex**. Information about forms and patterns is channeled primarily from V2 to **inferotemporal visual areas** (i.e., situated inferiorly in the temporal lobe). How far the specialization goes within each of these areas is not clear, however. The numerous interconnections among the extrastriate areas suggest that they cooperate extensively. Accordingly, single neurons in area V5, for example, are sensitive not only to movement but also to certain other visual features. Similarly, neurons in area V4 are not purely color-specific.

Color Vision and Color Opponency

We discussed parts of the elements responsible for color vision—namely, the three kinds of **cones** with sensitivities for light of different wavelengths (Fig. 16.6). We also emphasized that the brain must compare the degree of stimulation of three kinds of cone to "know" the wavelength composition of the light (and therefore the color of an object). Figure 16.6 shows the large overlap between the sensitivity curves of the three kinds of cone, especially between those with sensitivities in the red and green parts of the spectrum, respectively. How can we then perceive so many nuances of each color? Part of the explanation is found in how the cones are coupled to the next links in the pathway to the cortex. Thus, **retinal ganglion cells** and neurons in the **lateral geniculate body** have narrower sensitivity curves than the cones, making them better at discriminating wavelengths. Many ganglion cells and lateral geniculate cells respond to light of different wavelengths but with opposite signs—one wavelength exciting the cell, the other inhibiting it. This phenomenon is called **color opponency** and must be due to convergence on one ganglion cell (or lateral geniculate cell) of signals from cones with different wavelength sensitivities. Some neurons are excited (ON response) by red light in the central zone of the receptive field (Fig. 16.8) and inhibited (OFF response) by green light in the peripheral zone; others are inhibited by red light centrally and excited by green peripherally, and so forth. Such combinations improve the ability to **discriminate** wavelengths in the red–green part of the

5 Although behavioral studies suggest that the "parietal" pathway be made nonfunctional by destruction of the magnocellular layers of the lateral geniculate nucleus, the "temporal" pathway is not correspondingly affected by destruction of the parvocellular layers. Thus, whereas selective lesions of the parvocellular layers affect color vision, acuity, and contrast sensitivity, destruction of the temporal visual areas primarily affects form recognition and discrimination. Selective lesions of the magnocellular layers produce reduced perception of contrasts with fast-moving stimuli, while this defect does not occur after lesions of the parietal visual areas. Further, experiments with lesions of the magnocellular layers suggest that depth perception does not depend on information from M cells alone.

spectrum. Some neurons exhibit color opponency to blue and yellow light (a combination of red and green), others to white light (stimulation of all three kinds of cones) and darkness.

Even more complex kinds of color opponency are found among neurons in the **visual cortex**. For example, a neuron may respond with an ON response to red light and an OFF response to green light in the center of its receptive field, whereas the reverse responses are evoked from the peripheral zone (double opponency). Such neurons are found in the cytochrome-rich patches in laminas 2–3 of the striate area (Fig. 16.24). Together, all the color opponency neurons provide accurate information of the wavelength composition of the light hitting a spot on the retina.

Color Constancy

We are used to, and take for granted, that an object has a certain color, regardless of whether we see it in direct sunlight, in the shadow, or in artificial light. For example, we consistently identify a banana as yellow, an apple as red, the grass as green, and so forth (although we perceive differences in nuances). This property of our visual system, called **color constancy**, is by no means self-evident. Thus, the wavelength composition of the light reflected from an object depends not only on the physical properties of the surface but also on the light shining on the object. Different light sources produce light with quite different wavelength composition. The light received by the eye from an object thus differs markedly under different lighting conditions.

Color constancy is obviously of great **biologic importance**. The color of an object gives us essential information as to its nature, but only if the color is an invariant, typical property. For example, we know that a yellow banana is edible, whereas green or brown ones are not. Even under quite different illuminations, we easily make this kind of choice based on color.

We do not fully understand how the brain accomplishes this remarkable task, although it must depend on processing at the cortical level. Color constancy occurs only if the object we look at is part of a **complex, multicolored scene**. Experiments with patterned, multicolored surfaces show that the composition of the light reflected from one part of the visual scene may be changed considerably without changing the color perceived by an observer. If the same square is seen against an evenly dark background, however, the perceived color changes according to the composition of the reflected light—for example, from green to white. This must mean that under natural conditions the brain determines the color of an object by comparing the wavelength composition of the light from its surface with the composition of light from all other surfaces in the visual field.

Afterimages

If we look at a red surface for a few seconds and then move to a white, we see a green surface where we just saw the red. This is called an **afterimage**. The afterimage of yellow is blue, and for white it is black. This phenomenon can be partly explained by selective bleaching of a particular kind of cone. For example, a red light bleaches mainly the cones with wavelength sensitivity in the red part of the spectrum. When the eye then receives white light, the "red" cones are, for a short while, less sensitive than the others. This creates a relative dominance of signals from "green" cones, and the surface is perceived as green. What we have said so far might suggest that the color of the afterimage depends only on the light first hitting the retina. It is not that simple, however. The afterimage depends on the color perceived by the subject, not the absolute wavelength composition—that is, **color constancy** occurs also for after images. The afterimage effect can also occur when looking for a while at a moving object and then at a stationary one. We then perceive an **illusory movement** of the stationary object in the opposite direction.

What Is Color?

Even this fragmentary discussion of color vision may give some thoughts as to the real meaning of the term *color*. Color is, strictly speaking, not a property of an object but a subjective experience of a person seeing the object. The experience is based on how the brain processes information about the wavelength composition of the light reflected from the object (and from all other objects in the same visual scene). That we also can **imagine** colors raises the question of where and how colors (as percepts) are represented in our memory. Now we can only give fragmentary answers to this and other questions about how the brain creates colors or even visual images at all. Nevertheless, the considerations discussed here might serve to emphasize that there is no absolute correlation between a visual stimulus and the perception it evokes. Of course, this is not specific to seeing but pertains to the other senses as well. Fortunately, relationships between certain patterns of stimuli and external events are reasonably constant. Therefore, we usually take the right decisions by relying on our brain's interpretation (our percept) of the stimuli (the color of a traffic light, the movements of a snake, the contours of a horse, and so forth).

Lesions of the Extrastriate Areas: Visual Agnosia

Humans with lesions of the temporal extrastriate areas show various forms of reduced ability to **recognize objects** (agnosia). A patient may be unable to recognize faces, another may have no problem with faces but cannot recognize fingers (finger agnosia), and so on (see Chapter 34, under "Lesions of the Association Areas: Agnosia and Apraxia"). High-resolution fMRI in humans and recording from single neurons in monkeys indicate that a small region in the **fusiform gyrus** contains a particularly high proportion of **face-specific** neurons (Fig. 16.26). Nevertheless, recordings with multiple surface electrodes in patients (to localize epileptic foci) suggest that several, separate small areas in the inferior temporal cortex participate in **face recognition.** These areas appear to be parts of a mosaic of areas with different specializations. This agrees with observations after lesions of extensive parts of the inferotemporal extrastriate areas: such patients are deficient in several specific kinds of object recognition and suffer from not only **prosopagnosia** (inability to recognize faces; from Greek, *prosopon* = face). Selective loss of **color vision** (**achromatopsia**) after lesions restricted to a region below the calcarine sulcus (in the **lingual gyrus**) has been convincingly documented (Fig. 16.26). This corresponds most likely to **area V4** in monkeys. Patients with unilateral lesions in this region are reported to see everything in the opposite half of the visual field in black and white, whereas the other half has normal colors.

Damage at the junction between the occipital and the parietal lobes can produce selective impairment of the ability to recognize **movements** (**akinetopsia**). One patient with a bilateral lesion of this region could not see moving objects; when the same objects were stationary,

however, he could easily describe their form and color, and he could judge depth in the visual scene.

Patients with selective loss of **depth perception** after cortical damage have been described. To such patients other people look completely flat, as made from cardboard; patients can recognize their color, contours, and shading, however. The exact site of the lesion in such patients has not been determined, but PET studies indicate that tasks requiring depth perception activate several areas in the cerebral cortex (and in the cerebellar hemispheres), and that these areas overlap with areas involved in other visual tasks.

Integration of Visual Information: One Final Area?

The fact that there is much evidence of separate processing in the visual cortex of different aspects of visual information must not make us forget that at some level a synthesis has to occur. Information about form, position, movement, and color must in some way be linked together. After all, the color "belongs" to a certain object, with a certain form and position and with a certain speed and direction of movement. Our percept is unitary, although the brain first has "dissected" out and analyzed the bits and pieces of information in the light falling on the retina. What does integration of information mean in the context of sensory processing? One might think that there must exist one final, site (area) in which all aspects of visual information are brought together, but **anatomic** data do not favor the existence of such cortical areas. Even in the **prefrontal cortex,** visual information about "what" and "where" is treated separately (in conjunction with coupling of visual features of objects to voluntary movements).

There are also theoretical problems with the notion of a **final integrative area.** Thus, although our conscious experience is unitary, it consists of components to which we have separate, conscious access. For example, a car may be characterized by its color, by its shape, or by its movements. The components are kept separate yet linked in such a way that we perceive them as belonging together. Another theoretical problem with a final integrative area is where to "place" awareness of the visual image. As expressed by the British neurobiologist Semir Zeki (1993): "If all the visual areas report to a single master cortical area, who or what does that single area report to? Put more visually, who is 'looking' at the visual image provided by that master area?"

Role of the Striate Area in Visual Awareness and Visual Imagery

We mentioned patients with **blindsight** above (under "Visual Information Can Reach the Cortex via the Superior Colliculus and the Pulvinar"). Such patients have no awareness of having seen anything, yet they

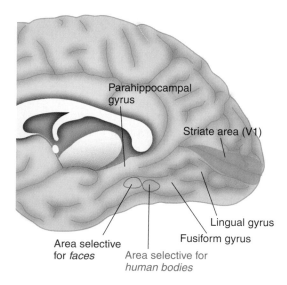

FIGURE 16.26 *Subdivisions of the extrastriate visual areas that are selective for recognition of human faces and human bodies, respectively.* Surface marking is based on high-resolution fMRI from normal persons. These two areas could not be discerned with standard fMRI with lower resolution. (Based on data published by Schwarzlose et al. 2005.)

can respond to movement in the visual field. In such cases, visual information reaches the extrastriate areas that are specialized for analysis of movements without going through the striate area. We may then ask whether conscious visual experience requires that visual information first go through the **striate area**—in other words, that activation of the striate area is necessary for visual awareness. One approach to this question is to study brain activity with the PET technique while subjects imagine visual scenes, such as a red car or their home street. In such situations, the subject has retrieved the information from memory and "sees" the scene with closed eyes. Which parts of the brain are then specifically activated? It appears that largely the same extrastriate areas are activated during **visual imagery** as when seeing. The PET data are conflicting as to whether the striate area is activated with visual imagery, but the fact that patients with cortical blindness (damage to the striate area) are able to imagine visual scenes strongly suggests that the striate area is not necessary for visual imagery. Also, clinical observations suggest that visual imagery and seeing may not use identical cortical structures. Thus, a few patients have been reported who could recognize objects when seeing them but could not imagine the same objects. The reverse situation has also been described.

Visual Awareness and Synchronized Network Activity

We have treated integration at early stages of the visual processing, such as cells in the striate area responding to contours with a certain orientation regardless where it occurs within a larger part of the visual field. Further integration produces more complex properties, so that cells respond only when several characteristics coincide (such as a contour with a specific orientation moving in a certain direction). Such and more complex integration of data need not occur on single cells, however; it may also occur by coordinated activity in separate neurons that are synaptically linked (neuronal networks). As mentioned, it is noteworthy that the many visual areas are so extensively interconnected. For example, the striate area receives connections from most of the areas to which it projects, and the same holds for many extrastriate areas and their relations to other cortical areas. Presumably, our **conscious visual image** is a product of the total pattern of impulses in many, interconnected cortical areas at any moment. **Synchronized activity** of neuronal groups receiving the same kind of information (e.g., about the direction of movement) may play an important part, and has been shown to occur in cortical areas.

fMRI studies suggest that an extended **network** connecting ventral (temporal) visual areas and parts of parietal and prefrontal areas is especially active in conjunction with visual **awareness**. A possible common denominator for awareness of sensory information in general, was formulated as follows by Zeman (2004, p. 324): ". . . awareness occurs as the result of physiologically appropriate interactions between neural systems which serve sensation, memory, and action; activity which remains within a single system . . . can influence behavior but will not enter awareness".

In conclusion, both clinical and brain imaging studies clearly show that extensive parts of the cerebral cortex are involved in conscious visual experience. It should be noted, however, that visual information that is not consciously perceived can nevertheless be used for preparation of voluntary (conscious) movements.

Subconscious Use of Visual Information

A striking example was published by Goodale and Milner in 1992. A woman suffered damage to parts of her occipital lobes (with sparing of the striate cortex) because of carbon monoxide poisoning. Afterward she was unable to recognize objects (**visual agnosia**). For example, she could not decide whether an object was oriented vertically or horizontally, nor could she show the size of the object with her fingers. When asked to grasp it, however, she accomplished this easily and with normal preparatory adjustment of the fingers. Thus, she could adapt her grip to specific visual features, yet she had no awareness of these features. Obviously, the parts of the brain preparing voluntary, **goal-directed movements** have access to information about shape, size, and orientation, no matter whether these features are consciously perceived or not.

Development of Normal Vision Requires Proper Use

There may be other causes than a squint for lack of normal visual development. For example, if the eye does not receive proper stimulation because errors of refraction produce a retinal image that is out of focus or because light for some reason does not reach the retina, vision is not developed normally. In humans, the first 2 to 3 years (in particular the first year) are especially important in this respect; lack of **meaningful use** of the eye even for a short period may then give permanently reduced visual acuity (as discussed in Chapter 9). Animal experiments furthermore show that, contrary to what might be expected, vision is better preserved if both eyes are covered for a period than if only one is covered. This is so because the two eyes "compete" during the early development of the visual system. If only one eye is used, it acquires an advantage and takes over neurons in the visual cortex that normally would have been used by the other eye.

17 | The Auditory System

The sense of hearing is of great importance in higher animals—not least in humans, for whom speech is the most important means of communication. The adequate stimulus for the auditory receptors is **sound waves** with frequencies between 20 and about 20,000 Hz. The sensitivity is greatest, however, between 1000 and 4000 Hz and declines steeply toward the highest and the lowest frequencies; that is, a tone of 15,000 Hz must be much stronger than a sound of 1000 Hz to be perceived. The range of frequencies to which the ear is most sensitive corresponds fairly well to the range of frequencies for human speech. The **frequency** of sound waves determines the pitch, whereas the **amplitude** of the waves determines the intensity. Many animals can perceive sound over a much wider range of frequencies than humans can. For example, dogs can hear a whistle hardly noticed by humans, and bats use extremely high-pitched sounds for echolocation. Sound waves pass through the air to the tympanic membrane, which transmits them via a chain of three tiny bones to the **cochlea.** The sensory cells—the **hair cells**—of the cochlea are low-threshold mechanoreceptors sensitive to the bending of stereocilia on their surface. From the cochlea, the signals are conducted to the **cochlear nuclei** in the brain stem through the eighth cranial nerve, the **vestibulo-cochlear nerve.** This nerve also carries signals from the sense organ for equilibrium—the vestibular apparatus—that anatomically and evolutionarily is closely related to the cochlea. Functionally, however, these two parts have little in common, and we describe the sense of equilibrium together with other aspects of vestibular function in Chapter 18.

From the cochlear nuclei, the **auditory pathways** carry signals to **the inferior colliculus** (and some other brain stem nuclei). Neurons in the inferior colliculus send their axons to the **medial geniculate body** of the thalamus. Thalamocortical axons reach the **primary auditory area** (A1) situated on the upper face of the temporal lobe (buried in the lateral sulcus). The auditory pathways from one ear reach both hemispheres, in contrast to the almost complete crossing of somatosensory pathways. Further processing of auditory information takes place in cortical areas surrounding A1 in the temporal lobe. Outward connections from these areas ensure integration of auditory information with other sensory modalities. Nuclei in the brain stem receiving

signals from both ears with a time difference are crucial for our ability to **localize sounds.**

THE COCHLEA

The Cochlea Is Part of the Labyrinth

The **labyrinth** consists of an outer bony part surrounding an irregular canal in the temporal bone, and an inner **membranous part** following and partly filling the canal (Figs. 17.1, 17.2, and 17.3). The membranous canal is filled with a fluid called the **endolymph** (Figs. 17.1 and 17.4). Between the membranous and the bony parts is a space filled with a fluid called the **perilymph.** The composition of the endolymph and of the perilymph differs: the concentrations of sodium and potassium ions in the perilymph are similar to those in the cerebrospinal fluid (i.e., similar to those in the extracellular fluid), whereas the concentrations of these ions in the endolymph are like those found intracellularly. Thus, the cilia of the sensory cells—surrounded by the endolymph (Fig. 17.5)—are embedded in an unusual extracellular fluid with K^+ as the dominating cation. The protein concentration, however, is much higher in the perilymph than in the endolymph and the cerebrospinal fluid. The high K^+ concentration creates a potential of about 90 mV between the endolymph and the perilymph, called the **endocochlear potential** (the endolymph is positive in relation to the perilymph). The special composition of the endolymph and the endocochlear potential are of crucial importance for the transduction mechanism of the hair cells, as discussed later in this chapter.

The labyrinth has two main parts. One is the cochlea and the other is the vestibular apparatus consisting of three semicircular ducts and two round dilatations (Fig. 17.2). Here we consider only the organ of hearing, the cochlea. The **membranous part** of the cochlea—**the cochlear duct**—forms a thin-walled tube with a triangular shape (in cross section), surrounded by the bony part of the cochlea. The duct forms a spiral with two and a half to three turns (Figs. 17.2, 17.3, and 17.4). The lowermost wall of the cochlear duct is formed by the **basilar membrane** (membrana basilaris), which is suspended between the two facing sides of the bony canal (Figs. 17.4 and 17.5). At the inner side of the turns, the basilar membrane is attached to a bony

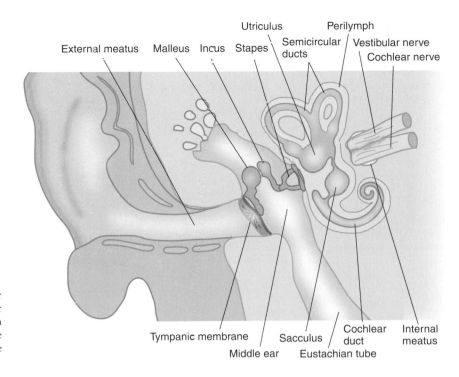

FIGURE 17.1 *The ear.* The middle ear has three ear ossicles, and the inner ear has the membranous labyrinth (located in the temporal bone). The eustachian tube connects the middle ear with the pharynx.

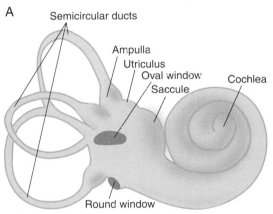

FIGURE 17.2 A: *The membranous labyrinth with its vestibular part (the semicircular ducts, the saccule, and the utricle) and the auditory part (the cochlea). The stapes is attached in the oval window.*

B: The fluid in the labyrinth visualized via three dimensional reconstruction of MRIs. (Courtesy of Dr. Einar Hopp, Rikshospitalet University Hospital, Oslo, Norway.)

prominence—the **bony spiral lamina** (lamina spiralis ossea)—which follows the cochlea in its spiraling course (Figs. 17.4 and 17.5). The sensory epithelium, forming the **organ of Corti**, rests on the basilar membrane (Figs. 17.4, 17.5, and 17.6). The length of the cochlear duct, and thus of the basilar membrane, is about 3.5 cm (Fig. 17.7). The thin **vestibular membrane** forms the upper wall of the cochlear duct (Figs. 17.4 and 17.5). The third, lateral, or outer wall of the cochlear duct lies on the bony wall of the canal and is formed by a specialized, stratified epithelium, the **vascular stria** (Fig. 17.6). As the name implies, there are **capillaries** among the

epithelial cells. The vascular stria is responsible for the high K$^+$ of the endolymph and the positive electric potential between the endolymph and the perilymph.[1]

The room outside the cochlear duct consists of two parallel canals. The one situated below the basilar membrane is the **scala tympani**; the one above the

1 In experimental animals, atrophy of the vascular stria causes hearing loss, and the severity seems to be proportional to reduction of the endocochlear potential. There is evidence that—in addition to loss of hair cells—atrophy of the vascular stria can contribute to presbyacusis (age-related hearing loss) in humans.

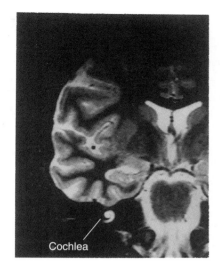
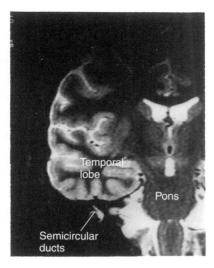

FIGURE 17.3 *The labyrinth*. Two closely spaced, frontal MRIs. The fluid-filled cochlea (**left**) and semicircular canals (**right**) are clearly seen just below the temporal lobe (the image is weighted so that water appears white).

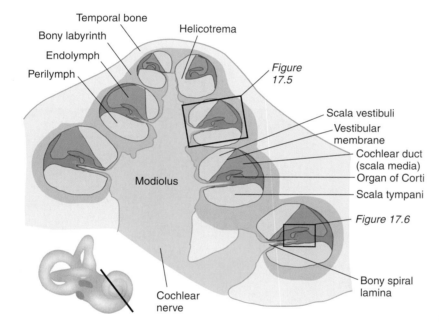

FIGURE 17.4 *Section through the cochlea.*

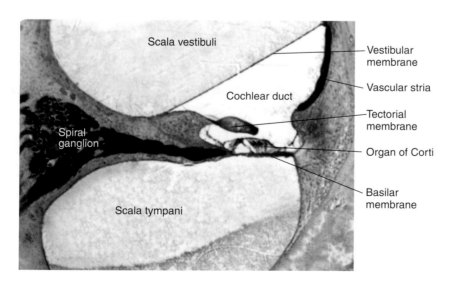

FIGURE 17.5 *Section through the cochlea.* Photomicrograph. Cf. Fig. 17.4.

A

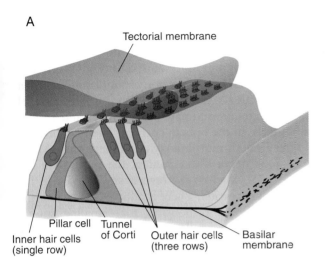

B

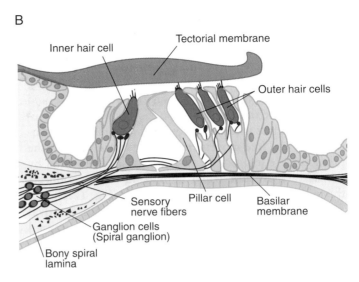

FIGURE 17.6 *The organ of Corti.* **A:** Three-dimensional representation of a short segment of the organ of Corti (the whole organ extends the full length of the cochlear duct). The inner hair cells are in a single row, and the outer hair cells are in three parallel rows. The pillar cells appear to change their form in relation to loud sounds, possibly to prevent damage of hair cells. **B:** Cf. Fig. 17.4. Note that only the tallest stereocilia of the outer hair cells are in contact with the tectorial membrane.

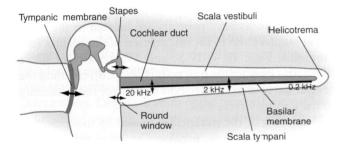

FIGURE 17.7 *The middle ear and the cochlea.* The cochlear duct is pictured as if straightened (length about 3.5 cm). The oscillations of the stapes are transmitted to the fluid in the scala vestibuli and from there to the cochlear duct. Different tone frequencies set different parts of the basilar membrane in motion. Note that the highest frequencies stimulate the hair cells near the base of the cochlea, whereas the lowest frequencies stimulate hair cells near the apex (near helicotrema). (Based on Fettiplace and Hackney 2006.)

vestibular membrane is the **scala vestibuli** (Figs. 17.4 and 17.5). Both have openings or windows in the bone facing the middle ear (Figs. 17.2 and 17.7). The **oval window** (fenestra vestibuli) is situated at the end of the scala vestibuli, whereas the **round window** (fenestra cochleae) is at the end of the scala tympani. The stapes and a thin membrane of connective tissue close the windows, respectively (Fig. 17.7).

How Sound Waves Are Transmitted to the Sensory Cells in the Cochlea

Conduction of sound waves from the air to the receptor cells in the cochlea occurs through the **external ear** (the auricle and the external auditory meatus) and the middle ear or **tympanic cavity** (Fig. 17.1). Sound waves hitting the skull can also be transmitted through the bone directly to the receptors. This kind of transmission, however, is very inefficient with regard to airborne sound waves and therefore plays no role in normal hearing (bone conduction of sound waves is used for testing the function of the cochlea and also for certain hearing aid devices).

Sound waves hit the eardrum or **tympanic membrane** located at the bottom of the external meatus (Fig. 17.1). The eardrum consists of a thin, tense connective tissue membrane covered by a thin layer of epithelium on both sides; it is richly supplied with **nociceptors**, like the tight skin of the inner part of the external meatus. The three **ossicles** form a chain through the middle ear and connect the eardrum with the oval window (Figs. 17.1, 17.2, and 17.7). The **malleus** (the hammer) has a shaft that is attached to the inner side of the eardrum. The head of the malleus connects to the **incus** (the anvil) by a joint, and the incus is further connected to the **stapes** (the stirrup) by a joint. The basal plate of the stapes inserts in the oval window, thus closing the scala vestibuli (Fig. 17.7). The sound waves make the eardrum and the ossicles vibrate with the frequency of the waves, and thus the movement transmits to the fluid in the cochlea. Because the area of the eardrum is so much larger than that of the basal plate of the stapes, the **pressure** per square unit increases 20 times. This amplification mechanism increases the sensitivity for sound dramatically, compared to a situation without the ossicles. Normally, even the slightest movement of the eardrum is sufficient to cause stimulation of the receptors in the cochlea: sound waves with **amplitude** of only 0.01 nm suffice to produce the weakest perceptible sound with the frequency to which the ear is most sensitive. If the sound waves

outer hair cells move the basilar membrane, producing both an **amplification** of the vibrations and a narrowing of the vibrating part, which sharpens the **tuning** of the **frequency curve**. Together, these changes ensure more precise signal transmission. Whether the amplification is due solely to deformation of the outer hair cell body (elongation and shortening) or whether movements of the cilia also contribute, is not settled.

The **efferent fibers** ending on the outer hair cells release **acetylcholine** (and most likely ATP) that hyperpolarizes the cells by binding to muscarinic receptors. This reduces the active movements of the stereocilia leading to less amplification and broader tuning of the frequency curve.

Otoacoustic Emissions

The ear actually emits faint sounds—**otoacoustic emissions**—that appear to be produced by the contractions of the outer hair cells. A microphone in the external meatus can record such sounds, which can occur spontaneously or be evoked by a click. The hearing system works in reverse, as it were: the outer hair cells move the basilar membrane, which in turn moves the fluid in the cochlea; this moves the ossicles, which then move the tympanic membrane that produces the sound. The phenomenon is used diagnostically—for example, in infants—to decide whether the cochlea functions normally.

Different Frequencies are Registered at Different Sites along the Basilar Membrane: Tonotopic Localization

The ordered arrangement of neurons and nerve fibers signaling different pitches of sound (frequencies) is called **tonotopic localization** (compare with somatotopic localization in the somatosensory system and retinotopic localization in the visual system). As discussed later, the auditory pathways are tonotopically organized all the way from the cochlea to the cerebral cortex. The tonotopic localization in the cochlea has been demonstrated in several ways. After receiving lesions restricted to a small part of the organ of Corti (which extends along the full length of the basilar membrane), experimental animals no longer react to sound in a certain, narrow range of frequencies (pitches), whereas they react normally to sounds of other frequencies. In humans, similar selective deafness may occur after prolonged exposure to noise, for example, in factories. Anatomic examination of the cochlea after death in such persons has shown that the hair cells have disappeared in a restricted region on the basilar membrane, the position of the region differing with the frequency to which the person was deaf. The tonotopic localization has been determined in detail by recording the response of single hair cells to sounds of different frequencies.

Each hair cell is best activated by tones within a very narrow range of frequencies. Together, the hair cells and the sensory fibers leading from them cover the total range of frequencies we can perceive.

The **tonotopic** localization is such that the tones with the **highest pitch** (highest frequencies) are registered by the hair cells closest to the oval window (i.e., on the basal part of the basilar membrane), whereas the lowest frequencies are registered at the top of the cochlea (i.e., at the apical part of the basilar membrane). This can be explained, at least partly, by the physical properties of the basilar membrane, as proposed by the German physicist Hermann Helmholtz in the nineteenth century. The basilar membrane is most narrow basally and becomes progressively wider in the apical direction. The fibers of the basilar membrane are oriented transversely to the long axis of the basilar membrane (Fig. 17.6) and are therefore longer apically than basally. In analogy with the strings of an instrument (e.g., a piano), basal parts would be expected to vibrate with a higher frequency than apical parts. This is the main basis of the **resonance theory** of Helmholtz, which postulates that each position along the basilar membrane corresponds to a certain frequency. Although later research has shown that even a pure tone makes large parts of the basilar membrane vibrate, the region in which the maximal amplitude occurs is very narrow. This appears to be caused by the amplification produced by contractions of the outer hair cells, as discussed in the preceding text. Thus, the hair cells differ in accordance with their position on the basilar membrane, so that their thresholds are lower for certain frequencies than for others.

Cochlear and Brain Stem Implants to Restore Hearing

When deafness is due to loss of hair cells without affection of the afferent nerve fibers, hearing can be restored by a so-called **cochlear implant**. During surgery, a thin, isolated electrode is inserted along the basilar membrane. The isolation is removed at around 20 points, enabling electric stimulation of the cochlear nerve fibers at these sites. Hence, a range of frequencies can be transmitted to the brain; in accordance with the tonotopic localization along the basilar membrane (the frequency resolution is of course inferior to what is possible with a normal number of hair cells). A microphone and microprocessor transform the sound waves to electric signals that are sent to the electrode.

In **children** who are **born deaf**, a cochlear implant can enable development of speech and speech comprehension. Most of the children are able to attend normal school classes. However, the implant must be inserted as early as possible, and not later than 3 to 4 years of age. If the cortical networks necessary for analysis and use of sounds are not developed before this age, they cannot develop later, probably because the auditory cortex has been taken over by other systems. Indeed, there is evidence from functional magnetic resonance imaging (fMRI) studies that visual stimuli may activate the auditory cortex in congenitally blind persons. This corresponds to the situation in children who are born blind and later regain sight (e.g., by removing a cataract), as discussed in Chapter 9. In **deaf adults**, who have had normal hearing earlier, a cochlear implant can restore hearing so they can comprehend speech. In this situation, the networks responsible for sound processing were presumably established in early childhood and remained essentially intact even after a period without hearing. However, intense training is required after surgery, in order to make sense of the foreign sounds provided by the implant. Further, the longer the time from loss of hearing to implantation, the poorer is the prospect of a satisfactory result.

When deafness is due to destruction of the **cochlear nerve**, a cochlear implant will of course have no effect. In some such patients, restoration of hearing has been attempted by implanting an array of electrodes over the ventral **cochlear nucleus**. Otherwise, the strategy is similar to that used in cochlear implants. The success so far has been much more limited than with cochlear implants, however.

THE AUDITORY PATHWAYS

Distinctive Features of the Central Auditory System

The anatomic organization of the central auditory pathways has some unusual features, different from other sensory systems we have dealt with. More nuclei are intercalated in the auditory pathways, and these nuclei have extensive and complicated interconnections. In addition, some fibers cross the midline at several levels of the auditory pathways. These features have made the auditory pathways more difficult to study than other sensory pathways. The crossing at several levels also renders hearing examinations of limited practical value for determining the site of lesions in the CNS.

Conduction Deafness and Sensorineural Hearing Loss

The most common causes of hearing loss are diseases of the middle ear, either because they compromise the conduction of sounds to the cochlea or because they destroy the neural elements of the cochlea or the eighth nerve. The first kind is called **conductive deafness**, the second **sensorineural (or nerve) deafness**. Transmission of sound to the cochlea can be reduced or abolished by middle ear infections that damage the eardrum or the ossicles. In **otosclerosis**, the basal plate of the stapes becomes fixed in the oval window and therefore cannot transmit sounds. Less frequently, lesions of the central

auditory pathways cause hearing loss; this kind, called **central deafness**, is considered later in this chapter.

To **distinguish** between conductive and sensorineural deafness, one can compare the threshold for sounds conducted through the air with sound conducted through the bones of the skull. In the **Rinne test**, a vibrating tuning fork is first applied to the mastoid process and then a little away from the external ear. Normally, the sound is heard much better when it is conducted through the air than through the bone; however, in conductive deafness, caused by destruction of the eardrum or the ossicles, the bone-conducted sound is heard best. In the **Weber test**, the vibrating tuning fork is applied to the forehead in the midline. Normally, the sound is heard equally in both ears; in conductive deafness, it is heard best in the deaf ear, whereas in sensorineural deafness it is heard best in the normal ear. The reason for the lateralization to the deaf ear in conduction deafness is not clear. It is possible that the airborne sound masks the bone-conducted sound on the normal side.

Destruction of the cochlear nerve or the cochlear hair cells, that is, **peripheral lesions**, produces hearing loss of the ear on the same side (the same happens, of course, with a lesion of the cochlear nuclei). The **hair cells** may be damaged by noise and by certain drugs. There is also a steady loss of hair cells with **aging**, particularly near the base of the cochlear duct (high frequencies). Destruction of the **cochlear nerve** may be caused by a tumor in the internal auditory meatus (Fig. 17.1, called **acoustic neuroma** (arising from the Schwann cells of the eighth cranial nerve). As the tumor grows, it compresses the cochlear, the vestibular, and the facial nerves (all passing through the internal meatus). Symptoms may therefore be caused by irritation (in the early phase) or destruction of all of these nerves. Thus, the first symptoms may be due to irritation of the cochlear nerve, causing ringing in the ear (tinnitus) and sometimes vertigo due to irritation of the vestibular nerve, but gradually deafness develops. As the tumor grows, it compresses the brain stem with additional symptoms from the trigeminal nerve and ascending and descending long tracts. The cochlear nerve may also be compressed or torn by **skull fractures** passing through the temporal bone. Peripheral lesions of the auditory system, in addition to causing unilateral deafness, also reduce or eliminate the ability to **localize** the source of a sound.

The Cochlear Nerve and the Cochlear Nuclei

The part of the eighth cranial nerve conducting signals from the cochlea is called the **cochlear nerve**. Most of the fibers are afferent and have their cell bodies in the **spiral ganglion**, which is located in the bony spiral lamina (Figs. 17.4–17.6). From the spiral ganglion the fibers pass through the midportion of the cochlea (the modiolus,

separated by no more than 2 degrees. To do this, central parts of the auditory system must be able to detect temporal differences of 11 µsec (microseconds) between sounds reaching the two ears.

Unilateral damage to the **auditory cortex** reduces the ability of experimental animals to locate sounds coming from the opposite side. Thus, a cat with such a lesion does not move toward its prey sending out a brief sound (e.g., a mouse). The head and eyes, however, move toward the prey—even after bilateral damage of the auditory cortex—showing that nuclei at lower levels of the auditory pathways can locate the sound and elicit appropriate reflex movements.

Concerning location of sounds in the **horizontal plane**—that is, to the right or left of the midsagittal plane—basic computations occur in the first synaptic relay after the cochlear nuclei, the **superior olive** (Fig. 17.10). We are less certain regarding mechanisms for location of sounds in the vertical plane, although the **dorsal cochlear nucleus** is probably involved. Neurons in the **inferior colliculus** respond specifically to sound from a certain direction, and the inferior colliculus probably contains a **map** of our **auditory space**.

The Superior Olive and Sound Localization

The **superior olivary complex** (superior olive) is located in the lower part of the pons, in the trapezoid body (Fig. 17.10). A striking feature is that most neurons are influenced from both ears, which led to the assumption that the superior olive is particularly important in localizing the origin of a sound. When a sound hits the head from the right side, it will reach the right ear slightly before it reaches the left, because the head is in the way. The sound will also be slightly weakened before reaching the left ear. Psychophysical experiments in humans indicate that side differences in both time and intensity are used by the auditory system to localize sounds. The time difference is most important for localizing sounds of low frequencies, whereas intensity differences are most important for sounds of higher frequencies (above 4000 Hz).

The superior olivary complex consists of several, tonotopically organized subdivisions. The lateral part receives afferents from the cochlear nuclei of both sides and projects bilaterally to the inferior colliculi. Most cells in the lateral part are excited by signals from the ear of the same side and inhibited by signals from the contralateral ear (via interneurons). The cells respond best when the sounds hitting the two ears are of different intensities. Consequently, the **lateral part** of the superior olive is assumed to use intensity differences for the analysis of sound localization.

The **medial part** of the superior olive appears to be particularly important in localizing **low-frequency sounds**. It receives afferents from a particular subdivision of the ventral cochlear nucleus of both sides (Fig. 17.10B). Each cell has two long dendrites oriented transversely. One dendrite receives signals from the right ear, the other from the left. These cells are very sensitive to small time differences in synaptic inputs to the two dendrites and are most sensitive to sounds with low frequencies. The efferent fibers of the medial part pass to the central nucleus of the inferior colliculus on the same side.

Descending Control of the Auditory Pathways

There are descending fibers at all levels of the auditory pathways. Numerous fibers pass from the auditory cortex to the medial geniculate body (like other thalamic nuclei) and to the inferior colliculus. Other fibers descend from the inferior colliculus to the nuclei at lower levels. As mentioned, efferent fibers in the cochlear nerve end in contact primarily with the outer hair cells of the cochlea; such fibers come from the **superior olivary complex** and form the **olivocochlear bundle**. The descending connections are, at least in part, precisely organized and can therefore be expected to selectively control subgroups of neurons in the auditory pathways (e.g., neurons transmitting information about a certain frequency).

There are many inhibitory **interneurons** in the nuclei of the auditory pathways, and both γ-aminobutyric acid (**GABA**) and **glycine** are used as transmitters for such interneurons. Physiological experiments show that the central transmission of auditory signals can be inhibited, probably at all levels from the cochlea to the cerebral cortex. The censoring of the sensory information that is allowed to reach consciousness is perhaps even more pronounced in the auditory system than in other sensory systems. Selective suppression of auditory information is necessary if we are to **select** the relevant sounds among numerous irrelevant ones. Such mechanisms are most likely at work when, for example, at a cocktail party with numerous voices we nevertheless are able to select and pay attention to only one of them.

The brain must be able to distinguish between sounds that are generated externally and sounds we produce ourselves. Indeed, auditory neurons are inhibited during **vocalization**. Although the exact mechanisms are unknown, this most likely involves interpretation of **corollary discharge**—that is, copies of the motor commands producing the sounds are sent to (most likely) the auditory cortex. Descending connections may ensure specific inhibition at several levels of the auditory pathways.

Auditory Reflexes

The ascending auditory pathways convey signals that enable the conscious perception of sounds. Auditory information is also used at a subconscious level to elicit reflex responses. The **reticular formation** receives collaterals from the ascending auditory pathways, and such connections mediate the sudden muscle activity provoked by a strong, unexpected sound—that is, a **startle response**. Other auditory signals pass to the nuclei of the facial and trigeminal nerves, which innervate two small muscles in the middle ear: the **stapedius** and **tensor tympani muscles**. Contraction of these muscles dampens the movements of the middle ear ossicles and thereby protects the cochlea against sounds of high intensity. Paresis of the **facial nerve** often is accompanied by hypersensitivity to sounds, or **hyperacusis**.

Other, more complex, reflex arcs mediate automatic **movements of the head and eyes**, and even the body, in the direction of an unexpected sound. The centers for such reflexes are probably located in the **inferior** and **superior colliculi**. The inferior colliculus sends fibers to the superior colliculus, which has connections with the relevant motor nuclei in the brain stem and spinal cord. Further, in the superior colliculus **integration** of auditory, visual, and somatosensory information takes place, so that the final motor response is appropriate for the organism as a whole.

THE AUDITORY CORTEX

The cortical auditory areas are less studied than the visual areas, and important aspects of human hearing are still poorly understood. While the auditory cortical areas are organized according to the same general principles as the other sensory areas, notable differences exist. Thus, the auditory system shows a more pronounced parallel organization than, for example, the visual system. This is particularly evident in the auditory pathways and intercalated nuclei but concerns also the cortical areas. Further, more information processing takes place at lower levels in the auditory than in other sensory systems. While the auditory cortex is not crucial for the ability to identify single sounds, it is required when different sounds are to be put together to a meaningful whole.

Core and Belt Areas

The **primary auditory area (AI, core region)** appears to consist of several tonotopically organized subdivisions (in contrast to the striate area that consists of one retinotopically organized representation of visual field).[6]

---

6 In monkeys, three areas in the superior temporal gyrus receive tonotopically organized projections from the ventral part of the medial geniculate body. One is the 'classical' AI area, the two others adjoin AI rostrally (termed R and RT). The reason to include them in the term primary auditory cortex is that all three show structural features typical of primary sensory areas, such as a well-developed lamina 4 consisting of densely packed, small neurons (see Fig. 33.4), and dense afferent projections from a specific thalamic nucleus. The tonotopic arrangement in AI is such that the highest frequencies are represented caudally and the lowest rostrally, whereas the opposite arrangement appears to exist in area R.

AI is situated on the upper face of the temporal lobe in a region called the **temporal plane** (Fig. 17.11). In humans, Brodmann's **area 41** is thought to correspond to area AI of monkeys and other animals. Several other auditory areas are arranged concentrically around AI (in monkey about 15 such areas have been identified; cf. organization of extrastriatal visual areas). The areas closest to AI form a belt-like region, and have therefore been termed the **auditory belt**. The belt region receives thalamocortical afferents from other parts of the medial geniculate body than AI, while its main afferents appear to come from AI. Outside the auditory belt, we find additional auditory areas that receive processed auditory information from the auditory belt, but no afferents from the medial geniculate body. Here starts integration of auditory and other sensory modalities. These areas are probably located within area 22 of Brodmann (Fig. 17.11; see also Fig. 33.3). There appears to be several **parallel channels** from the core region to the belt region, and further on to area 22 (similar to the organization of parallel pathways out of the striate area)—each conveying different aspects of auditory information. There are, however, numerous interconnections among areas suggesting that the functional segregation cannot be absolute.

Properties of Neurons in Primary Auditory Cortex

Fibers from the **medial geniculate body** end with precise tonotopic localization in the AI (Figs. 17.10 and 17.11). Accordingly, single neurons in AI respond to sounds with a narrower frequency range than neurons in other auditory areas (sharper tuning). Although many neurons in AI depict **simple**, physical features of sounds (such as pitch and amplitude), others have surprisingly **complex** properties. Some respond, for example, best to a sound when the frequency is increasing or decreasing. Other cells are influenced from both ears, but often such that they are excited by signals from one ear and inhibited from the other. Further, the response of many neurons (as in other primary visual areas) depends on the **context** of a stimulus. It even seems that the **object** with which a sound is associated modulates the activity of many AI neurons.

Asymmetrical Organization of the Auditory Cortex in the Temporal Plane

The auditory cortical areas appear to be asymmetrical in most humans. Thus, according to several MRI and postmortem studies the so-called **Heschl's gyrus**—containing the AI—is larger on the left than on the right side, and the same holds for regions (**area 22**) adjacent to AI in the temporal plane (some studies did not find such asymmetries, however). Intrinsic (horizontal) connections in area 22 show a higher number of separate

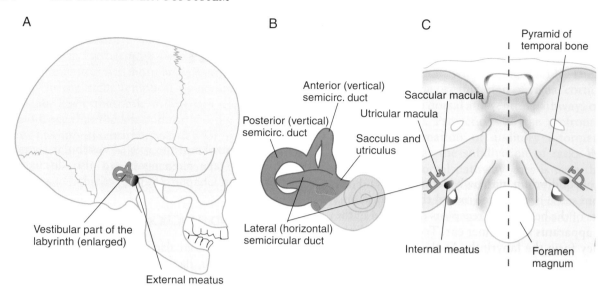

FIGURE 18.1 *The vestibular apparatus.* **A:** The position of the labyrinth in the temporal bone. **B:** The vestibular part of the labyrinth is colored more darkly than the auditory part. Note the orientation of the semicircular ducts in relation to the conventional planes of the body. **C:** The base of the skull, as viewed from above, with the vestibular apparatus projected to the surface of the pyramid of the temporal bone. Note the orientation of the saccular and utricular maculae.

More about Vestibular Hair Cells

The vestibular and cochlear hair cells have the same basic properties (see Chapter 17, under "The Inner Hair Cells and Mechanoelectric Transduction"), although there are some structural differences. On the apical end of the cells there are 50 to 110 **stereocilia** and one longer and thicker **kinocilium** (Fig. 18.6). The stereocilia are unusually long microvilli and contain actin filaments like other microvilli. The kinocilium contains microtubuli (like cilia of the respiratory epithelial cells). The stereocilia are arranged regularly in accordance with their height (Figs. 18.2, 18.4, and 18.6; see also Fig. 17.8). This structural **polarization** of the receptor cells corresponds with the functional polarization mentioned above. Thus, bending of the stereocilia toward the kinocilium increases the firing frequency of the sensory fibers in contact with the cell, whereas bending in the opposite direction reduces the firing frequency. This is because the receptor cell is depolarized or hyperpolarized by bending of the cilia. The receptor potentials of the hair cells induce release of **glutamate**, which depolarizes the afferent nerve fibers. Deflection of the cilia perpendicular to the direction of the polarization produces no response, whereas oblique displacements give a reduced response compared with a stimulus that is properly aligned with the polarization. This means that a given **firing frequency** of an afferent fiber is **ambiguous**; it can be caused by a weak stimulus in the direction of the polarization or a stronger obliquely oriented one. Further, a given firing frequency may be caused by moving the head forward (e.g., walking) or tilting the head backwards. This may be why the hair cells in the maculae are arranged differently with regard to the orientation of the polarization axes, so that all the cells together cover 360 degrees (Fig. 18.6B). This ensures that the information received by the brain about head position in space is unambiguous. This requires, of course, that the brain is able to compare the magnitude of the signals from various parts of the maculae to reach a conclusion.

Electron microscopic studies showed more than 50 years ago that there are two kinds of vestibular receptor cells, which are found both in the cristae of the semicircular ducts and in the maculae of the saccule and utricle (Fig. 18.6A). One kind, the **type 1** cell, is bottle-shaped, whereas the **type 2** cell is slender. The sensory fibers (the peripheral process of the vestibular ganglion cells) end differently on the two cell types (Fig. 18.6A). The functional significance of the two types of hair cells is still unknown.

The Adequate Stimulus for the Semicircular Ducts Is Rotation of the Head

Flow of the fluid (the endolymph) inside the semicircular ducts displaces the cupula, thereby bending the cilia (Fig. 18.3). This activates or inhibits the sensory cells, depending on the direction of bending. Rotational movements of the head produce flow of the endolymph in the semicircular ducts. This is explained by the inertia of the fluid: when the head starts to rotate, the fluid "lags behind," and when the rotation stops, the fluid continues to flow for a moment (like the water in a bowl that is rotated rapidly for a couple of turns). If the head rotation continues at even velocity, the fluid and

A

UTRICULAR MACULA

Otolith membrane

Otoliths

Cilia

Vestibular
nerve fibers   Hair cell

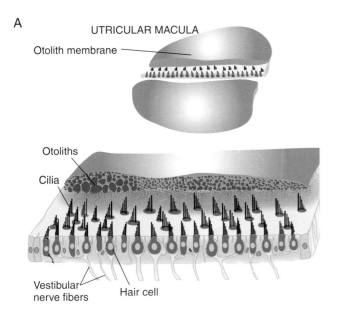

B

Endolymph   Otoliths   Hair cells

Vestibular
nerve

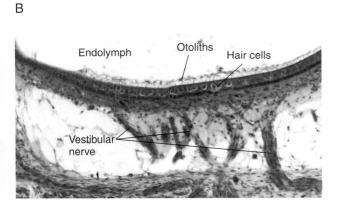

FIGURE 18.2 *The utricular and saccular maculae.* **A:** The utricular macula. Note the polarization of the hair cells. The otoliths are embedded in a gelatinous substance that covers the hair cells (otolith membrane). (Based on Lindeman 1973.) **B:** Photomicrograph of a section through the sacculus with the macula.

the head will after a short time move with the same speed and in the same direction, which means that the cilia are not bent. Thus, it is clear that not every rotational movement is recorded by the receptors of the semicircular ducts: alteration of the velocity of the rotational movement—that is, positive or negative **angular acceleration**—is the adequate stimulus for the semicircular duct receptors. Thus, these receptors have **dynamic sensitivity**. Linear acceleration does not affect (or affects only slightly) the semicircular ducts. By linear displacement of the head (a translatory movement) without concomitant rotation, there is no stimulation of the semicircular duct receptors. An example of linear acceleration is a car that starts or brakes on a flat, straight road. If the road goes up and down and is curved, rotational accelerations of the car (and the heads of its passengers) are superimposed on the linear ones.

The orientation of the semicircular ducts ensures that rotation of the head in any conceivable plane produces change of activity of the receptors in one or more of the ducts. The brain monitors the rotational movements of the head by reading the pattern of activity produced by all the receptors. The semicircular ducts of both sides must function normally to supply the brain with the necessary information. A pair of ducts (e.g., the right and left lateral ones) gives **complementary signals** to a given rotation—that is, increased signal frequency from the one and reduced from the other.

Sacculus and Utriculus Signal the Position of the Head and Linear Acceleration

The small **otoliths** have higher specific weight than the endolymph and the substance in which they are embedded and are therefore more influenced by gravitational forces. Taking as an example the utricular macula, which in the neutral head position is oriented horizontally (Fig. 18.1), a change of head position tilts the macula, and the otoliths pull the cilia in that direction. Different angles of tilt produce different patterns of activity of the macular hair cells. Owing to their different orientations in space, the utricular and saccular hair cells together provide information about all possible head positions. The **utricle** records especially **lateral tilt** (i.e., head positions that vary around a sagittal axis), whereas the **saccule** probably records mainly flexion–extension of the head (i.e., movement in the cervical joints around a transverse axis). Its ability to provide information about the position of the head at any one time (in the absence of movement) shows that the vestibular apparatus has **static sensitivity**. This property depends on the presence of receptors that adapt slowly or not at all, so that they give a constant signal as long as a certain position is maintained. The static sensitivity of the vestibular apparatus depends, as we have seen, on the force of gravity and disappears in a state of weightlessness (such as in space travel). Because the static sensitivity is a property of the utricle and the saccule, these parts of the vestibular apparatus are called the **static labyrinth**. We will see, however, that this part of the labyrinth also has dynamic properties.

The **dynamic sensitivity** of the utricle and the saccule is seen when their activity is recorded during **linear acceleration**. The response increases (i.e., the firing frequency of the afferent fibers) with increasing acceleration. This is again explained by the inertia of the otoliths. On linear displacement of the head with changing velocity, as in a car that is accelerating, the otoliths lag behind and thereby bend the cilia backward (in relation to the direction of the movement). The opposite happens when the car slows down; the otoliths continue to move for a moment and bend the cilia forward (compare with the forces acting on a loose object in a car when the car speeds up or slows down).

four major nuclei: the **superior**, the **lateral** (or nucleus of Deiters), the **medial**, and the **descending** (or inferior).

Primary afferent vestibular fibers divide into an ascending and a descending branch when entering the brain stem. Together, they end in large parts of the vestibular complex and in parts of the cerebellum (see Fig. 24.4). Although terminations of fibers from the ampullar cristae and the maculae **overlap** in the vestibular nuclei, they also show notable differences in distribution. Thus, afferents from the **cristae** (that is, from the semicircular ducts) end in the **superior nucleus** and the rostral part of the **medial nucleus** but not in the lateral nucleus, whereas the fibers from the **utricular and saccular maculae** end in the **lateral nucleus** but not (or only sparsely) in the superior nucleus. In agreement with the distribution of primary afferents, neurons in the superior nucleus respond best to rotational head movements (angular acceleration), whereas the cells in the lateral nucleus are particularly sensitive to static head position. Nevertheless, physiological studies show that a substantial proportion of neurons in the vestibular nuclei integrate information about angular acceleration and static position/linear acceleration.[2]

The Vestibular Nuclei Receive Afferents from Regions Other than the Labyrinth

The physiological properties of neurons in the vestibular nuclei are not copies of those of the primary afferent fibers. This is due to convergence on the cells of various kinds of afferents (such as fibers from the semicircular ducts and the utricle) and by interconnections between the nuclei (e.g., commissural fibers linking the two sides). Further, the vestibular complex receives afferents from other parts of the central nervous system (CNS), especially the **spinal cord**, the **reticular formation**, certain mesencephalic nuclei, and the **cerebellum**. Afferents from the mesencephalon arise, for example, in the **superior colliculus**, and the cerebellar fibers come from both the flocculonodular lobe and the anterior lobe (Fig. 18.7; see also Fig. 24.4), and contribute to adaptation of vestibular reflexes to changed conditions for example during growth of the head, wearing of glasses, and so forth.

The vestibular nuclei receive signals from the **cerebral cortex** (mainly indirectly via the reticular formation but also some direct fibers). The corticovestibular fibers arise in parts of the cortex, such as the **SI** (areas 2 and 3a) and the **insula**, which receive converging information from the labyrinth and proprioceptors. The vestibular nuclei are also influenced from the **posterior parietal cortex**, which

is concerned with spatial orientation and goal-directed movements. Presumably, these cortical regions are important for building internal representations of the position and movements of the body, necessary for the control of movements. Accordingly, physiological experiments show that **vestibular reflexes**—the vestibulospinal ones in particular—are modulated in conjunction with voluntary movements. In this way, the reflex responses are subordinated to the overall plan for the movements, presumably by way of corticovestibular connections (among others).

Efferent Connections of the Vestibular Nuclei

Schematically, the vestibular nuclei (and therefore also the vestibular receptors) act on three main regions (Figs. 18.7 and 18.8), namely **motoneurons** in the **spinal cord**, motoneurons in the **nuclei of the extraocular muscles**, and the **cerebellum**. Accordingly, information from the vestibular apparatus is used primarily to influence muscles that maintain our **upright position** (equilibrium) and muscles that produce **eye movements**. The latter movements ensure that the retinal image is kept stationary when the head moves.

Most of the fibers to the **spinal cord** come from the **lateral vestibular nucleus** and form the **lateral vestibulospinal tract**. The fibers descend in the ventral funiculus on the same side as the nuclei from which they come. In the ventral horn they end—in part monosynaptically—on α and γ **motoneurons** (Fig. 18.8A). The tract is somatotopically organized, so that various body parts can be selectively controlled. The vestibulospinal tract has strong effects on the muscles that contribute to equilibrium and posture (see also Chapter 22, under "Vestibulospinal Tracts"). As mentioned, the lateral nucleus receives afferents from the utricular macula; these provide information about the static position of the head in space and thereby indirectly about the position of the body. Change of body position also changes its center of gravity, with a resulting need to adjust muscle tone to maintain equilibrium.

A smaller, **medial vestibulospinal tract** arises in the **medial vestibular nucleus**. It also descends in the ventral funiculus and acts on motoneurons. The fibers do not reach below the upper thoracic segments, however, and are thought to be of importance primarily for **head movements** elicited by the vestibular receptors. The so-called **vestibulocollic reflex** serves to stabilize the position of the head in space.

Fibers to the **nuclei of the extraocular muscles** arise mainly in the **superior** and **medial nuclei**, which receive many primary afferent fibers from the semicircular ducts (Fig. 18.8B). The fibers leave the nuclei medially and join to form a distinct fiber bundle, the **medial longitudinal fasciculus**, which is located close to the midline below the floor of the fourth ventricle (Figs. 18.7 and 18.8; see also Fig. 6.18). Some of the fibers cross to the

---

2 For example, a study in the cat with electric stimulation of separate divisions of the vestibular nerve found that about one-third of all neurons received convergent inputs from the vertical semicircular canal and sacculus/utriculus. Another one-third received convergent input from sacculus and utriculus, and one fifth from the horizontal canal and sacculus/utriculus.

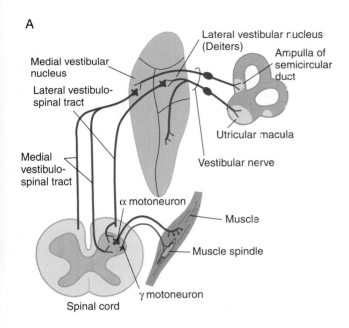

A

Medial vestibular nucleus

Lateral vestibulo-spinal tract

Medial vestibulo-spinal tract

Lateral vestibular nucleus (Deiters)

Ampulla of semicircular duct

Utricular macula

Vestibular nerve

α motoneuron

Muscle

Muscle spindle

γ motoneuron

Spinal cord

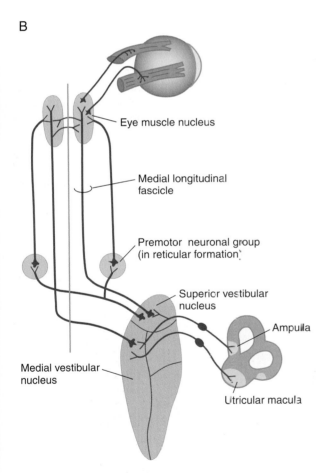

B

Eye muscle nucleus

Medial longitudinal fascicle

Premotor neuronal group (in reticular formation)

Superior vestibular nucleus

Ampulla

Medial vestibular nucleus

Utricular macula

FIGURE 18.8 *Main features of vestibular connections.* **A:** Descending connections acting on α and γ motoneurons in the spinal cord. The medial vestibulospinal tract reach only cervical levels. **B:** Ascending connections controlling eye movements.

other side as they ascend. They end in the abducent, the trochlear, and the oculomotor nuclei and are precisely organized. In addition to the direct connections in the medial longitudinal fasciculus, there are **indirect pathways** from the vestibular nuclei to the eye muscle nuclei via the **reticular formation** (Fig. 18.8B). We return to this below when discussing vestibular reflexes.

Vestibulocerebellar fibers (arising in the medial and descending vestibular nuclei) end primarily in the **vestibulocerebellum** (Fig. 18.7; see also Fig. 24.4). Fibers from the vestibulocerebellum to the vestibular nuclei can adjust the gain (sensitivity) of the **vestibulo-ocular reflex**, as will be discussed next (see also Fig. 25.4).

Connections to the **thalamus** from the vestibular nuclei have been demonstrated anatomically and end in the VPL and nearby nuclei. Physiologically, scattered neurons in a fairly large regions respond to signals from the vestibular apparatus. This probably explains why vestibular signals reach several, discrete regions of the cerebral cortex.

VESTIBULAR REFLEXES: CONTROL OF EYE MOVEMENTS AND BODILY POSTURE

The special problems encountered in space journeys aroused great interest in the mechanisms that underlie vestibular reflexes. As with other parts of the brain being comprehensively investigated, conditions turn out to be more complex than initially thought. We will discuss only a few salient points. There are two kinds of reflexes that are elicited from the vestibular apparatus: **vestibulo-ocular reflexes** that control eye movements and so-called **labyrinthine reflexes** mediated by the vestibulospinal tracts controlling bodily postures (especially the upright position). In general, signals from the utricle and the saccule elicit **tonic** reflex effects, whereas **phasic** reflex responses are caused by signals from the semicircular ducts when the stimulus is rotation of the head (angular acceleration) and from the utricle or saccule when the stimulus is linear acceleration. Because the vestibular receptors inform only about the head, other receptors must inform about the movements and positions of other bodily parts. To control our upright position, the brain must integrate these various sources of information and issue commands that are appropriate for the whole body. Therefore, the labyrinthine reflexes must operate in concert with other postural reflexes, and we will treat these together below.

Vestibulo-Ocular Reflexes

There are several vestibulo-ocular reflexes, mediated by reflex arcs of various complexities. This topic is also discussed in Chapter 25 dealing with the control of eye movements. In general, the vestibulo-ocular reflexes ensure that the **image is kept stationary** on the retina when the head moves (rotates).

The simplest vestibulo-ocular reflex is mediated by a chain of three neurons (Fig. 18.8; see also Fig. 25.4):

1. Primary afferent fibers from the cristae of the semicircular ducts
2. Neurons in the vestibular nuclei that send their axons to the nuclei of the extraocular muscles (passing in the medial longitudinal fasciculus)
3. Motoneurons in these nuclei, which send their axons to the extraocular muscles

In addition, there are other pathways from the vestibular nuclei to the nuclei of the extraocular muscles that are synaptically interrupted in the reticular formation and some other brain stem nuclei (Fig. 18.8B).

A movement of the head in any direction is accompanied by a **compensatory movement** of the eyes in the opposite direction and with the same velocity as the head movement. Rotation of the head produces movement of the endolymph inside the semicircular ducts. Taking a rotation in the horizontal plane (turning the head from one side to the other) as an example, mainly the lateral semicircular duct records the movement and elicits a compensatory eye movement in the horizontal plane.

When the head movement is relatively small, the eyes move with exactly the same velocity as and in the opposite direction of the head, and the image is kept in the same position on the retina all the time. When the head movement becomes larger, so that it becomes impossible to keep the image stationary even with maximal excursion of the eyes, a fast, or **saccadic**, movement occurs in the same direction as the head movement. Then the gaze is fixed again on the object, and another slow movement follows (as long as the head continues to move in the same direction). Such an alternation between slow and fast, saccadic eye movements is called **nystagmus**. In this case, the nystagmus was produced by stimulation of the semicircular ducts (rotation of the head) and is therefore called **vestibular nystagmus**. Movement of the surroundings can also elicit nystagmus when the head is stationary. This **optokinetic nystagmus** occurs, for example, in a train-passenger watching the landscape pass by.

Vestibular Signals Must Be Integrated with Other Sensory Modalities for Control of Eye Movements

As mentioned, the vestibular nuclei receive afferents from sources other than the labyrinth, such as nuclei in the mesencephalon, the reticular formation, and the cerebellum. Some of these sources mediate visual information that can modify the vestibular reflex responses. This convergence of various inputs seems logical. Thus, to achieve optimal control of the eye movements, the responsible neural cell groups must receive and integrate vestibular information about movements of the head, visual signals about movements of the image on the retina, and proprioceptive signals about movements of the eyes relative to the head.

Vestibular Stimulation Produces Nystagmus and Falling Tendency

When an upright person rotates fairly rapidly a few times around his axis and then stops, the eyes can be seen to move rapidly one way (saccade) and slowly the other for some seconds afterward. Obviously, the rotation has induced **nystagmus**. By using special instruments, it can be seen that there is nystagmus also at the start of the rotation, but in the opposite direction of that occurring after the rotation has stopped. When the person rotates to the right, the saccade movement is to the right and the slow movement is to the left, as if the person fixes her gaze on a stationary point and then moves the eyes rapidly when this point is slipping out of the visual field. The eyes then move to a new fixation point, and the same sequence of events is repeated. This **postrotatory nystagmus** is caused by stimulation of the receptors in the semicircular ducts. As mentioned, at the start of the movement the inertia of the endolymph makes it lag behind, thereby bending the cilia of the receptor cells, whereas the endolymph continues to flow for a moment after the rotation has stopped. The person who had just stopped rotating feels as if he were still rotating, but now in the opposite direction. The direction of the nystagmus corresponds to the **illusion** of such a rotation—that is, with the saccade phase to the left after a rotation to the right. If the rotation of the body continues for some time, the nystagmus disappears and the person gets dizzy (compare with ballet dancers who deliberately ensure that the head does not move with even velocity during pirouettes; this way they have sufficient time for fixation so that the brain gets information to determine the orientation of the body in space).

After stopping the rotation, the person is also unsteady and tends to fall to one side, especially if he is asked to keep his eyes closed. Further, the arm deviates to the right if the person is asked to point straight ahead (with his eyes closed). This is called **postrotational past pointing**. After the rotation stops, the illusion of the opposite movement (i.e., the person feels he is turning to the left) causes the past pointing to the right: the person feels that the room is moving to the right.

The postrotational effects on postural muscles are mediated via the **vestibulospinal tracts** (Fig. 18.8A) and show that the receptors of the semicircular ducts also influence the spinal cord and the postural muscles, not just the cranial nerve nuclei and the extraocular muscles.

Nystagmus, falling tendency, and past pointing can also be produced by irrigation of the external auditory meatus with hot or cold water. The change of temperature makes the endolymph flow in the semicircular ducts and thus produces stimulation of the receptors. Such a **caloric test** is used clinically to examine the function of the vestibular labyrinth and the conduction of signals to the brain stem.

Various **diseases** affecting the vestibular receptors or the signal pathways to the motoneurons of the extraocular muscles (the vestibular nerve, the vestibular nuclei, the medial longitudinal fasciculus, and the cerebellum) can produce nystagmus in the absence of vestibular or visual stimulation. This is called **spontaneous nystagmus.** In certain cases, the nystagmus may be present only in certain positions of the head (positional nystagmus).

Neck and Labyrinthine Reflexes

The vestibular receptors inform about the position and movements of the head in space, whereas neck proprioceptors can inform about the position and movements of the body in relation to the head. Based on information from both kinds of receptors, the brain can decide whether the head is moving in isolation or whether it moves together with the rest of the body. Obviously, different kinds of postural responses are needed in these two situations. The **labyrinthine reflexes** are elicited by stimulation of the sensory receptors of the **semicircular ducts** and the **utriculus** of the labyrinth. In the **neck reflexes,** the response is a change of muscle tension, especially in the extremities supporting upright stance, induced by a change in the position of the head relative to the body (such movements take place primarily in the upper cervical joints). The labyrinthine reflexes when operating alone produce muscle contractions in the trunk and extremities that serve to keep the position of the head constant. The neck reflexes, as mentioned, serve to keep the position of the body constant in relation to the head. The latter is a prerequisite for the labyrinthine reflexes to function properly; the vestibular apparatus can provide information only about the position of the head in space and not about its position in relation to the body. Thus, the labyrinthine reflexes work on the assumption that the head has a constant position relative to the body, and the neck reflexes ensure that this position is constant.

The reflexes may be either **tonic** or **phasic.** A phasic neck or labyrinthine reflex consists of a rapid, transient change of muscle tension in postural muscles as a response to a change of posture (usually a disturbance of the equilibrium). We experience phasic labyrinthine reflexes when we trip over and a coordinated set of compensatory movements occur before we consciously perceive what is going on. In a tonic reflex, the change of muscle tension lasts as long as the new position is maintained.

Vestibulospinal tracts are the most likely candidates for mediation of the labyrinthine reflexes. The **reflex center** of the neck reflexes is located in the medulla, and the effects on the motoneurons are most likely mediated by both the **reticulospinal** and vestibulospinal tracts.

More about the Neck and Labyrinthine Reflexes

Studies of **decerebrate,** four-legged animals have elucidated the neck and labyrinthine reflexes (the brain stem is transected just below the red nucleus in the mesencephalon). To demonstrate clearly the **neck reflexes** in decerebrate animals (mostly cats have been studied), the vestibular receptors must have been eliminated. When then the head is bent backward (extension of the neck), the muscle tension is increased in the extensor muscles of the forelimbs and decreased in the extensors of the hind limbs. Forward bending of the head (flexion) induces the opposite pattern of changes (extension of the hind limbs and flexion of the forelimbs). Tilting the head sideways increases the extensor tone on the same side and reduces it on the other side, as does turning the head sideways. These changes of the muscle tone aim at reestablishing the position of the body relative to the head. The receptors for these reflexes are located near the upper cervical joints, because they disappear after transection of the upper three cervical dorsal roots. **Muscle spindles** are the most likely candidates, but joint receptors may also contribute. As mentioned, the functional role of the neck reflexes cannot be understood when observed in isolation, however. Only in conjunction with the labyrinthine reflexes are their effects appropriate for the whole body.

To demonstrate clearly the **labyrinthine reflexes,** the neck reflexes must have been eliminated by cutting the upper dorsal roots (in a decerebrate animal). It then appears that the effects produced by the labyrinthine reflexes are the opposite of those of the neck reflexes when the latter act alone. Thus, bending the head backward elicits flexion of the forelimbs and extension of the hind limbs, and vice versa when the head is bent forward. The purpose of these changes of muscle tone is to bring the head back to the position held before the movement—that is, to keep the position of the head in space constant. Provided the neck reflexes ensure that the body stays in a constant position relative to the head, the labyrinthine reflexes will serve to maintain both the position of the head in space and the upright position of the whole body. The labyrinthine reflexes are shown clearly when the experimental animal stands on a platform that can be tilted in various directions. Tilting the platform forward increases the extensor tone in the forelimbs and decreases the tone in the hind limbs. Tilting the platform sideways increases the muscle tone in the extensors on the side to which the tilt is directed. Both responses are obviously appropriate for the maintenance of body balance. When the platform is moved quickly in one direction and then back, the reflex response is transient (**phasic reflex**). When the platform is maintained in the new position, the altered muscle tone is upheld (**tonic reflex**).

When **both reflexes work together** in an intact organism, backward bending of the head, for example (with movement taking place only in the upper cervical joints and no change of body position), produces no change in muscle tension of the extremities. The tendency of the labyrinthine reflexes to produce forelimb flexion and hind limb extension is canceled by the opposite tendency of the neck reflexes. In contrast, when the same movement of the head is produced by a backward movement of the whole body (with no movement of the head relative to the body, like a horse that is rearing), the labyrinthine reflexes act alone to produce extension of the hind limbs and flexion of the forelimbs. Another example is an animal standing on a platform tilting forward with no movement of the head relative to the body. In that case, the labyrinthine reflexes produce forelimb extension and hind limb flexion. This is an appropriate response to maintain balance when standing on a downhill slope. However, if the position of the head in space is kept constant and the body is moved in relation to the head, the neck reflexes act alone. An example is a cat jumping down from a table: the neck is extended (keeping the head position constant), producing extension of the forelimbs, which is appropriate for landing.

Postural Reflexes: Various Receptors Contribute

In order to control posture and balance, the CNS must receive sufficient information about positions and movements in various body parts as well as the nature of the support surface. This information enables the brain to compute the position of the center of gravity and the movements needed to keep it in the right position relative to our supporting base. Many sense organs can provide relevant information (visual, proprioceptive, cutaneous, and vestibular). The signals are analyzed in the CNS, which in response initiates **postural reflexes**, that is, automatic, coordinated contractions of muscles that maintain our upright position. Postural reflexes can be elicited from the labyrinth, from proprioceptors and by vision. The contribution of various receptors to control of the upright position is not static, however. This is because the contribution of each receptor type varies with the nature, magnitude, and context of a postural perturbation.[3] For example, somatosensory information from the sole of the foot is less reliable when the support surface is slippery than when it is firm and

even. Further, visual information may be unreliable if we are in an environment with moving objects, because it may be difficult to distinguish own movements from those of the surrounds. Persons with loss of vestibular function manage well as long as they can see but they have serious problems in maintaining the body's equilibrium in the dark. If one source is unreliable, its contribution tends to be ignored, and information from other sources becomes more important. We also treat postural reflexes in Chapter 22 in conjunction with the control of automatic movements.

More about Receptor Types and Their Contribution to Postural Control

Persons standing on a platform that can be tilted or moved forward or backward have been much used in studies of postural control. In this situation, the experimenter can control the direction, speed, and amplitude of perturbations, and specific kinds of sensory information can be removed temporarily. In addition, patients with loss of one or the other kind of receptor have been much studied.

Signals from **muscle spindles**—providing rapid informing about joint position and movements—are important for postural control. This is, for example, evident from persons who lose the proprioceptive sense (cf. Chapter 13, under "Clinical Examples of Loss of Somatosensory Information"). Further evidence that muscle spindles play a role for posture comes from experiments with **vibration** (activating Ia afferents) of leg muscles and neck muscles. Such vibration elicits postural adjustments, which are appropriate, considering that the brain "believes" that the muscles are being stretched. The signals are obviously interpreted as if the center of gravity were moving. In this case, the muscle spindle information is not primarily used at the segmental level for quick postural responses but is integrated with other inputs at higher levels. Platform experiments further support that the contribution of muscle spindles to postural control does not depend mainly on simple, **spinal reflexes** (i.e., reflex contractions in response to muscle stretch that do not depend on higher levels). When the platform is suddenly displaced backward (without tilting), the body first sways forward with movement primarily at the ankle joints. The balance is regained mainly because the calf muscles at the back of the leg contract (muscles of the hip, the back, and in the neck also contribute, especially if the displacement is large). The first part of the contraction of the leg muscles occurs so early after the perturbation that a reflex must mediate it. (Somewhat later there is also a voluntary contraction, which contributes to the final outcome of the postural adjustment.) In this case, a reflex elicited by stretch of muscle spindles in the calf muscles would seem appropriate. In another situation, however, such a reflex would worsen

---

3 There furthermore seems to be individual variation among normal subjects with regard to which kind of information they rely on for the reflex adjustments in quiet standing. In a study of healthy volunteers, only half of the subjects increased their body sway when the eyes were closed. This suggests that persons differ with regard to how much they rely on visual information to stabilize the quiet standing position.

the balance: if the platform is suddenly tilted backward, the calf muscles are stretched (as in the former example) but the center of gravity is now displaced backward instead of forward. Consequently, a contraction of the calf muscles would worsen the imbalance. To regain balance, the muscles at the front of the leg have to contract as rapidly as possible, in spite of being shortened by the tilting of the platform, and this is what happens. Thus, whether a segmental, spinal reflex is elicited depends on the situation, and inappropriate reflex responses to stretch are generally suppressed. Indeed, for the functionally important reflex response in the leg muscles (starting about 90 msec after the balance perturbation), signals from proprioceptors around the **vertebral column** may be more important than signals from leg muscle spindles. Thus, the contraction of the leg muscles correlates less with their own length change than with the displacement of the trunk.

Signals from **cutaneous** low-threshold mechanoreceptors in the **sole of the foot** seem to contribute to the reflex contractions of the leg muscles in platform experiments. The dorsal column–medial lemniscus pathway transmits such signals very rapidly. Presumably, the brain determines the center of pressure by calculating the difference between the pressure applied to the heel and the forefoot. The center of pressure informs about the position of the body center of mass. Patients with **neuropathies** who have reduced sensibility in the sole of the foot witness the importance of this input for postural control and for normal gait.

Vision also contributes to adjustment of muscle tone with the purpose of maintaining body equilibrium. Platform experiments indicate that the muscle contractions in response to a movement of the platform depend on whether the subject can see that the body moves in relation to the surroundings. If the experimental setup is such that it appears as though the surroundings do not move (i.e., they are made to move in the same direction as the head), the earliest reflex contractions of the legs are weaker than when the sense of vision also informs about the movement. We do not fully know the pathways involved, but the final commands are probably sent from the vestibular nuclei in the vestibulospinal tract.

In platform experiments with moderate postural perturbations, signals from **vestibular receptors** seem not to be essential for the corrective contractions of leg muscles (ankle strategy). With larger perturbations, however, vestibular information contributes to contractions of hip muscles (hip strategy). When visual information is eliminated, signals from the utricle and the saccule are indeed necessary for the proper orientation of the body in space, as can be shown in animals whose otoliths have been removed. **Unexpected fall** from some height elicits a postural reflex that depends on information from the vestibular apparatus. The fall initiates a contraction of the muscles of the leg as an appropriate preparation to the landing. The contraction begins about 75 msec after start of the fall and can therefore occur before landing (and thus before a stretch reflex can be elicited). The latency is also too short for the contraction to be voluntary. Animal experiments indicate that the receptors of this reflex are located in the labyrinth (probably in the saccular macula).

Postural Reflexes Are under Central Control

Reflex responses occur too early after a balance perturbation to be caused by conscious, high-level decisions. Indeed, the main advantage of a reflex response is that it occurs so rapidly. Nevertheless, even automatic movements are subject to central control. The response to a perturbation challenging our upright position is strongly modulated by expectation and the context in which the perturbation occurs. For example, a contraction of the triceps surae muscle in response to dorsiflexion in the ankle joint may restore balance in one situation while worsen it in another. In general, the individual reflex responses are subordinate an overall, coordinated motor plan designed to attain a certain goal.

In **infants**, comprehensive, high-level motor programs have not yet developed and accordingly, some postural reflexes operate "on their own." This concerns some vestibular reflexes, the grasp reflex, and others. In comatose patients with lesions of the upper brain stem, exaggerated postural reflexes may appear spontaneously—usually with a strong dominance of extensor tone. This condition is called **decerebrate rigidity**.

CORTICAL PROCESSING OF VESTIBULAR SIGNALS

Several Areas Receive Vestibular Signals

Vestibular signals reach several small areas in the cortex, as shown electrophysiologically in monkeys and with imaging methods in humans (Fig. 18.9). The **parietal insular vestibular cortex—PIVC**—is of particular interest (as the name implies, it lies at the junction between the parietal lobe and the insula).[4] The PIVC contains neurons that are activated by signals from both the semicircular canals (head rotation) and from proprioceptors around the upper cervical joints. Because, in addition, the neurons are influenced by visual signals it seems likely that they integrate all kinds

---

4 Imaging studies in humans place the PIVC and other presumptive vestibular-activated areas somewhat differently. For example, some find that PIVC includes posterior parts of the insula, while others limit it to a region just posterior to the insula. Such discrepancies are most likely due to differences in experimental conditions. It is very difficult to rule out that cortical activation evoked by caloric, galvanic, or optokinetic stimuli—applied to stimulate vestibular receptors—are due to concomitant stimulation of somatosensory or visual systems.

19 | Olfaction and Taste

The chemical senses of smell and taste enable us to recognize a vast number of different molecules in our surroundings. Obviously, this gives us information of great importance that triggers a range of responses—from avoiding poisonous food to enjoying the fragrance of a rose. Both senses depend on binding of molecules to specific **chemoreceptors**. These receptors are very sensitive, thus permitting recognition and discrimination of molecules in extremely low concentrations (in air or in fluids). Stereospecificity—that is, the shape of the ligand determines which receptor it binds to—is another common property of the chemoreceptors for taste and smell. The transduction mechanisms—that is, how the stimuli translate to graded receptor potentials—are similar for receptors for taste and smell because they (with some exceptions) are coupled to **G proteins** (as are photoreceptors and many neurotransmitter receptors).

The **olfactory system** differs from other sensory systems in certain respects: the **sensory cells**—located in the upper nasal cavity—are neurons with an axon going directly to the **olfactory bulb** (part of the central nervous system (CNS). Further, the signals in the **olfactory tract** destined for the cerebral cortex are not synaptically interrupted in the thalamus but goes directly to the **primary olfactory cortex** the medial temporal lobe near the uncus.

The taste (gustatory) receptor cells are found in taste **buds** scattered over most of the tongue. The sensory cells are equipped with receptors identifying four basic **taste qualities** (sweet, salty, sour, and bitter). In addition a fifth quality called umami (Japanese: savory, meaty) is evoked by glutamate binding to specific receptors. Signals from the taste buds are transmitted in the **facial** (intermediate) and **glossopharyngeal** nerves to the **solitary nucleus** in the upper medulla. From there signals are distributed to other brain stem nuclei important for food intake and digestion, and to higher levels such as the **hypothalamus**, the **amygdala**, and the primary taste area in the anterior part of the **insula**. Integration of olfactory and gustatory information takes place in the **orbitofrontal cortex** (and some other places). Here, information from the chemical senses is processed in a broader context with the aim to facilitate appropriate behavior.

THE OLFACTORY SYSTEM

The sense of smell does not play the same important role for adult humans as the senses of hearing and vision. This does not mean that the sense of smell is insignificant in daily life. The perception of odors is special by its close association with memories and with emotions and moods. Presumably, this explains why we usually remember odors so well. An enormous industry devoted to producing perfumes and other fragrances shows that for humans the sense of smell has an important role in interpersonal communication.

Going back in the evolution of the species, we find that smell is the most primitive of the senses. It is also the most important one at the early stages of evolution. To understand the evolution of the brain, knowledge of the "olfactory brain" or **rhinencephalon** has been important because in the early, primitive vertebrates almost the whole cerebrum is devoted to the processing of olfactory signals. In higher vertebrates, new parts of the cerebrum emerge that gradually and completely overshadow the phylogenetically old parts. The organization of the central pathways and nuclei that process olfactory information reflects the fact that this system developed earlier than the parts of the cortex (the neocortex) that treat other sensory modalities. The term olfactory brain for these old parts is unfortunate, however. In higher vertebrates, large parts of the regions corresponding to the rhinencephalon in lower animals have nothing to do with the sense of smell but have taken on other important functions, the hippocampus (Chapter 32) being the most striking example. This is a common occurrence during evolution: structures that are no longer used for one function may form the basis for the development of new capacities. Thus, the parts treating olfactory signals have not developed in pace with the rest of the brain during evolution and are therefore relatively much smaller in humans than in, for example, cats and dogs. In absolute terms, however, the differences are not so marked.

Receptor Cells for Smell

The special receptor cells for smell are located in the mucous membrane of the upper part of the nasal cavity,

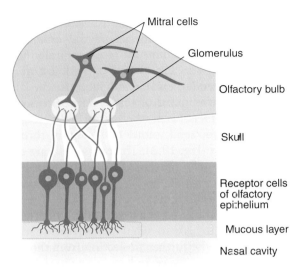

Mitral cells

Glomerulus

Olfactory bulb

Skull

Receptor cells of olfactory epithelium

Mucous layer

Nasal cavity

FIGURE 19.1 *The olfactory epithelium and connections to the olfactory bulb.* Neurons (receptor cells) in the olfactory epithelium have cilia embedded in mucus. The central process (axon) of the receptor cells end on mitral cells in the glomeruli of the olfactory bulb. The axons from neurons sharing odorant specificity tend to converge on one or a few glomeruli in the olfactory bulb. Thus, the glomeruli show some odorant specificity. (Based on Mombaerts 1996.)

the **olfactory epithelium**.[1] The total number of receptor cells has been estimated to about 10 million in humans, and the cells are constantly renewed. Because they are in fact primitive neurons, they are exceptions to the rule that neurons that die are not replaced. The olfactory epithelium is pseudostratified and consists of supporting cells and so-called basal cells besides the receptor cells (Fig. 19.1). The **supporting cells** probably insulate the receptor cells electrically, so that signals are not propagated from one cell to another. The **basal cells** divide mitotically and probably give rise to the receptor cells. The **receptor cells** are bipolar and send a dendrite-like branch toward the epithelial surface, and an axon through the base of the skull to the olfactory bulb. The dendrite ends with an expansion densely covered with **cilia** (Fig. 19.1). Because the cilia are embedded in the **mucus** that covers the epithelium, only substances dissolved in the mucus can act on the receptor cells. Many

odorous substances are hydrophobic, however; that is, they do not dissolve easily in water. Therefore, we assume that there exist mechanisms—such as transport proteins—to bring hydrophobic odorants through the mucus. Several families of **odorant-binding proteins** (OBPs) have in fact been identified in the mucus. It is probable that each protein binds specifically to certain odorants and may serve to concentrate the odorant in the proper part of the olfactory epithelium (i.e., the part containing the receptors specific for the particular odorant). The odorant-binding proteins may also help remove the odorant so that the receptors quickly regain their sensitivity. Specialized glands produce the mucus, which consists of several layers.

Transduction Mechanism

Experiments with a large number of odorants suggest that the shape of the molecule, rather than its chemical composition, determines how it smells (stereospecificity). This **stereochemical theory** of smell proposes that the receptor sites on the receptor cells have different shapes and that only molecules with a complementary shape fit into the receptor site. Binding of the molecules (odorants) to specific **odorant receptor proteins** (ORs) in the membrane of the cilia evokes a **receptor potential**. This involves activation of G proteins and cyclic AMP. Increased intracellular cyclic AMP opens Na^+-selective cation channels and thus depolarizes the cell. The ORs share structural features with photoreceptors and β adrenergic receptors. In contrast to photoreceptors, however, the olfactory receptors produce action potentials. The action potential arises in the initial segment of the axon and is transmitted to the olfactory bulb.

The Olfactory Receptor Cells Express an Enormous Repertoire of Receptor Molecules

What is the basis of our ability to discriminate several thousand different odors? The olfactory system is special by the expression of a large number of specific **odorant receptor proteins** (ORs), coded by the largest vertebrate gene family comprising around 1000 genes (only the immune system can recognize more different molecules). Human ORs express "only" about 350 different ORs on the surface of the cilia, while rodents and lower primates express many more, probably because a large fraction (60%–70%) of the human odorant-receptor genes appears to be **pseudogenes** (genes that are not expressed). In rodents, the proportion of pseudogenes is only about 5%. Presumably, this evolutionary increase in the number of pseudogenes may reflect diminished importance of olfaction in higher primates.

1 The **area of the olfactory epithelium** is obviously not easy to determine in humans. Thus, figures in the literature vary from 1 to 5 cm^2. This variation may at least partly be due to a patchy distribution of the epithelium and age-related loss. Thus, while in the fetus the epithelium is continuous and covering a large proportion of the nasal cavity, it is gradually replaced by respiratory epithelium in a patchy fashion. Further, the epithelium may be more anteriorly located than formerly believed. A combined histological (biopsies) and electrophysiological study located the anterior border of the olfactory epithelium at the level of the anterior end of the middle turbinate—1 to 2 cm anterior to what was formerly believed (Leopold et al. 2000).

amygdala and highly processed information that has been analyzed regarding its meaning for the organism.

The olfactory nuclei (not the olfactory bulb) on the two sides are interconnected by fibers running through the **anterior commissure** (Fig. 19.2). Thus, olfactory information from both sides of the nasal cavity is treated in each hemisphere.

Olfactory Signals and Behavior

Olfactory connections to the hypothalamus—both direct and indirect ones via the amygdala—are important for eating and for behavior directed at **acquiring food**. **Sexual** reflexes and sexually related behavior are also influenced by olfactory signals, although more so in lower mammals than in humans. The structural basis for such reflexes and behavior is very complex and not known in detail. Olfactory connections to the amygdala are most likely of importance, not only because the amygdala acts on the hypothalamus but also because it acts on parts of the prefrontal cortex involved in control of emotions and emotional behavior.

Olfaction and Learning

Olfactory sensations in certain **sensitive** (critical) periods of development can induce lasting changes of behavior; that is, learning. This phenomenon is called **olfactory imprinting**. One example concerns **sheep** that establish a strong bond to the lamb shortly after the birth. This depends on odors of the lamb that are present in the amniotic fluid. The mother must be exposed to the odor(s) during the first 4 to 12 hours for the bond to develop. The migration of **salmons** for thousands of miles is an almost incredible example of how memory of odors can control behavior. At 2 years of age, the salmon is imprinted by odors at its birthplace, and these odors guide it when returning "home" several years later. Imprinting by smell or taste can occur also before birth. If **pregnant rabbits** are fed a diet with certain aromatic substances, their offspring prefer foods containing these substances. This happens even if they grow up with a substitute mother on a different diet.

Olfactory imprinting is related to synaptic changes in the **olfactory bulb** (and most likely other places as well). Simultaneous arrival of olfactory signals and signals in **norepinephrine**-containing afferents seems to be necessary for lasting synaptic changes to occur. In the example with sheep mentioned above, more mitral cells responded to odors from the lamb after imprinting.

Pheromones

The term pheromone was introduced by Karlson and Lüscher in 1959 (p. 55), and defined as ". . . substances which are secreted to the outside by an individual and received by a second individual of the same species, in which they release a specific reaction, for example, a definite behaviour or a developmental process." Now the term is often used more broadly about all kinds of inborn, chemical communication between individuals of the same species. In animals—rodents have been most studied—several substances in body fluids (such as urine and saliva) have pheromone activity and influence a wide range of social interactions, such as sexual behavior, aggression, recognition of other individuals, and so forth. After destruction of the sense organ for pheromone recognition, rodents show, for example, reduced sexual activity and territorial defense. Pheromones may be volatile substances (small molecules) that move easily with the air, or they may be heavier molecules (peptides) that are exchanged among individuals only by close contact. In general, it seems that the volatile pheromones act as signals for sexual attraction or warning impending danger, whereas the peptide pheromones are of special importance for recognition among individuals.

The **vomeronasal organ** is a tubular structure in the nasal septum with an anterior opening. It is well developed in rodents, whereas it seems to disappear before birth in humans. It contains sensory cells like those in the olfactory epithelium, expressing a distinct class of receptor molecules (In higher primates, the genes coding for these receptors have become nonfunctional). In rodents, the sensory cells send their axons to the **accessory olfactory bulb** and from there connections to cortical structures that partly overlap those treating signals from the olfactory epithelium.

Even though the vomeronasal organ is lacking, there is evidence of pheromone-like actions in humans, where pheromones presumably act via receptors in the olfactory epithelium (in rodents pheromones act via both the vomeronasal organ and the olfactory epithelium). Synchronization of the menstrual cycle in women living close together is believed to be mediated by pheromones. Especially volatile substances present in armpit sweat seem to act as pheromones in humans. For example, some studies suggest that male armpit sweat may influence female menstrual cycle and mood. Mothers (but not fathers) seem to be able to recognize their babies by smell.

The significance of pheromones for human social behavior and development is controversial. It is safe to say, however, that they would play a minor role compared with their effects in rodents and other animals. In a broader context, pheromones are just one means of social communication. As concluded by Swaney and Keverne (2009, p. 239): ". . . the evolution of trichromacy [color vision] as well as huge increases in social complexity have minimised the role of pheromones in the lives of primates, leading to the total inactivation of the vomeronasal organ . . . while the brain increased in size and the behavior became emancipated from hormonal regulation."

GUSTATORY SYSTEM (THE SENSE OF TASTE)

The sense of taste is not among the most important of the special senses in humans, and much of what we usually call taste experience is in reality brought about by stimulation of **olfactory receptors**. This happens primarily by expiratory airflow through the nose while eating (compare the reduced sense of taste during a common cold). We nevertheless interpret this olfactory stimulation as taste (a further example of the importance of central interpretations of sensory signals for our conscious perception). In addition, signals from oral **thermoreceptors** and **mechanoreceptors** contribute to what we experience as a unitary sensory phenomenon. Finally, **nociceptors** activated by spicy food (such as chili peppers) contribute to taste perception.

The Taste Receptors and Taste Qualities

The true taste signals come from **chemoreceptors** in the taste buds that are located primarily in the epithelium of the tongue (Fig. 19.4). The taste buds are concentrated along the lateral margins of the tongue and the root of the tongue and are found in small elevations of the mucous membrane called **papillae**. The largest (vallate)

papilla lies along a transverse line posteriorly on the tongue (Fig. 19.5).[2] The **taste buds** are composed of approximately 100 elongated sensory cells and supporting cells (Fig. 19.4). The **sensory cells** of the taste buds are constantly renewed; each cell lives probably only about 10 days. They have long **microvilli** at their apical surface, protruding into a small opening in the epithelium, the **taste pore**. Here, substances that are dissolved in the saliva contact the membrane of the sensory cell. Terminal endings of sensory (afferent) axons contact the basal ends of the sensory cells. Binding of the tasty substances to receptors in the membrane of the sensory cells depolarizes the cell and thus produces a **receptor potential** (as in other sensory cells).[3] **ATP** released from the basal aspect of the sensory cell binds to ionotropic **purinoceptors** (P_{2x}) in the sensory nerve endings and produces action potentials.

2 There are also some taste buds on the soft palate, which are innervated by the intermediate nerve. The few taste buds present on the most posterior part of the tongue and on the upper side of the epiglottis are innervated by the vagus nerve. Extralingual taste receptors are believed to protect the airways from aspiration of fluids.

3 There are two kinds of receptor cell in the taste buds. Unexpectedly, it seems that the kind that expresses taste receptors in high concentrations do not contact sensory fibers, whereas the other kind, expressing fewer taste receptors, makes direct contact. Therefore, several taste cells probably work together as a unit with some cells being responsible for transduction while others transmit signals to the sensory fibers. Indeed, the taste cells seem capable of mutual communication by way of gap junctions and release of neurotransmitters (ATP, serotonin, and others).

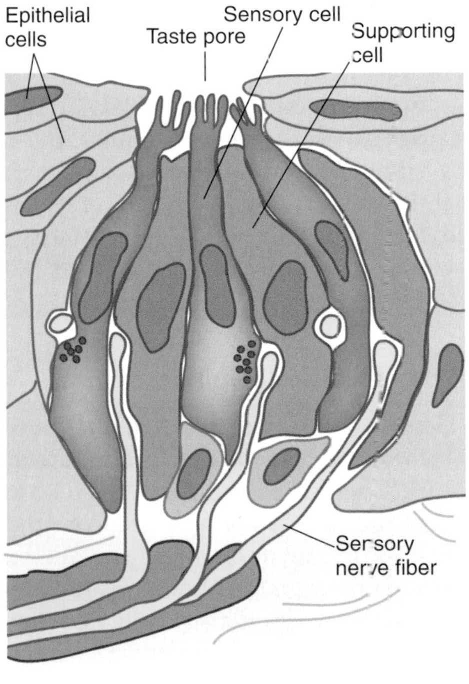

FIGURE 19.4 *Taste bud.* Semischematic drawing based on electron micrographs. The receptor molecules for taste substances sit in the membrane of the receptor cell cilia. In the taste pore, the receptors are exposed to substances dissolved in fluids.

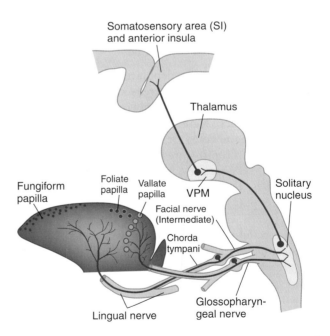

FIGURE 19.5 *Pathways for taste signals.* The various kinds of papilla contain taste buds. In the solitary nucleus, taste information is integrated with somatosensory signals from the oral cavity. The solitary nucleus receives addition input from the viscera via the vagus nerve (not shown in the figure).

the tongue (see Fig. 14.8) and the anterior part of the **insula**. Together, these areas comprise the **primary taste area** (Fig. 19.6). Sensory units responding to the elementary taste qualities are, as mentioned, to some degree segregated in the first link of the taste pathways. However, a considerable convergence occurs in the **solitary nucleus**. Most neurons respond to several taste qualities, although a few respond specifically to sweet or bitter substances. In the primary taste area, even fewer neurons appear to be specific. Further, many neurons receive convergent inputs of taste and other sensory modalities, so that integration of taste and, for example, olfaction starts at the first cortical station. For example, **chemotopic localization** in the primary taste area (topographically organized representation of different flavors) has not been documented in neurophysiologic studies of primates. Nevertheless, we have no problems discriminating the basic taste qualities and innumerable other nuances of taste. How can a high level of discrimination be achieved if there are no "labeled lines" keeping apart signals from different kinds of receptor (as in the somatosensory system)? One view is that discrimination occurs by simultaneous analysis of the activity pattern in many sensory units—so-called **population coding**. The temporal pattern of signals from different receptors is crucial, not their spatial segregation. Nevertheless, the "labeled line" view received support recently from evidence of chemotopic localization in the primary taste area of rodents. This was shown by transsynaptic transport to the cortex from bitter and sweet receptors in the taste buds.[4] Possibly, there may be elements of both mechanisms—that is, labeled lines and population coding—in the central processing of gustatory signals. It is fair to say, however, that the mechanisms responsible for taste discrimination are not fully understood.

Signal Transmission from Taste Buds Is Modulated in the Brain Stem

The response of neurons in the solitary nucleus to signals from taste buds depends on several other inputs to the solitary nucleus. For example, the response is inhibited by distension of the **stomach**. This is mediated by signals transmitted from the stomach by the **vagus nerve**. Further, solitary neurons respond to alterations in blood levels of **insulin** and **glucose** (presumably by

way of descending fibers from the hypothalamus). The solitary nucleus receives descending fibers from the **amygdala**, probably mediating conditioned **aversion** to certain flavors. Finally, the cortical taste area sends fibers to the rostral part of the solitary nucleus, enabling that the signal traffic is modulated by **context** and **expectation** already at the brain-stem level.

Further Cortical Processing

Our **conscious experience** of taste is due not just to stimulation of taste receptors, as mentioned. Furthermore, numerous taste cells with different specificities are presumably always stimulated while eating or drinking. The synthesis in the cerebral cortex of all these varied signals forms the basis of our subjective experience of taste. Convergence of olfactory and taste signals takes place in the anterior part of the insula. A higher level of integration occurs in the **orbitofrontal cortex** where taste, smell, and other sensory modalities meet (Fig. 19.6). Thus, responses of neurons in the orbitofrontal cortex to flavors depend on whether the animal is hungry or not. This may be caused by connections from cortical areas related to **motivation**—that is, areas that may inform about the significance of a sensory stimulus. That our subjective sensory experience is determined not only by the stimulus holds for all sensory systems. Nevertheless, the emotional influence on the sensory experience is probably more marked for taste and smell than for other modalities. We know from everyday experience, for example, how the same smell or taste may be experienced as pleasant in one situation and nauseating in another.

Conditioned Taste Aversion

Taste is an important learning signal; it may be of vital importance to learn rapidly the association between a taste and its significance—that is, whether it signals something edible or poisonous. Survival of wild animals depends upon their ability to learn such association at the first trial, establishing a stable **conditioned taste aversion** to dangerous foods. Nausea is a very efficient learning signal when evoked by food intake. By just trying a small portion of the food, the animal usually can survive and learn to never again try the same potential food. The close coupling in the solitary nucleus of gustatory information with signals from the stomach most likely is involved in establishing the associations between flavors and their significance. Other neuronal groups believed to participate in conditioned taste aversion are found in the **parabrachial area** (pons), the **amygdala**, and the **orbitofrontal cortex**.

---

4 An functional magnetic resonance imaging (fMRI) study of six persons reported slightly different locations of cortical responses to different flavors. The interpretation of such data is uncertain, however, because the distribution of response may have been influenced by other factors than taste that varied during the experimental sessions.

IV | MOTOR SYSTEMS

THE cell groups and tracts in the central nervous system that control the activity of the skeletal muscles compose the **motor systems**. We may also use the term **somatic** motor systems to distinguish them from the systems that control smooth muscles and glands.

Although the motor systems consists of several interconnected parts,we first discuss some general aspects (Chapter 20). Then we treat the peripheral (**lower**) **motor neurons** (Chapter 21) and the **central** (**upper**) **motor neurons** (Chapter 22). These parts are directly involved in mediating the commands from the motor centers to the muscles, and are necessary for the initiation of voluntary movements; paralysis ensues when they are damaged. Then we treat the **basal ganglia** (Chapter 23) and the **cerebellum** (Chapter 24), which have their main connections with the central motor nuclei and are necessary for the proper execution of movements rather than for their initiation. Finally, in Chapter 25 the **control of eye movements** is treated separately due to the distinctive features of this system.

Indeed, the hand is a sensory organ in its own right. For example, we use delicate, exploratory finger movements to judge the form, surface, consistency, and so forth of objects. Losses of muscle coordination or of hand sensation have equally devastating consequences for hand function. In addition, eye movements are entirely devoted to assist the brain in the acquisition of visual information, and head movements aid the auditory system. As aptly formulated by the Israeli neuroscientist Ehud Ahissar (2008, p. 1370) "Without eye movement, the world becomes uniformly gray; without sniffing, only the initial changes in the odor environment are sensed; and without finger or whisker motion, objects cannot be identified."

Motor Systems and Self-Recognition

Movements play an important role in the experience and ownership of our bodies. For example, experiments in human volunteers show that self-recognition (e.g., the hand belongs to me) is significantly better during a self-generated movement than when depending on proprioceptive and visual information alone. Our body scheme and body image (cf. Chapter 18) depend on regular updating by sensory information provided by our own, purposeful movements. If there is a mismatch between movement commands and sensory feedback, misconceptions of the body regularly occur (e.g., after amputation, deafferentation, immobilization of joints, and so forth).

CLASSIFICATION OF MOVEMENTS

Stabilizing and Moving

Before we describe the motor systems, some comments on movements in general are pertinent. First, muscle contraction may not necessarily elicit movement (i.e., alter the position of one or more joints); just as often, muscle activity is used to prevent movement—for example, muscles maintain our **posture** by counteracting the force of gravity. In preventing movement, the muscles may be said to **stabilize** a joint (against external forces) and to have a postural function. Further, movement in one part of the body—for example, in an arm—requires that muscles in other parts contract to prevent the body balance from being upset. Therfore, a muscle in one situation may be used as a mover and in another situation as a stabilizer.

Contractions: Concentric, Isometric, and Eccentric

Whether or not a movement is to occur depends on the magnitude of the force produced by the muscle contraction and the external forces acting on the joint. When the

external force is smaller than the muscle force, the muscle shortens and a movement occurs; this is called **concentric** or **isotonic contraction**. When the external forces equal the force of the muscle contraction, no movement occurs; this is called **isometric contraction**. When the external force is greater than the opposing force produced by the muscle contraction, the muscle lengthens; this is called **eccentric contraction**. Eccentric contraction occurs, for example, with the thigh muscles when we walk down a staircase, as the muscles brake the movement produced by the weight of the body.

Ramp and Ballistic Movements

Movements may be classified by the **speed** with which they are performed. **Ramp movements** are performed relatively slowly. The crucial point is that the movement is slow enough to enable sensory feedback information to influence the movement during its execution. **Ballistic movements** are very rapid, and their characteristic feature is that they are too fast to enable feedback control: the name derives from analogy with a bullet shot out of a gun.

Automatic and Voluntary Movements

Movements may also be classified according to whether they are **voluntary** or **automatic**; automatic movements take place without our conscious participation. In reality, this is much too crude a distinction: there is a gradual transition from what Hughlings Jackson in the past century termed the most automatic to the least automatic movements. The **most automatic** movements are basic, simple reflexes, such as the retraction of the arm from a noxious stimulus. Locomotion is an example of a semiautomatic movement—that is, the basic pattern is automatic, but starting and stopping and necessary adjustments may require conscious (voluntary) control. The **least automatic** movements are precision grips with the fingers and delicate manipulatory or exploratory movements such as writing, drawing, playing a musical instrument, and so forth. Equally precise voluntary control exists for the muscles of the larynx, the tongue, and some of the facial muscles. We know that the degree to which a movement is automatic changes with **learning**: in the beginning a new movement requires full voluntary control, and in the process of learning the movement becomes more automatic. When playing a well-rehearsed musical piece on the piano, for example, we do not need to pay attention to the fingers and their movements.

As a rule, the most automatic movements require only the use of relatively simple **reflex arcs** at the spinal level; participation of higher motor centers is not necessary. Somewhat less automatic and more complex movements such as ventilation, locomotion, and postural control depend, in addition, on the participation of neuronal groups in the brain stem. Such movements do not require our attention directed toward them but can be subjected to voluntary control. The least automatic movements depend on the participation of the highest level—the **cerebral cortex**—to coordinate and control the activity of motor centers in the brain stem and spinal cord. The vast number of neurons and the plasticity of the human brain enable learning of an almost infinite repertoire of voluntary movements. Also, these features ensure great **flexibility** in how motor tasks are solved. The same task may be solved in different ways, and we can continuously adapt to novel challenges. The great adaptability and flexibility of movements distinguish humans from most animals. Most animals are highly specialized for a limited number of motor tasks, controlled by stereotyped motor programs that develop according to a fixed pattern.

21 | The Peripheral Motor Neurons and Reflexes

OVERVIEW

The peripheral or lower motor neurons (motoneurons) constitute the final and only connection between the central nervous system (CNS) and the muscles. If they are destroyed, paralyses of the muscles ensue. There are two types of lower motor neurons—**α motoneurons** innervating the extrafusal muscle fibers and **γ motoneurons** supplying the muscle spindles. The motoneurons are arranged in **columns** in the spinal cord; each column supplying one or a few muscles with synergetic actions. Each column extends through two or more segments, so that each muscled receives fibers from at least two spinal segments. An α motoneuron and all the muscle fibers it innervates is called a **motor unit**. Large muscles consist of a few hundred to more than a thousand motor units. Muscle fibers are classified according to ATPase activity into **type 1** and **type 2** fibers. In general, type 1 fibers have the highest endurance whereas the type 2 fibers contract with the highest velocity and force. The muscle fibers of one motor unit are all of the same fiber type.

A **reflex** is an involuntary response to a stimulus, which is mediated by the nervous system. The motoneurons are parts of **reflex arcs**, consisting of receptors that capture the stimulus, sensory neurons conducting signals to the CNS, a reflex centrum (e.g., in the spinal cord), and an effector (muscle or glandular cells). In this chapter, we discuss the **flexion reflex** and **stretch reflexes** in particular. Stretch reflexes are of two main kinds: the **monosynaptic** stretch reflex (routinely tested by a tendon tap) and the polysynaptic, **long-latency** stretch reflex. Both consist of a muscle contraction in response to muscle stretch (the muscle spindle is receptor). We also discuss the **resting tone of muscles** (muscle tone), and how it may vary in health and disease. Finally, we treat the ability of peripheral nerves to **regenerate** after severance.

MOTONEURONS AND MUSCLES

The **peripheral motor neurons** are nerve cells that send their axons to skeletal muscles. Another term is **lower motor neurons**. These are the motoneurons in the ventral horn of the spinal cord and in the somatic motor cranial nerve nuclei. There are two kinds: α **motoneurons** innervate the extrafusal muscle fibers, whereas the **γ motoneurons** innervate the intrafusal muscle fibers of the muscle spindle (see Figs. 13.6 and 13.7).

The motoneurons of the ventral horn (Fig. 21.1) and in the cranial nerve nuclei are easily recognized in microscopic sections because of their large size and the big clumps of rough endoplasmic reticulum (rER) in the cytoplasm of their cell bodies (see Fig. 1.2). The rich content of rER indicates that the neurons have a high protein synthesis. These proteins are, for example, enzymes for transmitter synthesis and metabolism and various kinds of membrane proteins. The vast surface of the motoneurons with their large dendritic tree and long axons presumably explains why motoneurons contain more rER than most other neuronal types.

Ventral Roots and Plexuses

The axons of the motoneurons leave the spinal cord through the **ventral roots** and continue into the **ventral** and **dorsal branches** (rami) of the spinal nerves to innervate skeletal muscles of the trunk and the extremities (see Figs. 6.5 and 6.7). Correspondingly, the axons from the **cranial nerve motor nuclei** supply the muscles of the tongue, pharynx, palate, larynx, and face, as well as the extraocular muscles. The axons of all the motoneurons located in one spinal segment leave the cord through one ventral root and continue into one spinal nerve. The ventral branches of the spinal nerves form **plexuses** so that the motor axons from one spinal segment are distributed to several peripheral nerves (Fig. 21.2).

The Final Common Path and Synaptic Contacts on Motoneurons

Contraction of skeletal muscles can be elicited only by signals conducted in the axons of motoneurons. If these axons are interrupted, the muscles become **paralyzed**. The peripheral motor neurons thus constitute the **final common path** for all signals from the CNS to skeletal muscles (the term "final common path" was introduced by the British neurophysiologist and Nobel laureate

A

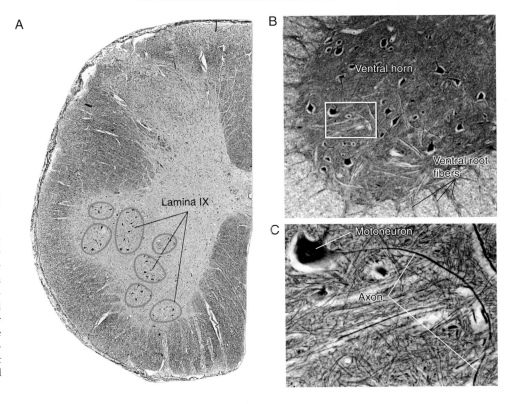

B

C

FIGURE 21.1 *Motoneurons.* **A:** Photomicrograph and drawing of a transverse section of the (lumbar) spinal cord. The motoneurons are collected in groups (columns) that together form the lamina IX of Rexed (outlined in orange). **B:** Photomicrograph of a transverse section through the human lumbar enlargement, Bodian's silver impregnation method. Cell bodies and axons are black. Due to shrinkage, the cell bodies are surrounded by a light zone. Bundles of motor axons can be seen penetrating the white matter. **C:** Higher magnification of a motoneuron and the first part of its axon; from the framed area in **B**.

Sir Charles Sherrington). The motoneurons may be compared with the keys of a piano on which higher levels of the CNS can play. As we describe later in this chapter, many parts of the CNS cooperate in determining the activity of the motoneurons and thus the contraction of our muscles.

Each motoneuron probably receives about 30,000 nerve terminals—some forming excitatory synapses, others inhibitory; some with fast synaptic actions, others with slow modulatory ones. The sum of these influences determines whether and with what frequency the motoneurons will send action potentials to the muscles. That we can

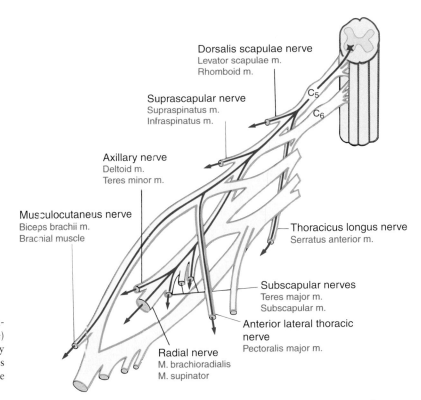

FIGURE 21.2 *The brachial plexus.* Axons of motoneurons in one spinal segment (C_5 is used as an example) are distributed to several peripheral nerves to supply various muscles of the arm. Each muscle also receives motor fibers from other segments, although they are not shown here.

perform such a wide variety of movements is due to the ability of the CNS to select precisely, by way of the motoneurons, the combinations of muscles to be used and to determine the speed and force with which they are to contract.

Neurotransmitters

The motoneurons use **acetylcholine** as transmitter, and the synthesizing enzyme **choline acetyltransferase** (ChAT) can be demonstrated immunohistochemically in the motoneurons and in their terminals. Motoneurons also contain the neuropeptide calcitonin gene-related peptide (**CGRP**). The level of CGRP in the motoneurons is under the influence of descending connections from higher levels of the CNS; when such connections are transected, the level of CGRP drops. There is experimental evidence that CGRP influences the synthesis of acetylcholine receptors of the muscle cells. If so, this may be one (of several) means by which the CNS can influence the properties of muscle cells.

Motoneurons Are Collected in Columns

The motoneurons are collected in groups, which form **Rexed's lamina IX** in the spinal cord (Fig. 21.1; see also Fig. 6.10). The dendrites of the motoneurons do not respect the boundaries of lamina IX, however, and extend far in the transverse and in the rostrocaudal directions—for example, into lamina VII, where many interneurons are located (see Fig. 6.12). The rostrocaudal (longitudinal) extension of the dendrites enables dorsal root fibers from several segments to act on each motoneuron. The dendritic tree increases the surface of the motoneurons enormously, and, not surprisingly, the vast majority of the nerve terminals contacting motoneurons are axodendritic.

Three-dimensionally, the motoneurons are collected in longitudinally oriented **columns** (Fig. 21.3). Each column contains the α and γ motoneurons to one muscle or a few functionally very similar (synergistic) muscles. Within a column supplying more than one muscle, the motoneurons to each muscle are at least partly segregated. As a rule, each column extends through more than one segment of the cord. Consequently, each muscle receives motor fibers through more than one ventral root and spinal nerve.[1] **Destruction of one root** or spinal

nerve only—for example, by disk protrusion in sciatica or by a tumor growing in the spinal canal—will not produce paralysis of a muscle but only a more or less pronounced paresis (weakness).

The anatomic organization of motoneurons has been studied via transection of muscle nerves in experimental animals. A retrograde reaction, which is easily seen through a microscope, occurs in the cell bodies of the motoneurons. Studies using retrograde transport of tracer substances have detailed the picture considerably. Study of patients with **poliomyelitis** has provided information about conditions in the human cord (the poliovirus infects and kills motoneurons). Because the distribution of paralyzed muscles usually has been determined before death, it can be compared with the distribution of cell loss among the motoneuron groups in the cord and brain stem.

Motoneuron Columns Are Somatotopically Distributed in the Ventral Horn

Groups of motoneurons that supply **axial muscles**—that is, muscles of the back, neck, abdomen, and pelvis—are located most medially within the ventral horn, whereas motoneurons supplying muscles of the **extremities** lie

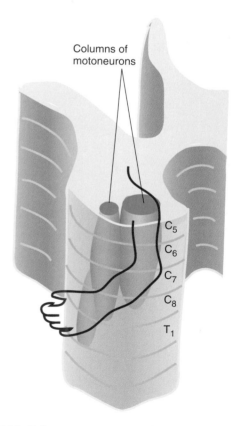

Columns of motoneurons

C_5
C_6
C_7
C_8
T_1

FIGURE 21.3 *Columnar arrangement of motoneurons.* Schematic of the somatotopic localization of the motoneuronal columns innervating the arm, located in the spinal segments C_5–T_1. Motoneurons supplying the intrinsic muscles of the hand are located most caudally (C_8–T_1) and most dorsally in the ventral horn.

---

1 About 20 *Hox* genes control the specification of motoneurons with regard to their peripheral target (muscle). In addition, expression of recognition molecules and guidance receptors in the peripheral tissues is required for axons to find their target. When looking at the intricate trajectory of branches from motoneurons in one segment (Fig. 21.2) the task of creating a precise topographic relationship between spinal cord motoneurons and muscles seems daunting. It should be recalled, however, that at the time of outgrowth in early embryonic life, the distances are small and trajectories of axonal growth are usually fairly straight. The complicated structure of the plexuses (Fig. 21.2) arises later in development.

more laterally. This explains why the ventral horn is broader (extends more laterally) in the segments of the cord that send fibers to the extremities (i.e., C_5–T_1 and L_1–S_2; compare Figs. 6.8, 6.10, and 6.11). There is also a further somatotopic organization: motoneurons supplying **proximal muscles** of the extremities (the shoulder and hip) are located more ventrally than those supplying the **distal muscles** (the hand and foot). This is shown in Figure 21.3, which also shows that the proximal muscles are supplied from motoneurons located more rostrally than those supplying the distal muscles. For example, the shoulder muscles are mainly innervated by the upper parts of the brachial plexus (C_5–C_6), whereas the lowermost segments (C_8–T_1) innervate the intrinsic muscles of the hand.

Motoneurons Are of Functionally Different Kinds

As mentioned, the α and γ motoneurons supplying one muscle lie together within one column in the ventral horn. In a microscopic section of the cord it can be seen that the motoneuron cell bodies vary in size (Fig. 21.1; see also Fig. 1.2). As in other parts of the nervous system, the neurons with the largest cell bodies have the thickest (and thus the fastest conducting) axons. The γ **motoneurons** are the smallest within a group, while the α **motoneurons**—although larger than the γ motoneurons— vary considerably in size. Such **size** differences are related to differences among the muscle cells supplied by the α motoneurons. Briefly stated, the smallest α motoneurons control delicate movements with little **force**, whereas the largest motoneurons come into play only when a movement requires great force. The large α motoneurons also have a much higher maximal **firing frequency** than the small ones, and the large ones tend to fire in brief bursts with a high frequency, whereas the small α motoneurons tend to go on firing for a long time with a low frequency. These differences in **firing pattern** reflect that the large motoneurons are used for forceful, rapid movements of short duration, whereas the small motoneurons can uphold a moderate muscular tension for a long time. For these reasons, we apply the term **phasic** α motoneurons to the large ones, and **tonic** α motoneurons to the small ones. The properties of the α motoneurons are discussed further when we deal with the motor units.

The Motor End Plate and Neuromuscular Transmission

After entering the muscle, the α-motoneuron axon divides into many thin branches or collaterals. Each of these terminal branches contacts one muscle cell only. Each muscle cell is thus contacted by only one branch from one α motoneuron. Such a branch ends on the muscle cell approximately midway between its ends, forming the **motor end plate**, where the signal transfer

from nerve to muscle takes place (Figs. 21.4 and 21.5). Within the end-plate region, the axonal branch divides further and forms up to about 50 nerve terminals (boutons), each establishing synaptic contact with the muscle cell. The postsynaptic side at this **neuromuscular junction** is somewhat special compared with synapses in the CNS, as **junctional folds** and a thin **basal lamina** are intercalated between the presynaptic and postsynaptic membranes (Fig. 21.5B). The boutons contain **acetylcholine**, and the postsynaptic membrane contains **acetylcholine receptors** of the **nicotinic** type. The density of acetylcholine receptors is much higher in the end-plate region than elsewhere on the muscle cell surface, which is appropriate because only at the end plate is the muscle cell normally exposed to acetylcholine. During embryonic **development**, however—before the nerve fibers growing out from the cord have reached the muscle cells—the acetylcholine receptors are evenly distributed all over the muscle membrane. Only after establishment of properly functioning synaptic contacts are the receptors redistributed to attain the mature pattern. During development, spinal motoneurons transiently express the neuropeptide **galanin**, which presumably influences the synapse formation at the motor end plate.

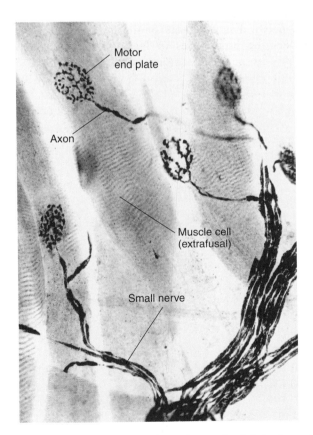

FIGURE 21.4 *Motor end plates.* Photomicrograph of skeletal muscle cells and a small bundle of nerve fibers innervating the cells. The tissue is stained with gold chloride to darken the nerve fibers and their terminal boutons. Each motor end plate consists of numerous small boutons. Four end plates are seen here. Magnification, ×500.

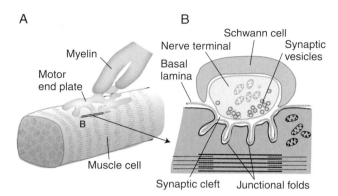

FIGURE 21.5 *The motor end plate.* **A:** Schematic showing how the myelinated nerve fiber loses the myelin sheath before it ramifies in the end-plate area, each terminal branch ending in a nerve terminal. Each muscle cell has only one end plate. **B:** Section through one of the nerve terminals in **A**, based on electron microscopic observations. The synaptic cleft contains a thin basal lamina, and the postsynaptic membrane is thrown into deep folds (junctional folds).

An action potential propagated along the axon of the motoneuron depolarizes all the boutons and elicits release of acetylcholine. The transmitter binds to the acetylcholine receptors, and, as at other excitatory synapses, this depolarizes the postsynaptic membrane. This change in the membrane potential is called the **end-plate potential**. Because of the large number of nerve terminals formed by one terminal fiber, enough transmitter is released by a single nerve impulse to depolarize the muscle cell membrane to the threshold for an action potential. The action potential is propagated over the whole surface of the muscle cell and elicits a brief contraction. The enzyme **acetylcholinesterase** rapidly terminates the action of acetylcholine by degrading it. The enzyme is present in the synaptic cleft and the junctional folds.

Neuromuscular Transmission Can Be Disturbed by Poison and Disease

Various drugs and naturally occurring poisonous substances can influence the signal transmission at the neuromuscular junction and produce involuntary muscle contractions or muscle paralysis. The South American Indian poison **curare** and similar synthetic substances paralyze the muscle cells by blocking the acetylcholine receptors. Such drugs are often used during abdominal surgery to obtain sufficient muscle relaxation. Several kinds of **snake poisons** act by blocking acetylcholine receptors and thereby paralyze the victim. The **botulinum toxin** (produced by a microorganism growing in certain kinds of spoiled food) paralyzes the muscles by preventing the release of acetylcholine from the nerve terminals at the motor end plate. A similar mechanism sometimes produces muscle weakness in patients with **cancer**; apparently, substances preventing release of acetylcholine are produced in the body.

The disease **myasthenia gravis** is characterized by excessive fatigability of striated muscles, which is caused by **autoantibodies** binding to the acetylcholine receptors. Thus, there are fewer than normal acetylcholine receptors available at the neuromuscular junction and release of acetylcholine opens fewer ion channels, leading to less than normal depolarization. The probability of evoking an action potential in the muscle cell membrane is consequently reduced. Drugs that inhibit the acetylcholine esterase (**neostigmine, physostigmine**) may lessen the symptoms. With this inhibition, the transmitter gets a longer time to act, and the probability of evoking an action potential is increased. Typically, most severely affected are the muscles of the head, producing symptoms such as double vision (due to paresis of extraocular muscles) and involuntary lowering of the upper eyelids (ptosis). The voice becomes weaker while speaking and swallowing may become difficult. In addition, the respiratory muscles are usually affected.

The Force of Muscle Contraction Is Controlled by the Motoneurons

A single presynaptic action potential at the motor end plate elicits only a brief contraction, a **twitch**, of the muscle cell (Fig. 21.6). The twitch lasts only for about one-tenth of a second. However, if another action potential follows shortly after the first one—that is, before the tension produced by the first twitch is over—the tension produced by the muscle is upheld and, furthermore, may increase considerably. This is called **summation**. Up to a limit, the tension produced by the muscle cell increases with increasing frequency of action potentials; that is, the **force** produced by the muscle cell is determined by the **firing frequency** of the motoneuron. Whereas the twitch is the response of the muscle cell to a single nerve signal, **tetanic** contraction is the term used of the muscle response to a train of signals with the highest frequency to which the muscle cell can respond (Fig. 21.6). The tetanic tension is thus the maximal force the muscle cell can produce. (One may, as shown in Fig. 21.6, differentiate between unfused or incomplete tetanus at submaximal firing frequencies and fused or complete tetanus at the maximal firing frequency. The term "tetanus," as used here, refers to the complete tetanus.)

There Are Functionally Different Kinds of Striated Muscle Fiber Types

In both animals and humans, the skeletal muscles are composed of different kinds of muscle cells or muscle fibers (these terms are used interchangeably). The most clear-cut evidence is provided by the fact that in some species certain muscles have a dark color ("**red**" muscles), whereas other muscles are light ("**white**" muscles)—for

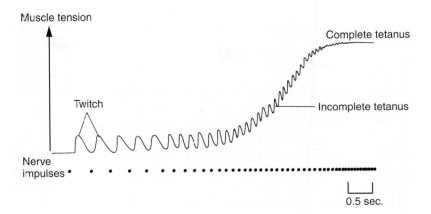

FIGURE 21.6 *Muscle contraction.* The muscle tension increases with increasing firing frequency of the motoneurons innervating the muscle cell. (Redrawn from Kandel and Schwartz 1985.)

example, the almost white breast muscles and the dark leg muscles of the chicken. Such muscles are composed of muscle fibers of only one (or predominantly one) kind, and we classify the muscle cells as either white or red. The color difference is due to differences in the content of **myoglobin,** which is red (closely related to hemoglobin) and transports oxygen within the muscle cell. Further study showed that white and red muscle cells differ with regard to **endurance**—that is, how long they can maintain tension. This is mainly due to differences in the capacity to take up oxygen and to **aerobic ATP production** (oxidative phosphorylation). As one would expect, the red muscles have the highest endurance. In addition to containing more myoglobin than the white muscle fibers (cells), the red ones also contain more mitochondria, which are responsible for the aerobic ATP production. There are also other important differences: the white muscle fibers contract more rapidly and develop greater force than the red fibers. With physiological methods, muscle cells can be classified as **fast twitch** (FT), corresponding largely to white fibers, and **slow twitch** (ST), corresponding to the red fibers.

The differences with regard to **contraction velocity** and maximal force development are related to differences in the amount and type of **myosin ATPase** (enzymes cleaving ATP, thus providing the energy for the muscle contraction). With histochemical staining methods, muscle fibers are classified in accordance with their ATPase activity (Fig. 21.7). On the basis of ATPase staining, human muscle fibers are classified as **type 1,** corresponding largely to the red and the ST fibers mentioned above, and **type 2** fibers, corresponding largely to the white and FT fibers. The type 2 group is heterogeneous, however, and consists of **type 2A** fibers, which resemble the type 1 fibers in having a relatively high oxidative capacity, and the **type 2B** fibers, which are the most typical white fibers with low oxidative capacity.

The CNS thus can **select** muscle fibers in accordance with the requirement of the **task:** one fiber type is best suited for contractions of moderate force that last for a

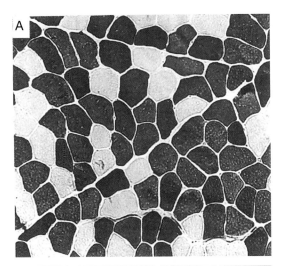

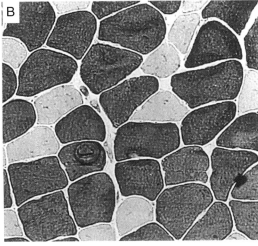

FIGURE 21.7 *Muscle fiber types.* Photomicrographs of cross sections of skeletal muscle (human). The sections are treated so that the color intensity of the muscle fibers depends on their myosin-ATPase activity. With this particular treatment, the type 1 fibers are light and the type 2 fibers are dark. A: From the quadriceps muscle of a "normal" person. B: From the same muscle of a weight lifter. Note the difference in muscle fiber thickness. Magnification, ×200. (Courtesy of Dr. H.A. Dahl, Norwegian University of Physical Education and Sport, Oslo.)

Although a reflex response is mediated each time by the same set of neurons, the **excitability** of these neurons can be modified from higher levels of the CNS. This is necessary to adapt individual reflexes to the overall plan for bodily movements. Reflex movements that operate on their own would disturb normal voluntary movements. **Modulation** of the excitability of the reflex center can be exerted by presynaptic inhibition of primary afferent fibers, by postsynaptic excitatory of inhibitory actions on interneurons and motoneurons, and by efferent control of the sensitivity of some kinds of receptor (cf. γ motoneurons).

We first discuss two different spinal reflexes with skeletal muscles as effectors. The first—the **flexion** or **withdrawal reflex**—serves to protect the body; the second, so-called **stretch reflex** (or rather stretch reflexes since there are several varieties), automatically adjusts muscle tension during postural tasks and voluntary movements.

The Flexion Reflex

This reflex is evoked by activation of **nociceptors** in the skin and underlying tissues. For example, when a foot hits a sharp object while walking, the whole leg is immediately withdrawn away from the object (Fig. 21.10). In this case, one or more interneurons are intercalated between the terminals of the afferent sensory fiber and the motoneurons producing the response—that is, the reflex is **polysynaptic**. That this is a reflex is clear from, among other things, the fact that it may be elicited even when the spinal cord is transected above the reflex center. The flexion reflex disappears in deep unconsciousness. For surgery, anesthesia has to be sufficiently deep to abolish flexion reflexes.

As mentioned, the **receptors** for the flexion reflex are nociceptors. The **stimulus** usually hits a small spot on the skin, whereas the **response** involves a complex array of muscles (such as extensors of the ankle, flexors of the knee and the hip; Fig. 21.10). Contraction of the muscles in the leg that is withdrawn, however, is not sufficient. Muscles of the other leg must also contract (primarily extensor muscles) to prevent loss of balance. Thus, the stimulus must be distributed to motoneurons in many segments of the cord. This happens by way of ascending and descending collaterals of the primary sensory fibers and by way of spinal interneurons (Fig. 21.10). In response to a simple stimulus, a purposeful, harmonious movement occurs, requiring that all the muscles contract at the right time and with the right force. The synaptic couplings in the cord underlying this response must be both complex and precise.

A Flexion Reflex Can Be Evoked from Low-Threshold Receptors

Under certain circumstances, several kinds of receptor in the skin, around the joints, or in muscles can elicit a flexion reflex. Common to these receptors is that their signals converge on **interneurons** that excite **flexor motoneurons**. The sensory fibers from such receptors were therefore termed **flexor reflex afferents** (FRAs). Their effects have been most studied in so-called spinal animals (the cord is transected and isolated from the rest of the CNS). Many FRAs lead from low-threshold mechanoreceptors (e.g., group II muscle afferents), while others lead from nociceptors. Normally, the convergence of FRAs on interneurons is believed to ensure necessary **feedback** during ongoing movements—perhaps rhythmic movements in particular. The term "flexor reflex afferents" is therefore not quite appropriate because many of the FRAs do not normally evoke the protective flexion reflex. In patients with **transverse lesions of the cord** the situation is different, however.

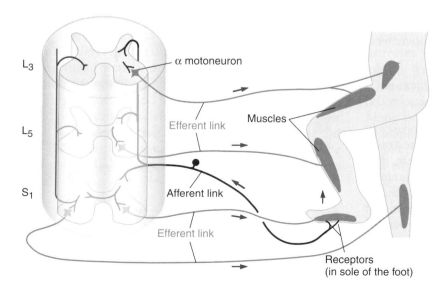

FIGURE 21.10 *The flexion (withdrawal) reflex.* The diagram is highly simplified. In this case, several synapses are intercalated between the afferent and the efferent links of the reflex arc. Here nociceptors in the sole of the foot are activated (by walking on a sharp object). The signals are conducted centrally in a sensory fiber (red), which sends out several collaterals and, via interneurons and propriospinal fibers, activates α motoneurons at several segmental levels of the cord. In turn, the motoneurons make many muscles contract to lift the foot off the ground (away from the painful stimulus). At the same time, extensor muscles are activated in the other leg to maintain balance.

Reflex changes occur in body parts that have been innervated from the cord below the lesion, including forceful and long-lasting contractions of flexor muscles. Such contractions are elicited by innocuous stimuli, including stimulation of low-threshold mechanoreceptors and thermoreceptors. Most likely, this is due to abnormal excitability of interneurons in receipt of FRA inputs produced by the lack of supraspinal control (see also Chapter 22, under "Mechanisms Responsible for Development of Spasticity").

Stretch Reflexes

Under certain circumstances a muscle responds with a contraction when it is being stretched. (It is easy to find out by oneself that stretching a muscle does not always produce a contraction.) When the latency of the contraction is too short to be voluntary, we call this a **stretch reflex**. The most obvious purpose of such a reflex might be to keep the muscle length constant. **Receptors** for stretch reflexes are the **muscle spindles**. Stretch reflexes have been much studied due to their relation to movement control.

We speak of different stretch reflexes because muscle contraction occurring as a result of muscle stretching usually consists of several phases of contractions, each with a different latency as recorded by EMG. The reflex **latency** is the time between the stimulus and the response (between stretch and contraction). It results from the conduction time from the muscle spindles to the spinal cord; the delay at the synapse(s) intercalated between the muscle spindle afferent fibers and the α motoneurons; the conduction time from the motoneurons to the muscle; and, finally, the synaptic delay at the motor end plate. Measurement of the latency between the stimulus and the response makes it possible to decide whether a muscle contraction is the result of a **monosynaptic** stretch reflex, or whether other—**polysynaptic**—pathways are involved. The monosynaptic stretch reflex, with only one synapse intercalated between the afferent and the efferent link, is the simplest reflex with the shortest latency (Fig. 21.11). Each intercalated synapse increases the latency with a few milliseconds. Thus, muscle contractions occurring with longer latencies after stretching the muscle indicate that there are more neurons intercalated between the afferent link (the sensory fibers) and the motoneurons. That some stretch reflex responses have longer latency than others may not only be due to more synapses intercalated in the reflex center, however. Thus, while the fast monosynaptic reflex depends on signals in the thick group Ia fibers (see Figs. 13.6 and 13.7), slower conducting group II muscle spindle afferents may contribute to reflex responses with longer latencies.

We discuss the monosynaptic and the polysynaptic stretch reflexes separately next. Much remains to be clarified, however, concerning the role of the stretch reflexes in movement control.

The Monosynaptic Stretch Reflex

The **patellar reflex** (Fig. 21.11)—tested routinely as part of a clinical examination—is probably the best-known example of a stretch reflex. The **stimulus** is a tap on the patellar ligament (the tendon of the quadriceps muscle). The **response** is a contraction of the quadriceps muscle, thus producing a brief extension movement at the knee joint. The reflex arc is shown schematically in Fig. 21.11, and it can be seen that only one synapse is intercalated in the reflex center—that is, the reflex is **monosynaptic**. The **receptors** are the muscle spindles in the quadriceps muscle that is stretched; the **afferent link** is constituted by the Ia fibers, which end in the spinal cord with some collaterals ending directly (monosynaptically) on the α motoneurons supplying the quadriceps muscle. The axons of the α motoneurons constitute the **efferent link**, which at the motor end plate activates the extrafusal fibers of the quadriceps muscle (the effector). For the patellar reflex, the **latency** between the stimulus and the start of the contraction (as recorded with EMG) is about 30 msec, and a slightly shorter latency pertains

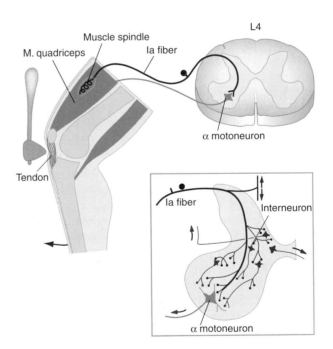

FIGURE 21.11 *Stretch reflex.* The patellar reflex is used here as an example of a monosynaptic reflex—that is, with only one synapse intercalated between the afferent and the efferent link. The stimulus is a tap on the patellar ligament below the patella, which stretches the muscle. The response is a brief muscle contraction. **Bottom right:** The Ia fiber from the muscle spindle contacts the motoneurons monosynaptically, but it also contacts many interneurons. Some of these are excitatory, mediating a polysynaptic activation of some motoneurons; other interneurons are inhibitory, mediating inhibition of other motoneurons.

(Fig. 21.11), establishing **polysynaptic** routes from the muscle spindle afferents to the motoneurons. Rapid stretching of the biceps muscle may elicit two or three reflex responses, as determined with EMG in human subjects. In addition to an early EMG activity with a latency of about 25 msec (the monosynaptic stretch reflex, or **M1** response), another reflex contraction (**M2**) starts at about 50 msec and sometimes a new phase of contraction (M3) at about 70 to 80 msec. These are not voluntary responses, since the earliest voluntary muscle contractions occur at about 100 msec after the stretch (in the upper arm). These reflex responses constitute the **long-latency stretch reflex** (other names are the functional stretch reflex, the polysynaptic stretch reflex, and the long-loop stretch reflex).

A striking property of the long-latency stretch reflex is that the strength of the response depends to such a high degree on whether the muscle is relaxed or **active** at the time of stretching. If the muscle is relaxed or only slightly active when stretched, there is usually no long-latency reflex response at all. Further, the strength of the response depends on **prior instruction** to the subject with regard to whether to resist the imposed stretch or to let go. When the person is asked to let go when an imposed movement (at an unpredictable time) stretches the muscle (e.g., an imposed extension at the elbow that stretches the biceps muscle), the reflex response is much smaller than when the person is asked to resist the imposed movement. Thus, the magnitude of the reflex response can be adapted to what is functionally appropriate in a particular situation.

A further characteristic of the long-latency stretch reflex is that the strength of the response may change during **learning** of a motor task. Thus, by repeated trials, the reflex response becomes weaker in muscles in which a contraction in response to stretching is functionally inappropriate and stronger in muscles in which a contraction is appropriate. This learning effect, or adaptation of the stretch reflex, occurs only in connection with the particular learned movement; in connection with other movements, the reflex response of the muscle is unaltered. As mentioned, the monosynaptic stretch reflex is also subject to similar learned, task-related modulation, but the changes appear to be smaller than those obtained with the long-latency reflex.

Is the Long-Latency Stretch Reflex Mediated by the Cerebral Cortex?

The exact central pathway followed by the impulses mediating the long-latency stretch reflex has been much debated. Indirect data indicate that the reflex pathway may involve the motor cortex of the cerebral cortex (therefore, the term "long-loop stretch reflex" is often used). In support of a **transcortical** route are the observations that the reflex is weakened or abolished by lesions of the descending motor pathways or by lesions of the dorsal columns (presumably carrying the signals from the muscle spindles to the cerebral cortex). Further, the reflex is often weakened after lesions of the **cerebellum**. But such findings may also be explained by a purely spinal reflex that is under strong supraspinal control.

More decisive evidence of a transcortical route for the long-latency stretch reflex—at least regarding certain muscle groups—comes from observations in a few patients with a peculiar inborn abnormality of the pyramidal tract. These persons always perform **mirror movements** of the hands; asked to flex the index finger of the left hand, they always flex the right index finger as well (more proximal movements, e.g., of the shoulders, are performed normally). This behavior appears from electrophysiological studies to be caused by branching of individual pyramidal tract axons to supply motoneurons of both sides of the spinal cord. Thus, stimulation of the hand region of the motor cortex of one hemisphere causes symmetrical movements of both hands (unlike the normal situation, in which such stimulation always cause movements of the opposite hand only). When eliciting stretch reflexes in such subjects, the monosynaptic reflex occurs only on the same side as the stretch is applied (as normal), whereas the long-latency stretch reflex occurs in both hands after a unilateral stimulus. The latter observation is hard to explain unless the reflex arc of the long-latency reflex involves the pyramidal tract.

These findings may not pertain to long-latency stretch reflexes in all muscle groups. For example, the long-latency stretch reflexes appear to be transcortical for distal arm muscles but not (or to a lesser degree) for proximal arm muscles and muscles in the foot. For these latter muscles, the long-latency reflex may be elicited by **group II muscle afferents**, which conduct with about half the velocity of group Ia fibers.

The Function of Stretch Reflexes

One might think that the stretch reflexes—which, after all, are relatively simple—are well understood with regard to their functional roles. For example, the muscle spindles and the motoneurons are among the best-characterized receptors and central neurons, respectively. Nevertheless, we still do not fully understand the role of the stretch reflexes in the control of voluntary movements and in the control of posture and muscle tone. We discuss here only some possible functions.

As mentioned, one likely task of the stretch reflex is to ensure that the **length** of a muscle is kept constant. In many situations, this is of obvious importance—for example, in the upright position when some external perturbation threatens the **body balance**. The sudden displacement of the center of gravity forward stretches the extensor muscles of the back and thus might elicit a stretch reflex tending to resume the former position. It is furthermore an obvious advantage that such a corrective contraction occurs as quickly as possible. Making such an adjustment depend only on voluntary contraction would lengthen the latency fourfold, with the danger of the corrections occurring too late. Also while **walking**—when external perturbations may disturb the programmed pattern of muscular activity—stretch reflexes may contribute to rapid adjustments. Nevertheless, it is not clear to what extent stretch reflexes really participate in such adjustments. (See also Chapter 18, under "More about Receptor Types and Their Contribution to Postural Control.")

Another situation in which stretch reflexes may be of importance is during slow, **precise voluntary movements** when the external opposing forces change unpredictably. Again, the advantage would be that the adjustment of muscle tension occurs much earlier than can be achieved by voluntary action alone. (See also Chapter 13, under "Proprioceptors and Voluntary Movements")

Stretch Reflexes May Correct for Change in External Resistance during Precision Movements

Studies of slow movements of the thumb by the British neurologist David Marsden have shed light on the contribution of stretch reflexes during precision movements. The subject is asked to flex the thumb with a constant speed against an external opposing force of constant magnitude. The EMG of the flexor pollicis longus muscle is recorded continuously. The external force is then changed suddenly at unpredictable times during the movement—either increased or reduced. When the external force is increased, the movement is immediately slowed down. Because of the α–γ coactivation (see Chapter 13, under "Muscle Spindles in Humans and α–γ Coactivation"), the frequency of signals from the muscle spindle increases. The α-γ coactivation ensures that, as the muscle shortens owing to the activation of the α motoneurons, the spindle midportion is stretched. This upholds the firing of muscle spindle afferents in spite of the shortening, which otherwise would have led to reduced firing. To keep up with the steadily shortening muscle, the firing of the γ motoneurons must also increase steadily. When the movement is suddenly halted or slowed down, the firing frequency of the γ motoneurons continues increasing, in anticipation of further shortening of the muscle. Thus, for a moment, the firing of the muscle spindle afferents increases more than what is appropriate with regard to the actual length of the muscle. This increases the excitation of the α motoneurons, and their firing increases, thus increasing the force of the muscle contraction. The result is that the increased external force is rapidly compensated for, and the original speed of the movement is resumed.

When the opposing external force is suddenly reduced, the opposite events take place. The speed of the flexion movement of the thumb increases, and the firing frequency of the spindle afferents decreases for a moment, thus reducing the firing of the α motoneurons and the force of contraction. The speed of movement is adjusted.

It is probable that the stretch reflex functions in this manner especially during **slow precision movements** when we cannot accurately predict the external force at all times. The sensitivity of the muscle spindles is kept at a high level, so that they may record even the slightest perturbations and ensure that the activity of the α motoneurons is adjusted appropriately.

Cutaneous Receptors and the Precision Grip

In some situations, stimulation of low-threshold skin **mechanoreceptors** causes reflex muscular contraction. For example, when (during a precision grip with the fingers) the object slips, a reflex increase of the grip force occurs. The latency from the start of the slip to the muscular response is only 60 to 80 msec—that is, too short to be mediated by a voluntary command. Examination of patients with reduced cutaneous sensation but normal motor apparatus suggests that loss of such rapid, reflex adjustment of the grip force is partly responsible for their difficulties with precision movements (see Chapter 13, under "Clinical Examples of Loss of Somatosensory Information").

Central Modulation of Reflexes

It should be clear from the preceding discussing that stretching of a muscle does not necessarily elicit a reflex contraction. Many factors influence whether there will be a response, such as the velocity of stretching and whether the muscle is active when being stretched. Further, the response depends heavily on whether a reflex contraction is functionally appropriate. Such **gain modulation** of the stretch reflex is mediated by descending connections from higher levels of the CNS (e.g., from the motor cortex). It appears to be exerted mostly by a precise control of the excitability of specific sets of **spinal interneurons**, which are intercalated in particular reflex arcs. In addition, **presynaptic inhibition** may very selectively "switch off" the input from specific sets of receptors. Thus, reflex arcs may be "opened" or "closed" in accordance with the need of the overall plan for movements (Fig. 21.15). Obviously, the motor programs in the cerebral cortex and the brain stem specify not only the muscular activity but also the gain of spinal reflex arcs at any moment.

Reflex modulation has been studied most during **locomotion** in humans and is found in several muscle groups. Thus, the strength of reflex contractions in many leg muscles depends on whether the leg is in the

many years ago that the kinds of cramp mentioned here are caused by high-frequency **firing of α motoneurons** (other kinds of cramp may be caused by altered conditions in the muscle itself). An interesting possibility is that cramps arise because of the motoneurons' ability to form **plateau potentials**, as characterized by a stable depolarized state (see also Chapter 22, under "Monoaminergic Pathways from the Brain Stem to the Spinal Cord," and "Mechanism Responsible for the Development of Spasticity"). In this state, a brief excitatory input can trigger a train of action potential lasting for many seconds or even minutes. Experimentally, a brief train of signals in Ia fibers from the muscle spindles can cause sustained motoneuron firing and cramps, possibly because of induction of plateau potentials, but any excitatory input would presumably have the same effect. The plateau potential can be terminated by a brief hyperpolarizing synaptic input. Whether plateau potentials occur in muscle cramps in humans is unknown, but if they do, why they are induced at rest in some healthy persons needs nevertheless to be explained. Conceivably, increased extracellular K⁺ due to intense motoneuronal firing during endurance exercise may elicit plateau potentials. Another possibility is that plateau potentials are triggered by altered inputs to motoneurons during muscular fatigue—for example, by increased muscle spindle afferent activity and reduced presynaptic inhibition. That stretching and sometimes massage terminate cramps might be due to stimulation of afferent inputs that inhibit motoneurons (via interneurons). Ia afferents are unlikely to be activated in this situation, as they respond poorly to slow stretching of the muscle. Electrical stimulation of the tendon inhibits experimentally evoked muscle cramp, suggesting that stretching of the cramped muscle works by activation of 1b afferents from the tendon organ.

So-called **writer's cramp** is a task-specific **focal dystonia** of the hand. The cramp usually occurs when trying to do a task that requires fine-motor movements. In this case, it is believed that basal-ganglia dysfunction lies behind the abnormal motoneuronal firing.

Changes of Muscle Tone in Disease

Pathologically changed muscle tone is called hypotonia when it is lower than normal and hypertonia when higher than normal. Of course, to recognize abnormal muscle tone one must first be able to decide what is normal, but from the preceding discussion, it should be clear that "normal muscle tone" is not a precise, well-defined concept. The decision as to whether a muscle has a normal tone is based largely on the subjective judgment of the examiner. This judgment, of course, depends on experience. Whereas hypertonia may be identified with reasonable certainty and even measured in semiquantitative terms by stretching the muscles, the

decision as to whether a muscle has abnormally low tone is more difficult. As mentioned, a normal, fully relaxed muscle will have a very low tension when tested by stretching. Some authors believe that when paretic or paralytic muscles feel softer and more flaccid than normal muscle, it is because of lack of voluntary contraction, which probably occurs to some extent during passive movements and palpation. Indeed, experiments measuring the resistance to passive stretching of normal and alleged hypotonic muscles did not show consistent differences. The experiments were performed by measuring the falling time of the leg (passive flexion of the knee) in healthy persons with the ability to relax fully (determined with EMG) and in patients with pareses of the quadriceps muscle (clinically judged as hypotonic). On the other hand, the individual differences in falling time—that is, muscle tone—among the normal subjects were fairly large, presumably because of differences in the passive viscoelastic properties. Nevertheless, with peripheral pareses, rapid changes of the passive viscoelastic properties of the muscles may occur, which may help explain why the paretic muscles feel softer on palpation. After damage to peripheral motoneurons, the muscles waste rapidly, reducing the muscle volume to sometimes only 20% to 30% of normal in about 3 months. The metabolism of muscle cells is obviously dramatically altered by loss of contact between nerve and muscle.

Abnormally increased muscle tone, **hypertonia**, would imply that the muscles continuously have an increased tone, in spite of attempts to relax. As mentioned, many healthy persons are not able to relax completely, at least not in an examination situation, and the border between normal and pathologically increased muscle tone may not be easy to draw. Fairly characteristic disturbances of muscle tone do occur in certain diseases of the CNS, however.

Spasticity and Rigidity

The term **spasticity** is used in clinical neurology of a condition in which there is increased resistance against rapid stretching of muscles. By palpation, the muscles may feel normal or hypotonic, and there may not be increased resistance against slow, passive movements. Spasticity occurs after damage to the descending motor pathways from the cerebral cortex to the motoneurons and is probably due primarily to changed spinal-interneuron excitability. The increased resistance to rapid stretch is most likely caused by abnormally brisk monosynaptic stretch reflexes, whereas the long-latency stretch reflexes are weaker than normal.

Rigidity is the term used to characterize the increased muscle tone occurring in **Parkinson's disease** (Chapter 23). Even with very slow, passive movements, an increased, "cogwheel"-like resistance is felt by the examiner. This may be caused by increased **long-latency stretch reflexes** that are elicited by abnormally slow movements.

Also with rigidity and spasticity, there is evidence of changed passive **viscoelastic properties** (in addition to the changed stretch reflexes). Thus, in patients with moderately severe Parkinson's disease, increased resistance to slow elbow extension was found, even though there was no EMG activity of the biceps muscle (which was being stretched). In some spastic patients, increased resistance even to slow stretching of relaxed leg muscles was present, but only when the spasticity had lasted for more than a year. Thus, it seems as though an altered pattern of signals from the motoneurons—like those occurring in diseases with rigidity or spasticity—may change the passive, viscoelastic properties of the muscles.

INJURY OF PERIPHERAL MOTOR NEURONS AND REGENERATION

When all motoneurons (or their axons) supplying a muscle are destroyed, the muscle cannot be made to contract: it is **paralyzed**. Both voluntary and reflex movements are abolished. If not all of the motoneurons (or their axons) supplying a muscle are destroyed (Fig. 21.16), the muscle can still contract, although with less speed and force than normal. This is called a partial paralysis, or **paresis**. Typically, the paretic muscle feels soft and flaccid, and there is a marked reduction in the muscle mass. This is called muscle **atrophy** or wasting and is more marked with more complete destruction of the motoneurons. The muscle cells that no longer receive signals from the motoneurons become thinner and eventually disappear if no reinnervation takes place (see later).

Peripheral and Central Pareses

The muscle weakness caused by the loss of the α motoneurons or their axons (**lower motor neurons**) is called a **peripheral paralysis** (paresis), to distinguish it from a **central paralysis** caused by interruption of the central motor pathways (the upper motor neurons). Central pareses are discussed in Chapter 22. Suffice it here to mention that in central pareses the spinal reflex arcs are intact (Fig. 21.16). Characteristic of peripheral pareses—apart from the weakened or abolished voluntary contractions—is that the muscles are flaccid, reflex movements are weakened or abolished, and muscle wasting progresses rapidly and becomes marked.

In cases of peripheral pareses, the **distribution** of affected muscles may tell us where the disease process is located. For example, the distribution will differ, depending on whether the lesion is located in the spinal cord, in the plexuses formed by the spinal nerves, or in the peripheral nerves more peripherally (Fig. 21.2). As a rule, one muscle is supplied with motor fibers from two or more spinal segments, as discussed above (Fig. 21.3). Therefore, damage restricted to one spinal segment or

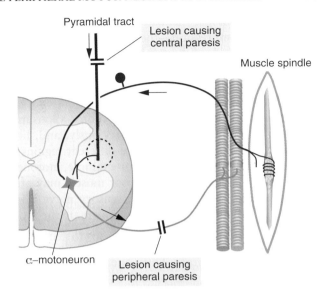

FIGURE 21.16 *Peripheral and central pareses.* Lesions of the motoneurons produce peripheral pareses, characterized by loss of both voluntary and reflex contractions. Central pareses—characterized by loss of voluntary movements but retained reflex contractions—ensue when descending corticospinal pathways are interrupted.

its ventral root (e.g., the C_5 root as in Fig. 21.2) produces only a paresis, not a complete paralysis of a muscle. Alternatively, several muscles become paretic because each segment contains motoneurons supplying several muscles, but if the peripheral nerve (e.g., the thoracicus longus nerve in Fig. 21.2) supplying a muscle (the serratus anterior) is severed, the muscle becomes paralytic.

Peripheral Axons Can Regenerate

When a **peripheral nerve** is **injured** so that the axons are interrupted, the distal parts of the axons degenerate and are gradually removed (by macrophages). The cell bodies (of the motoneurons and the spinal ganglion cells) show **retrograde** changes and, even though some of the cells die, many survive. The proximal parts of the axons of the surviving neurons start to grow (in contrast to what happens in the CNS; see Chapter 11, under "Can We Help Restitution?"). When possible, the growing axons follow the canals in the nerve left by the degenerated axons. The **Schwann cells** do not die and form a lining of the canals for the growing axons. The axons grow 1 to 2 mm per day, although the growth gets slower the farther peripherally the axon grows.

Factors that Influence Regeneration

The outcome of this regeneration of the axons depends on several factors, among them the conditions at the site of injury and the age of the person. If the continuity

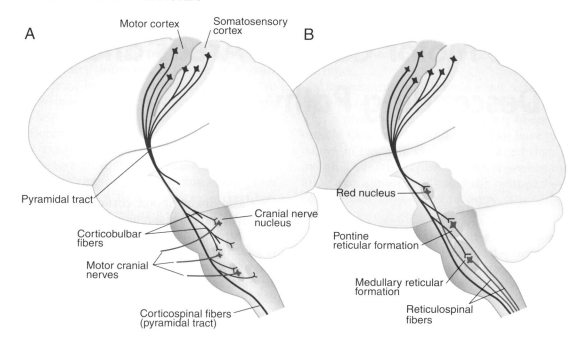

FIGURE 22.1 *Direct and indirect motor pathways to the spinal cord.* **A:** The pyramidal tract passes directly from the cerebral cortex to the motoneurons in the brain stem (corticobulbar fibers) and in the spinal cord (corticospinal fibers). **B:** Nuclei in the brain stem with efferent connections acting on motoneurons. Indirect corticospinal pathways are established by corticofugal connections to the brain stem nuclei.

of the medulla and continue downward in the lateral funicle of the cord, to finally establish synaptic contacts in the spinal gray matter.

Fibers also leave the pyramidal tract on their way through the brain stem, to reach cranial nerve motor nuclei (Figs. 22.1 and 22.3). Such fibers form part of the **corticobulbar tract** (other corticobulbar fibers reach the red nucleus, the pontine nuclei, the reticular formation, the colliculi, the dorsal column nuclei, and other nuclei).

The pyramidal tract derives its name from the **pyramid** of the medulla, which is formed by the fibers of the corticospinal tract (see Figs. 6.15 and 6.16). Strictly speaking, therefore, the term "pyramidal tract" encompasses only the fibers destined for the spinal cord and not those destined for the cranial nerve motor nuclei.

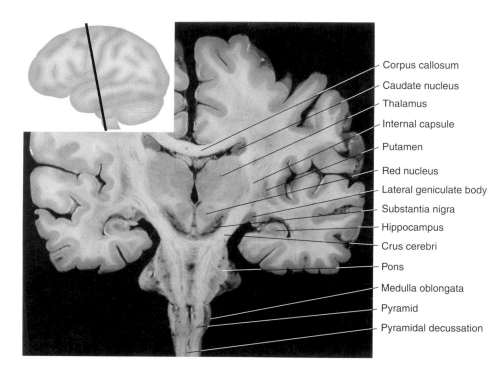

- Corpus callosum
- Caudate nucleus
- Thalamus
- Internal capsule
- Putamen
- Red nucleus
- Lateral geniculate body
- Substantia nigra
- Hippocampus
- Crus cerebri
- Pons
- Medulla oblongata
- Pyramid
- Pyramidal decussation

FIGURE 22.2 *Course of the pyramidal tract through the internal capsule and the brain stem.* Longitudinal bundles of myelinated fibers are evident in the crus, the pons, and the medullary pyramid. Compare with Fig. 22.13.

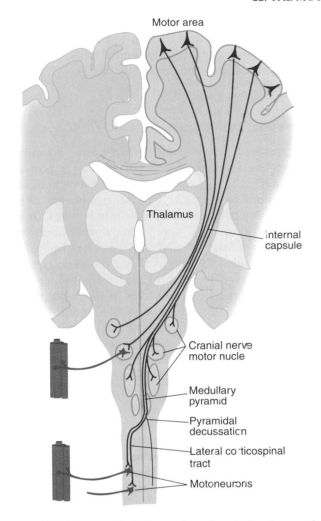

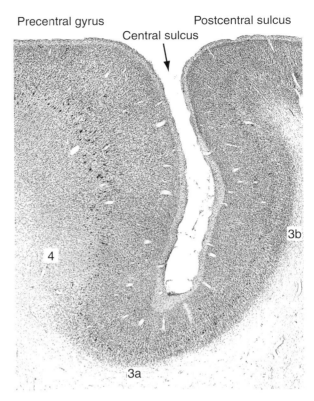

FIGURE 22.4 *The central region with MI (primary motor area) and SI (somatosensory area)*. Photomicrograph of a section perpendicular to the central sulcus (monkey). There is a notable difference in thickness between the MI and the SI. The dark dots in the deep parts of the cortex (in layer 5) are the cell bodies of pyramidal tract cells that have been retrogradely labeled by an injection of a tracer substance (horseradish peroxidase) in the spinal cord. There are more labeled cells in the MI than in the SI.

FIGURE 22.3 *Direct corticobulbar and corticospinal pathways (the pyramidal tract)*. The corticospinal tract is mainly crossed, whereas many of the cranial nerve nuclei receive crossed and uncrossed corticobulbar fibers. Note the crossing of the corticospinal tract in the lower medulla.

Nevertheless, for practical reasons both groups are usually included in the term.

Origin of the Pyramidal Tract

A large proportion of the fibers of the pyramidal tract comes from neurons with their cell bodies in the **precentral gyrus**—that is, **area 4** of Brodmann (Figs. 22.4, and 22.5; see also Fig. 33.3). This region was called the **primary motor area** (MI), because muscle contractions could most easily (with the weakest current) be elicited from this part of the cerebral cortex. The **somatotopical organization** of MI (Fig. 22.5) has been verified in humans with various kinds of stimulation and imaging techniques (electric and magnetic stimulation, positron emission tomography [PET], functional magnetic resonance imaging [fMRI]). It corresponds roughly to the somatotopical pattern in SI (see Fig. 14.8). We return to MI later in this chapter.

It was originally thought that all fibers of the pyramidal tract came from area 4 and, furthermore, only from the cells with the largest cell bodies, the **giant cells of Betz**. The number of Betz cells, however, is much too low to account for the number of axons in the pyramidal tract (about 1 million in humans). More recent studies with retrograde transport of tracer substances (Fig. 22.4) have largely clarified the origin of the pyramidal tract in various animals. In the monkey, numerous cells in area 4, in addition to the Betz cells, contribute to the pyramidal tract, as do also many cells in areas outside area 4. Although the relative contribution from various areas differ among authors, it seems that about two-thirds of all fibers arise in front of the central sulcus—that is, in area 4 and **area 6** (PMA and SMA in Fig. 22.6), whereas the rest comes from **SI** (areas 3, 1, 2), **SII**, and parts of the **posterior parietal cortex** (area 5). A considerable fraction of the fibers from SI arise in **area 3a**—that is, the part of SI adjacent to area 4 (Fig. 22.4) that receives an input from muscle spindles. Muscle contractions can also be elicited from the areas outside MI, like SI, by electrical stimulation, but the stimulation has to be more intense than in area MI. This reflects

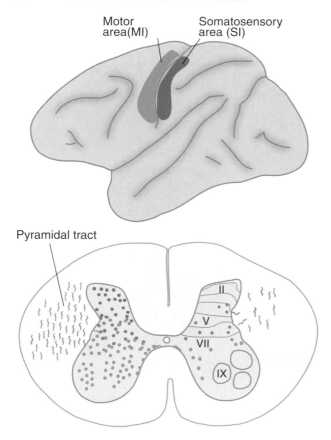

FIGURE 22.8 *Terminal regions of the pyramidal tract.* Based on experiments in monkeys with anterograde transport of radioactively labeled amino acids after injections in various parts of the motor cortex (MI) and the somatosensory cortex (SI). Corticospinal fibers from the MI end more anteriorly in the gray matter of the cord than those from the SI. The uncrossed fibers end predominantly medially in the ventral horn—that is, in contact with the motoneurons that supply axial and proximal muscles. (Based on Ralston and Ralston 1985.)

This asymmetry presumably arises because a larger proportion of the fibers from (usually) the left hemisphere cross than from the right hemisphere. Thus, the lateral (crossed) tract becomes larger on the right side than on the left, whereas the ventral (uncrossed) tract becomes smaller on the left side.

Such individual variations would influence the severity of motor symptoms after damage to the brain or spinal cord and may help explain why symptoms vary so much among patients with very similar lesions. Thus, occasionally an infarct of the internal capsule produces most severe ipsilateral pareses (on the same side), and lesions of the cord may give motor symptoms that are unexpected from their location.

Conduction Velocity and Termination of the Pyramidal Tract

The pyramidal tract fibers vary considerably in thickness, from the thickest myelinated kind to unmyelinated ones. Most are rather thin; with **conduction velocities**

between 5 and 30 m/sec. Corticospinal neurons are **glutamatergic**, exerting excitatory effects. In general, the thickest (and thus fastest conducting) fibers come from MI.

In accordance with the **somatotopic pattern** within MI (Fig. 22.5), fibers from the medial parts of the precentral gyrus (leg representation) end in the lumbosacral part of the cord, whereas fibers from more lateral parts (arm representation) end in the cervical and upper thoracic cord. Fibers from **MI** and **SI** also terminate differently in the cord (Fig. 22.8). Thus, fibers from SI end predominantly in the dorsal horn, whereas fibers from MI end in the intermediate zone and the ventral horn (laminae VII–IX).

Monosynaptic Cortico-Motoneuronal Connections

Anatomic and physiologic data show that some of the pyramidal tract fibers coming from MI end **monosynaptically** on the motoneurons. This concerns primarily motoneuron groups that control the **distal muscles** of the extremities—in particular, the intrinsic muscles of the **hand**. During evolution, the pyramidal tract has increased in size and with regard to monosynaptic connections with the motoneurons. This change has taken place in parallel with increased versatility and precision of the movements of the hand (which, in turn, depend on increased brain volume). In the rat and the rabbit, for example, the pyramidal tract is only slightly developed. It is more prominent in the cat, but there are no monosynaptic connections between pyramidal tract neurons in the motor cortex and motoneurons in the cord—all connections are with spinal interneurons. In monkeys, there is a modest proportion of monosynaptic connections, but the proportion is larger in the anthropoid apes (e.g., the chimpanzee) and still larger in humans. Even some shoulder muscles, like the deltoid, receive some monosynaptic connections in humans. The monosynaptic connections are of particular importance for the movements that require the highest degree of voluntary control—the **least automatic movements**—such as independent or **fractionated finger movements**. This relationship is witnessed by the fact that in certain subprimate mammals with an exceptional manual dexterity (and the ability to use the fingers individually), some monosynaptic motoneuronal connections are present.

Distribution and Actions of Single Corticospinal Fibers

A corticospinal neuron in MI usually has strong **excitatory** actions on some motoneurons and weaker excitatory actions or **inhibitory** actions (via interneurons) on many others. Accordingly, anatomic data from tracing of single fibers show **widespread ramifications** of a single pyramidal tract axon, enabling it to contact numerous motoneurons in different segments of the cord that supply several muscles. This may appear surprising in light of the very discrete and precise movements the pyramidal tract is capable of producing. However, as a rule, the various muscles contacted from one corticospinal neuron have similar actions—that is, they are synergists. Further, the strength of the influence of one pyramidal tract cell probably varies greatly among the motoneurons it contacts, depending on the number and location of synaptic contacts. For example, corticospinal fibers terminate on both proximal and distal parts of the dendrites. Contacts with **inhibitory interneurons** further increase the specificity of actions. In many voluntary movements, commands from the motor cortex elicit **reciprocal inhibition** in the cord. Such varied effects of the pyramidal tract fibers fit with the motor cortex being organized to initiate **purposeful movements**, requiring coordinated activity of multiple muscles around several joints (rather than the contraction of muscles in isolation). This topic is discussed further under "Functional Organization of the Primary Motor Area."

The Pyramidal Tract Controls Flexors More than Extensors

Experiments with transcranial magnetic stimulation (TMS) of the motor cortex show that **flexors** of the thumb have a **lower threshold** for activation than the extensors. Corresponding findings pertain to the biceps muscle (flexor) and the triceps muscle (extensor) of the upper arm. At least concerning finger movements, it seems reasonable that the flexors require somewhat more precise control than the extensors, although both certainly are necessary for manual dexterity (e.g., holding and manipulating small objects). Interestingly, fMRI studies indicate that a smaller part of MI is activated during simple finger flexions than during finger extensions. Presumably, this may be due to more monosynaptic connections to the flexor motoneurons.

The functional flexors of the ankle joint (the tibialis anterior muscle and others that dorsiflex the ankle) are more influenced by the pyramidal tract than are the plantar flexors (the triceps surae and others). This would seem to fit with clinical observations in patients with **hemiplegia**: ankle dorsiflexion is more reduced in power than plantar flexion (the foot droops). However, the typical posture of the hemiplegic arm (Fig. 22.11)—with tonic flexion at the elbow—can obviously not be explained in this way.

The Pyramidal Tract Controls Sensory Neurons in the Spinal Cord

The effects of SI (via fibers traveling in the pyramidal tract) on neurons in the dorsal horn are quite specific. Thus, projections differ from individual cytoarchitectonic subdivisions within SI: area 3b—receiving input from cutaneous low-threshold mechanoreceptors—sends fibers primarily to laminae III and IV, which receive the same kind of sensory input (through the dorsal roots). Fibers from area 3a end deeper in the dorsal horn, where primary afferents from proprioceptors end. Physiological experiments confirm that SI influences sensory cells in the dorsal horn. Most often, SI inhibits neurons that are excited from low-threshold mechanoreceptors. As discussed in Chapter 14 (under "The Transmission of Sensory Signals Can Be Controlled from the Brain"), suppression of certain kinds of sensory information may be important, for example, during movements.

The Pyramidal Tract Fibers Open and Close Spinal Reflex Arcs

Even in humans, a large proportion of the pyramidal tract fibers end in synaptic contact with **interneurons** in laminae VII and VIII (Fig. 22.8; see also Fig. 6.12). Many—perhaps most—of these interneurons make synaptic contacts either on motoneurons or on other interneurons, which, in turn, contact motoneurons. In this manner, the pyramidal tract may mediate varied effects on the motoneurons. This is true of both the α motoneurons and the γ **motoneurons**, so that the pyramidal tract can control the sensitivity of the **muscle spindle**. Because many of the interneurons contacted by pyramidal tract fibers are intercalated in reflex arcs, the motor cortex can ensure that the various spinal reflexes are adapted to the overall aim of the movements. For example (as described in Chapter 21), the strength of the **long-latency stretch** reflex can be increased or decreased, depending on what is appropriate during motor learning. The interneurons mediating **reciprocal inhibition** during stretch reflexes (see Fig. 21.13) are also controlled by the pyramidal tract. Likewise, the **Renshaw cells** (see Fig. 21.14) are subject to supraspinal control, so that the strength of the recurrent inhibition can be increased or decreased selectively in various motoneuronal groups. A final example is the interneurons that mediate inhibition of motoneurons evoked by stimulation of **tendon organs** (in the same muscle as supplied by the motoneurons). This reflex arc can also be "opened" or "closed" by the pyramidal tract. Thus, the **autogenic inhibition** elicited by stimulation of tendon organs can be reversed to excitation during voluntary contraction of the muscle (whereas at the same time the inhibition of other muscles may be enhanced).

Function of the Pyramidal Tract as Judged from Functional Deficits after Lesions

To clarify the function of a tract, two approaches have mainly been used: studying (1) the properties of single neurons and (2) the deficits that ensue when the entire tract is eliminated. We discussed in the preceding text

colliculus and form the **tectospinal tract**. The descending fibers cross the midline shortly below the superior colliculus, and most terminate at **cervical levels** of the cord. The superior colliculus receives numerous fibers from the retina, the visual cortex, and from the so-called **frontal eye field** (area 8 in Fig. 25.7), which are of particular importance for control of conjugate eye movements. Efferent fibers from the superior colliculus do not act solely on the cord; motoneurons in the brain stem innervating extraocular muscles are also influenced (although indirectly via the reticular formation). In agreement with these anatomic data, electrical stimulation of the superior colliculus in experimental animals produces coordinated movements of the **eyes** and the **head**. The tectospinal tract is of particular importance for movements of the **head** and the **eyes** as parts of **optic reflexes**: that is, the head and the eyes are directed toward something in the visual field. (Auditory signals also reach the superior colliculus via the inferior colliculus and can thus elicit head movements.)

The superior colliculus also receives afferents from nonvisual parts of the cortex, like the **SI** and **MI**. Thus, a **corticotectospinal pathway** may perhaps play a part in voluntary movements.

Vestibulospinal Tracts

Primary sensory fibers from the vestibular apparatus terminate in the **vestibular nuclei**, which is located in the pons and medulla (see Fig. 9.7). Vestibular signals about the position and movements of the head also indirectly provide information about the position of the body and about disturbances in balance. Two tracts, issued from the vestibular nuclei to the spinal cord, can contribute to the maintenance of body balance and posture. The largest is the **lateral vestibulospinal tract**, which comes from the lateral vestibular (Deiters) nucleus and reaches all levels of the cord. The tract lies in the **ventral funicle**. The fibers exert an **excitatory** action on both α and γ **motoneurons**. Like the reticulospinal fibers, the vestibulospinal ones act primarily on motoneurons in the medial parts of the ventral horn—that is, **axial muscles** and **proximal muscles** of the extremities. Thus, the lateral vestibulospinal tract can adjust the contraction of muscles that oppose the force of gravity (antigravity muscles).

The other vestibulospinal tract is much smaller and reaches only the cervical and upper thoracic segments of the cord. This **medial vestibulospinal tract** is therefore primarily important for mediation of **reflex head movements** in response to vestibular stimuli. This conclusion is also supported by physiological experiments. Unlike the lateral vestibulospinal tract, many of the neurons of the medial tract are **inhibitory** (probably using **glycine** as a transmitter).

In contrast to the other cell groups in the brain stem sending fibers to the cord, the vestibular nuclei receive few afferents from the cerebral cortex. The vestibulospinal neurons are therefore more independent of the cerebral cortex than, for example, the reticulospinal neurons. The vestibular nuclei mediate primarily **automatic, reflex movements** and adjustments of muscle tone. Nevertheless, the activity of the vestibular nuclei may be influenced indirectly from the cortex, as they receive afferents from the reticular formation. For example, the influence of vision on automatic adjustments of posture appears to be mediated via the vestibular nuclei.

The Red Nucleus and the Rubrospinal Tract

The red nucleus (nucleus ruber) in the mesencephalon (see Figs. 6.20 and 6.21) consists of a caudal **magnocellular** part (large, motoneuron-like neurons) and a rostral **parvocellular** (small-celled) part. In monkeys the magnocellular part is quite small, and in humans it contains even fewer neurons. The large parvocellular part receives its main afferents from the **cerebellum** (especially from the dentate nucleus, receiving its main afferents from the cerebellar hemispheres). Many (most?) of the efferents from the **parvocellular** part goes to the **inferior olive** (which sends its efferent fiber to the cerebellum). By way of cerebellar pathways to the motor cortex, it appears that the parvocellular red nucleus influences movements primarily through its interplay with the cerebellum and the motor cortex, not by sending fibers to the spinal cord.

The **magnocellular** red nucleus sends fibers to the spinal cord, forming the **rubrospinal tract**. The tract crosses the midline just below the red nucleus and descends in the lateral funicle, mixed with the fibers of the pyramidal tract. The rubrospinal tract is somatotopically organized. In the cat and the monkey, the fibers terminate in largely the same parts of the spinal gray matter as the pyramidal tract and have their most marked effect on **flexor motoneurons** of distal muscles (also like the pyramidal tract). The red nucleus receives fibers from the motor cortex of the same side. A **corticorubrospinal** pathway is thus established from the cerebral cortex to the spinal motoneurons. In the cat and monkey this pathway supplements the pyramidal tract in the control of voluntary movements (although it is of greater functional importance in the cat than in the monkey). Whether it plays such a role in humans seems unlikely because the magnocellular part is so small, and the parvocellular part does not appear to project to the spinal cord (in monkey and humans). In monkeys, the ratio of rubrospinal to corticospinal fibers has been estimated to about 1:100, and this ratio is most likely even lower in humans.

Monoaminergic Pathways from the Brain Stem to the Spinal Cord

Although they are often included among the reticulospinal pathways, descending monoaminergic fibers to the cord from the **raphe nuclei** (Fig. 22.9; see also Figs. 26.6 and 26.7), the **locus coeruleus** (see Fig. 15.6), and scattered cell groups in their vicinity have distinct properties. Such monoaminergic fibers terminate in the ventral horn (in addition to in the dorsal horn). Many of the **raphespinal** fibers contain **serotonin**, whereas the **coeruleospinal** fibers contain **norepinephrine**. In addition, several **neuropeptides** coexist with the monoamines. Both these tracts end rather diffusely in the spinal gray matter and can hardly mediate information related to specific movements. More likely, they exert general, widespread **facilitatory** influences on the motoneurons, as judged from the effects on spinal motoneurons of microinjections of serotonin and norepinephrine. Thus, the excitability of most motoneurons may be enhanced, so that they react more vigorously to an input from the pathways that mediate specific motor commands (such as the pyramidal tract). At the same time, the descending monoaminergic connections to the **dorsal horn** may prevent "disturbing" signals from nociceptors from reaching consciousness. In deep **sleep** (REM sleep), all movements are suppressed, and the descending monoaminergic neurons show their lowest activity.

It is possible that these monoaminergic pathways contribute to the effects of **motivation** on the performance of voluntary movements when the muscle contractions occur with increased speed and force. This may be related to the ability of the monoamines (serotonin in particular) to alter the excitability of the motoneurons by inducing a so-called **plateau potential** (see Chapter 21, under "Muscle Cramps and Plateau Potentials"). Thus, serotonin (and other transmitters) can bring the motoneuron from a state of stable hyperpolarization with low excitability to stable depolarization (plateau potential). In this state, a brief excitatory input elicits tonic firing from seconds to minutes. Plateau potentials may also be an efficient means to control the activity of muscles used for **postural tasks** because they exhibit long periods of tonic contractions (at least in experimental animals). A brief inhibitory input suffices to terminate the tonic firing.

CONTROL OF AUTOMATIC MOVEMENTS

In this section, we treat the control of two kinds of automatic movement: the postural reflexes and locomotion. Postural control and control of movements, either automatic or voluntary, are not independent, however, since postural control is a prerequisite for proper execution of virtually every purposeful movement. Postural reflexes were treated in more depth in Chapter 18 in conjunction with the control of body balance.

The Cerebral Cortex Coordinates Brain Stem and Spinal Networks

Brain stem and spinal networks can on their own control quite complex movement sequences; the contribution of the cerebral cortex being restricted to start and stop signals. In general, however, the cerebral cortex, the basal ganglia, and the cerebellum are needed to incorporate the activity of the lower networks in an overall plan. To achieve this, the **indirect corticospinal pathways** are instrumental in coordinating the various automatic responses initiated from the lower levels. This happens mainly by modulating the excitability of brain stem and spinal interneurons. Further, most purposeful movements challenge our balance by moving the center of gravity. When learning a sequence of movements, the higher levels make internal models that, among other things, anticipate the postural perturbations caused by the desired movements. Thus, such **anticipatory control** is an important characteristic of skilled and of harmonious movements.

Postural Reflexes

To maintain equilibrium we need rapid corrections of muscle tension in various parts of the body. Postural reflexes produce the automatic movements that help us regain equilibrium quickly—for example, when slipping on ice. It is a common experience that these compensatory movements happen so rapidly that only afterward are we aware of which movements we performed. The tasks of the postural reflexes are to maintain an appropriate posture of the body, to help regain equilibrium when it is disturbed, and to ensure optimal starting positions for the execution of specific movements. Large perturbations may require additional voluntary movements (coming later than the automatic ones). To issue the right motor commands, the brain must receive immediate and reliable information as soon as something threatens our upright position—that is, information from receptors that detect joint movements and movements of the whole body. Because our **upright position** is **labile**—with a small supporting area and a high center of gravity—constant corrections are necessary. For example, we sway a little back and forth in quiet standing, as an expression of imperceptible postural corrections (reflex responses).

Receptors that provide information used for postural control are **proprioceptors** in the legs, the spine, and the neck; **cutaneous** receptors on the sole of the foot; **vestibular receptors** in the inner ear; and photoreceptors in the **retina**. The more demanding the challenge to the

are usually recognized: the medially situated **supplementary motor area** (SMA), and the lateral **premotor area** (PMA). Besides sending fibers to the spinal cord, thus contributing to the corticospinal tract, both the SMA and the PMA send many fibers to the MI. They can therefore act on motoneurons in two fairly direct ways. Usually, however, the effect on MI has been considered most important, and, consequently, the SMA and PMA are often placed above the MI in a **hierarchy of motor areas**. The SMA and PMA—sometimes termed **supramotor** areas—are believed to instruct the MI in what to do. Several observations support this assumption—for example, that the SMA and PMA usually become active in advance of MI during voluntary movements. Clinical observations of patients with complete or partial lesions suggest that **SMA** and **PMA** are important for **sequential movements**, especially performance of rhythmic sequences (there are no pareses). A pianist suffering from such a lesion could no longer play because he was unable to keep even intervals between the keystrokes. The great Russian neuropsychologist Alexander R. Luria used the term loss of **movement melodies** to describe symptoms after lesions of area 6. Among typical

symptoms are difficulties with coordination of **bilateral movements**, such as swinging the arms in opposite directions.

The **posterior parietal cortex** and the **prefrontal cortex** are also concerned with motor control, although less directly than the MI, SMA, and PMA. In certain respects, the parietal and prefrontal areas are higher up in the hierarchy of motor areas. The posterior parietal cortex is important for the transformation of somatosensory and visual information into appropriate motor commands. The prefrontal cortex shows increased activity before self-initiated movements (i.e., movements that are not a response to external stimuli). The functions of these cortical regions are multifarious, however, and certainly not restricted to motor control. They are discussed more fully in Chapter 21.

During execution of well-rehearsed, routine movements, only relevant parts of the MI increases its activity, as judged from fMRI studies (Fig. 22.11). Apparently, "higher" motor areas are only minimally engaged; their contribution restricted to mediating the intention to move. Presumably, "motor program" is located in the motor cortex, the basal ganglia, and the cerebellum.

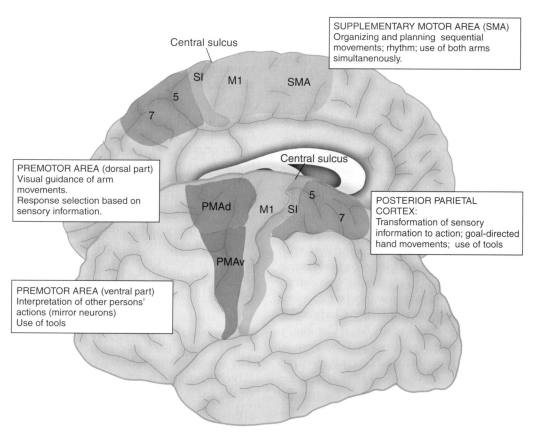

FIGURE 22.10 *Areas of special importance for the control of voluntary movements.* The borders of the various areas are not exact. They are partly based on cytoarchitectonic maps (Brodmann), partly on PET and fMRI studies. Areas in the prefrontal cortex are engaged in cognitive aspects of motor control (selection of goal, choice of strategy, and so forth), but are not shown.

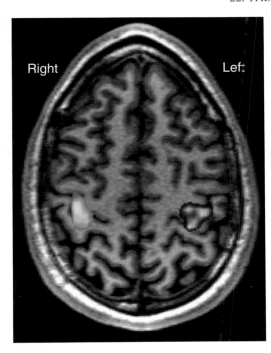

FIGURE 22.11 *Parts of the motor cortex activated by finger tapping.* T1-weighted fMRI. Areas with increased blood flow are colored (red: left motor cortex, activated by tapping the right index finger, green: right motor cortex activated by tapping the left index finger). Movements that are more complex activate addition areas. (Courtesy of Dr. S.J. Bakke, Rikshospitalet University Hospital, Norway.)

The Connections of MI

The physiologically defined MI corresponds fairly closely to Brodmann's area 4.[5] It receives main **afferents** from **SI, SII, SMA, PMA,** and **the posterior parietal cortex**, in addition to afferents from "motor" parts of the **thalamus** (the ventrolateral nucleus, VL; see Figs. 6.21 and 14.16). The **cerebellum**, especially, sends important information about movement performance to MI via VL (the basal ganglia mainly influence the MI via connections to area 6).

Although a large fraction of the pyramidal tract fibers arise in MI, these nevertheless constitute only a minority of all **efferents** from MI. The motor cortex sends, for example, **feedback** connections to the cortical areas from which it receives afferents. Further, numerous fibers pass to subcortical regions involved in motor control, such as the **basal ganglia**, the **cerebellum**

(via the pontine nuclei), the **red nucleus**, the **reticular formation**, and the "motor" **thalamus**. This means that a copy of the motor commands that are issued to the motoneurons—an **efference copy**—reaches the basal ganglia and the cerebellum. Such information helps them to assist in the control of ongoing movements and in learning new ones. Efference copies also reach cortical regions that are responsible for the **sense of effort** (see Chapter 13, under "Perception of Muscle Force"), and regions that enable us to distinguish sensory information that arises as a result of our own movements from such that is due to external events. Efference copies are also important for updating the **body scheme** and for our perception of bodily **ownership** (see Chapter 18, under "Distributed Networks, Body Image, and Body Scheme"). Consequently, damage to the motor cortex is not identical to damage of the pyramidal tract—many neuronal groups besides the motoneurons lose crucial information.

Most if not all **pyramidal tract** fibers ending monosynaptically on the motoneurons come from MI, which explains why the threshold for eliciting movements by electrical stimulation is lower here than in any other part of the cortex.[6] Accordingly, the movements evoked by very weak electrical stimulation of the motor cortex are mediated by the pyramidal tract. Such movements occur in the opposite body half and can be limited to a few muscles in distal parts of the extremities and the face. Increasing stimulus strength recruits more muscles, and ones that are more proximal. These effects are most likely mediated by polysynaptic pyramidal tract connections (via spinal interneurons) and by **corticoreticulospinal** pathways. Muscles that are often used simultaneously on both sides of the body, like the muscles of the back and the abdomen, can be relatively easily activated on both sides (bilaterally) by stimulation of the MI of one side. Movements of the fingers, however, can be evoked only from the opposite (contralateral) MI, which reflects that the fingers are used independently and usually differently on the two sides. The anatomic basis of this is the complete crossing of the pyramidal tract fibers that control distal muscles, as mentioned earlier. Similar conditions pertain to the **commissural fibers** that interconnect the MI of the two hemispheres: only parts of the MI representing the trunk and the proximal parts of the extremities are interconnected. The large areas representing the distal muscles are devoid of commissural connections, presumably as an expression of the independent use of the two hands (see Fig. 33.12).

---

5 It is not clear whether there is complete coincidence between the physiologically defined MI and area 4, which is defined cytoarchitectonically. Some authors maintain that the MI extends anteriorly somewhat into area 6 with the representation of axial and proximal muscles. Such disagreement may be caused by lack of clear-cut cytoarchitectonic changes when moving anteriorly from area 4 into area 6. Cytoarchitectonic borders, as depicted so confidently in maps like that in Fig. 33.3, are in reality seldom unequivocal. The considerable differences between maps published by different authors witness this point.

6 Near the end of the nineteenth century, electrical stimulation of area 4 in dogs produced the first firm evidence of specializations within the cerebral cortex. Before that, the existence of functional localization in the cerebral cortex was hotly debated.

with the **reticular formation**, the **red nucleus**, the **basal ganglia**, and the **cerebellum**. As with the SMA, however, the connections from the PMA to the **MI** are probably those most directly related to the motor functions of the PMA. As indicated in Fig. 22.10, the PMA consists of a dorsal (PMd) and a ventral (PMv) subdivision that differ with regard to connectivity and functional properties. Experiments in monkeys indicate that the PMA is important for the control of **visually guided** movements, such as the proper orientation of the hand and fingers when they approach an object to be grasped. The PMA thus performs **visuomotor transformations** of signals coming especially from the posterior parietal cortex. In monkeys, many cells in the PMA change their activity about 60 msec after a light signal that the monkey is trained to respond to with a certain movement. The activity of the PMA neurons continues until just before the movement starts, even when the monkey is trained to wait for many seconds after the signal before actually performing the movement. Thus, the PMA appears to hold the intention to move and the motor plan in standby until it is appropriate to start.

Monkeys with lesions of the PMA also have difficulties with moving the hand around a transparent obstacle to reach an object: They persistently use the direct approach, bumping into the obstacle. After damage to the MI, the handling of an object is clumsy and insecure, but the ability to avoid an obstacle is not lost. Connections from the **extrastriate areas** in the occipital lobe to the PMA are necessary for the ability to perform such **circumventive goal-directed movements**. Obviously, the PMA is important for the ability to adapt a goal-directed movement to altered external conditions.

Damage of the PMA often produces a peculiar tendency to continue a certain movement when first started, even though the movement is unsuccessful in achieving its goal. Thus, when the hand in one of the examples mentioned above bumps into an obstacle (in this case, a transparent plate), the monkey nevertheless repeats the same movement repeatedly. This phenomenon is called **perseveration** and occurs in humans after damage to the frontal lobes.

Mirror Neurons

In the ventral part of the **PMA** (PMv) and in the **posterior parietal cortex** certain neurons are active not only when the person performs a certain movement but also when she watches another person performing the same movement. Such **mirror neurons** respond particularly well to use of tools, and they may respond to the sound produced by an action. Although identified with certainty only in monkeys, mirror neurons probably exist also in the human brain, as judged from fMRI studies.

It is believed that the perceived action of the other person is automatically simulated by the mirror system without being actually carried out. The system of mirror neurons is probably involved in **learning by imitation** and in the "reading" of other persons' **motor intentions**. Some argue that the mirror system also is responsible for mind reading in a wider sense, that is, perception of others' intentions and the communicative content of movements (called **social cognition**). Others question this so-called "motor theory of social cognition." As said by Jacob and Jeannerod (2005, p. 22) ". . . we grant that simulating an agent's movements might be sufficient for understanding his motor intention, but we . . . argue that it is not sufficient for understanding the agent's prior intention, his social intention, and communicative intention." Certainly, identical movements may result from very different intentions and for different purposes. Another system, collecting much more varied information than the mirror system does, seems necessary for social cognition (notably association areas in the superior temporal sulcus, the amygdala, and the orbitofrontal cortex).

Motor Imagery

Do we use the same parts of the brain when we imagine a movement as when we perform it? Many studies with brain-imaging methods, such as PET and fMRI have addressed this question. Most agree that largely the same **cortical networks** are activated in both situations. This holds for the PMA, parts of the prefrontal cortex, the basal ganglia, lateral parts of the cerebellum, and the posterior parietal cortex. Some studies also show increased activity in MI, although considerably less than in relation to movement execution. In agreement with such data, magnetic stimulation of MI most easily evokes contraction of the muscles involved in the imagined movement (data are conflicting, however, whether spinal motoneurons also show similar facilitation during motor imagery). Dissimilarities concern SMA, where somewhat different subregions are active in motor imagery than in real movements. Further, inferior parts of the prefrontal cortex are active only during imagery, so perhaps this region is responsible for the **suppression** of movements. The same neuronal processes seem to underlie imagined and real movements, as indicated by the fact that they take equal time from start to end. Patients with **lesions** of the **motor cortex** can still imagine movements in the paretic side, but just as the real movements the imagined ones are slower than normal. Patients with **Parkinson's disease** likewise exhibit similar slowing and reduced amplitude of real and imagined movements. After lesions of the **posterior parietal cortex**, however, the imagination of movements seems to be more affected than their execution.

Learning and the Motor Cortex

Brain-imaging studies show that higher association areas in the prefrontal and posterior parietal cortices are active during learning of new motor skills. As movements become more automatic, the activity decreases in these areas, presumably because of use-dependent plastic changes. We mentioned that the pre-SMA might be particularly engaged in learning new sequential movements. Further, animal experiments and human brain-imaging data indicate that plastic changes occur also in the MI during motor learning. Both **LTP** and **LTD** can be induced in the cerebral cortex, and motor learning appears to be associated with strengthening of **horizontal connections** within MI thereby coupling functionally related neurons. Thus, pyramidal cells in laminas II and III strengthen their synaptic couplings with neurons in other parts of the motor cortex during skill learning in rats. Further, the connections are specific for the body parts that are used in the motor performance.

In humans, the finger representation in MI increases during 1 week of intense **piano training** of a specific sequence, as judged from threshold changes to magnetic stimulation of various parts of the motor cortex. Changes were obtained both with real movements and with mental training (motor imagery), although the effect was largest with real movements. In a group of right-handed elite **badminton** players, the stimulation threshold was lower and the hand area was larger in the left than in the right motor cortex (such differences were not found in a group of recreational players).

The Posterior Parietal Cortex and Voluntary Movements

Area 5 is of particular importance for processing somatosensory information (received from SI), whereas **area 7** also receives information from visual cortical areas (see Figs. 21.9 and 21.10). Many neurons in these areas are active in relation to movements, as shown by Vernon Mountcastle (1975) and others. One kind of neuron is active before goal-directed, reaching movements, such as when a monkey stretches its hand toward a banana. Such neurons do not become active, however, in relation to a movement in the same direction but without a specific aim, or in relation to a passive movement. Other kinds of neurons increase their activity in relation to exploratory hand movements, such as when a monkey studies a foreign object. In area 7, some neurons increase their activity only when the monkey stretches the hand toward an object that it also looks at. As there are ample connections from the posterior parietal cortex to the SMA and PMA), it is likely that the posterior parietal cortex in part determines the behavior of cells in these motor areas.

Indeed, **damage** to the posterior parietal cortex also produces motor disturbances. There are no pareses, however, but rather difficulties with the execution of more complex movements. Patients with such lesions may be unable to open a door or to handle previously familiar tools like a screwdriver or a can opener. They also have difficulties with proper orientation of the hand in relation to an object, and they easily miss an object even though they see it clearly. This kind of symptom is called **apraxia** (see also Chapter 34). Interestingly, similar symptoms may occur after lesions of the frontal lobes in front of the MI, presumably reflecting the intimate connections between the posterior parietal cortex and the frontal lobes.

SYMPTOMS CAUSED BY INTERRUPTION OF CENTRAL MOTOR PATHWAYS (UPPER MOTOR NEURONS)

The term **central paresis** is used for a muscle weakness that is caused by interruption of the central motor pathways that conduct signals from the cerebral cortex (especially the MI) to the motoneurons. Only the pyramidal tract goes directly; the other pathways are indirect, with synaptic interruption in the brain stem. We have discussed that the various pathways take care of somewhat different aspects of motor control. The term **upper motor syndrome** is often used for the clinical picture resulting from interruption of the central motor pathways, to differentiate it from the **lower motor syndrome** (peripheral pareses) resulting from destruction of the motoneurons (including their axons; see Fig. 21.16).

Mechanisms underlying recovery after damage to the upper motor neurons was discussed in Chapter 11, under "Studies of Recovery after a Stroke in Humans."

"Negative" and "Positive" Symptoms

Although pareses are present in both, peripheral and central pareses differ in other respects. In peripheral pareses, the symptoms are all **negative**, in the sense that they represent **loss of function**, like reduced or abolished muscle power, resting tone, and reflex contractions. There is also marked and rapid wasting. In central pareses **positive symptoms** also occur—that is, there are symptoms caused by hyperactivity of neurons, such as increased reflex responses and resting muscle tone. Such differences are understandable when considering that the peripheral motor neurons are still functioning in central paresis (see Fig. 21.16). The motoneurons can be activated by signals from various receptors through the dorsal roots, from spinal interneurons, and from any remaining descending pathways, even though they cannot be brought into action voluntarily. Because the feature of pareses in hemiplegia is that the **velocity** with which voluntary movements can be performed is reduced more than the isometric force (i.e., speed of movements is reduced more than strength). This is called **retardation** and concerns particularly fine finger movements and movements of the lips and tongue, whereas larger movements are less severely affected. Writing, tying, buttoning, and similar delicate movements may be impossible for a patient with capsular hemiplegia, or the movements are performed only very slowly and clumsily. This **loss of dexterity** is due to the loss of direct corticospinal fibers (the pyramidal tract), which are necessary for independent finger movements. Movements lose their rhythm and fluency. The **fatigability** is also abnormally great—that is, the muscular force drops quickly when a voluntary movement is repeated several times. The patient experiences a dramatic increase in the **mental effort** needed for voluntary movements: movements that before the stroke required no mental effort can afterward be performed only with the utmost concentration and strain.

Changes in the **contractile properties** of the paretic muscles also occur in hemiplegic patients. Thus, in the intrinsic muscles of the hand, the fatigability of type 1 muscle cells is increased and the contraction velocity of the type 2 fibers is reduced. Such changes will presumably contribute to the slowness and increased fatigability in patients with central pareses. Further, the passive,

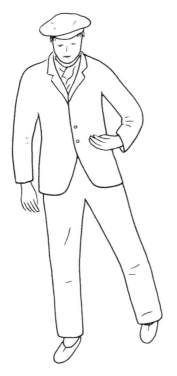

FIGURE 22.14 *Hemiplegia of the left side.* Note the characteristic position of the arm with flexion in the elbow and wrist. The paretic leg is moved laterally in a semicircle during the swing phase to keep the foot off the ground (circumduction).

viscoelastic properties of muscles can change gradually after damage to the upper motor neurons. That is, resistance to stretch may be increased without concomitant muscle contraction, and the range of joint motion may be restricted. The latter phenomenon is called **contracture** and is due to change of connective tissue elements in muscle, tendons, and joint capsules that are kept in a shortened position. Drugs used to treat spasticity such as **baclofen** (reducing the excitability of motoneurons) or **botulinum toxin** (paralyzes muscles) cannot treat this kind of reduced joint mobility.

The Plantar Reflex and Other Reflexes that Are Changed in Upper Motor Neuron Lesions

Interruption of descending central motor pathways, as in capsular hemiplegia, also produces changes of reflexes other than the stretch reflexes. The so-called **plantar reflex**, elicited by stroking with a pointed object in a forward direction along the sole of the foot (especially the lateral margin), is inverted (Fig. 22.15). Instead of the normal response, which is a flexion movement of the great toe (and the other toes), the great toe extends (moves upward). This phenomenon, with extension instead of flexion of the great toe, is called the **sign of Babinski** and is a sensitive indicator of damage of corticospinal pathways.[12] For example, increased intracranial pressure and unilateral herniation with compression of the descending motor fibers in the mesencephalon may invert the plantar reflex at an early stage (this will occur with the foot contralateral to the herniation, owing to the crossing of the pyramidal tract in the lower medulla). An inverted plantar reflex may also occur during general anesthesia and in other conditions with reduced cerebral activity. In patients with central pareses, the threshold for eliciting the plantar reflex is lowered and it can be elicited from a wider area than normally. Further, the response may include a complete flexion reflex of the lower extremity with flexion in the hip and knee and dorsiflexion in the ankle.[13]

In **newborn children**, the plantar reflex is inverted and can remain so until the age of 2 (although most infants respond with plantar flexion of the big toe by 12 months). This is most likely due to the dependence of the "normal" reflex on the integrity of the pyramidal tract, which is not fully myelinated until between 12 and 24 months after birth.

12 Studies of patients subject to cordotomy (cutting parts of the lateral funicle to achieve analgesia) indicate that the sign of Babinski occurs only if the lesion affects the pyramidal tract.
13 Electrophysiological studies indicate that Babinski's sign is due to hyperexcitability of the reflex center in the cord, so that the extensor hallucis longus muscle is recruited together with the ankle extensors. EMG recordings and experiments with nerve blocks show that the flexors of the great toe are still active but that they are overcome by the greater force exerted by the extensors.

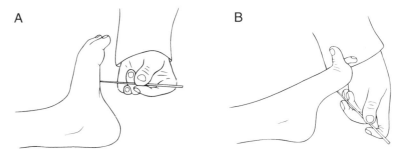

FIGURE 22.15 *Inverted plantar reflex in central pareses (sign of Babinski)*. **A:** The normal plantar reflex is plantar flexion of all the toes when a pointed instrument is moved along the sole of the foot (from the heel to the toes). **B:** In a patient with central pareses (damage of the pyramidal tract) the big toe moves upward (dorsiflexion).

Reduction or absence of the so-called **abdominal reflex** is also typical of upper motor neuron lesions. The normal reflex response is a unilateral contraction of abdominal muscles upon stroking the skin with a pointed object. The so-called **clasp-knife reflex** or phenomenon occurs in some patients: when the patient contracts a muscle isometrically against resistance for some time, it suddenly yields. The involuntary stop of contraction is due to stimulation of high-threshold muscle afferents that inhibit the motoneurons (signals from tendon organs were formerly believed to be responsible, but this was not confirmed in animal experiments).

The "Pyramidal Tract Syndrome"

Formerly, all of the motor symptoms occurring in capsular hemiplegia were thought to be caused by damage to the pyramidal tract, and the term "pyramidal tract syndrome" is still widely used. Closer study suggests, however, that not all symptoms can be explained by damage to the pyramidal tract. Both in monkeys and humans with **lesions restricted to the medullary pyramid**, difficulty with fractionate finger movements is the only constantly remaining symptom after some time. Otherwise, the recovery is almost complete—a patient with an infarction limited to the right medullary pyramid even learned to play the cello afterward (see caption to Fig. 22.13). In monkeys, spasticity ensues after lesions of the motor and premotor cortex but not after complete lesions of the medullary pyramid. To complicate matters, however, hyperreflexia and spasticity have been reported in a few patients with (most likely) pure lesions of the pyramid. Nevertheless, the weight of evidence favor the view that in capsular hemiplegia motor symptoms other than loss of dexterity arise from destruction of other corticofugal pathways than the pyramidal tract. It seems likely that interruption of the **corticoreticulospinal pathways** is important for the more severe symptoms after a capsular lesion than after one limited to the medullary pyramid, including the development of spasticity.

We should also keep in mind that a lesion of the internal capsule might interrupt tracts of importance for motor control other than the corticospinal and corticoreticular ones. Thus, many fibers acting (directly or indirectly) on the **cerebellum** and on the **basal ganglia** will usually be destroyed, and this probably contributes to the clumsiness of voluntary movements. Further, many patients with capsular hemiplegia have **sensory symptoms** in addition to the motor ones, either because the thalamus itself is affected or because the ascending fiber tracts conveying sensory signals from the thalamus to the cortex are interrupted (e.g., visual field defects). Reduced or altered cutaneous sensation and kinesthesia may therefore also contribute to the motor symptoms.

23 | The Basal Ganglia

OVERVIEW

In Chapter 22, we discussed descending pathways from the cerebral cortex, which (directly and indirectly) influence the motoneurons and thereby are crucial for the initiation and control of movements. As mentioned, the basal ganglia form a side loop to the descending motor pathways, and diseases affecting the basal ganglia lead to characteristic disturbances of voluntary movements and of muscle tone but no pareses.

Broadly speaking, the basal ganglia are intercalated in a loop of fiber connections from the cerebral cortex and back to the cerebral cortex through the thalamus. In this respect, the basal ganglia resemble the cerebellum. The basal ganglia process information from large parts of the cerebral cortex before "answers" are sent back to the cortex. Different parts of the basal ganglia assist different subdivisions of the cerebral cortex in their specific tasks. In this way, the basal ganglia are organized in several anatomically and functionally different, **parallel circuits**.

Striatum, composed of the **putamen** and the **caudate nucleus,** is the receiving part of the basal ganglia. The striatum receives excitatory (glutamate) connections from not only motor parts of the cortex but also from association areas and so-called limbic parts of the cortex (e.g., orbitofrontal cortex). In addition, the striatum receives strong connections from the thalamus. Among striatal afferents, the **nigrostriatal** pathway has a special position; it is **dopaminergic** and exerts strong modulatory control of striatal activity. Most of the striatal neurons are **GABAergic,** and send their axons to the **globus pallidus** and the **substantia nigra.** These nuclei send their GABAergic efferent connections to the **thalamus** and certain cell groups in the **brain stem.** From the thalamus, excitatory (glutamate) connections reach especially motor and prefrontal parts of the cortex, whereas the brain stem nuclei (especially the **pedunculopontine nucleus [PPN]**) influence reticulospinal pathways engaged in control of posture and locomotion.

It is noteworthy that the pathway from the striatum to the thalamus contains two inhibitory neurons in a row. Thus, increased activity of striatal projection neurons (driven from the cortex) leads to **disinhibition** in the thalamus, and hence increased excitation in the cortical areas receiving the thalamic input. This has led to the suggestion that the basal ganglia serve, as it were, to release a brake on voluntary movements, facilitating **switching** from one movement (or mental task) to another. In addition, the basal ganglia are important for the establishment of habits and **learning** of automatic movement sequences. The tasks of the basal ganglia are not restricted to motor control, however. Even though the most obvious symptoms in diseases of the basal ganglia are related to the motor system, both clinical and experimental evidence indicates that the basal ganglia also play a role in **cognitive functions.** Further, the most ventral parts of the basal ganglia—termed the **ventral striatopallidum**—contribute to control of **motivation** and **emotions.**

The multifarious connections and tasks of the basal ganglia serve to remind us that classification of parts of the brain into rigid functional categories such as "motor," "sensory," and "cognitive" must not be taken literally but rather as a didactic oversimplification.

STRUCTURE AND CONNECTIONS OF THE BASAL GANGLIA

Figure 23.1 gives a simplified account of the how the basal ganglia are intercalated in a **side loop** of the direct and indirect descending motor pathways. It also shows that the basal ganglia connect with motor centers in the brain stem. Figure 23.2 gives a schematic presentation of the main connections of the basal ganglia, emphasizing the circuit cortex–striatum–globus pallidus/substantia nigra–thalamus–cortex.

On an anatomic basis the term "basal ganglia" usually includes the **caudate nucleus,** the **putamen,** and the **globus pallidus** (Figs. 23.3–23.5; see also Fig. 6.29).[1] Here we use the term "basal ganglia" of a set of functionally related cell groups rather than in a strictly topographic sense. Therefore, we also include the **substantia nigra** and the **subthalamic nucleus** because both are intimately connected with the anatomically defined basal ganglia (Figs. 23.3 and 23.4). Because of their

---

1 The **claustrum** (Fig. 23.4) and the **amygdala** (amygdaloid nucleus) were also included in the term "basal ganglia" by the early anatomists. The function of the claustrum is still largely unknown, even though it is known to receive its main afferents from the cerebral cortex and to send efferents directly back to the cortex. The amygdala differs with regard to both connections and functions from the other parts of the basal ganglia, and is now usually considered a part of the so-called limbic structures (Chapter 31).

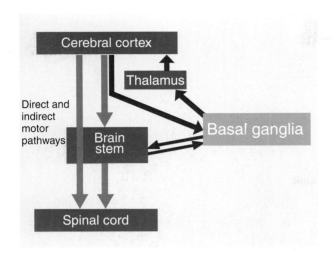

FIGURE 23.1

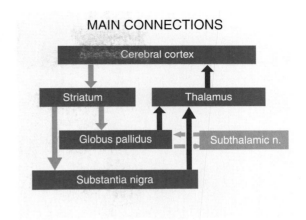

FIGURE 23.2

macroscopic shape, the putamen and globus pallidus together are called the **lentiform nucleus**. The caudate nucleus and the putamen are similarly built, with predominantly small neurons. They are also functionally related and are collectively termed the **striatum** or **neostriatum**. The neostriatum contains several neuronal types that differ with regard to where they send their axons and to which neurotransmitters they use. Most of the neurons, however, send their axons out of the striatum (projection neurons); only a minority is interneurons with axons ramifying locally within the striatum. The presence of several kinds of interneuron is consistent with the fact that the striatum is not simply a relay station but also performs considerable processing of information.

The **globus pallidus** has a different internal structure than the striatum, with larger, more "motoneuron"-like cells, and is also called the **paleostriatum** or **pallidum**. It consists of two parts, an **internal segment** (**GP$_i$**) and an **external segment** (**GP$_e$**) (Figs. 23.3 and 23.4). The term **corpus striatum** includes both the pallidum and the neostriatum. Phylogenetically, the caudate nucleus and the putamen developed together and are younger than the pallidum (thus the names neostriatum and paleostriatum). As we will see, these two main divisions of the basal ganglia differ also with regard to connections.

Cell groups that join the corpus striatum ventrally without sharp transitions—such as the **nucleus accumbens** and the olfactory tubercle—are now collectively termed the **ventral striatum**, and thus included in the

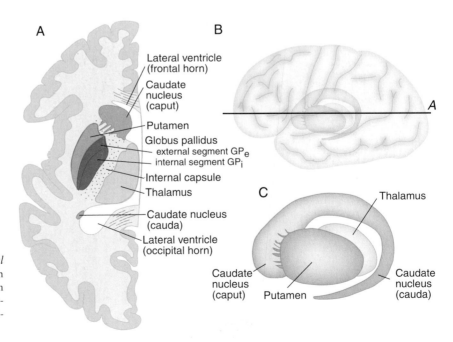

FIGURE 23.3 *Shape and position of the basal ganglia.* **A:** Part of a horizontal section through the hemisphere, as shown (**B**) with a line in drawing of the hemisphere (cf. Fig. 6.30 showing the whole section). **C:** Left putamen and caudate nucleus; lateral aspect.

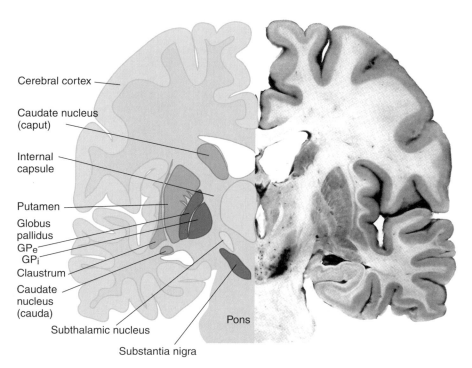

Cerebral cortex

Caudate nucleus
(caput)

Internal
capsule

Putamen

Globus
pallidus
GP$_e$
GP$_i$

Claustrum

Caudate
nucleus
(cauda)

Subthalamic nucleus

Substantia nigra

Pons

FIGURE 23.4 *The basal ganglia seen in the frontal plane.*

basal-ganglia concept. There is also a ventral extension of the globus pallidus, called the **ventral pallidum**. The ventral striatum differs in some respects from the rest—that is, from the **dorsal striatum**—and is treated separately in this chapter. The connections of the **ventral striatopallidum** correlate with its importance for behavior governed by emotions.

The Striatum Is the Receiving Part of the Basal Ganglia

Most of the information to be processed in the basal ganglia first reaches the striatum. It is characterized by three major sources of afferents: the **cerebral cortex**, the **intralaminar thalamic nuclei**, and **dopamine-containing cell groups in the mesencephalon** (Fig. 23.6).

Amygdala   Putamen   Globus
pallidus   Caudate 3d ventricle Internal
nucleus   capsule

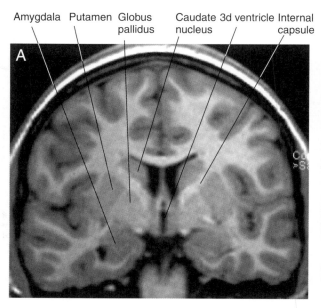

Amygdala   Caudate
nucleus   Putamen   Thalamus   Lateral ventricle

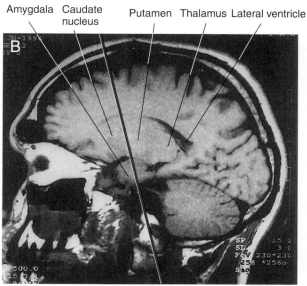

FIGURE 23.5 *Magnetic resonance images (MRI) of the basal ganglia.*
A: Frontal plane; red line in **B** shows approximate position of

the section. **B:** Parasagittal plane. (Courtesy of Dr. S. J. Bakke, Rikshospitalet University Hospital, Oslo, Norway.)

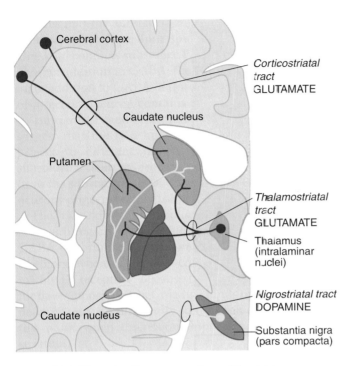

FIGURE 23.6 *The main afferent connections of the striatum.*

The largest contingent of afferents comes from the **cerebral cortex**. Almost all areas of the cortex send fibers to the striatum, but the caudate nucleus and the putamen receive from different parts (Fig. 23.7).

The **putamen** is dominated by somatotopically organized inputs from the **SI** and **MI**. The **caudate nucleus**, in contrast, receives fibers predominantly from the **association areas**—that is, regions that are less directly concerned with motor control than with cognitive functions and emotions. Whereas the putamen receives relatively "raw," or unprocessed, information from sensory receptors via the SI and from upper motor neurons in the MI, the caudate nucleus receives information that is a result of integration of signals from many sources. Such information reaching the caudate nucleus may concern, for example, earlier stages in the chains of neural events leading to a decision about which movements are appropriate in the situation.

The striatal afferents from the **intralaminar thalamic nuclei** (Fig. 23.6; see Fig. 6.22) are numerous and are believed to transmit information to the striatum about stimuli that need special attention.

Dopaminergic striatal afferents to the dorsal striatum arise in the **pars compacta** of the **substantia nigra**, whereas the ventral striatum receive such fibers from more scattered dopaminergic cells in the **ventral tegmental area** (VTA) dorsal to the substantia nigra (Fig. 23.8). VTA also sends dopaminergic fibers to the prefrontal cortex.

Additional, quantitatively minor afferent contingents to the striatum come from the serotonergic **raphe nuclei** in the brain stem, among several other sources.

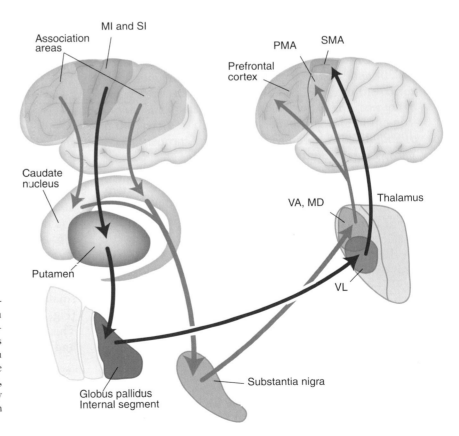

FIGURE 23.7 *Parallel circuits cortex–basal ganglia–thalamus–cortex.* Highly simplified. The putamen receives fibers primarily from the motor and somatosensory areas (red), whereas the caudate nucleus is dominated by inputs from the association areas in the frontal, parietal, and temporal lobes (blue). The figure further shows that sensorimotor information, after processing in the basal ganglia, ends primarily in the SMA, whereas information from the association areas reaches large parts of the prefrontal cortex.

Dopaminergic terminals of nigrostriatal neurons contact the projection neurons and the cholinergic interneurons (Fig. 23.9). In agreement with this, both cell types express mRNA for dopamine receptors.

Compartments in the Striatum: Islands, Striosomes, and Matrix

The various cell types, neurotransmitters and afferent connections are not evenly distributed throughout the striatum. First, the striatal neurons form clusters, called **islands**. Further, a **mosaic** pattern appears after staining to demonstrate **acetylcholine esterase**. Poorly stained patches called **striosomes** are embedded in a heavily stained **matrix**. The matrix can be further subdivided by visualization of various transmitters and their receptors. Cholinergic interneurons and GABAergic projection neurons are found within both the matrix and the striosomes, and the two main kinds of projection neurons do not appear to be clearly segregated, either. However, corticostriatal fibers terminating in the striosomes and in the matrix come from deep and superficial parts of layer 5, respectively. Thus, cortical information to neurons in the two compartments would be expected to differ slightly, even when coming from the same cortical area. Further, the further projections also appear to differ with regard to exact termination and patterns of arborizations. Finally, striatal afferent connections terminate in patches within the matrix. Each small part of the cortex, for example, projects divergently in many patches. These data have been taken as evidence that the striatum is organized in numerous minor compartments or **modules**, each presumably representing a functional unit. It is fair to say, however, that in spite of a wealth of data, the functional significance of striatal compartmentalization is still a matter of speculation (and the interpretation of data is made more difficult by the existence of species differences).

Efferent Connections of the Basal Ganglia: Acting on Premotor Networks in Thalamus and Brain Stem

The efferent connections of the basal ganglia may be summarized as follows. The internal segment of the globus pallidus and the substantia nigra send the information processed in the basal ganglia to premotor networks in the thalamus, the mesencephalon, and the superior colliculus. Here we use the terms premotor and **premotor networks** in a rather loose sense about neuronal groups acting either directly on motoneurons or on the motor cortex. Such premotor networks are found in the spinal cord, the reticular formation, and the thalamus. Neurons of the thalamic VL nucleus, for example, are considered premotor due to their direct projection to the motor cortex. Premotor networks organize the activity of motoneurons to produce purposeful

actions, not merely isolated movements. Thus, the effects exerted by the basal ganglia on other parts of the nervous system are mediated primarily by efferent fibers from the **pallidum** and the **substantia nigra**. These nuclei receive their main afferents from the striatum (Figs. 23.7 and 23.10). In this manner, the pallidum and nigra process information from the striatum before it is sent to premotor networks. The efferents from the striatum are **topographically organized**, so that subdivisions of the striatum are connected with specific parts of the pallidum and the nigra.

The Substantia Nigra

The substantia nigra and some of its connections have been mentioned several times, and we will also return to it when dealing with Parkinson's disease, in which the nigra plays a crucial role. A collective treatment of the main features of the substantia nigra may therefore be pertinent at this stage

The substantia nigra can be divided anatomically into two parts, the **pars compacta** and the **pars reticulata** (Figs. 23.8A and 13.11A). The compacta is richer in cells than the reticulata, whereas the latter (as the name implies) is dominated by dendritic arborizations. The reticulata also contains numerous neurons, however. The compacta neurons contain pigment (neuromelanin), which makes the nigra visible as a dark band in the cut human mesencephalon (see Fig. 23.4). The pars

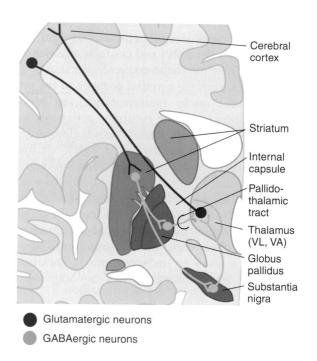

- ● Glutamatergic neurons
- ● GABAergic neurons

FIGURE 23.10 *The loop cortex–basal ganglia–thalamus–cortex contains two inhibitory neurons in series.* This means that increased signal traffic out of the striatum leads to less inhibition in the thalamus (disinhibition). Cf. text.

reticulata, located ventral to the compacta, is lighter. The dopaminergic nigrostriatal neurons are located in the pars compacta, whereas the GABAergic nigrothalamic neurons are located primarily in the pars reticulata (Fig. 23.8C).

The **efferent** connections of the **pars compacta** (Fig. 23.11A) pass primarily to the striatum (with a smaller contingents to the subthalamic nucleus and some other nuclei). This is the largest dopaminergic pathway in the brain, and nigra is the largest collection of dopamine-containing neurons. **Pars reticulata** send GABAergic fibers to the thalamus (VA, MD). In addition, it projects to the superior colliculus (Fig. 23.11A), which control coordinated eye and head movements, and to the pedunculopontine nucleus (PPN) involved control of gait and posture. The nigral neurons sending their axons to the thalamus and the superior colliculus are found in largely separate parts of the pars reticulata.

The **afferent** fiber connections of the nigra (Fig. 23.11B) arise in numerous cell groups, but quantitatively the most important input comes from the **striatum**. This projection shows some topographic organization; for example, afferents from the putamen and caudate nucleus end differently. Even though most striatonigral fibers terminate in the pars reticulata, cells in the compacta can also be influenced because their long dendrites extend into the reticulata (Fig. 23.8). GABA is the transmitter for the striatonigral fibers, exerting

inhibitory effects on the cells in the nigra. **Excitatory** afferents to the nigra arise in the subthalamic nucleus and the pedunculopontine nucleus (PPN) in the mesencephalon (glutamate). Afferents with **modulatory** effects come from the locus coeruleus (norepinephrine) and the raphe nuclei (serotonin). Additional afferents arise in the **ventral striatum** and the **bed nucleus of the stria terminalis** (BST), presumably mediating signals related to motivation, attention, and mood. An important link in the latter pathways is the **habenula** (especially the lateral nucleus). Electric stimulation of the lateral habenula effectively suppresses activity of dopaminergic neurons, presumably by activating inhibitory interneurons.

Pathways from the Globus Pallidus and the Substantia Nigra to the Cerebral Cortex

As mentioned, the **globus pallidus** consists of two parts, an **external** (GP$_e$) and an **internal** (GP$_i$) segment (Figs. 23.3 and 23.4). Both segments receive their main **afferents** from the striatum, with additional inputs from the subthalamic nucleus. Whereas the fibers from the striatum exert inhibitory actions in the GP$_i$, the subthalamic afferents are excitatory. The balance between these two inputs therefore to a large extent determines the activity of the GP$_i$ neurons. The main part of the **efferents** from GP$_i$ goes to the thalamus and the substantia nigra (pars reticulata), whereas the GP$_e$ projects

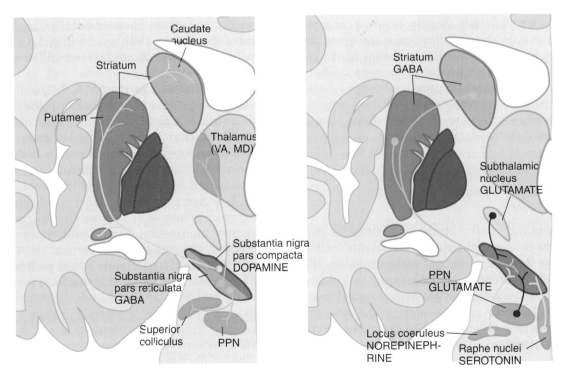

FIGURE **23.11** *Main connections of the substantia nigra.* **A:** Efferents. Dopaminergic neurons in the pars compacta send fibers to the striatum, whereas GABAergic neurons in the reticulata act on premotor neurons in the thalamus and the brain stem. **B:** Afferents. Inhibitory (GABAergic) afferents come from the striatum, whereas excitatory (glutamate) fibers com from the subthalamic nucleus and the PPN. Modulatory afferents arise in the raphe nuclei (serotonin) and the locus coeruleus (norepinephrine).

premotor neurons in the thalamus and the brain stem in a state of inhibition when the animal is not moving. Commands from the cortex to the basal ganglia in relation to the preparation or execution of movements would release the **premotor neurons** from this inhibition. Indeed, electrophysiological experiments show that increased striatal activity reduces the activity of many pallidal and nigral neurons, followed by increased firing of thalamocortical neurons.

It has been proposed that the disinhibition of premotor neurons by the basal ganglia is a **gating mechanism** to control the access of other inputs (e.g., sensory) to the motor cortex. As the connections of the basal ganglia are topographically organized at all levels, this would be a specific and focused gating rather than a diffuse one, varying with the nature of the motor task. Such focused effects might serve to reinforce wanted movements while suppressing unwanted ones.

The Subthalamic Nucleus Regulates Pallidal and Nigral Activity

While efferents of the internal pallidal segment (GP$_i$) end primarily in the thalamus (and the nigra), the GABAergic fibers from the GP$_e$ are directed toward the subthalamic nucleus (Fig. 23.13). The subthalamic nucleus also receives excitatory afferents from the **motor cortex**, thus constituting a cortical input to the basal ganglia in addition to the major corticostriatal pathway. Most of the **efferents** from the subthalamic nucleus go back to both segments of the pallidum and to the pars reticulata of the substantia nigra. As mentioned, the **subthalamopallidal** fibers exert excitatory actions.

The efferents of the subthalamic nucleus are **topographically** organized, as shown with axonal transport methods. Thus, different neuronal populations project to the substantia nigra and the pallidum, and there are differences with the regard to projections to minor parts of the pallidum. Fibers from the subthalamic nucleus and the striatum converge on the same neurons in the GP$_i$. These data suggest that the activity of the GABAergic neurons in GP$_i$ are determined largely by the sum of synaptic influences from the striatum (–) and the subthalamic nucleus (+). Because GP$_i$ neurons inhibit thalamocortical neurons, increased subthalamic activity would be expected to produce reduced excitation of the motor cortex—that is, inhibition of voluntary movements. Thus, the subthalamic nucleus is believed to control or **stop ongoing movements**, rather than to select and initiate movements. Considering the somatotopical organization of its connections, the subthalamic nucleus presumably exerts specific actions rather than a diffuse inhibition of all motor activity.

Loss of influence from the subthalamic nucleus would produce **disinhibition** of thalamocortical neurons.

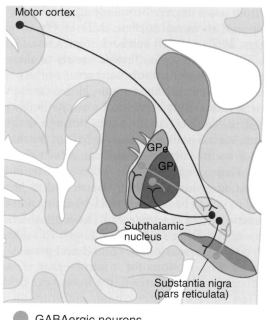

FIGURE 23.13 *Main connections of the subthalamic nucleus.* Inhibitory afferents arise in the globus pallidus and substantia nigra, whereas excitatory connections come from (among other sources) the motor cortex. Glutamatergic neurons in the subthalamic nucleus excite the GABAergic neurons in the globus pallidus and the substantia nigra. Especially the connections from GP$_e$ to the subthalamic nucleus and from there to GP$_i$ have been postulated to be of special significance for the symptoms in Parkinson's disease.

Thus, the violent involuntary movements of the opposite body half after destruction of the subthalamic nucleus—**hemiballismus**—might be caused by hyperactivity among the thalamocortical neurons. In a yet unknown way, disturbed activity of subthalamic neurons (abnormal high-frequency firing and oscillatory activity) appears to be crucial to the symptoms in **Parkinson's disease**. Indeed, "switching off" the subthalamic nucleus by lesion or by electric stimulation has produced marked symptomatic relief in many patients.

Actions of Dopamine in the Striatum

The connections and transmitters described so far are concerned with fast transmission of specific information, mediated by glutamate and GABA. In addition, modulatory transmitters have important roles in the functioning of the basal ganglia. This concerns **dopamine** in particular. Indeed, the most studied basal ganglia connection is the dopaminergic **nigrostriatal pathway**, which is the most massive dopaminergic pathway in the central nervous system (CNS). Many dopaminergic nerve terminals are strategically placed on spines close to the corticostriatal nerve terminals

(Fig. 23.9B).[9] This is a pathway of great clinical interest because several diseases are related to disturbed dopamine-mediated synaptic transmission (Parkinson's disease, schizophrenia, Tourette's syndrome, and others).

Striatal neurons express, not unexpectedly, **dopamine receptors**. Dopamine alters the response of striatal neurons to specific inputs from the cerebral cortex and the thalamus. In more detail, however, actions of dopamine on neuronal excitability in the striatum are multifarious and not fully understood.

There are two main kinds of dopamine receptor—D_1 and D_2, with subtypes of each. Common to the D_1-like receptors (D_1 and D_5) is that they increase the synthesis of intracellular cyclic AMP, whereas D_2-like receptors (D_2–D_4) have the opposite effect. Dopamine receptors are present both pre- and postsynaptically in the striatum, and dopamine influences, among other things, several kinds of ion channel. The actions of the D_1 receptor is most studied, whereas more remains to be known about the D_2 receptor.

Although there is, as mentioned previously, physiological evidence that the major effect on striatal projection neurons of D_1-receptor activation is excitatory and that of D_2-receptor activation is inhibitory, the actions of dopamine is not properly described by this simple dichotomy. One factor complicating the analysis is that dopaminergic neurons fire in two characteristic modes, **tonic** and **phasic**, with either a sustained or transitory rise in dopamine concentrations. There is some evidence that phasic release of dopamine acts on D_1 receptors (excitatory, LTP induction) whereas tonic release activates D_2 receptors (inhibitory, LTD induction). Because the two main types of medium spiny neurons express different dopamine receptors (Fig. 23.14), this would imply the neuronal target of dopamine depends on the firing mode of the nigrostriatal neurons. Another factor making it difficult to generalize dopamine actions is that the effect of dopamine depends on the **state** of the postsynaptic neuron. For example, D_1 receptors may produce depolarization or hyperpolarization, depending on the membrane potential of the postsynaptic neuron. In one state, the neuron is depolarized and fire bursts of action potentials; in the other state it is hyperpolarized and inactive. In the inactive state, activation of D_1 receptors depolarizes the cell (by closure of K^+ channels) so that it reacts more easily with burst to an excitatory input from the cortex. If the neuron is in the active state, however, D_1 receptor activation closes a Na^+ channel that keeps the neuron depolarized by leakage of cations into the cell. Closing this channel would

stabilize the membrane potential, perhaps to avoid excessive activation by glutamate from the cortex.

In conclusion, dopamine probably serves to keep the membrane potential in the range where the postsynaptic neuron is apt to fire in **bursts**—that is, in a state suited for efficient signal transmission. Some data suggest that D_1 receptor activation enhances the activity of neurons that receive a strong and **focused excitatory input** (from the cerebral cortex), while reducing the activity of neurons receiving weak inputs. This would help in focusing striatal activity, in accordance with other data indicating that the basal ganglia assists in the **selection of behavior**, such as the choice of specific movements.

The "Indirect Pathway," the Subthalamic Nucleus, and Parkinson's Disease

The signal pathway we described above—cortex-striatum-GP_i-thalamus-cortex—are often said to establish a

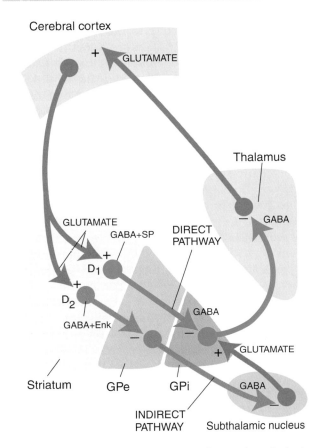

FIGURE 23.14 *"Direct" and "indirect" pathways through the basal ganglia.* One pathway goes directly from the globus pallidus to the thalamus; the other goes indirectly via the subthalamic nucleus. Excitation of striatal projection neurons from the cerebral cortex would produce disinhibition in the thalamus via the direct pathway, while producing inhibition via the indirect pathway. Disturbance of the balance between these two pathways is postulated to explain some of the symptoms in Parkinson's disease. However, anatomic data speak against that the division between the direct and indirect pathway is as sharp as shown in this figure.

9 **Dopamine depletion** in the striatum is associated with loss of dendritic arborizations and spines (in Parkinson's disease and in animal experiments). Therefore, dopamine probably has a direct growth-promoting effect on neurons, or it protects against the harmful effects of strong glutamatergic excitation (or both).

no matter whether the drug is amphetamine, cocaine, or morphine. The addictive behavior is reduced by lesions of the nucleus accumbens or by removing its dopaminergic innervation. Thus, after giving a dopamine antagonist, the experimental animals stop self-administration of cocaine (they could easily obtain an intravenous dose by a movement). Further, dopaminergic activity is increased in paranoid **psychoses** elicited by amphetamines or cocaine (see also Chapter 5, under "GABA Receptors Are Influenced by Drugs, Alcohol, and Anesthetics," "Nicotinic Addiction," and "Drugs Altering Monoamine Activity in the Brain").

However interesting these observations are, they provide only limited insight. By focusing on one transmitter and one part of the brain, one may even give the impression that there is a simple biologic explanation to complex mental phenomena. Indeed, many parts of the brain other than the nucleus accumbens show altered activity in the conditions discussed here (see Chapter 34 for some comments on mental illness and the cerebral cortex). In drug addiction, for example, changes of neuronal activity occur in the locus coeruleus (norepinephrine) and in the intralaminar thalamic nuclei, amygdala, and parts of the basal forebrain adjoining the nucleus accumbens. It is not clear whether the nucleus accumbens or the ventral tegmental area is the primary target of narcotic drugs in the brain; neither is it known how such drugs alter the properties of dopaminergic neurotransmission.

FUNCTIONS OF THE BASAL GANGLIA

In spite of enormous research activity during recent years, the functions of the basal ganglia are still far from fully understood. One reason is that recent research has made us realize that the basal ganglia participate in much more than just motor control; they also provide important contributions to cognitive and emotional processing. Further, their role in various aspects of learning attracts increasing interest.

Movement Planning and Learning

Taking the **connections** of the basal ganglia as a starting point (leaving out the ventral striatum for the time being), it is noteworthy that their major output goes to the SMA, PMA, and the prefrontal cortical areas. The properties of these areas suggest that the basal ganglia would be important in the **planning** phase of a movement, such as when several single-joint movements have to be put together to produce a complex movement, or when sensory stimuli or stored information has to be translated into an adequate motor response. Observations of symptoms in monkeys with lesions of the globus pallidus indicate that learned movements are slower than

normal, whereas the manner in which the task is performed is not significantly altered. Therefore, neither the movement command nor the movement program appears to be located within the basal ganglia themselves. There is also evidence that the basal ganglia participate when movements are **learned by repetition** and not by gaining insight into the nature of the task and, furthermore, that the basal ganglia enable **automatic** performance of well-rehearsed movements by the use of motor programs located elsewhere in the CNS. We also discussed earlier the role of the basal ganglia (and dopamine in particular) with regard to **associative learning**.

Motivation

Some experimental evidence shows that the basal ganglia contribute to the linking of **motivation** and **emotions** to the execution of movements. Thus, recording the activity of single cells in the striatum indicates that many respond best when a stimulus is linked with memory of an event that has a particular significance for the animal. For example, certain cells in the substantia nigra are active just before a rapid eye movement, but only when the movement is directed toward a target whose location the animal must remember in order to obtain a reward. As mentioned, the nigrostriatal dopaminergic fibers appear to provide information about the relevance of a stimulus. Further, motivation (expectation of reward) influences strongly how sensory information is processed in the striatum.

Shift of Behavior

A central theory, trying to unite several lines of investigation, proposes that the basal ganglia are important for the **selection** and **shift** of **behavior** in particular. This appears to concern both movements and cognitive functions. In response to unexpected changes in the environment, it is often necessary to switch attention quickly from one target to another. At the same time, the behavior might need to be shifted on the basis of a decision of what is appropriate in the new situation. Thus, a new behavior is selected, and the current behavior must therefore be stopped.[11] The **evaluation** (giving priority to a certain behavior) probably requires cooperation between the prefrontal cortex and limbic structures, while the **execution** of the behavioral switching may depend on the basal ganglia (regardless of whether it concerns change of movements or thoughts).

---

11 Because the activity of most GP$_i$ neurons *increases* in relation to a movement (thus increasing inhibition of thalamocortical neurons), one would think that the basal ganglia were concerned primarily with stopping ongoing movements rather than helping to initiate new ones. Such stopping is of course a prerequisite for starting anew.

Interval Timing

Finally, the basal ganglia seem to be involved in **interval timing**, underlying the ability to judge intervals and duration. This is the basis of our ability to form **temporal expectations** and predictions about ongoing and future events (the expected time of movement sequences and cognitive processes). Striatal neurons may monitor oscillatory patterns in large areas of the cortex. Thus, human functional magnetic resonance imaging (fMRI) studies of persons performing timing tasks show altered activity in the striatum and the substantia nigra, in addition to in areas such as the prefrontal cortex, the cingulate gyrus, SMA, parietal cortex, and the insula. There is some evidence that these regions functions as a network in relation to interval timing. However, also other parts of the brain may be of importance in this respect, notably the **cerebellum** (see Chapter 24, under "The Timing Theory: Does the Cerebellum Perform a Basic Operation Used in All Its Functions?"). It should be emphasized, however, that it is not settled whether the "sense of time" is represented by specific modules and networks, or whether it is an ubiquitous property of neuronal activity in itself.

Symptoms after Focal Lesions of the Basal Ganglia in Humans

Studies of patients with destruction (vascular lesions in particular) confined to parts of the basal ganglia have given limited insight in their normal functions. A meta-analysis of 240 such patients found that **dystonias**—that is, abnormal positions of body parts due to persistently increased muscle tone—were most frequently encountered. Parkinsonism or choreatic movements occurred in only very few patients. Motor symptoms were most frequent, after lesions comprising the putamen and the globus pallidus, which is in agreement with the connections of these parts. Most frequent among behavioral changes was **apathy**, with loss of initiative, spontaneous thought, and emotional responses (**abulia**). Such symptoms were most frequent after lesions affecting the caudate nucleus, in agreement with its extensive connections with the prefrontal cortex. Nevertheless, on further analysis, many observations could not be fitted into the current theories of basal ganglia functions, and the symptoms varied considerably, even among patients with very similar localization of their lesions.

DISEASES OF THE BASAL GANGLIA

As the functions and internal operations of the basal ganglia are still incompletely known, it should come as no surprise that we have only partial explanations of the relationships between certain symptoms and the elements responsible within the basal ganglia.

As mentioned, the most obvious symptoms in diseases of the basal ganglia are motor ones. As a rule, there is a mixture of symptoms due to **loss of neuronal activity** (compare with pareses after destruction of central motor pathways) and symptoms due to abnormally **increased neuronal activity** (compare with spasticity occurring after lesions of central motor pathways). The most frequent diseases of the basal ganglia impede the initiation of movement and lead to **akinesia**. When started, the movements are slower and of smaller amplitude than normal (**bradykinesia**). Because movements are difficult to initiate, there is also a conspicuous paucity of movements, usually implied in the term "akinesia" but sometimes termed **hypokinesia**. In addition, there are more or less pronounced **involuntary** movements (**dyskinesia**).

The diseases of the basal ganglia fall into two broad groups: those characterized by akinesia and rigidity (Parkinson's disease is the most common example), and those dominated by dyskinesia (e.g., Huntington's disease). The first group is also characterized by loss of dopamine effects in the basal ganglia, whereas the second group shows signs of dopaminergic hyperactivity. Some authors use the terms **hyperkinetic** and **hypokinetic** disorders to distinguish the two main kinds of basal ganglia diseases. The hypokinetic disorders are usually combined with rigidity and tremor (i.e., signs of neuronal hyperactivity), whereas the hyperkinetic disorders are often combined with muscular hypotonia.

The most frequent disease affecting the basal ganglia is **Parkinson's disease**, mentioned several times already in this chapter. Typically, voluntary movements are hard to initiate (akinesia) and they are slower and smaller than normal (bradykinesia). In addition, there is an increased muscular resting tone in the form of **rigidity** (cf. Chapter 21) and **resting tremor**—that is, involuntary, rhythmic, alternating movements. Patients with Parkinson's disease have regularly been found to have a pronounced **neuronal loss** in the **substantia nigra** and a corresponding decrease of dopamine in the striatum.

In **Huntington's disease**, in which there is a marked cell loss in the striatum, the most pronounced symptom is involuntary, jerky, often "dance-like" movements (chorea).

Violent, large involuntary movements of one side of the body, called **hemiballismus**, occur typically after damage to the subthalamic nucleus of the opposite side. Other diseases are also dominated by sudden, involuntary muscular contractions, occurring with uneven intervals, called **tics**. One example is **Tourette's syndrome**, believed to be caused by dysfunction of the basal ganglia. The symptoms can be partially relieved by dopamine antagonists.

Parkinson's Disease

This disease of unknown etiology usually starts during the fifth or sixth decade of life. The syndrome includes, as mentioned, **akinesia, bradykinesia, tremor,** and **rigidity.** In addition, there are disturbances of **postural reflexes.** Notably, the body balance during walking is disturbed, so that the patient appears to be "running after his center of gravity." The steps are typically very short, which is due to the bradykinesia (the movements are not only slower than normal but also reduced in amplitude). When being pushed from behind, the patient has difficulty stopping and continues to move forward. The normal pendulum movements of the arms during walking are absent. There is also a conspicuous loss of facial expression (the face becomes like a mask). There are disturbances of the **autonomic nervous system,** such as increased salivation and secretion from sebaceous glands of the skin. We do not know how the basal ganglia would influence the autonomic nervous system, and the autonomic symptoms perhaps may be caused by a more general disturbance of monoamine metabolism (not only dopaminergic cell groups are affected in Parkinson's disease).

The **tremor** is typical, with its frequency of 3 to 6 per second, and it is most pronounced at rest. When the patient uses the hand, the tremor disappears or is reduced in amplitude. The increased muscle tone, the **rigidity,** is different from the spasticity that occurs after lesions of central motor pathways. The resistance to passive movements is equal in extensors and flexors and is independent of whether the muscle is stretched slowly or rapidly. There is no clear-cut increase in the strength of the monosynaptic stretch reflex (such as the patellar reflex), whereas the long-latency stretch reflexes are increased, and this may perhaps contribute to the difficulties with balance and locomotion. The rigidity is apparently not caused by hyperactivity of γ motoneurons but by descending influences that increase the excitability of the α motoneurons so that they fire continuously—perhaps like the situation in a nervous person who is unable to relax his muscles. The **plantar reflex** is normal in patients with Parkinson's disease, indicating that there is no damage to the central motor pathways. It is indeed an old clinical observation that the tremor and rigidity disappear if a patient with Parkinson's disease has a capsular hemiplegia, and corresponding observations are made in experimental animals. The last central link in the pathways mediating the tremor and rigidity must therefore be pathways from the cerebral cortex to the motoneurons.

The most pronounced structural change in the brain of patients with Parkinson's disease is a profound loss of pigmented (melanin-containing) neurons in the pars compacta of the **substantia nigra** (Fig. 23.8). These are the dopamine-containing neurons. As a consequence of the loss of dopaminergic nigrostriatal fibers, the dopamine content of the striatum is reduced. Symptoms first appear, however, when the dopamine content of the striatum is reduced by 80% to 90%. Another striking change is loss of 20% to 30% of the spines on striatal projection neurons. As mentioned, this may be due to loss of a possible growth-promoting effect of dopamine. Another possibility is that spine loss is due to glutamatergic overactivity in corticostriatal synapses. The latter explanation is suggested by the observation that loss of dopamine indeed increases activity in glutamatergic synapses, and by the close proximity of dopaminergic and glutamatergic synapses on the spines (Fig. 23.9B).

Can We Explain the Symptoms in Parkinson's Disease?

Increased firing of neurons in the subthalamic nucleus is the most striking electrophysiological finding in Parkinson's disease. There is also increased activity in the GP_i, presumably due to the increased excitatory input from the subthalamic nucleus. As discussed earlier ("The "Indirect Pathway," the Subthalamic Nucleus, and Parkinson's Disease"), it is not clear how loss of dopamine in the striatum leads to subthalamic hyperactivity. Even if we ignore that problem, the relationship between the subthalamic hyperactivity and the symptoms is not obvious. True enough, increased GP_i activity would increase thalamic inhibition and thus reduce excitation in the motor cortical areas, and this fits with positron emission tomography (PET) studies that show reduced blood flow in the SMA in Parkinsonian patients. Although reduced thalamocortical activation of motor areas thus helps to explain bradykinesia/akinesia, it is nevertheless puzzling that **thalamotomy** (a stereotaxic lesion of VL/VA) mainly improves rigidity and tremor with less effect on the akinesia and bradykinesia, and neither is voluntary movement made more difficult by the surgery. Further, thalamic infarcts affecting the VL/VA do not produce Parkinson-like symptoms, even though thalamocortical activation of motor areas must be severely reduced. Like thalamotomy, **pallidotomy** improves rigidity and tremor; in addition, it improves the akinesia. Because loss of dopamine in the striatum produces such devastating motor disturbances, it seems paradoxical that thalamotomy and pallidotomy—which eliminate the major effects of the basal ganglia on other parts of the brain—do not worsen control of voluntary movements. It may be mistaken, however, to try to explain the symptoms simply in terms of more or less excitation or inhibition at stations in the cortex-basal ganglia-cortex loop. There is evidence, for example, that thalamic neurons (both in the lateral nucleus and in the intralaminar nuclei) in Parkinsonian patients show various forms of abnormal, partly **rhythmic** firing. Further, their activity—in contrast to that in normal persons—shows no modulation in relation to movements. In addition, the hyperactivity in the subthalamic nucleus takes the form of high-frequency oscillations (which appear to be reduced by dopaminergic medication). We furthermore know that hyperpolarization of thalamocortical neurons can induce **oscillatory** activity under certain circumstances (cf. Chapter 26, under "Thalamocortical Neurons and EEG"). Perhaps the abnormal inhibition from the GP$_i$ in some way releases the thalamic neurons from normal control. As proposed by Marsden and Obeso (1994), the Parkinsonian symptoms may arise mainly because the basal ganglia outputs become "noisy" and thus disrupt the activity of their targets. Some neurons fire rhythmically while others become very difficult to activate. The oscillatory (20 Hz) firing of large populations of neurons may be abnormally synchronized. Presumably, such states are labile, with rapid shifts between oscillatory activity and inactivity. Neuronal networks might shift from one functional state to another in milliseconds. Conceivably, such shifts produce the rapid fluctuations in symptoms sometimes observed in Parkinson's disease. The motor system may be better off when the disruptive basal ganglia outputs are removed (be it by thalamotomy, pallidotomy, or deep brain stimulation)—leaving it in "peace" to compensate for the loss of basal ganglia inputs.

Therapeutic Approaches to Parkinson's Disease

The finding of reduced striatal dopamine led to attempts to alleviate the symptoms by giving the patients dopamine, to substitute for the loss of dopaminergic neurons. For various reasons, a precursor of dopamine—**levodopa** (L-dopa)—has to be used. This is converted to dopamine in the brain. This treatment has a beneficial effect on the symptoms, particularly on the very troublesome bradykinesia. Even though L-dopa has proved to be a very helpful drug, the first hopes turned out to be unrealistic. The drug does not affect the course of the disease, and the therapeutic effect decreases as the disease progresses. There probably must be a certain number of remaining dopaminergic neurons in the nigra for L-dopa to be converted to dopamine in the striatal dopaminergic boutons. More profound changes of the striatal neurons and their ability to react to dopamine may also occur. One might think that when the brain is unable to produce enough dopamine itself, it would not be able to produce dopamine from a supplied precursor, either. However, enzymes converting L-dopa to dopamine are present not only in dopaminergic neurons in the nigra but also in glial cells and in other types of neurons.

The L-dopa treatment has **side effects**, as one might expect when giving a drug that acts not only in the striatum but also in many cell groups in the brain.

For example, altered dopamine functioning in the hypothalamus might explain side effects such as nausea, loss of appetite, and reduced control of blood pressure. Other side effects are sleep disturbances and changes of mood. In some cases, the treatment can precipitate a psychosis that might be due to actions of dopamine on the prefrontal cortex limbic structures. Long-term treatment may provoke motor symptoms that are different from those caused by the disease, such as chorea-like and **athetoid dyskinesias** (athetosis is used of slow, "wormlike," involuntary movements of the fingers and toes).

Stereotaxic surgery has now been replaced by **deep brain stimulation** (DBS) of the subthalamic nucleus or the GP$_i$. Such treatment gives considerable improvement to many patients (the effect is better on positive than on negative symptoms). It appears that improvement occurs regardless of whether the subthalamic nucleus is destroyed or stimulated electrically. Although this might seem to support the hypothesis that DBS removes a disturbing influence (rather than normalizing basal ganglia functioning), the mechanism whereby DBS achieves its effect is poorly understood.

Replacement of lost dopaminergic neurons by **transplantation** has now been tried for some years in patients with Parkinson's disease, with marked improvement in at least some patients. The basis for this approach is animal experiments—pioneered by, among others, the Swedish neurobiologist Anders Björklund—showing that transplantation can eliminate virtually all symptoms produced by lesions of the substantia nigra in adult rats. The transplanted cells must be embryonic or transformed stem cells to avoid rejection, and are injected into the striatum of the recipient. The surviving cells synthesize and release dopamine. Neurons for transplantation can be developed from stem cells in culture, and this approach might be used in the future (thus avoiding ethical and practical problems with the use of human embryos).

Huntington's Disease

This disease is dominantly inherited and usually starts in the fourth decade of life. It is caused by expansion of trinucleotide (CAG) repeats in the *huntingtin* gene (for mechanisms of neuronal death in neurodegenerative diseases, see Chapter 10, under "Common Molecular Mechanisms in Neurodegenerative Diseases"). The disease has a steadily progressing course, and is characterized by rapid, jerky, involuntary movements of the face, arms, and legs. In advanced stages, the patient is never at rest. The dance-like quality of the movements led to the terms **chorea** and **choreatic movements** (Greek: *chorea*, dance). The most prominent pathological change involves the **striatum**, with a marked loss of GABAergic projection neurons.

Observations suggest that in **early stages** of the disease, mostly neurons projecting to the GP_e degenerate (the "indirect pathway"; see earlier). This would produce reduced inhibition of GP_e neurons and, by that, increased inhibition of the subthalamic nucleus. (Animal models support that reduced activity of the subthalamic nucleus may be crucial for development of choreatic movements.) This in turn leads to reduced excitation of GP_i, and thereby to less inhibition (disinhibition) of thalamocortical neurons in VL and VA. Thus, the choreatic movements might be causally related to increased excitatory input to motor cortical areas.

In **later stages** of the disease, the striatal neurons projecting to the GP_i also die (as do many neurons in other parts of the brain). This leads to reduced inhibition of GP_i, with subsequent increased inhibition of thalamocortical neurons (as in Parkinson's disease). This is taken to explain why bradykinesia develops in later stages of Huntington's disease, while the choreatic movements continue. This is not obviously logical, however, if the effects of both the direct and indirect pathways are mediated by the GP_i. Another explanatory model focuses on dopaminergic hyperactivity in the striatum, caused by loss of GABAergic inhibition in the substantia nigra. Although there are problems also with this model, it fits with the observation that L-**dopa** worsens the choreatic movements of patients with Huntington's disease. The disease also leads to mental deterioration with **dementia**, which probably may be explained by cell loss occurring also in the cerebral cortex (particularly the frontal lobes).

The genetic defect is located on the short arm of **chromosome 4**, and this makes it possible to decide whether a person is a carrier of the disease long before the symptoms occur. This is of importance regarding the choice whether or not to have children. However, to provide individuals with such knowledge as long as there is no effective treatment poses obvious ethical questions.

Tourette's Syndrome

This is a peculiar and multifarious condition with multiple **tics** (quick involuntary movements that are repetitive at irregular intervals) associated with involuntary vocalization as central manifestations. It has a strong heritable component but responsible genes have not been identified. The condition is probably caused by a functional disturbance of the basal ganglia and the prefrontal cortex, although the mechanisms are not known. Volumetric studies with MRI indicate that the caudate nucleus is smaller than normal, and fMRI studies show altered activity in the striatum and related cortical regions. It has been postulated that the tics are caused by abnormal activity in small groups of striatal projection neurons (cf. striosomes and matrix discussed in the preceding text). Involvement of both motor and limbic circuits has been proposed to explain both the motor and associated behavioral and emotional symptoms. Dopaminergic hyperactivity may play a role in the disease, but other transmitters, such as serotonin and GABA, have also been implicated.

The disease starts during childhood, usually between the ages of 5 and 10 years, and it affects boys more frequently than girls. Often the symptoms diminish before or during adolescence. Many patients have a repertoire of **repetitive behavior**, such as touching others, repeating their own words, or echoing the words or movements of others. Vocalizations (vocal tics) commonly include explosive cursing or compulsive utterance of obscenities, which interrupt normal speech. Many patients describe that an inner tension builds up, and this is temporarily relieved by the tic. Some people with Tourette's syndrome appear to have unusual energy and creativity. As children, they often show hyperactive behavior. This may lead to serious social problems, especially when, as often happens, the disease is misdiagnosed as a behavioral disorder of social origin.

Treatment with **dopamine antagonists** (especially haloperidol, a D_2-receptor antagonist) may reduce the involuntary movements and other troublesome symptoms. However, the patient's mental energy and self-perception may be severely affected by the treatment. As vividly described by Oliver Sacks in *The Man Who Mistook His Wife for a Hat*, this may be experienced by some patients as worse than the symptoms. Since 1999, **deep-brain stimulation** has been used in some patients with severe symptoms and poor response to conventional treatments. Beneficial results have been reported with different sites of stimulation (the GP_i, the accumbens, and the intralaminar thalamic nuclei).

24 | The Cerebellum

OVERVIEW

The cerebellum and the basal ganglia have in common that they are involved in motor control without being responsible for the initiation of movements, and both are built into "side loops" of the motor cortical areas and the central motor pathways. Both contribute to motor learning, although in different ways. Although the major fiber connections of the cerebellum suggest a motor function, some connections are compatible with a cerebellar contribution to cognitive functions. A brief account of the cerebellum was given in Chapter 6.

Damage to the cerebellum produces characteristic symptoms primarily with respect to the execution of **voluntary movements**. Our normal movements are always **coordinated**—that is, the various muscles participating contract at the proper time and with the proper force. This is a prerequisite for our ability to hit a nail with a hammer, for writing even and rounded letters, for the words to follow each other with proper loudness and rhythm during speech, and so forth. After cerebellar damage, such coordination is lacking, and the movements become uncertain and jerky.

The cerebellum **receives information** from many sources. Sensory signals come from the skin, joints, muscles, vestibular apparatus, and eye. In most instances, this sensory information appears to be related to aspects of movement, such as signals from muscle and joint receptors about positions and ongoing movements. Information is also coming from other parts of the central nervous system (CNS), especially from the cerebral cortex—primarily from cortical areas treating information about movements or involved in planning or initiation of movements. The cerebellum **sends information** primarily to cell groups that give origin to the central motor pathways, like the motor cortical areas and the reticular formation of the brain stem.

A striking feature of cerebellar organization is that the number of fibers leading to the cerebellum is much larger than the number of fibers leading out; the relationship is about 40:1 in humans. The high degree of **convergence** shows that considerable integration and processing of information takes place in the cerebellum before an answer is issued.

The **afferent fibers** end in segregated regions of the cerebellar cortex, and the efferents from these regions are also largely segregated. As a general rule, the cerebellum sends signals to same regions from which it receives afferents. In contrast to the cerebral cortex, the cerebellar cortex has no association and commissural connections: different parts of the cerebellum do not "talk" to each other. Consequently, the cerebellum consists of many functional units or **modules**, each carrying out a specific task. The cerebellum can be subdivided in three main parts based on connections: **vestibulocerebellum**, **spinocerebellum**, and **cerebrocerebellum**. Within each of these major divisions numerous small modules have been identified. The cerebrocerebellum—receiving large number of afferents from the cerebral cortex via the pontine nuclei—comprise about 90% of the human cerebellar volume. The spinocerebellum receives afferents from the spinal cord informing about sensory events and the state of premotor networks and act back by way of reticulospinal and vestibulospinal pathways.

Owing to the structural **homogeneity of the cerebellar cortex**, all modules have the same kind of machinery and, presumably, perform the same kind of information processing. Among several possibilities, the cerebellum may be specially designed for accurate **timing** of events, not only for movements but also for certain cognitive tasks carried out by the cerebral cortex. Further, the cerebellum is involved in aspects of **motor learning**.

SUBDIVISIONS AND AFFERENT CONNECTIONS OF THE CEREBELLUM

The macroscopic anatomy of the cerebellum is described in Chapter 6 (see Figs. 6.1, 6.13, and 6.32), but some points bear repetition here. Figure 24.1 shows how the cerebellum resides in a "side loop" of the motor cortical areas and the central motor pathways. Figure 24.2 shows how all afferent and efferent connections pass through the cerebellar peduncles. The thickness of the arrows indicates the relative number of afferent and efferent fibers. The external part of the cerebellum is a thin, highly convoluted sheet of gray matter, the **cerebellar cortex** (Fig. 24.3). The folds are arranged transversely and form numerous **folia**. If the cerebellum were unfolded completely in the anteroposterior direction, it would measure 2 m! The cerebellar cortex is thinner and of a simpler build than the cerebral cortex, consisting only of three layers (Fig. 24.2). The total number of neurons is nevertheless much higher than in the cerebral cortex due to the dense packing of tiny neurons in the granular layer. All signaling out of the cerebellum is

Afferents from the Labyrinth and the Vestibular Nuclei

Primary vestibular afferents bring sensory signals from the vestibular apparatus in the inner ear. They enter the cerebellum through the inferior cerebellar peduncle (Fig. 24.1) and end in the flocculonodular lobe and adjoining parts of the vermis (Fig. 24.5). Although most of the primary vestibular afferents end in the **vestibular nuclei,** many neurons in the latter send axons to the cerebellum. In this manner, the cerebellum receives vestibular information also via **secondary vestibular afferents.** The vestibular input provides the cerebellum with information about the position and movements of the head. **Efferents** from the flocculonodular lobe end in the vestibular nuclei and can thereby influence the body equilibrium (via the vestibulospinal tracts) and eye movements via the medial longitudinal fascicle (Fig. 24.5 and see Fig. 18.9).

Afferents from the Spinal Cord

Several pathways bring signals from the spinal cord to the cerebellum (Fig. 24.6). Some of these pathways go uninterrupted from the cord to the cerebellum and are called **direct spinocerebellar tracts,** whereas others are synaptically interrupted in brain stem nuclei and are

therefore termed **indirect spinocerebellar tracts** (not shown in Fig. 24.6). The spinocerebellar tracts originate from neurons with their cell bodies located in different lamina of the spinal cord (Fig. 24.7). They are therefore influenced by different kinds of **sensory receptors** and spinal **interneurons** and bring different kinds of information to the cerebellum. The spinocerebellar axons end mostly in the spinocerebellum of the same side (as their cell bodies). Some pass uncrossed; other fibers cross twice (first in the spinal cord and then back again in the brain stem). The fibers are located in the **lateral funicle** as they ascend (Fig. 24.7). The tracts are **somatotopically** organized, so that signals from different body parts are kept segregated. The somatotopic pattern is maintained within the cerebellum (Fig. 24.8) so that the leg is represented anteriorly within the anterior lobe, with the arm and the face represented successively more posteriorly. In the posterior lobe, the arrangement is the reverse, with the face represented anteriorly.

Direct Spinocerebellar Tracts

Functionally, the direct spinocerebellar tracts consist of two main groups. One group of tracts conveys information from **muscle spindles, tendon organs,** and **cutaneous low-threshold mechanoreceptors.** Physiological studies show that many of the neurons of the direct spinocerebellar tracts are activated monosynaptically by primary

VESTIBULOCEREBELLUM

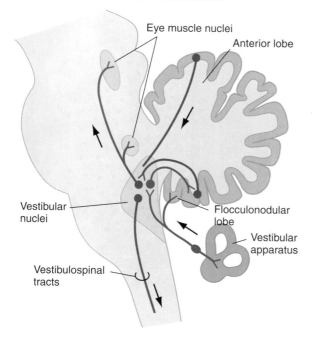

FIGURE 24.5 *Main connections of the vestibulocerebellum.* Afferents are shown in black and efferents in blue in a schematic of a sagittal section through the brain stem. Also shown are primary and secondary vestibulocerebellar fibers and the projection back to the vestibular nuclei. In addition to afferents from the vestibulocerebellum, the vestibular nuclei receive cerebellar afferents from the anterior lobe vermis and from the fastigial nucleus (not shown).

SPINOCEREBELLUM

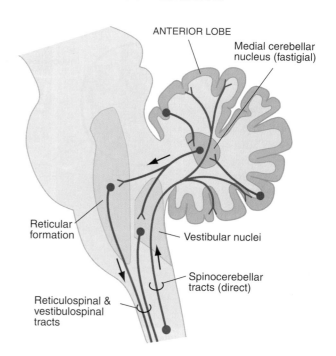

FIGURE 24.6 *Main connections of the spinocerebellum.* The spinocerebellum can influence spinal motoneurons by both the reticulospinal and vestibulospinal pathways.

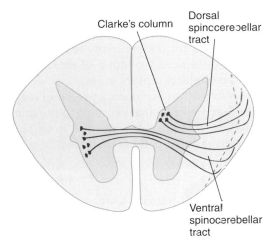

FIGURE 24.7 *The dorsal and ventral spinocerebellar tracts.* Transverse section through the thoracic cord, showing the position of the cell bodies in the gray spinal matter and the tracts in the white matter. Most of the fibers of the ventral spinocerebellar tract cross twice (once in the cord and once in the brain stem), so that most spinocerebellar signals reach the cerebellar half on the same side as the cell bodies are located.

afferent (sensory) fibers. The tracts conduct very rapidly and appear to give precisely timed information about movements.

Another group of direct spinocerebellar tracts does not convey signals from receptors but provides information about the level of activity among specific groups of **spinal interneurons**. As a rule, such interneurons are intercalated in spinal reflex arcs and between descending motor pathways and motoneurons forming **premotor networks**. Information about their activity is therefore presumably highly relevant for cerebellar operations.

Together, the direct spinocerebellar tracts provide the cerebellum with information about the activity both *before* and *after* the motoneurons—that is, about the

commands issued to the motoneurons and the movements they produce. The cerebellum can probably judge whether the command led to the desired result. When, for example, an unexpected increase of external resistance to a movement reduces the velocity compared with what was intended, the cerebellum would be informed immediately. By means of its connections to the spinal cord, the cerebellum can then help to adjust the firing of the motoneurons to the new situation, so that the correct velocity is regained.

Indirect Spinocerebellar Tracts

There are several indirect spinocerebellar tracts, but here we will only mention the largest one, which is synaptically interrupted in the **inferior olive** in the medulla (see Fig. 6.17). Neurons at all levels of the cord send fibers to the inferior olive of the opposite side. The **spino-olivary** fibers end in parts of the inferior olive that project to the spinocerebellum of the opposite side; thus, like the direct spinocerebellar tracts, the spino-olivocerebellar tract conveys information mainly from one side of the cord to the cerebellar half of the same side. This pathway, too, is precisely **somatotopically** organized. The kind of information conveyed by the spino-olivocerebellar tract appears to be different from that conveyed by the other spinocerebellar tracts. We return to the inferior olive later in this chapter, because it has a unique role among the cell groups that send fibers to the cerebellum.

The Dorsal, Ventral, and Some Other Spinocerebellar Tracts

Originally, two direct spinocerebellar tracts were described, differing with regard to the position of their fibers in the lateral funiculus of the cord. The fibers of one of the tracts are located dorsally, and the tract was called the dorsal spinocerebellar tract; the fibers of the ventral spinocerebellar tract are located more ventrally (Fig. 24.7).

The **dorsal spinocerebellar tract** comes from a distinct cell group with fairly large cells at the base of the dorsal horn, forming the **column of Clarke** located in the spinal segments from T_1 to L_2 only. The axons of the cells in the column of Clarke ascend on the same side and enter the cerebellum through the inferior cerebellar peduncle (Fig. 24.1). Primary afferent fibers entering the cord through spinal nerves below the L_2 ascend in the dorsal columns before entering the lowermost part of the column of Clarke. The dorsal spinocerebellar tract conveys information only from the trunk and the lower extremities and ends in the corresponding parts of the spinocerebellum. Another cell group, the **external cuneate nucleus**, located laterally in the medulla oblongata, mediates the same kind of information from

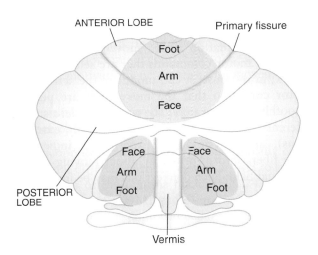

FIGURE 24.8 *Somatotopic localization of the cerebellar cortex.* Based on experiments with electrical stimulation of peripheral nerves and of somatotopic subdivisions of the SI and the MI.

The Intermediate Zone Is a Meeting Place for Signals from the Cord and the Cerebral Cortex

The intermediate zone (Fig. 24.4) is mainly defined on the basis of its efferent connections (projecting to the interposed intracerebral nuclei; Fig. 24.11). It also has special features with regard to afferents, however (Fig. 24.11). Whereas the lateral parts of the hemispheres are strongly dominated by inputs from the cerebral cortex, and the vermis is dominated by spinal inputs, the intermediate zone receives connections from both the cerebral cortex and the spinal cord (Fig. 24.4). Animal experiments indicate that the cortical input to the intermediate zone comes primarily from the MI and SI. Single neurons in the intermediate zone can be activated from both the cerebral cortex and the spinal cord. For example, in the "arm region" of the anterior lobe, intermediate-zone neurons receive converging input from the arm region of the MI and SI and from sensory receptors in the arm. Perhaps the cerebellum in this case **compares** copies of the motor commands sent from the cerebral cortex with the signals from the periphery providing information about the actual movement that was produced by the command (signaled by the spinocerebellar tracts).

THE CEREBELLAR CORTEX AND THE MOSSY AND CLIMBING FIBERS

Before discussing the efferent connections of the cerebellum, we need to know something about the cerebellar

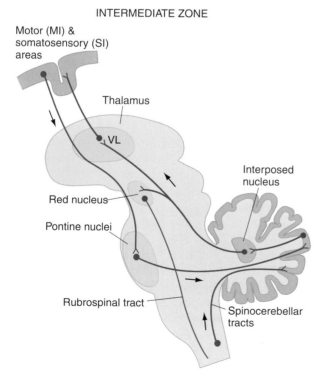

INTERMEDIATE ZONE

cortex. Here, the vast amount of information provided by all of the afferents is processed. To some extent, different kinds of information are integrated, and then "answers" are issued to various motor centers of the brain and spinal cord. As mentioned, the cerebellar cortex has the same structure all over (it cannot be subdivided into cytoarchitectonic areas, differing also in this respect from the cerebral cortex), and it lacks association fibers that interconnect different regions. The structural arrangement of the neuronal elements is strictly **geometric**, so the individual elements can be distinguished fairly easily. This helps explain why the structure and internal connections of the cerebellar cortex are much better known than that of the cerebral cortex.

The Cerebellar Cortex Consists of Three Layers

The superficial, outermost layer is the **molecular layer** (Figs. 24.2 and 24.12). It contains mainly dendrites and axons from cells in the deeper layers and only a few cell bodies. The middle layer is dominated by the large Purkinje cells, arranged in a monolayer, and is called the **Purkinje cell layer.** The deepest, lowermost layer is the **granular layer,** named so because it is packed with tiny **granule cells.** The axons of the granule cells ascend through the Purkinje cell layer into the molecular layer, where they divide at a right angle into two branches running parallel with the surface of the cortex (Figs. 24.12 and 14.13). These branches are called **parallel fibers** and run in the direction of the long axis of the folia. The parallel fibers form numerous synapses with the Purkinje cell dendrites. The **Purkinje cell dendritic tree** is unusual: first, it has an enormously rich branching pattern; second, the dendritic tree is compressed into one plane, forming an espalier oriented perpendicular to the long axis of the folia and the parallel fibers. This arrangement ensures that each parallel fiber forms synapses with many Purkinje cells (the parallel fibers can be several millimeters long). At the same time, an enormous number of parallel fibers contact each Purkinje cell: it has been estimated that each Purkinje cell receives about 200,000 synapses. Considering that there are approximately 100 billion granule cells but only 30 million Purkinje cells, each Purkinje cell would integrate signals from about 3000 granule cells.[3]

In addition to granule cells and Purkinje cells, the cerebellar cortex contains **inhibitory interneurons** (Fig. 24.13) that serve to limit the activity of the Purkinje cells and probably increase the spatial precision of the

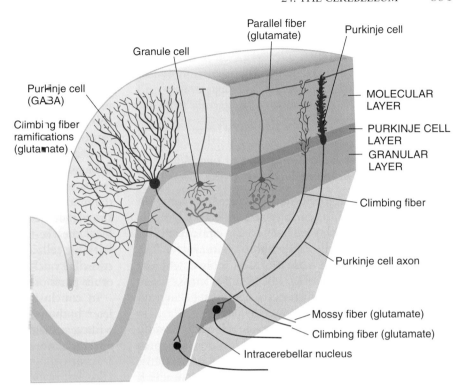

FIGURE 24.12 *Structure of the cerebellar cortex.* The three layers and the main cell types are shown schematically in a piece of cerebellar folium. The Purkinje cell dendrites are arranged perpendicular to the long axis of the folium and the parallel fibers. The two main kinds of afferent fibers (mossy and climbing fibers) are also shown. The mossy fibers end on the granule cells, whereas the climbing fibers enter the molecular layer to end on the Purkinje cell dendrites.

incoming signals (cf. inhibitory interneurons in sensory systems; see Fig. 13.4).

As mentioned, the **Purkinje cells** are the only ones that send their axons out of the cerebellar cortex and thus constitute the efferent channel. The Purkinje cells contain γ-aminobutyric acid (**GABA**), and they inhibit their target cells, as shown physiologically. The **granule cells** have an excitatory action on the Purkinje cells, releasing **glutamate**.

The Cerebellar Cortex Contains Three Kinds of Inhibitory Interneurons

All cerebellar interneurons contain GABA (some may also contain glycine, another inhibitory neurotransmitter). One main type of interneuron is the **stellate cell**, located in the molecular layer (Fig. 24.13). It receives afferent excitatory input from the granule cells (parallel fibers), and its axons form synapses with the Purkinje cell dendrites. Another kind of interneuron, the **basket cell**, is located close to the Purkinje cell layer. Basket cells are also contacted by parallel fibers, whereas their axons end with synapses around the initial segment of the Purkinje cell axons—a location that enables the basket cells to inhibit the Purkinje cells very efficiently. The axonal branches of the basket cells are arranged perpendicular to the long axis of the folia, so that they inhibit Purkinje cells lateral to those that are being activated by parallel fiber excitation. Activation of a group of granule cells would lead to a narrow band of excitation of the Purkinje cells along the folium, flanked by a zone of basket-cell mediated inhibition on each side. Thus, it appears to be a kind of lateral inhibition, which is common in sensory systems to increase the spatial precision. Correspondingly, the extent of the cerebellar cortical region activated by each mossy fiber is reduced. The third kind of inhibitory interneuron, the **Golgi cell**,

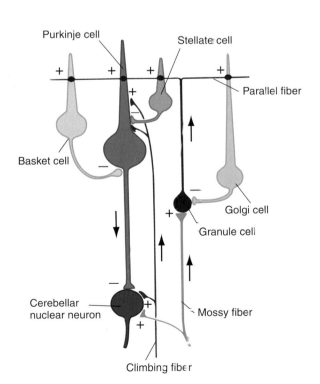

FIGURE 24.13 *The cerebellar cortex.* Schematic of the main cell types and their synaptic arrangements. The three types of GABAergic interneurons are colored green. (Redrawn from Eccles et al. 1967.)

Further, the same body part is usually represented in several widely separated patches. This arrangement of the mossy fibers was termed **fractured somatotopy** by Welker. It presumably is a means to integrate various inputs sharing relevance for a certain movement. How this pattern of mossy fiber inputs is coordinated with the climbing fiber inputs is not clear. As discussed later (Fig. 24.18), the climbing fibers terminate in narrow sagittal strips or zones, and one such strip is often related to one body part only.

EFFERENT CONNECTIONS OF THE CEREBELLUM

As previously mentioned, the three main subdivisions of the cerebellum act largely on the parts of the nervous system from which they receive afferent inputs. The vast majority of the Purkinje cell axons end in the cerebellar nuclei (corticonuclear fibers). The neurons of these nuclei forward the information to the various targets of the cerebellum.

The Cerebellar Nuclei and the Corticonuclear Connections

The cerebellar nuclei are located in the deep white matter of the cerebellum, just above the roof of the fourth ventricle (Figs. 24.2 and 24.14). In humans, there are four nuclei on each side. Close to the midline, under the vermis, lies the **fastigial nucleus** (medial cerebellar nucleus); then follow two small nuclei; and most laterally lies the large, folded **dentate nucleus** (lateral cerebellar nucleus). The two small nuclei have specific names in humans (the **globose** and the **emboliform** nuclei) and correspond to the anterior and posterior **interposed nuclei** in animals.

The **corticonuclear connections** are precisely, topographically organized, so that, as a rule, fibers from the anterior parts of the cerebellar cortex end in anterior parts of the nuclei, fibers from medial parts of the cortex end medially, and so forth. There is in addition a marked **longitudinal localization**, with the vermis sending fibers to the fastigial nucleus, the intermediate zone to the interposed nuclei, and the hemispheres to the dentate nucleus (Fig. 24.15). There is also somatotopic localization within each of the nuclei so that different parts influence movements in different parts of the body. Overall, signals from different parts of the cerebellum are kept segregated through the nuclei and further on to other parts of the brain. Thus, each of the nuclei sends efferent fibers to a separate target region, as shown in a very simplified manner in Figs. 24.6, 24.9, and 24.11.

Direct Projections from the Cerebellum to the Vestibular Nuclei

Parts of the vestibular nuclei correspond in certain respects to the cerebellar nuclei. Thus, the Purkinje cells of the **vestibulocerebellum** send their axons directly to the vestibular nuclei as **corticovestibular** fibers (Fig. 24.5). These fibers end primarily in vestibular nuclei that send ascending connections to the nuclei of the external ocular muscles (the medial longitudinal fasciculus; see Fig. 18.8) and, to a lesser extent, in parts of the nuclei sending fibers to the spinal cord. The vestibular nuclei also receive direct projections from Purkinje cells of the vermis of the **anterior** and the **posterior lobes**—that is, outside the vestibulocerebellum as defined here. These fibers end primarily in the lateral vestibular nucleus (nucleus of Deiters; see Figs. 18.7 and 18.8), which projects to the spinal cord. Thus, the cerebellar vermis

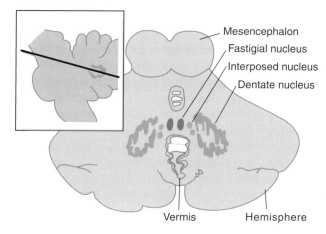
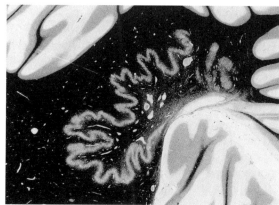

FIGURE 24.14 *The cerebellar nuclei.* **Left:** Drawing of an oblique section through the cerebellum and the brain stem. **Right:** Photomicrograph of a myelin-stained section placed slightly more dorsally than the drawing. Therefore, only the dentate and the interposed nuclei are seen in the photomicrograph.

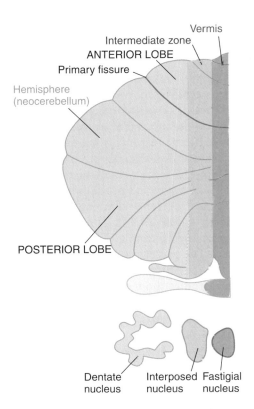

FIGURE 24.15 *Sagittal arrangement of corticonuclear connections.* Purkinje cells in the hemispheres project to the dentate nucleus, whereas Purkinje cells in the intermediate zone and the vermis project to the interposed and fastigial nucleus, respectively. In addition, Purkinje cells in the anterior and posterior vermis project to the vestibular nuclei.

can influence spinal motoneurons via the lateral vestibulospinal tract, besides its effects mediated by means of the fastigial nucleus to the reticular formation and the lateral vestibular nucleus. The vestibulocerebellum thus contributes to the control of eye movements, whereas the vermis via the vestibular nuclei primarily controls posture and equilibrium.

Cerebellar Nuclear Neurons Are Spontaneously Active

The nuclear cells fire with a high frequency even in an animal sitting quietly. When neurons fire without any obvious excitatory input, they are said to be **spontaneously active**. Indeed, in vitro studies of cerebellar slices show that the nuclear neurons have intrinsic properties that depolarize the membrane even in the absence of an excitatory input (**pacemaker** properties). Because all Purkinje cells are inhibitory (GABA), a continuous firing of the nuclear cells is a prerequisite for the information from the cerebellar cortex to be passed on (increased Purkinje cell activity leads to reduced nuclear cell firing). In addition to their tendency for spontaneous depolarization, the nuclear cells receive some excitatory inputs, namely the spinocerebellar and olivocerebellar projections that give off collaterals to the cerebellar nuclei.

Increase or decrease in the firing frequency of the Purkinje cells immediately causes change in the activity of the nuclear cells. A prerequisite for this is synchronous firing of many Purkinje cells with axons converging on a few nuclear cells. Then even minute changes of the activity of each Purkinje cell changes the signals issued from the cerebellum to its target nuclei. Indeed, there is evidence that **synchronous firing** of assemblies of functionally related Purkinje cells is a fundamental feature in cerebellar functioning.

In conclusion, the outputs of the cerebellar nuclei reflect with high temporal precision even very weak inputs to the cerebellar cortex. This is presumably important for, among other tasks, the cerebellar role in control of rhythm, as we discuss later in this chapter.

Organization of Efferent Connections from the Cerebellar Nuclei

The fibers from the **dentate nucleus** leave the cerebellum through the superior cerebellar peduncle (Fig. 24.2). They cross the midline in the mesencephalon, and some fibers end in the red nucleus of the opposite side. Most fibers continue rostrally, however, to end in the thalamus. Here, the dentate fibers end primarily in the **ventrolateral nucleus, VL** (some also reach the VA) (Fig. 24.16). These nuclei also receive fibers from the basal ganglia, but they end in different parts than the cerebellar fibers (as shown schematically in Fig. 24.16), in agreement with physiological studies showing that the basal ganglia and the cerebellum do not influence identical parts of the cortex. Signals from the cerebellar hemispheres pass primarily to the **MI**, whereas the basal ganglia via the thalamus act mainly on premotor areas and the prefrontal cortex. In addition, the cerebellum influences parts of the **SMA** and **PMA** that apparently differ from the parts influenced from the basal ganglia. There is also anatomic and physiological evidence of connections from the dentate nucleus (via the thalamus) to area 9 in the dorsolateral **prefrontal cortex**. Even though such connections most likely are modest compared to those reaching the motor areas, they are suggested to be of decisive importance for the cerebellar influence on cognitive tasks.

As mentioned, the efferents from the intermediate zone reach the **interposed nuclei**. These send their efferents both to the contralateral **thalamus** (to the VL mainly, like the dentate) and the **red nucleus** (Fig. 24.11). This enables the interposed nuclei to influence motoneurons via both the rubrospinal tract and the pyramidal tract. Because the rubrospinal tract is crossed, the interposed nucleus (and the intermediate zone) acts on the body half of the same side. The human rubrospinal tract is, however, most likely too small to be of much functional significance (cf. Chapter 22, under "The Red Nucleus and the Rubrospinal Tract").

Eye movements may also be disturbed in humans with cerebellar lesions that affect the vestibulocerebellum.

Damage to the **anterior lobe** in experimental animals primarily produces a change of **muscle tone**. In decerebrate animals, the decerebrate rigidity increases, as do the postural reflexes. This fits with the observation that electrical stimulation of the anterior lobe reduces the decerebrate rigidity (as mentioned, the Purkinje cells inhibit the cells of the cerebellar nuclei, whereas the nuclear cells have excitatory actions on reticulospinal and vestibulospinal neurons).[8] In addition, some Purkinje cells in the anterior lobe vermis send axons directly to the vestibular nuclei, and removal of this inhibitory action would also tend to increase the activity of the vestibulospinal neurons and thus the decerebrate rigidity. In **humans**, it is doubtful whether lesions of the anterior lobe produce increased muscle tone. More marked is **gait ataxia** (unsteadiness of walking) in patients with damage that mainly affects the anterior lobe vermis and the intermediate zone (this occurs in cerebellar degeneration caused by alcohol abuse). The anterior lobe vermis, by means of its efferent connections to the fastigial nucleus and from there to the reticular formation, must therefore be assumed to have a role in coordination of the half-automatic movements of walking and postural adjustments. Similarly, selective lesions of the fastigial nucleus in monkeys cause difficulties with walking, sitting, and maintaining the upright position.

Cerebellar Lesions and Eye Movements

As mentioned, lesions of the flocculonodular lobe can cause nystagmus. This may manifest itself as **spontaneous nystagmus** (i.e., nystagmus occurring in a person at rest with no kind of stimulation) or only when the patient tries to keep the gaze in an eccentric position (paralysis of gaze nystagmus). Conceivably, these symptoms are due to the loss of Purkinje cells that normally inhibit the vestibular nuclei (especially the medial nucleus) sending fibers to the nuclei of the extrinsic eye muscles (see Fig. 18.8). In addition, the patients with lesions of the flocculonodular lobe may have difficulties with slow **pursuit movements** (tracking a moving object with the gaze). Pursuit movements may also be impaired after lesions restricted to lateral parts of the **pontine nuclei** or the **cerebellar hemispheres** (impaired to the side of the lesion). Finally, lesions of the cerebellar hemisphere may cause so-called **saccadic dysmetria**—that is,

---

8 Electrical stimulation with electrodes surgically implanted at the cerebellar surface has been used in patients with neurological disorders such as **epilepsy** and **cerebral palsy**. The theoretical basis is the inhibitory action of the Purkinje cells with subsequent reduction of abnormally increased neuronal excitability and muscle tone. Even though some report favorable results with such stimulation, there is no agreement as to whether the effect is due to the cerebellar stimulation or to some other factor.

the rapid eye movements overshoot the target and are followed by several correcting movements before the gaze is finally fixed. The role of the cerebellum in the control of eye movements is further discussed in Chapter 25, under "The Cerebellum Controls Both Saccades and Pursuit Movements."

The Neocerebellar Syndrome

The neocerebellum plays a different functional role than the phylogenetically older parts of the cerebellum: it is primarily concerned with the coordination of the (least automatic) voluntary movements. This stands to reason, since the cerebellar hemispheres send their main output to the MI (via the dentate nucleus and the thalamus) and thus influence the neurons of the pyramidal tract (Figs. 24.9 and 24.18). After removal of one cerebellar hemisphere in a monkey, the voluntary movements become uncertain on the same side of the body: they become **uncoordinated** or **ataxic**. The same effect can be produced by cooling the dentate nucleus (by the use of a cooling electrode) in a monkey that is performing a well-rehearsed movement (as soon as the cooling is reversed, the movements again become normal). Movements that were performed quickly and smoothly become unsteady and jerky by the cooling. The monkey misses repeatedly when trying to grasp an object, even though it knows perfectly well where it is and what is demanded. Sometimes the hand is moved too far in relation to the object, sometimes too short. The movements tend to be **decomposed**; that is, instead of occurring simultaneously in several joints, they take place in one joint at a time, and the **velocity** is uneven—sometimes too high and sometimes too low. Selective damage or transient "uncoupling" of the dentate nucleus in monkeys indicates that the cerebellar hemispheres are particularly important when movements must take place in **several joints** at the same time. Picking up a raisin, for example, became impossible because the monkey could no longer coordinate the movements of the joints of the wrist, thumb, and index finger. Precise movements of one finger at the time could be done normally, however. Difficulties with hitting an object when trying to grasp it with the hand can probably be attributed to the same basic defect; that is, difficulties with coordinating the movements of the wrist, shoulder, and elbow joints.

Ataxia of this kind is also the most prominent symptom in **humans** with damage to the cerebellar hemispheres. For example, difficulty with the **precision grip** similar to that described in monkeys has recently been observed in patients with unilateral infarcts of the cerebellar hemispheres. The increase of force when grasping an object is slower than normal and the adjustment of the grip force is deficient when grasping and lifting at the same time. In clinical neurology, the various elements of ataxia have particular names, such as **dysmetria** (movement is not stopped in time), **asynergia** (decomposition of complex movements), **dysdiadochokinesia** (reduced ability to perform rapidly alternating movements of, for example, the hand), and **intentional tremor** (tremor arising when trying to perform a movement, such as grasping an object). Speech is also often disturbed in cerebellar diseases. It has been called **speech ataxia**, to emphasize that it also appears to be caused by incoordination (in the respiratory muscles, the muscles of the larynx, and others), making the strength and velocity of the speech uneven.

All the elements of ataxia have been attributed to a fundamental defect in control of the force and of the exact timing of the **starting** and **stopping** of movements.[9] As mentioned, the **temporal** aspect appears to be central to the cerebellar contribution to motor control. This is evidenced by patients with cerebellar damage who are unable to perform sequences of finger movements in a particular **rhythm**. The movements are done by each finger without a fixed temporal relation to movements of the other fingers.

In acute damage to the cerebellar hemispheres in humans, the muscle tone often appears to be reduced when tested by passive stretch (the symptom is transient). This is called **cerebellar hypotonia**. The underlying mechanism is not clear, although experiments in anesthetized animals suggested that it is caused by reduced γ motoneuron activity. Recent experiments in awake animals and in humans, however, show that the muscle-spindle sensitivity to stretch is not significantly altered by cerebellar lesions (even when they include the dentate and interposed nuclei).

The Timing Theory: Does the Cerebellum Perform a Basic Operation Used in All Its Functions?

Even though the study of cerebellar symptoms provides reasonable insight into the functions of the cerebellum, we are far from understanding how the cerebellum performs its tasks. The striking uniformity and strictly geometric structure of the cerebellar cortex has led to comparison with a **computer**, which can perform the same kinds of computations on various kinds of information. The subdivision of the cerebellum into numerous, apparently independent units or modules may fit such a concept. Several theories have been put forward to explain how the cerebellum operates. None of them has so far been universally accepted, however, and there is disagreement with regard to interpretation of some experiments said to support one theory or the other.

9 It is not certain, however, that this suffices to explain why the symptoms are most marked when movements in two or more joints must be coordinated (such as moving the index finger quickly to the tip of the nose from a position with the arm stretched out).

The German neuroscientist Valentin Braitenberg proposed more than 50 years ago that the cerebellum functions as a kind of **clock**, measuring temporal intervals with great accuracy. The theory was subsequently modified to emphasize the cerebellar role in the control of **movement sequences** and perhaps other sequential behaviors. The theory is based on, among other things, the regular arrangement of the parallel fibers (Figs. 24.12 and 24.13). Action potentials conducted along the parallel fibers will excite the Purkinje cells in a fixed temporal sequence. We discussed that a timing function might be crucial in the cerebellar contribution to motor control, and recent data suggest that the cerebellar timing function may also be used in nonmotor tasks. Thus, patients with cerebellar damage were impaired not only in their ability to reproduce a certain rhythm by tapping their fingers but also in discriminating different sound rhythms—that is, not only impaired execution but also **perception of rhythm**. They had no problems with discriminating sounds of different intensities, however, which suggest that the defect is specific to discrimination of **temporal intervals**. Reduced ability to judge the velocity of visual stimuli has also been reported in patients with cerebellar lesions.

The **inferior olive** and the climbing fibers may have a crucial role in the timing function of the cerebellum. Thus, the olivary neurons fire rhythmically, and neurons that activate Purkinje cells within a narrow sagittal zone fire synchronously. Further, there is experimental evidence that the firing rhythm of olivary neurons and the rhythm of certain movements is correlated (see also the earlier section, "The Inferior Olive").

Another aspect of timing is the judgment of **duration**, for example, how long time has passed since I started a particular action (mental or physical)? Whether the cerebellum plays a role for this time function as well is not clear (see also Chapter 23, under "Interval Timing").

The Cerebellum and Motor Learning

Animal experiments indicate that long-lasting changes in synaptic efficacy may take place in the cerebellar cortex during motor learning. Much interest is devoted to theories that consider the cerebellum to be a learning machine. The cerebellum may help automation of movements and perhaps also of certain cognitive functions. There is considerable evidence that plastic changes occur in the cerebellum during motor learning. For example, the activation of the cerebellar hemispheres (as measured with fMRI) is higher when a new sequence of movements is learned than when the automated movement is performed afterward. We discussed the possible role of the **climbing fibers** in motor learning, and **LTD** as a likely cellular mechanism (see the earlier section, "Mossy and Climbing Fibers Mediate Different Kinds of Information"). Recent studies found that patients

25 | Control of Eye Movements

OVERVIEW

For the eye to provide useful information to higher visual centers, the picture must be held stationary on the retina. Further, the eyes must be positioned so that the most salient part of a visual scene falls on the central part of the retina with the highest visual acuity. Finally, to sample enough information, the eyes must be moved quickly from one point of salience to another. The control system must therefore be able to move the eyes quickly and precisely to make the image fall on the macula; such movements are called **saccades** (or saccadic movements). In addition, the control system must move the eyes so the retinal image is stationary even if the head or the object is moving. The latter are called **slow-pursuit movements**. The extraocular muscles responsible for moving the eyes receive their nerve supply from the nuclei of the **third, fourth, and sixth cranial nerves**. The control system coordinates the activity of the α motoneurons in these nuclei. **Premotor networks** interconnecting areas in the cerebral cortex, the brain stem, and the cerebellum carry out this task. To enable coordinated activity, the nuclei of the extraocular muscles are interconnected by numerous fibers forming the **medial longitudinal fascicle**. The control system uses **sensory information** from the retina, which informs about whether the retinal image is stationary or slipping, from the **vestibular apparatus** about the movements of the head, and from **proprioceptors** in the eye muscles about the movements of the eyes in the orbit. All this sensory information is integrated and transformed into a **motor signal** specifying the total activity of the extraocular muscles at any time. For control of **horizontal eye movements**—especially saccades—the most important premotor area, the **paramedian pontine reticular formation** (PPRF), lies close to the abducens nucleus on each side. The PPRF sends fibers to the abducens and oculomotor nuclei and coordinates their activities. A corresponding premotor area for **vertical eye movements** is found in the mesencephalic reticular formation close to the oculomotor nucleus.

There is an important difference between the control of eye muscles and of other muscles subjected to precise voluntary control (e.g., intrinsic hand muscles): the nuclei of the extraocular muscles—in contrast to spinal α motoneurons—receive no direct fibers from the cerebral cortex. The central control is exerted via premotor networks in the brain stem. At least two regions of the cerebral cortex are closely involved in the control of eye movements (Fig. 15.7): the **frontal eye field** is primarily related to initiation of saccadic movements, whereas several smaller areas in the **parietotemporal region** are mainly involved in the control of pursuit movements.

The third, fourth, and sixth cranial nerves and their nuclei are treated in Chapter 27, together with the light reflex and accommodation reflex mediated by the intrinsic eye muscles. Chapter 16 gives a brief account of the structure of the eye.

MOVEMENTS OF THE EYES AND THE EYE MUSCLES

Horizontal, Vertical, and Rotatory Movements of the Eye

The eye is a sphere, lying in the orbit, surrounded by fat. It can rotate freely in any direction around its center, whereas translatory movements are prevented. To describe the rotatory movements of a sphere, we define **three axes**, passing through the center and oriented perpendicular to each other. For convenience, we describe the movements as taking place in three planes: a **frontal**, **sagittal**, and a transverse or **horizontal** plane. A movement in the horizontal plane takes place around a vertical axis, and the anterior part of the eye—and therefore the gaze—moves from side to side. We perform **horizontal eye movements** when looking to one side; when looking to the left, the left eye rotates laterally and the right eye rotates medially. A movement in the sagittal plane takes place around a transverse axis, and the anterior part of the eye moves up and down. Such movements, directing the gaze up and down, are called **vertical eye movements**. Movements in the frontal plane take place around a sagittal axis, and the eye rotates without any horizontal or vertical movement. For practical reasons only, such movements around a sagittal axis are called **rotatory eye movements** (strictly speaking, all eye movements are rotations around the center of the eyeball).

The Extraocular Muscles and Their Actions

The six extraocular (extrinsic) muscles (Fig. 25.1) ensure that the **visual axes** of the eyes (see Fig. 16.2) can be directed precisely toward any point in the visual field. The scheme in Fig. 15.2 shows the main movements produced by each of the extraocular muscles if they were acting alone (this is a theoretical situation, because in reality they always work in concert). Most of the muscles produce combinations of vertical, horizontal, and rotatory movements. Further, the actions of each of the muscles change with the position of the eye because this changes the position and direction of the line of pull. The extraocular muscles (Fig. 25.1; see also Fig. 27.16) all **attach** to the sclera and originate from the wall of the orbit (a brief account of the structure of the eye bulb is given in Chapter 16). We analyze the **actions** of the extraocular muscles in relation to the above-defined three axes through the center of the eyeball. We then need to know the direction of the force exerted by the muscles in relation to the axis. We must furthermore know whether the muscle insertion in the sclera is anterior or posterior to the **equatorial plane** of the eye, a frontal plane dividing the eye in an anterior and a posterior half.

There are **four straight** and **two oblique extraocular muscles** (Fig. 25.1, see also Fig. 27.16). Figure 25.2 shows schematically the actions of each muscle if it acted alone. Most muscle produce movements that are composed of horizontal, vertical, and rotatory components. We can nevertheless simplify their functions by stating that two muscles produce predominantly horizontal movements (the medial and lateral rectus muscles), two produce predominantly vertical movements (the superior and inferior rectus muscles), whereas two muscles produce mainly rotatory movements (the superior and inferior oblique muscles). The straight ones (the rectus muscles) come from the posterior end of the orbit and run forward to insert in front of the equatorial plane. This means that the **lateral rectus** muscle pulls the front of the eye (the cornea) laterally, whereas the **medial rectus** muscle pulls it medially (these two muscles thus produce pure horizontal movements). Correspondingly, the

superior rectus muscle pulls the eye (the cornea) upward, whereas the **inferior rectus** muscle pulls it downward. These two therefore produce vertical movements. Because the superior and inferior rectus muscles run anteriorly in a lateral direction, however, they do not only produce vertical movements but also some horizontal movement (in the medial direction). Thus, when the superior rectus muscle acts alone, it produces an upward movement combined with a (smaller) medial— that is, an oblique movement. In addition, the muscle produces a small medial rotation of the eye (around the sagittal axis). The **superior oblique** muscle has a more complicated course than the other extraocular muscles (Fig. 15.1; see also Fig. 27.16). It originates posteriorly in the orbit and runs forward medially. Just behind the anterior margin of the orbit, it bends sharply around a small hook of connective tissue and continues in a posterolateral direction to insert posterior to the equatorial plane. The muscle has actions around all three axes: it rotates the eye around the sagittal axis so that the upper part moves medially and furthermore directs the gaze downward and laterally (Fig. 15.2). The **inferior oblique** muscle originates from the bottom of the orbit in its anteromedial part and runs, like the superior oblique, posterolaterally to insert behind the equator (Fig. 15.1). It directs the gaze laterally and upward and rotates the eye around the sagittal axis with its upper part laterally.

These considerations and the scheme in Fig. 15.2 concern movements starting from a **neutral position** of the eye—that is, when viewing a distant object straight ahead. Changing the position of the eye in the orbit also changes the action of the muscles (for some muscles the change is small, for others quite marked). For example, the superior rectus is a pure elevator when the eye is 23 degrees abducted. The oblique muscles perform pure vertical movements when the eye is about 50 degrees abducted (cf. Fig. 27.16 showing the line of action of the superior oblique). This is basis for the test of the extraocular muscles in Fig. 25.3, designed to test each muscle in isolation (as far as possible).

Natural Eye Movements Are Conjugated

Virtually every natural eye movement is a combination of the various movement directions described in the preceding text. By combining proper amounts of vertical and horizontal movements, any oblique movement can be produced. Further, all natural eye movements are **conjugated**—that is, the two eyes move together to ensure that the image always falls on corresponding points of the two retinas (see Fig. 16.3). **Double vision** (**diplopia**) results if the eye movements do not occur in conjugation. This is a typical symptom of pareses of the extraocular muscles.

Almost all eye movements require a complicated cooperation of numerous muscles, with activation of synergists

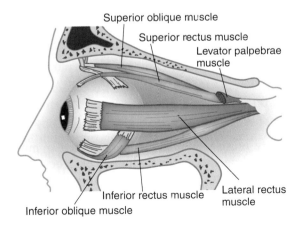

Superior oblique muscle
Superior rectus muscle
Levator palpebrae muscle
Inferior rectus muscle
Lateral rectus muscle
Inferior oblique muscle

FIGURE 25.1 *The extraocular muscles seen from the lateral aspect.* The lateral wall of the orbit is removed. The straight muscles insert in front of the equatorial plane of the eye, whereas the oblique muscles insert behind it (see also Fig. 27.16, which shows the orbit and the eye muscles from above).

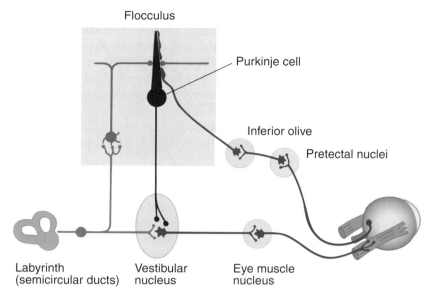

FIGURE 25.4 *Main structural elements of the vestibulo-ocular reflex.* Only excitatory connections are shown, even though there are inhibitory neurons in the vestibular nuclei that influence the motoneurons of the antagonists. The reflex arc consists of three neurons from the semicircular duct to the extraocular muscles. The cerebellar flocculus receives signals from the labyrinth and from the retina, and the output of the Purkinje cells can adjust the sensitivity of the vestibular neurons, if necessary, to avoid retinal slip. (Based on Ito 1984.)

reflex is three-dimensional in the sense that all directions of head rotation elicit specific compensatory eye movements.[1]

5. **Vergence** movements change the visual axes of the eyes in relation to each other when the point of fixation moves away from or toward the eyes. This is necessary to keep the image on corresponding points of the retina. Vergence movements are a prerequisite for fusion of the two images and for stereoscopic vision. **Convergence of the visual axes**, which takes place when an object is approaching the eyes, depends primarily on the activity of the medial rectus muscles, with some contribution also from the superior and inferior recti (Fig. 15.2). **Accommodation** and **pupillary constriction** accompany convergence movements.[2]

More about Voluntary Saccades and Scanning

When **reading** we fixate a point on the line for an average of 250 msec (60–500) before the gaze is moved on by a saccade. How far the gaze moves before reaching a new point of fixation varies greatly. There is a tendency to fixate on long "content" words rather than on short "functional" words. Native readers of English perceive about 4 letters to the left and 15 to the right of the point of fixation.

A woman with inborn **ophthalmoplegia** (inability to move the eyes) had surprisingly small problems and was able to live a normal life. She apparently used quick head movements to compensate for the lack of saccadic eye movements (Gilchrist 1997), and was thereby able to scan the visual scene with sufficient speed and accuracy.

The Cerebellum Can Adjust the Vestibulo-Ocular Reflex to Changing External Conditions

The magnitude of the reflex response (not the response itself) to a certain rotational stimulus depends on signals to the vestibular nuclei from the cerebellum (Fig. 25.4). The Purkinje cells of the vestibulocerebellum receive primary vestibular fibers (ending as mossy fibers) that provide information about direction and velocity of the head movement. In addition, the same Purkinje cells receive information, via the inferior olive and climbing fibers, about whether the image is stationary or slips on the retina. A retinal slip indicates that the velocity of the compensatory head movement is too high or too low. The cerebellum is then capable of adjusting the excitability (the gain) of the neurons in the vestibular nuclei—that is, in the reflex center of the vestibulo-ocular reflex. Such adaptive change of **gain of the reflex** is presumably needed continuously during growth and in situations of muscular fatigue. Experiments in which animals wear optic prisms that deflect the light so that it appears to come from another direction than it really does, show the remarkable capacity for adaptation (learning) in this system.

---

1 The VOR described here—the **rotational VOR** or RVOR—is not the only vestibulo-ocular reflex. Translatory (linear) accelerations of the head (stimulating the sacculus and utriculus) also elicit compensatory eye movements (**translational VOR**, or TVOR; **otolith-OR**, or OOR). In real life, both kinds of head movement occur, and the different sensory inputs from the labyrinth must be integrated centrally to yield a motor command that ensures a stable retinal image.

2 **Gaze holding** is sometimes included among the kinds of eye movement. It is the ability to stabilize the eye position (and the image on the retina) after a shift of gaze. Premotor neurons controlling gaze holding appear to rely on a partly separate premotor network, although located close to the paramedian pontine reticular formation (PPRF) and the rostral interstitial nucleus of the medial longitudinal fasciculus (riMLF).

Brain Stem Centers for Control of Eye Movements

Signals informing about desired eye position, actual position, retinal slip, and position of the head are integrated in the **reticular formation** close to the eye muscle nuclei. From these **premotor** neuronal groups commands are sent to the α motoneurons. By combining anatomic data on the fiber connections with physiological results (obtained by single-cell recordings, electrical and natural stimulation, and lesions) the preoculomotor networks have been described in detail.

A "center" for **horizontal eye movements** has been identified in the **paramedian pontine reticular formation** (PPRF). PPRF lies close to, and sends fibers to, the abducens nucleus (Fig. 25.5). It also sends fibers to the parts of the oculomotor nucleus that contains the motoneurons of the medial rectus muscle. Together with the lateral rectus (innervated by the abducens nucleus), the medial rectus participates in horizontal movements. In addition, there are so-called **internuclear neurons** in the abducens nucleus that send axons to the medial rectus motoneurons of the opposite side (Fig. 25.6). This premotor network ensures simultaneous activation of the lateral rectus on one side and the medial rectus on the other, along with inhibition of the antagonists.

A **lesion** in the region of the **PPRF** reduces horizontal conjugate movements to the side of the lesion. Especially marked is the reduction in saccadic movements. A unilateral lesion of the **medial longitudinal fasciculus** between the abducens and the oculomotor nucleus produces

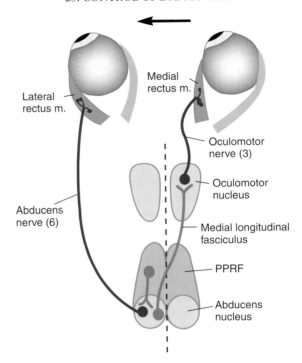

FIGURE 25.6 *Control of horizontal conjugate eye movements*. Highly simplified scheme to show some of the connections responsible. Only excitatory connections are included. The figure also shows how interruption of the medial longitudinal fascicle produces a paralysis of the gaze in the medial direction (internuclear ophthalmoplegia).

so-called **internuclear ophthalmoplegia** with abolished ability to adduct the eye on the same side (the medial rectus muscle). This may be understood based on the diagram in Fig. 25.6. However, **vergence** movements are possible even though the medial rectus is responsible also in that case. Thus, pathways other than the medial longitudinal fasciculus are responsible for the activation of the medial rectus muscle during vergence movements.

A center for **vertical** and rotatory eye movements has been identified in the reticular formation close to the oculomotor nucleus. This region includes a nucleus called the **rostral interstitial nucleus of the medial longitudinal fasciculus** (riMLF or RI) and probably another small cell group (the **interstitial nucleus of Cajal**). This region receives **afferents** from the vestibular nuclei, the pretectum (and thereby indirectly from the superior colliculus), and the frontal eye field. Physiologic studies indicate that there are monosynaptic connections from the region of the riMLF to the trochlear nucleus and to the motoneuron groups within the oculomotor nucleus that produce vertical eye movements.

The PPRF and the region of the RI are interconnected, indicating that they do not operate independently of each other. The fact that most natural eye movements are neither purely horizontal not purely vertical but combinations of both strongly suggests that the centers

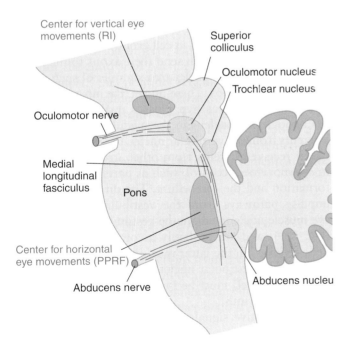

FIGURE 25.5 *Centers for vertical and horizontal eye movements*. Sagittal section through the monkey brain stem. (Based on Büttner-Ennever 1988.)

Pursuit Movements

With regard to cortical control of **smooth-pursuit movements**, several small areas in the parietal lobe, and at the temporo-occipital junction are of particular importance (Fig. 15.7; see also Figs. 16.25 and 34.2). This notion is based on, among other things, single-cell recordings. The **middle temporal area** (area **MT**, V5) is important for perception of movement. Neurons in MT respond to movement of the image on the retina (retinal slip), which is a strong stimulus to elicit pursuit movements of the eyes. The **middle superior temporal area** (area **MST**) lies close to area MT and is of special interest because it contains many neurons that respond preferentially to moving visual stimuli in a specific direction. The subcortical cell groups intercalated between these cortical regions and the eye muscle nuclei are not fully clarified. One important pathway seems to go from the cortex to the **pontine nuclei** (see Fig. 24.10), then to the **cerebellum**, further to the **vestibular nuclei** and the **reticular formation**, and thence to the eye muscle nuclei. In addition to in the parietal and temporal areas, neurons with activity related to pursuit movements occur in the frontal eye field and the supplementary eye field. Accordingly, impairment of pursuit movements has been reported in humans with frontal lesions including the supplementary eye field.

Gaze Fixation

The ability to **fix the gaze** is a prerequisite for voluntary slow-pursuit movements. A specific fixation center in the cerebral cortex has not been found; as with most other tasks carried out by the cerebral cortex the task is solved in a distributed network. In monkeys, single neurons that change their activity in relation to gaze fixation are present in the frontal eye field and in the posterior parietal cortex. PET studies in humans, however, indicate that frontal lobes are particularly important for the ability actively to fix the gaze. This includes the **frontal eye field**, the **anterior cingulate gyrus**, and parts of the **prefrontal cortex**. In general, these regions become active in conjunction with **directed attention**, and lesions in humans produce an impaired ability to fix the gaze.

Often the tendency to fix the gaze on an object is not voluntary (cf. the term fixation reflex), at least not in the strict sense (even though fixation depends on the person being conscious). **Optokinetic nystagmus** is an expression of the strong tendency to fix the gaze. When a screen with alternating black and white vertical stripes is moved horizontally in front of a person, nystagmus occurs. The gaze is fixed automatically on one of the stripes and follows it until it leaves the visual field. Then a quick movement resets the eyes to the starting position, and the gaze is fixed again on another stripe. This sequence repeats itself as long as the screen moves.

Miniature Eye Movements

Closer study shows that even during active fixation, the eyes are not completely still. Several kinds of **miniature movement** occur, such as a slow drift of the eyes, miniature saccades, and tremor. The amplitudes of these movements are very small, however, and are not normally perceived. Nevertheless, the phenomenon can be demonstrated by fixating a square pattern for about 20 seconds and then move the gaze to a white surface. The afterimage of the square pattern is then seen to move, because the eyes are not completely still (Ilg 1997).

V | THE BRAIN STEM AND THE CRANIAL NERVES

THE definition of the term brain stem varies. The widest definition—used in Chapter 6—includes the medulla oblongata, the pons, the mesencephalon, and the diencephalon. In this part of the book, and most often in clinical contexts, we restrict it to the **medulla**, the **pons**, and the **mesencephalon**, which together form a macroscopically distinct part of the brain. Which definition is used is of no great importance because the brain stem is a topographically and embryologically defined unit; it does not represent a functional "system." Neuronal groups within the brain stem take part in virtually all the tasks of the central nervous system.

Functionally, the brain stem may be said to have two levels of organization. On the one hand, most of the cranial nerves and their nuclei represent "the spinal cord of the head." On the other hand, many neuronal groups in the brain stem represent a superior level of control over the spinal cord and the cranial nerve nuclei. Examples are the vestibular nuclei and various premotor nuclei in the reticular formation. In addition, other neuronal groups—usually included in the reticular formation—exert ascending influences on the thalamus and the cerebral cortex related to consciousness, arousal, and sleep. This section deals with both levels of organization. Chapter 26 deals with the reticular formation, which represents the superior level of control. Chapter 27 describes most of the cranial nerves and their nuclei.

26 | The Reticular Formation: Premotor Networks, Consciousness, and Sleep

OVERVIEW

The reticular formation extends from the lower end of the medulla to the upper end of the mesencephalon. At all levels, it occupies the central parts and fills the territories not occupied by cranial nerve nuclei and other distinct nuclei and by the large fiber tracts. The **raphe nuclei** (serotonin) and the **locus coeruleus** (norepinephrine) are often included in the reticular formation, and are treated in this chapter. Although the reticular formation consists of many functionally diverse subdivisions, they all share some anatomic features. Thus, the neurons have wide dendritic arborizations and their long axons give off numerous collaterals. The afferent and efferent connections show only a rough topographic order. Efferent connections reach most parts of the central nervous system (CNS, from the cord to the cerebral cortex), while afferents bring all kinds of sensory information. These features show that the reticular formation is built for **integration**. Accordingly, the reticular formation attends primarily to tasks involving the nervous system and the organism as a whole. Subdivisions of the reticular formation form **premotor networks** that organize several complex behaviors. These behaviors include control of body **posture, orientation** of the head and body toward external stimuli, control of **eye movements**, and coordination of the activity of the **visceral organs**. These tasks fit with the reticular formation being phylogenetically old and present even in lower vertebrates. In addition, parts of the reticular formation (especially in the upper pons and mesencephalon) send ascending connections to the thalamus and the cerebral cortex. These connections form the **activating system of the brain stem**. The integrity of this system is a prerequisite for **consciousness**, and is closely linked to control of **awareness** and attention. Further, parts of the reticular formation, including cholinergic cell groups in the upper pons, are concerned with regulation of **sleep**.

STRUCTURE AND CONNECTIONS OF THE RETICULAR FORMATION

Structure and Subdivisions

The reticular formation extends from the lower end of the medulla to the upper end of the mesencephalon, where it gradually fuses with certain thalamic cell groups (Fig. 26.1).[1] At all levels it occupies the central parts and fills the territories not occupied by cranial nerve nuclei and other distinct nuclei (such as the dorsal column nuclei, the pontine nuclei, and the colliculi) and by the large fiber tracts (such as the medial lemniscus and the pyramidal tract). The reticular formation received its name from the early anatomists because of its network-like appearance in microscopic sections (Figs. 26.2 and 26.3). It is built of cells of various forms and sizes that appear to be rather randomly mixed. Between the cells, there is a wickerwork of fibers passing in many directions (Fig. 26.2). These fibers are partly axons and dendrites of the neurons of the reticular formation and partly afferent axons from other sections of the CNS. The reticular neurons have typically very long and straight **dendrites**, so that they cover a large volume of tissue (Fig. 26.3). This distinguishes the reticular neurons from those found in specific nuclei of the brain stem, such as the cranial nerve nuclei (see the hypoglossal nucleus in Fig. 26.3).

Medial Parts Are Afferent and Lateral Parts Are Efferent

A more detailed analysis of the reticular formation makes clear, however, that it consists of several **subdivisions**, among which the cells differ in shape, size, and arrangement even though the borders between such subdivisions are not sharp (Fig. 26.1). It is especially

---

1 Some authors include certain thalamic cell groups—especially the intralaminar nuclei—in the term "the reticular formation of the brain stem."

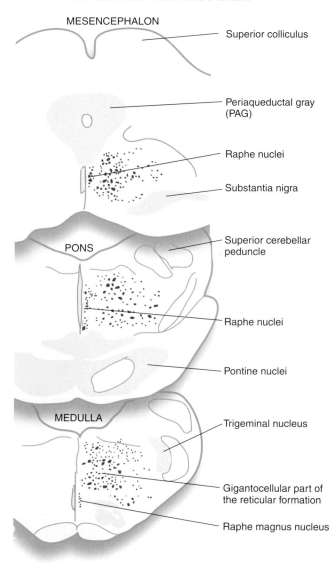

MESENCEPHALON

— Superior colliculus

— Periaqueductal gray (PAG)

— Raphe nuclei

— Substantia nigra

PONS

— Superior cerebellar peduncle

— Raphe nuclei

— Pontine nuclei

MEDULLA

— Trigeminal nucleus

— Gigantocellular part of the reticular formation

— Raphe magnus nucleus

FIGURE 26.1 *The reticular formation.* Transverse sections through various levels of the brain stem (cat) showing the position of the reticular formation. The size of the red dots indicates the size of the neurons, which varies considerably among subdivisions of the reticular formation. (Based on Brodal 1957.)

important that such cytoarchitectonically defined subdivisions also differ with regard to fiber connections, neurotransmitters, and functions. In the pons and the medulla, approximately the **medial two-thirds** of the reticular formation consists of many large cells, in part so-called **giant cells** (Figs. 26.1 and 26.2). The **lateral one-third** contains almost exclusively **small cells**. Tract-tracing methods have shown that the medial part sends out many long, ascending and descending fibers, whereas the lateral small-celled part receives most of the afferents coming to the reticular formation. In general, therefore, we may say that the lateral part is **receiving**, whereas the medial part is **efferent** (executive). The efferents convey the influence of the reticular formation to higher

parts, such as the thalamus, and lower parts, such as the spinal cord.

The Reticular Formation Is Built for Integration

Studies with the Golgi method and with intracellular tracers give evidence of how complexly the reticular formation is organized. The long ascending and descending efferent fibers give off numerous **collaterals** on their way through the brain stem (Fig. 26.4). As can be seen in Fig. 26.3, the collaterals run primarily in the transverse plane. Most dendrites of reticular cells have the same preferential orientation, so the reticular formation appears to consist of numerous **transversely oriented disks** (Fig. 26.3). The numerous collaterals of the axons from the cells in the medial parts ensure that signals from each reticular cell may reach many functionally diverse cell groups (such as other parts of the reticular formation, cranial nerve nuclei, dorsal column nuclei, colliculi, spinal cord, certain thalamic nuclei, and hypothalamus).

The Raphe Nuclei and the Locus Coeruleus: Common Features

The **raphe nuclei** (raphe, seam) together form a narrow, sagittally oriented plate of neurons in the midline of the medulla, pons, and mesencephalon (Figs. 26.1, 26.5, and 26.6). In many ways, these nuclei have similarities with the reticular formation proper and are often considered part of it. The **locus coeruleus** is small group of only about 15,000 strongly pigmented neurons located under the floor of the fourth ventricle (Fig. 26.7). It has clear borders except ventrally where it merges gradually with the adjoining reticular formation, which also contains many norepinephric neurons. This is one reason the locus coeruleus is often included in the reticular formation.

A characteristic feature of these two nuclei is that they contain only a small number of neurons, while their axons have extremely widespread ramifications, reaching virtually all parts of the brain and the spinal cord. Their synaptic actions are **modulatory**, although the effects vary among different targets due to different distribution of receptors. The raphe nuclei contain mainly **serotonergic** neurons, whereas the locus coeruleus neurons contain **norepinephrine** (cf. Chapter 5, under "Biogenic Amines"). Another special feature is that they send fibers directly to the cerebral cortex, that is, without synaptic interruption in the thalamus, as is typical of most cortical afferent pathways from lower levels. These features are shared with other cell groups, notably the dopaminergic neurons in the mesencephalon and the cholinergic cell groups in the pons and the basal forebrain (cf. Chapter 5, under "Modulatory Transmitter "Systems").

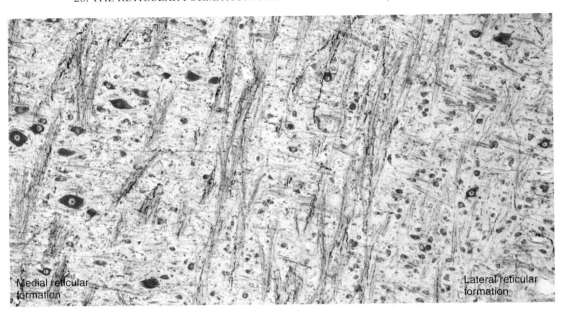

FIGURE 26.2 *The reticular formation.* Photomicrograph of section of the medulla, stained to show myelinated fibers (blue) and cell bodies (red). The cell bodies are distributed diffusely without clear nuclear borders and with small fiber bundles coursing in various directions. The photomicrograph shows the transition between the large-celled medial division and the small-celled lateral division. Magnification, ×300.

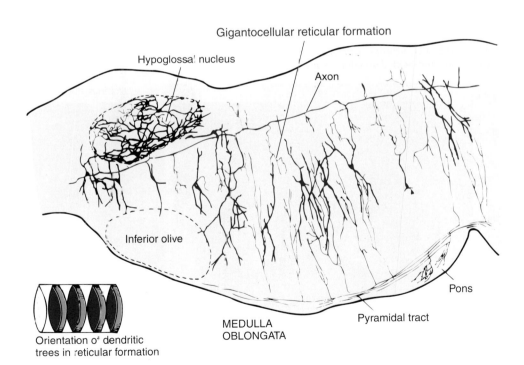

FIGURE 26.3 *Orientation of dendrites in the reticular formation.* Sagittal section through the medulla (rat). The long, straight dendrites are typical of the neurons of the reticular formation, in contrast to the neurons of a cranial nerve nucleus (the hypoglossal) and other specific brain stem nuclei. A long axon with numerous collaterals extending ventrally in the transverse plane is also shown. Collaterals of the pyramidal tract fibers enter the reticular formation. (Modified from Scheibel and Scheibel 1958.)

the hippocampus, and other limbic structures. Direct fibers also reach the spinal cord but only parts of the brain stem (especially sensory nuclei). The dense norepinephric innervation of the reticular formation and the motor nuclei must therefore originate from the scattered norepinephric neurons outside the locus coeruleus.

The **afferent** connections come mainly from a few regions. The locus coeruleus receives direct connections from the **cingulate gyrus** and the **orbitofrontal cortex** (in monkeys and presumably in humans as well). Subcortical afferents seem from recent studies to arise in the medullary part the reticular formation and in the amygdala. The medullary connections probably provide the locus coeruleus with integrated sensory information, while fibers from the amygdala might signal the emotional value of sensory information. **Single neurons** in the locus coeruleus respond preferentially to novel, "exciting" sensory stimuli. Because norepinephrine increases the response to specific stimuli and improves the signal-to-noise ratio of postsynaptic neurons, the locus coeruleus is believed to play a particular role in mediating **arousal** and **shifts of behavior**. One example is the facilitatory effect of norepinephrine on **spinal motoneurons** (see Chapter 22, under "Monoaminergic Pathway from the Brain Stem to the Spinal Cord"). Norepinephrine also has a special role in relation to synaptic **plasticity**. For example, it is especially concentrated in the cerebral cortex during sensitive periods of development.

Possible Tasks of the Raphe Nuclei and the Locus Coeruleus

The modulatory neurotransmitters—including serotonin and norepinephrine—influence virtually all brain functions. This is not surprising, considering the widely branching axons of the neurons containing these neurotransmitters. In view of the small and relatively homogeneous nuclei giving origin to the axons, it seems nevertheless possible that the multifarious actions are subject to a common aim or "plan." However, in spite of several unifying theories, none has obtained general acceptance. We here present just a few possible unifying concepts. One of the theories concerning **serotonin** views the raphe nuclei as especially important for **homeostatic control** (another theory tries to collect all serotonin actions under the heading of motor control). One of the facts favoring homeostatic control as a common theme is that many raphe neurons are **chemosensitive** and measure the CO_2 level in the blood (thus indirectly monitoring the pH of the nervous tissue). Chemosensitive neurons in the medulla participate in control of respiration (normalization of CO_2). Actions of serotonin on spinal motoneurons can perhaps have something to do with the fact that muscular activity is a major source of CO_2 production. Serotonergic actions

on pain transmission might be viewed in the perspective of pain as part of a homeostatic response, as discussed in Chapter 15. Further, chemosensitive neurons in the rostral raphe nuclei can increase wakefulness and alter cerebral circulation. They also seem to mediate signals that evoke anxiety associated with high blood CO_2 levels (a single inhalation of air with 35% CO_2 provokes acute anxiety).

An overarching function of the **locus coeruleus** may be to increase **arousal** and **attention** in response to salient sensory information. However, the task may be more specific than this, according to a theory put forward by Aston-Jones and Cohen (2005). During wakefulness, the locus coeruleus neurons alternate between phasic and tonic firing. The phasic state is proposed to optimize ongoing actions (help to maintain the focus on the present task). Tonic activity, on the other hand, allows shift of attention away from the ongoing activity to enable exploratory behavior to select a new (and more rewarding) behavior. Instruction to **shift behavior** appears to reach the locus coeruleus from parts of the prefrontal cortex (the cingulate and the orbitofrontal cortex). The gyrus cinguli, for example, seems to monitor errors during execution, and helps decide whether actions produce the expected results.

The Efferent Connections of the Reticular Formation

The reticular formation sends fibers to (and thereby acts on) four main regions: the **thalamus**, the **spinal cord**, **brain stem nuclei**, and the **cerebellum**. The cell groups giving off ascending axons are located somewhat more caudally than those emitting descending axons (Fig. 26.8). By means of the numerous collaterals of both the ascending and descending fibers in the reticular formation (Figs. 26.3 and 26.4), the two kinds of cell groups can influence each other. Further, there are also many interneurons connecting different parts of the reticular formation. Thus, a close cooperation is possible between the parts of the reticular formation that act on the cerebral cortex and those that act on the spinal cord. Collaterals of ascending and descending axons mediate actions on brain stem nuclei.

Parts of the reticular formation form **premotor networks**. Chapter 25 deals with premotor networks in the pons and mesencephalon controlling and coordinating the activity of the eye muscle nuclei. Other premotor networks in the reticular formation control rhythmic movements such as locomotion (Chapter 22) and respiration. Further, premotor networks coordinate the activity of the widely separated motoneurons responsible for the cough reflex and the vomiting reflex.

The **descending** fibers run in the ventral part of the lateral funicle and in the ventral funicle (Fig. 26.9), and are related to **motor control**. Such reticulospinal fibers end primarily on interneurons, which, in turn, can

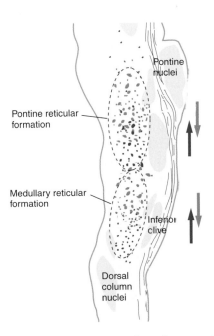

FIGURE 26.8 *Position of efferent reticular cell groups.* Drawing of sagittal section through the brain stem (cat). Neurons sending axons to higher levels (the thalamus) are red, while neurons with descending axons are green. The cell groups sending descending fibers are located somewhat more rostrally than the regions sending ascending fibers, providing opportunity for mutual influences by collaterals (as shown in Fig. 26.4).

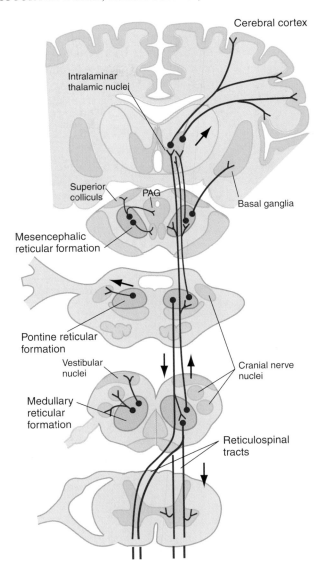

FIGURE 26.9 *Efferent connections of the reticular formation.* Various subdivisions of the reticular formation send fibers to higher levels, such the thalamus, the basal ganglia, and the cerebral cortex. Descending fibers end in the spinal cord. In addition, the reticular formation sends fibers to the cranial nerve nuclei and other brain stem nuclei, such as PAG and the superior colliculus, and the vestibular nuclei. Most of the long connections are both crossed and uncrossed, although this is not shown in the figure. Numerous shorter fibers interconnecting subdivisions of the reticular formation are not shown.

influence motoneurons. The ventral reticulospinal tracts are discussed in Chapter 22 ("More About Reticulospinal Tracts"). The **ventral reticulospinal tracts** are both crossed and uncrossed and mediate both inhibitory and excitatory effects on spinal motoneurons. The reticulospinal neurons are further characterized by their axonal branching pattern, with collaterals given off at several levels of the spinal cord. Thus, each neuron can influence muscles in different parts of the body. As discussed in Chapter 22, the ventral reticulospinal tracts are of particular importance for **postural control**, for the **orientation of the head and body** toward external stimuli, and for **voluntary movements of proximal body parts.** Connections from the **superior colliculus**—that mediate sensory information to the reticular formation—are crucial for orienting movements toward novel stimuli. Combined anatomic and physiologic studies of single cells have shown the importance of a tecto-reticulospinal pathway for such movements. The **dorsal reticulospinal fibers** concern primarily **control of sensory information.** Many of these fibers are monoaminergic and arise partly in the raphe nuclei and adjoining parts of the reticular formation (see Fig. 15.3).

The **ascending fibers** from the reticular formation end in the **intralaminar thalamic nuclei** (Fig. 26.9), unlike the specific sensory tracts that end in the lateral thalamic nucleus. Some fibers also end in the **hypothalamus.** We discuss the functional significance of the ascending

reticular connections later in this chapter; suffice it to say here that they are of particular importance for the general level of activity of the cerebral cortex, which, in turn, concerns consciousness and attention.

The Reticular Formation Receives All Kinds of Sensory Information

Various cell groups send fibers to the reticular formation (Fig. 26.10). **Spinoreticular fibers** are discussed in Chapter 14. These fibers ascend in the ventral part of the lateral funicle together with the spinothalamic tract, but diverge in the lower medulla. Among other destinations, the fibers end in the parts of the reticular formation that give off long ascending axons to the thalamus. This provides a **spino-reticulothalamic pathway** that is anatomically and functionally different from the major sensory pathways. Some of the spinoreticular fibers end in areas containing neurons that send axons back to the spinal cord, thus establishing **feedback** loops between the reticular formation and the cord.

In addition to spinal neurons that send their axons only to the reticular formation, many secondary sensory neurons send **collaterals** to the reticular formation. This concerns many of the fibers of the **spinothalamic tract,**

which, presumably, mediate **nociceptive** and **thermoceptive** signals to the reticular formation. Collaterals of ascending axons from the sensory (spinal) trigeminal nucleus supply the same kind of information from the face.[2] **Visceral sensory** signals reach the reticular formation by collaterals of ascending fibers from the **solitary nucleus** (which receives afferents from the vagus nerve, for example).

The **superior colliculus** sends fibers to parts of the reticular formation, as mentioned. These connections make it possible for **visual signals** to influence the reticular formation because the superior colliculus receives visual information directly from the retina and from the visual cortex. In addition, the superior colliculus receives somatosensory information from the cortex and integrates visual and somatosensory stimuli enabling orientation toward external stimuli.

Auditory signals reach the reticular formation by collaterals of ascending fibers in the auditory pathways. **Vestibular** signals come from the vestibular nuclei.

The preceding description of afferents indicates that signals from virtually all kinds of receptors can influence neurons of the reticular formation. This is verified by physiological experiments. Electrodes placed in the reticular formation can record potentials evoked by stimulation of receptors for light, sound, smell, and taste. Furthermore, stimulation of peripheral nerves carrying signals from cutaneous receptors and proprioceptors and of visceral nerves evokes activity. Whenever a receptor is stimulated, the signals reach not only the cortical areas important for the perception of the stimulus but also the reticular formation.

Afferents from Subcortical Nuclei and the Cerebral Cortex

Corticoreticular fibers arise mainly in the cortical areas that give origin to the pyramidal tract (Fig. 26.10). They end preponderantly in the regions of the reticular formation that send axons to the spinal cord. As discussed in Chapter 22, the **corticoreticulospinal pathway** is of special importance for the control of voluntary and automatic movements.

As discussed in Chapter 23, the **basal ganglia** (the substantia nigra) send efferents to the mesencephalic reticular formation (the locomotor region, or PPN). Fibers from the **hypothalamus** ending in parts of the reticular formation serve to coordinate the activity of different peripheral parts of the autonomic system. Limbic structures, notably the **amygdala**, also send fibers to the reticular formation. Such connections probably mediate emotional effects on autonomic and somatic motor

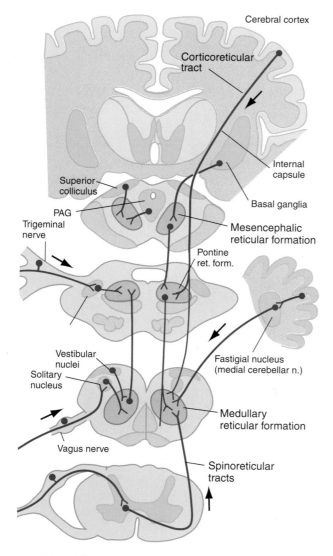

FIGURE 26.10 *Afferent connections of the reticular formation.* Several spinoreticular tracts mediate various kinds of sensory information. In addition, the reticular formation is influenced from sensory cranial nerve nuclei and other brain stem nuclei, such as the PAG, the superior colliculus, and the vestibular nuclei (not shown). The descending fibers from the cerebral cortex are links in indirect corticospinal pathways (cf. Fig. 22.1).

---

2 The medial lemniscus does not give off collaterals to the reticular formation. Information from low-threshold mechanoreceptors must therefore reach the reticular formation by means of spinoreticular neurons.

functions. The periaqueductal gray (PAG) is discussed in Chapter 15 in relation to suppression of nociceptive signals, but this mesencephalic complex of smaller nuclei has a wider specter of functions; for example, it helps initiate defensive reactions to external threats or other kinds of stress. This happens by way of its efferent connections to premotor networks in the reticular formation. The reticular formation receives afferents from the **cerebellum** (primarily the fastigial nucleus; see Fig. 24.6). This is an important pathway for the cerebellar influence on α and γ motoneurons. In addition, this pathway presumably mediates cerebellar influence of the autonomic nervous system. Thus, electric stimulation of the vermis can elicit changes in autonomic functions.

FUNCTIONS OF THE RETICULAR FORMATION

It follows from the preceding discussion of its efferent connections that the reticular formation can act on virtually all other parts of the CNS. We considered its effects on the spinal cord in Chapters 14 and 22, and we add more here on this point. In addition, we discuss the effects on the cerebral cortex, which are of particular importance. Parts of the reticular formation that are involved in the control of eye movements are discussed in Chapter 25, whereas the parts involved in the control of autonomic functions are described briefly in Chapter 28.

"The Activating System"

Electrical stimulation of parts of the reticular formation alters several functions mediated by the spinal cord, such as muscle tone, respiration, and blood pressure. In addition, the general activity of the cerebral cortex, which is closely related to the level of consciousness, can be altered by stimulation of the reticular formation. The **activating system of the brain stem** was therefore introduced as another name for the reticular formation. It should be emphasized, however, that these widespread effects are not served by the reticular formation as a whole but by relatively specific subregions. Further, stimulation of the reticular formation can also produce **inhibitory** effects on several processes. Therefore, the term "activating system" is not synonymous with "the reticular formation" but pertains to effects obtained from specific subregions only (to be discussed further later in this chapter).

There is continuous activity in the reticular formation maintained by a constant inflow of signals from various sources. The level of consciousness reflects the tonic activity in specific parts of the reticular formation. In particular, such activity is essential for the conscious awareness of sensory stimuli and for adequate behavioral responses to them. When a novel stimulus catches our attention, this is mediated by the reticular formation. At the same time, premotor networks in the reticular formation produces the motor responses that ensure automatic orientation of the head and the body toward the source of the stimulus. The motor apparatus is mobilized, together with alterations of respiration and circulation.

Actions on Skeletal Muscles

Animal experiments during the 1940s led to the identification of two regions within the reticular formation that influence muscle tone. Stimulation of a region in the medulla that sends particularly strong connections to the spinal cord (Fig. 26.9) could inhibit stretch reflexes and movements induced by stimulation of the motor cortex. This region was therefore called the **inhibitory region** (Fig. 26.11). A region with opposite effects, the **facilitatory region**, was found rostral to the inhibitory one. It extends rostrally into the mesencephalon and is located somewhat more laterally than the inhibitory region. The distinction between inhibitory and facilitatory regions is less sharp than originally believed, however. In several places, single neurons with inhibitory or facilitatory actions on muscles are intermingled.

The actions in the cord concern not only α but also γ **motoneurons**, so that the reticular formation can control the sensitivity of the muscle spindles. The activity

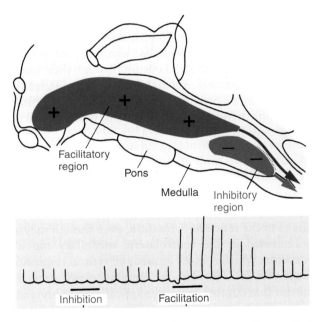

FIGURE 26.11 *Facilitatory and inhibitory regions of the reticular formation.* Schematic sagittal section through the brain stem (cat). The diagram at the bottom shows the amplitude of the patellar reflex (measured with EMG). In the period marked "Inhibition," the inhibitory region was stimulated electrically and the reflex response is almost abolished. In the period marked "Facilitation," the facilitatory region was stimulated and the patellar reflex response is markedly enhanced. (Modified from Kaada 1950.)

In humans with prolonged periods of unconsciousness after **head injuries**, there is often damage of the **mesencephalic reticular formation**. The lesion can be surprisingly small and yet produce deep unconsciousness. This fits with animal experiments showing that interruption of the ascending reticular connections in the mesencephalon produces loss of consciousness, in spite of normal conduction in the large sensory pathways (medial lemniscus, spinothalamic tract, and visual and auditory pathways).

Control of Sensory Information and Focusing of Attention

The main task of the ascending activating system is probably to **focus our attention** on certain stimuli or internal events, rather than to produce a diffuse awareness (if such a state is conceivable). To achieve this, it is necessary to prevent irrelevant stimuli from entering consciousness. Together with other mechanisms, inhibition from the reticular formation can ensure that, for example, we do not notice that someone is talking to us while we are absorbed in a book. In Chapters 14 and 15, we discussed how the central transmission of sensory signals is controlled from higher levels of the CNS, usually so that signals from certain kinds of receptor or parts of the body are inhibited. For example, descending connections to the spinal cord from the raphe nuclei and various (other) parts of the reticular formation suppress the central conduction of signals from nociceptors. Further, the central transmission of visual, auditory, and other sensory impulses is controlled by the reticular formation. Thus, even though it is not alone in this capacity, the reticular formation plays an important part in eliminating sensory signals that are considered irrelevant, so that our attention can be focused on salient signals.

Pathways and Transmitters Responsible for Cortical Activation

What are the pathways used by the reticular formation to influence consciousness, attention, and sleep? All of the major specific sensory pathways (the spinothalamic tract, the medial lemniscus, and the visual and auditory pathways) can be interrupted without affecting consciousness or the activation of the EEG produced by stimulation of the reticular formation. If these sensory pathways are left intact but the ascending connections of the reticular formation are interrupted by a cut in the mesencephalon, the animal becomes unconscious. Electrical stimulation of the reticular formation can no longer activate the EEG, even though stimulation of peripheral receptors evokes potentials in the cortical sensory regions. Thus, the sensory signals reach the cortex, but they are restricted to the sensory regions, and,

most importantly, they are unable to arouse the animal. Pathways other than the major sensory ones must therefore be responsible when the reticular formation activates the EEG over major parts of the cerebral hemisphere and produces behavioral changes indicating increased attention.

Connections from the reticular formation to the **intralaminar thalamic nuclei** are likely candidates. Thus, electrical stimulation of these nuclei can produce activation of the EEG similar to that seen after stimulation of the reticular formation itself. The intralaminar thalamic nuclei send widespread efferents to the cerebral cortex (cf. Chapter 33, under "The Intralaminar Thalamic Nuclei"). Therefore, a reticulothalamocortical pathway probably is important for the actions of the reticular formation on the cerebral cortex. Many of the reticulothalamic fibers to the intralaminar nuclei are **cholinergic** and come from a few small cell groups in the **dorsal part of the pons**.[5] In addition to this indirect reticulothalamocortical pathway, there are direct projections to the cerebral cortex from **monoaminergic** cell groups in the brain stem—usually considered parts of the reticular formation—such as the **raphe nuclei** (serotonin), the **locus coeruleus** (norepinephrine), and the **ventral tegmental area** in the mesencephalon (dopamine). These nuclei also project to the thalamus, however. Stimulation of each of these cell groups can produce synchronization of the EEG, even though they behave differently in other respects. For example, their activities differ with regard to sleep, as discussed below. Norepinephric neurons increase their firing rate shortly before and during periods with cortical activation and focused attention. Similarly, **serotonergic** raphe neurons and **histaminergic** neurons in the hypothalamus (tuberomammillary nucleus) are more active during wakefulness than during sleep.[6] As with the other modulatory inputs, activation of histaminergic fibers can bring thalamocortical neurons from a state of burst firing to single-spike firing.

Experiments in rats with selective elimination of various neurotransmitter systems suggest the following (very simplified) specializations with regard to tasks requiring focused attention: the **cholinergic** connections increase the precision of the performance, the **norepinephric** ones reduce the effect of distracting stimuli, the **dopaminergic** ones increase the speed of execution, and the **serotonergic** ones limit the frequency of impulsive response errors (see also "Possible Tasks of the

5 The largest pontine cholinergic cell groups are the **pedunculopontine nucleus** (PPN) and the **lateral dorsal tegmental nucleus** (LDT). The PPN consists of several subdivisions, however, and many neurons are glutamatergic; moreover, a part of the PPN has important connections with the basal ganglia and other parts of the brain stem.
6 Histamine-receptor antagonists, commonly used for allergy and motion sickness, block the activating effect of histamine, and this might explain why they have sleepiness as a side effect.

Raphe Nuclei and the Locus Coeruleus" earlier in this chapter).

To summarize, at least five cell groups, using as many transmitters, cooperate in the control of consciousness and attention. They exert their effects partly in the thalamus and partly in the cerebral cortex. Most likely, each of the cell groups and transmitters influence different aspects of wakefulness.

Coma, Vegetative State, and the Locked-in Syndrome

For clinical purposes, the definition of consciousness is practical: a condition of wakefulness in which the person responds appropriately to stimuli and, by his behavior, demonstrates awareness of himself and his surroundings. Patients with diseases or damage of the brain can exhibit states of consciousness ranging from full awareness to coma. A person in a coma appears to be sleeping, but cannot be awakened by any kinds of sensory stimulus. Purely reflex movements may be evoked, however (e.g., the withdrawal reflex). A coma may have several different causes but it is always a serious condition. The prognosis is poorer the longer a comatose state lasts. After acute head trauma, persistent unconsciousness suggests brain stem involvement, typically of the mesencephalic reticular formation.

After a few weeks, some comatose patients enter a persistent vegetative state in which they show some signs of wakefulness: they may open their eyes upon strong stimulation and after some time even spontaneously. They may briefly fix the gaze on a person or an object. They show no other signs of being aware of their surroundings, however, and they do not talk. Functional magnetic resonance imaging (fMRI) studies in such patients show activity patterns compatible with unconsciousness. For example, in 15 patients noxious stimuli activated expected parts of the brain stem, thalamus, and SI but not the rest of the "pain network," including the insula, the cingulate gyrus, and the SII. Nevertheless, doubt exists as to whether some patients in the vegetative state can perceive and respond adequately to external events. Thus, a patient showed activation (measured via fMRI) of relevant motor networks when asked to imagine playing tennis. Further, speech areas were activated when the patient was presented with spoken sentences. It is not clear, however, whether these observations mean that the patient was in fact conscious, or whether it just shows how much of cerebral processing that can occur without entering consciousness.

On rare occasions, a patient may appear unconscious yet be fully awake. This occurs typically after brain stem infarctions that damage the ventral parts of the pons with the pyramidal tract and corticobulbar tracts on both sides. The sensory pathways located more dorsally are spared, as is also the ascending activating system. This condition is called the locked-in syndrome. The patient is unable to move or talk but is otherwise fully conscious and mentally intact.

SLEEP

The necessity of sleep and its contribution to mental and physical health may seem self-evident. Yet, the more specific functions of sleep and its neurobiological basis are not fully understood. Indeed, control of sleep and its various phases has turned out be very complex, involving many neuronal groups and neurotransmitters. Here we provide only a brief and simplified treatment of this topic.

Sleep Phases

Sleep consists of several phases that can be distinguished based on differences in the EEG. The transition from alertness to drowsiness changes the EEG in the direction of synchronization. When a subject is falling into a deep, quiet sleep, the α waves disappear altogether and are replaced by irregular slow waves with greater amplitude (slow-wave sleep). After an initial light phase I, the sleep becomes gradually deeper, until phase IV. To waken a person in sleep phase IV requires relatively strong stimuli, whereas only weak stimuli are necessary in phase I. Phase V is special because the EEG is desynchronized, and there are conjugated movements of the eyes, much like a person looking at moving objects. Because of these rapid eye movements (REM), this phase is called REM sleep or paradoxical sleep. The eye movements appear to relate to the content of the dream. Thus, patients suffering from neglect of the left visual hemifield (after damage to the right hemisphere) have conjugated eye movements during REM sleep only to the right side; that is, the visual field they attend to when awake. Muscle tone is generally reduced, with occasional muscular twitches, and there are changes of blood pressure and heart rate. Dreaming occurs—at least mainly—during REM sleep. The various phases of sleep follow each other with the same order throughout the night. Usually, the first REM phase occurs after about 1.5 hours of sleep and lasts for about 10 minutes. Thereafter the REM phases return at intervals of 1 to 2 hours, and become gradually longer up to about 30 minutes. When waking up (or being wakened) just after a REM phase, a person remembers the content of the dream vividly.

The cerebral cortex is as active during REM sleep as when awake, but is partly uncoupled from the thalamus, which in the awake state delivers a constant stream of information about the external world. The EEG pattern during sleep is produced by complex interactions between neuronal firing patterns in the thalamus and

reduced by prevention of REM sleep a certain period after the learning situation. During REM sleep in certain animals, a particular pattern of electrical activity—**theta rhythm**—occurs in the hippocampus. Since the hippocampus plays a crucial role in learning, this has been taken to support the relationship between REM sleep and learning.

The view that dreams are psychologically meaningful, relating in a disguised form to inner conflicts and life events, is the basis for their central place in the psychoanalysis since Freud. Rather than emphasizing the role of dreams in learning, psychoanalytic tradition would stress their importance for the elaboration of inner conflicts that are not consciously accessible. These two possibilities might not be mutually exclusive, however. Perhaps a common purpose for all dreams is to help the individual develop **coping strategies,** as this requires the integration of new with old experiences, as well as ensuring that inner conflicts do not block learning and appropriate behavior.

27 | The Cranial Nerves

W e usually count 12 cranial nerves, even though neither the first (the olfactory nerve) nor the second (the optic nerve) are true nerves. These two and, in addition, the cochlear nerve and the vestibular nerve are dealt with in Chapters 16 to 19.

A brief survey of the cranial nerves is given in Chapter 6. The prenatal development of the cranial nerve nuclei is treated in Chapter 9 (see under "Cranial Nerves and Visceral Arches").

The cranial nerves connect the brain stem with structures in the head, neck, and in the thoracic and abdominal cavities. The cranial nerves are not as regularly built as the spinal nerves because some are purely motor, others are purely sensory, and some are mixed (like the spinal nerves). The cranial nerves contain four main fiber types. **Somatic efferent** fibers supply skeletal (striated) muscles, while **visceral efferent** fibers supply smooth muscles and glands and belong to the **parasympathetic** part of the autonomic nervous system. **Somatic afferent** fibers conduct sensory signals from the skin and mucous membranes of the face, from muscles and joints, and from the vestibular apparatus and the cochlea, while **visceral afferent** fibers bring sensory signals from the visceral organs. In early embryological development, the **cranial nerve nuclei** form longitudinal columns (cf. columnar arrangement of motoneurons in the cord), each column giving origin to only one of the four kinds of fiber. The columns are arranged so that, in general, motor cranial nuclei (somatic and visceral efferent) lie medially in the brain stem while sensory nuclei (somatic and visceral afferent) lie laterally. Later in development, the columns break up into discrete smaller nuclei but their mediolateral position and fiber composition remain the same (with some exceptions). The cranial nerve nuclei and the cranial nerves are links in various **brain stem reflexes** (e.g. the blink reflex and the vomiting reflex). The somatic motor nuclei receive innervation from the motor cortical areas, partly as collaterals of **pyramidal tract** fibers, partly as **corticobulbar** fibers destined only for the brain stem. Somatic sensory nuclei convey signals to the sensory areas of the cerebral cortex by joining the large **ascending sensory tracts** (e.g. the spinothalamic tract and the medial lemniscus).

A fair knowledge of the position of the various cranial nerve nuclei, the course of the nerves, and their main functions serve as a necessary basis for a topographic diagnosis of brain stem lesions.

GENERAL ORGANIZATION OF THE CRANIAL NERVES

Before dealing with specifics for each of the cranial nerves (Fig. 27.1), we discuss some features that are common to them all. Like the spinal nerves that connect the spinal cord with the body, the cranial nerves connect the brain stem with the peripheral organs. Several structural features are shared by the spinal cord and the brain stem, and thus also by the spinal and cranial nerves. Nevertheless, the brain stem is less regularly built and more complex in its organization than the spinal cord and the cranial nerves are not as schematic in their composition as the spinal nerves. Most of the cranial nerves, for example, lack a distinct ventral (motor) root and a dorsal (sensory) root. Some of the cranial nerves are purely sensory, others are purely motor, and others are mixed. Like the spinal nerves, several of the cranial nerves contain autonomic (preganglionic) fibers supplying smooth muscles and glands. Finally, some also contain afferent fibers from visceral organs.

The Cranial Nerves Can Contain Four Different Kinds of Nerve Fibers

The cranial nerves can contain the following kinds of fibers:

1. **Somatic efferent** fibers innervating skeletal (striated) muscles
2. **Visceral efferent** fibers supplying smooth muscles and glands and belonging to the parasympathetic part of the autonomic nervous system
3. **Somatic afferent** fibers with sensory signals from the skin and mucous membranes of the face, from muscles and joints, and from the vestibular apparatus and the cochlea
4. **Visceral afferent** fibers with sensory signals from the visceral organs

The **efferent fibers** of the cranial nerves have their cell bodies in brain stem nuclei corresponding to the columns of spinal motoneurons (see Fig. 21.3) and the intermediolateral cell column of the cord. We use the terms **somatic efferent** and **visceral efferent** cranial nerve nuclei of these cell groups (Figs. 27.2 and 27.3). The afferent fibers have their cell bodies in **ganglia** close to the brain stem, corresponding to the spinal ganglia. The central process of the ganglion cells enters the brain stem and ends on neurons in nuclei corresponding to

and their nuclei. It is helpful at the outset to remember the following general rule, evident from Figs. 27.2 and 27.3: the efferent (motor) nerve nuclei lie medially in the brain stem, whereas the afferent (sensory) nuclei are located laterally. Further, in most cases the nuclei are located at about the same rostrocaudal level as their nerves leave the brain stem. In clinical neurology it is important to know the approximate mediolateral and rostrocaudal level of each nucleus (Fig. 27.5).

Further on the Position of the Cranial Nerve Nuclei

The **somatic efferent** nuclei are in early embryonic life all arranged in a column close to the midline, but later some move away in a ventrolateral direction (Figs. 27.3 and 27.5). The nuclei remaining in the medialmost column are termed **general somatic efferent** and comprise (from caudal to rostral) the **nucleus of the accessory nerve** (11), the **nucleus of the hypoglossal nerve** (12), the **nucleus of the abducens nerve** (6), and the **nucleus of the oculomotor nerve** (3). (In the following, for practical reasons we use abbreviated names, such as the accessory nucleus and the hypoglossal nucleus.) All of these nuclei innervate **myotome muscles**—the muscles that are developed from the segmentally arranged somites of early embryonic life. The somatic efferent nuclei that have moved away from the medial column all innervate **branchial muscles**—the striated muscles developed from the branchial (visceral) arches (facial and masticatory muscles, and muscles of the pharynx and larynx). We call these nuclei **special somatic efferent** (although they most commonly are termed "special visceral efferent").[1] This group comprises the **ambiguus nucleus** (9, 10), the **facial nucleus** (7), and the **motor trigeminal nucleus** (5).

The **visceral efferent** (parasympathetic) column of cranial nerve nuclei is located immediately lateral to the somatic efferent column (Figs. 27.2, 27.3, and 27.5) and comprises the **(dorsal) motor nucleus of the vagus** (10), the small **inferior** and **superior salivatory nuclei** (9, 7), and the **parasympathetic oculomotor nucleus of Edinger-Westphal** (3). The **visceral afferent fibers** all end in one long nucleus, the **solitary nucleus**, which is located lateral to the visceral afferent column (Figs. 27.2, 27.3, and 27.5).

Most laterally, we find the **somatic afferent nuclei**. This group comprises the **sensory trigeminal nucleus** (5), the **vestibular nuclei** (8), and the **cochlear nuclei** (8). The sensory trigeminal nucleus consists of three functionally different parts (the spinal, the principal, and the mesencephalic nuclei). Together, the three parts form one continuous column, which extends from the upper cervical segments of the cord into the mesencephalon (Fig. 27.2).

The fibers of the vestibulocochlear nerve are often classified as **special somatic afferent** because they originate from special sense organs; the trigeminal fibers are then termed **general somatic afferent**.

Figure 27.4 and the discussion here show that fibers of one kind all come from one of the columns of nuclei only, even though the fibers peripherally may follow several of the cranial nerves. Thus, all (general) somatic afferent fibers end in the sensory trigeminal nucleus, whereas the fibers peripherally follow not only the trigeminal nerve but also the glossopharyngeal and the vagus nerves.

Brain Stem Reflexes

Like the spinal nerves that are links in spinal reflex arcs, the cranial nerves constitute afferent and efferent links of reflex arcs with reflex centers in the brain stem (Fig. 27.4). Some brain stem reflexes are simple, such as the monosynaptic stretch reflex—the **masseter reflex**—that can be elicited of the masticatory muscles. Often, however, the reflex centers are more complex, comprising neurons at several levels of the brain stem (for some, even at the cortical level). Thus, the afferent fibers may enter the brain stem at one level, whereas the efferent fibers leave at another. One example is the **corneal reflex** (touching of the cornea elicits an eye wink), in which the afferent fibers of the trigeminal nerve, entering at the midpontine level, descend in the brain stem and form synapses in the lower medulla (the spinal trigeminal nucleus). From the medulla, the signals travel by interneurons to the facial nucleus on both sides, located in the lower pons. The reflex center is in this case rather extensive; consequently, lesions at various levels of the brain stem may produce a weakened or abolished corneal reflex. Depending on the location of the lesion, however, the change of the corneal reflex will be accompanied by various other symptoms, which helps in determining the exact site of the lesion.

Several other brain stem reflexes are treated below in conjunction with the cranial nerves that mediate them.

The Cranial Nerve Nuclei Are Connected with Central Sensory and Motor Tracts

As mentioned, the cranial nerves and their nuclei are organized in accordance with the same general rules as

---

1 Both anatomically and functionally, however, "the special visceral efferent neurons" are more similar to the somatic efferents. First, branchial (visceral) arch striated muscles are among those subject to the most precise voluntary control (the mimetic muscles of the face and the muscles of the larynx) and should therefore not be mixed up with visceral (smooth) muscles. Second, the neurons are structurally like α motoneurons; that is, they are larger than the preganglionic, parasympathetic neurons. In addition, the visceral arch neurons contain the neuropeptide CGRP that occurs in spinal motoneurons but not in preganglionic parasympathetic neurons. Therefore, we find it preferable to use the term **special somatic efferent**. Otherwise, it is of no great importance which terms are used to group the neurons of the cranial nerves; the important thing is to know where the cell bodies of the various cranial nerves are located, the course of their fibers, and their functions.

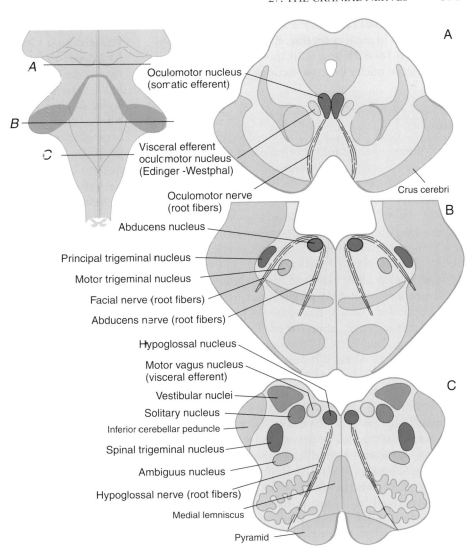

FIGURE 27.5 *Position of the cranial nerve nuclei at three levels of the brain stem.* **A:** Mesencephalon. **B:** Pons. **C:** Medulla oblongata. Compare with Fig. 27.2.

the spinal nerves (with some exceptions). This means that the cranial nerves are the first links in sensory pathways corresponding to the **dorsal column—medial lemniscus system** and the **spinothalamic pathway** (Fig. 27.4; see also Figs. 14.2 and 14.4). Further, as the nuclei involved in the sensory pathways conducting from the spinal cord, those of the brain stem are subjected to **descending control** of the sensory transmission. This concerns influences from parts of the reticular formation and from the cerebral cortex.

Several of the somatic efferent (motor) cranial nerve nuclei are influenced by the **pyramidal tract**—that is, by fibers forming the **corticobulbar tract** (Fig. 27.4, see also Fig. 22.1). An important difference between the corticospinal and corticobulbar fibers is that several of the cranial nerve nuclei receive both crossed and uncrossed fibers. Unilateral damage to the descending fibers (e.g., in the internal capsule) produces clear-cut pareses only in some of the muscle groups innervated

by the cranial nerves (most marked in the mimetic muscles).[2]

Examination of the cranial nerves is of great importance in clinical neurology because it can provide exact information about the site of a disease process. A prerequisite is that the examiner has reasonably precise knowledge of where the cranial nerves exit from the brain stem (Fig. 27.1; see also Fig. 6.16) and the position of their nuclei both rostrocaudally and mediolaterally (Figs. 27.2 and 27.5). Further, the functions of the various nerves must be known in sufficient detail as a basis for the necessary tests. On the basis of such knowledge, together with knowledge of the positions of the long motor and sensory tracts passing through the brain

---

2 The accessory, the hypoglossal, and the part of the facial nucleus supplying the lower part of the face—and often also the motor trigeminal nucleus—receive only crossed fibers, as judged from clinical observations (Monrad-Krohn 1954).

THE VAGUS NERVE

The vagus nerve is the **tenth cranial nerve** and is characterized by containing fibers of all four kinds described above. Correspondingly, it is connected with four different nuclei in the medulla. The root fibers emerge in a row at the lateral aspect of the medulla (Figs. 27.1 and 27.3) and join to form one nerve, which leaves the skull through the jugular foramen (Fig. 27.8). Embryologically, the vagus nerve belongs to the fourth, fifth, and sixth branchial arches, and this explains the peculiar course of some of its branches. In the **jugular foramen** and immediately below, the nerve has two swellings—the **jugular** and the **nodose ganglia** (Fig. 27.9)—that contain the pseudounipolar cell bodies of the sensory vagus fibers.

As implied by the name (Latin: *vagus,* wandering), the vagus nerve sends branches to widespread regions of the body. After leaving the skull, the nerve passes as a fairly thick cord downward in the neck together with the common carotid artery, further through the thorax, and into the abdomen through the diaphragm. It gives off branches in the neck, in the thorax, and in the abdomen.

Visceral Efferent (Parasympathetic) Vagus Fibers

The visceral efferent neurons belong to the parasympathetic part of the autonomic system. The cell bodies lie in the (dorsal) **motor nucleus of the vagus** (Figs. 27.2 and 27.6; see Fig. 6.17).[3] The fibers do not pass directly to the organs but end on a second set of neurons in parasympathetic ganglia close to or in the walls of the organs (Fig. 27.9), as is the case for all parasympathetic nerves. The neurons leading from the CNS to the ganglia are called **preganglionic,** and those leading from the ganglion to the organ are called **postganglionic** (see Fig. 28.1).

The vagus gives off visceral efferent fibers descending to the **heart** in the neck (Fig. 27.9). The cell bodies of the postganglionic neurons are located in the wall of the heart and around the great vessels near the heart, and the postganglionic fibers end among the muscle cells of the heart, especially those of the **sinus node,** which determines the heart rate.

Other branches from the vagus supply the **esophagus** and the **trachea** and, further down in the thorax, the **bronchi** of the lung. The postganglionic fibers innervate smooth muscles and glands in these structures.

---

3 Experiments with tracing techniques show that the neurons supplying the **heart** (and probably also the lungs) have their cell bodies in an external, distinct part of the **nucleus ambiguus**. The cell bodies are morphologically like those of the dorsal motor vagus nucleus, but they differ from the larger motoneurons in the main nucleus ambiguus, which innervate striated muscles (of the pharynx and larynx).

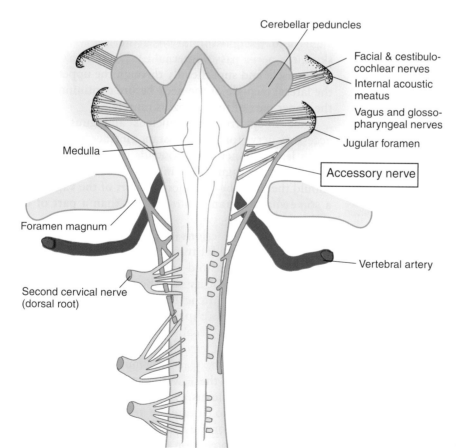

Cerebellar peduncles

Facial & cestibulo-cochlear nerves

Internal acoustic meatus

Vagus and glosso-pharyngeal nerves

Jugular foramen

Accessory nerve

Medulla

Vertebral artery

Foramen magnum

Second cervical nerve (dorsal root)

FIGURE 27.8 *The accessory nerve.* The lower part of the brain stem and the upper cervical cord, as viewed from behind. The cerebellum is removed. The fibers of the accessory nerve proper emerge from the three upper cervical segments and exit the cord between the ventral and dorsal roots (the ventral roots are not visible in the figure). Compare with the emergence of the vagus fibers in Fig. 27.1.

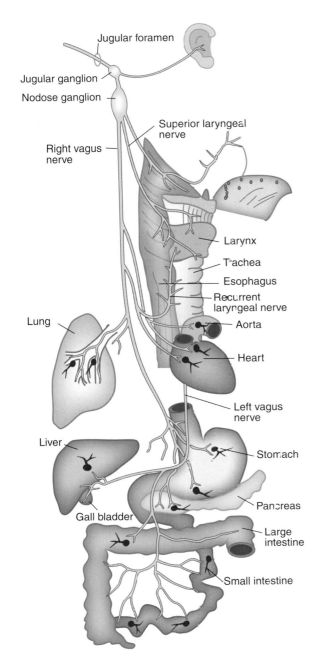

FIGURE 27.9 *Course and distribution of the vagus nerve.*

In the **abdomen**, the vagus sends fibers to the **stomach**, the **small intestine**, and the first half of the **large intestine**. The vagus also supplies the **liver**, the **gallbladder**, and the **pancreas** with parasympathetic fibers. To reach the various organs, the fibers follow the arteries and form plexuses around them together with sympathetic fibers.

Functionally, signals in the vagus nerve reduce the heart rate, constrict the bronchi, and increase bronchial secretion, whereas the peristaltic movements and secretion are increased in the stomach and intestine. The secretion of the pancreas is also increased.

Visceral Afferent Vagus Fibers

All branches of the vagus with visceral efferent fibers also contain afferent (sensory) fibers. These neurons have their pseudounipolar cell bodies in the large **nodose ganglion** (Fig. 27.9). When the fibers enter the brain stem, they form a small bundle that passes caudally: the **solitary tract** (this is not a true tract, however, but the central course of a nerve). The fibers establish synapses in the **solitary nucleus** (Figs. 27.2 and 27.6; see Fig. 6.17). The efferent fibers from this nucleus pass to the reticular formation and other cranial nerve nuclei in the vicinity and to higher levels such as the thalamus and the hypothalamus (Fig. 27.4).

All of the sensory fibers from the **larynx** and some from the **pharynx** follow the vagus. The sensory fibers from the larynx follow the **superior laryngeal nerve** (from the part above the vocal cords) and the **recurrent laryngeal nerve** (from the lower part of the larynx). On an **embryological** basis, all sensory fibers from the pharynx (and the posterior part of the tongue) should be classified as visceral afferent. There is evidence, however, that such fibers end in the somatic afferent trigeminal nucleus and not in the visceral afferent solitary nucleus. Functionally, they may therefore be considered somatic afferent rather than visceral afferent. Vagus may also carry nociceptive signals from parts of the **heart** (see Chapter 29, under "Central Pathways for Visceral Afferent Signals").

Visceral afferent signals in the vagus nerve most likely contribute to conscious **feelings** like hunger or satiety. There is also evidence that signals in the vagus nerve contribute to the feelings associated with infections (loss of appetite, tiredness, somnolence, and so forth) and the induction of **sickness behavior**. Together with other visceral afferent fibers, the vagus contributes to our general bodily feeling—also called the "sense of the physiological condition of the body" (Craig 2002). This is discussed further in Chapter 30, under "The Hypothalamus and the Immune System."

Visceral Reflexes

The visceral afferents in the vagus nerve are links in reflex arcs that control **secretion** and **peristaltic movements** of the gastrointestinal tract (and vomiting). Such reflexes also mediate alterations of **airway secretion** and of the **airway resistance** by changing the tone of the bronchial smooth muscles. The **reflex centers** of all these reflexes are located in the medulla, and the efferent links are visceral efferent fibers coming from the dorsal motor nucleus of the vagus.

Visceral afferents from **baroreceptors** in the wall of the large vessels provide information about the blood pressure in the aorta. Increased blood pressure gives rise to increased firing frequency of the afferent fibers. In turn, this produces increased firing of visceral efferent vagus fibers, which reduces the heart rate. The **reflex center** must involve connections from the solitary nucleus to the motor nucleus of the vagus (these two nuclei are close neighbors, as can be seen in Fig. 27.2).

The motor nucleus of the vagus can be influenced also by signals other than those coming from the viscera. For example, the sight, the smell, or even the thought of food can produce increased secretion of gastric juice. These are examples of **conditioned responses**, whereas the stimulation of taste receptors produces an unconditioned (true reflex) response.

Other examples of visceral reflexes are discussed in Chapter 29, under "Visceral Reflexes."

The Vomiting Reflex

Vomiting is usually caused by marked dilatation of the stomach or irritation of its mucosa. The biologic significance of the reflex is presumably to rid the stomach of potentially harmful contents. As we all know, however, vomiting can also be provoked by irritation of the pharynx (putting a finger in the throat) and by foul odors, strong emotions, and travel sickness. Several different afferent links to the reflex center must therefore exist. The emptying of the stomach is caused by coordinated contractions of the smooth muscles in the stomach wall and striated muscles in the diaphragm and the abdominal wall. In addition, laryngeal muscles (closing the airways) and muscles of the pharynx, the soft palate, and the tongue also participate. Thus, the reflex center must activate visceral efferent neurons and α motoneurons at several levels of the brain stem and the spinal cord in a specific sequence. The **reflex center** is actually quite widespread, but usually matters are simplified by restricting it to the medulla, including the **solitary nucleus**. This receives the visceral afferent fibers from the stomach, forming the afferent link when the reflex is elicited from the stomach itself. From the reflex center in the medulla, signals pass to the motor nuclei via synaptic interruption in the reticular formation and reticulospinal fibers. In addition, there are direct spinal projections from the solitary nucleus to the motoneurons of the diaphragm and abdominal wall.

Substances in the bloodstream cause vomiting by direct action at the **area postrema** of the medulla (see Chapter 8, under "Some Parts of the Brain Lack a Blood–Brain Barrier"). Neurons in the area postrema project to the solitary nucleus. **Apomorphine** and other alkaloids are given orally or subcutaneously to provoke vomiting.

Somatic Efferent Vagus Fibers

The somatic efferent vagus fibers come from the **ambiguus nucleus** (Figs. 27.2 and 27.5), which belongs to the

special somatic efferent nuclei. The fibers supply all striated muscles of the **larynx** and parts of the muscles of the **pharynx**. The fibers to the pharynx take off from the vagus as several small branches, whereas most of the fibers to the larynx are collected in the **recurrent laryngeal nerve** (Fig. 27.9). This nerve takes off from the main vagus trunk at the level of the aortic arch on the left side and the subclavian artery on the right. It then arches behind the vessels and ascends in the furrow between the trachea and the esophagus, to reach the larynx. One of the laryngeal muscles located on the outside, the **cricothyroid muscle**, receives motor fibers in the superior laryngeal nerve (which is a predominantly sensory nerve, as mentioned earlier). The vagus also innervates one of the muscles of the soft palate, the **levator veli palatini** muscle.

A **lesion** of the vagus nerve above the exit of the motor branches to the pharynx and the soft palate produces deviation of the uvula and the posterior pharyngeal wall to the normal side (as can be seen, e.g., when a patient is asked to say "aah"; Fig. 27.10). Pareses of the soft palate and the pharynx cause fluid and food to enter the nasal cavity when swallowing (owing to inadequate closure of the nasopharynx). Further, the voice becomes hoarse because the vocal cords cannot be properly adducted. Such a symptom will obviously also occur after a lesion of the recurrent laryngeal nerve anywhere along its course. In case of a unilateral lesion, the voice hoarseness will gradually disappear, because the muscles of the normal side adapt to the changed conditions.

The neurons of the nucleus ambiguus are influenced by, among other sources, the **pyramidal tract** during speech. They can also be activated involuntarily in the **cough reflex** by irritating stimuli of the respiratory tract.

Somatic Afferent Vagus Fibers

This is the smallest contingent of fibers in the vagus nerve. They have their cell bodies in the small **jugular**

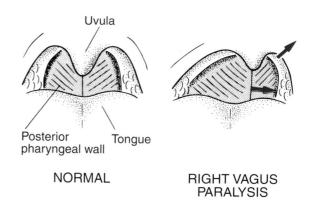

NORMAL   RIGHT VAGUS
                          PARALYSIS

FIGURE 27.10 *Paralysis of the right vagus nerve.* The uvula and the posterior pharyngeal wall are pulled toward the normal side when the patient says "aah." (Redrawn from Mumenthaler 1979.)

ganglion and come from a small region of the skin of the external ear—the **auricular ramus** (Fig. 27.9). The fibers terminate in the **trigeminal sensory nucleus**. Touching the innervated area, for example, by an otoscope in the external meatus may evoke a cough reflex and in some individuals even a vomiting reflex. The causes of these phenomena are unknown. They might be due to connections from the trigeminal nucleus to the solitary nucleus or by abnormal signal transmission between sensory fibers of the vagus nerve (**ephaptic transmission**).

THE GLOSSOPHARYNGEAL NERVE

The **ninth cranial nerve**, the glossopharyngeal, resembles the vagus but is smaller and innervates a more restricted region. The root fibers leave the medulla immediately rostral to the vagus fibers (Fig. 27.1). The root fibers fuse to form one trunk that leaves the cranial cavity through the **jugular foramen** (together with the vagus and the accessory nerves). The nerve follows an arched course (ventrally) lateral to the pharynx, which it penetrates to reach the base of the tongue. Close to the jugular foramen, the nerve contains two small **sensory ganglia** with pseudounipolar ganglion cells, the **superior** and **petrous ganglia**.

Of the peripheral branches, some innervate the muscles and the mucous membrane of the **pharynx** (together with the vagus, which appears to be the most important quantitatively); other sensory fibers reach the posterior part of the tongue, to innervate **taste buds**, and the mucous membrane (and also the mucous membrane of the soft palate and the tonsillar region). The glossopharyngeal nerve also contains **visceral efferent** (parasympathetic) fibers to the **parotid gland** and to the salivary glands in the posterior part of the tongue (see Fig. 28.11 for the course of the parasympathetic fibers).

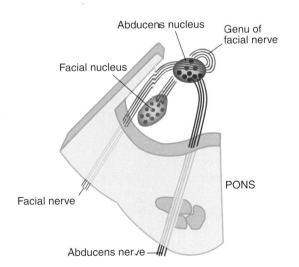

FIGURE 27.11 *Course of the facial nerve and its relation to the abducens nucleus.* Schematic cross section through the lower pons.

The Sinus Nerve and Baroreceptors

A special contingent of visceral afferent fibers in the glossopharyngeal nerve comes from the wall of the **carotid sinus** (the thin-walled, dilated part of the internal carotid artery). The fibers conduct signals from mechanoreceptors recording the tension of the arterial wall; that is, the receptors monitor the blood pressure and are therefore called **baroreceptors** (cf. the same kind of afferents from the aorta running with the vagus nerve). The afferent fibers end in the **solitary nucleus**, and from there the signals are conveyed to the **motor nucleus of the vagus**. Increased signal frequency of the cardiac vagus fibers reduces the heart rate, and thereby the blood pressure is reduced. When the blood pressure falls, there will be reduced firing of the cardiac vagus fibers, with increased heart rate and blood pressure. This is one of several mechanisms to keep the **blood pressure** within certain limits and that the cerebral blood flow is sufficient at all times.

The Nuclei of the Glossopharyngeal Nerve

The **somatic efferent** fibers to the striated pharynx muscles come from the **ambiguus nucleus**, whereas the **visceral efferent** fibers have their cell bodies in the small **inferior salivatory nucleus** (Fig. 27.2). The signals from this nucleus follow a somewhat complicated course to reach the parotid gland (as is the case for several of the parasympathetic fiber components of the cranial nerves). The preganglionic parasympathetic fibers from the inferior salivatory nucleus end in the small **otic ganglion** just outside the cranial cavity. The postganglionic fibers from the ganglion cells join one of the trigeminal branches—the **auriculotemporal nerve** that passes close to the ganglion—to reach gland (see Fig. 28.11).

The **visceral afferent fibers** carrying signals from the **taste** buds in the posterior third of the tongue end in the **solitary nucleus**. From there, the signals pass to the thalamus and further on to the cerebral cortex. The sensory fibers from the posterior part of the tongue, the tonsils, the soft palate, and the pharynx end in the **sensory trigeminal nucleus**.

THE VESTIBULOCOCHLEAR NERVE

The **eighth cranial nerve**, although consisting of only one trunk, is in reality two functionally different nerves: the **cochlear nerve** (see Chapter 17) and the **vestibular nerve** (described with the sense of equilibrium in Chapter 18). The nerves fuse after leaving the labyrinth (the cochlea and the vestibular apparatus) and follow the **internal acoustic meatus**. At the lower end of the pons, in the **cerebellopontine angle**, the nerve enters the brain stem. Most of the fibers in the vestibular nerve end in the **vestibular nuclei**; some end in the cerebellum. The cochlear nerve ends in the **cochlear nuclei** (Fig. 27.2). The cell bodies of the primary afferent fibers are located at the bottom of the internal meatus, forming the **vestibular ganglion** and the **spiral ganglion**. The main structural features of the labyrinth are described in Chapters 17 and 18.

THE FACIAL AND INTERMEDIATE NERVES

The **seventh cranial nerve** belongs to the **second branchial (visceral) arch** and innervates structures developed from this. The facial nerve is the motor nerve of the facial (mimetic) muscles, supplying them with **special somatic efferent** fibers. The small **intermediate nerve** follows the facial nerve and is usually considered to belong to it. Thus, parts of the intermediate nerve might be regarded as a sensory root of the facial nerve with its **visceral afferent** fibers. The intermediate nerve also contains **visceral efferent** (parasympathetic) fibers, however.

The facial nerve and the intermediate nerve leave the brain stem together laterally at the lower border of the pons, just ventral to the eighth nerve (Fig. 27.1). They then follow the eighth nerve to the bottom of the internal auditory meatus, where the intermediate nerve leaves the facial nerve. The facial nerve proper (with the somatic efferent fibers) then arches first posterolaterally and thereafter downward in the facial canal. It leaves the skull through the **stylomastoid foramen** immediately medial and anterior to the mastoid process. The nerve then passes forward through the parotid gland and divides into several branches, spreading out like a fan to all the facial muscles.

The **visceral efferent** (parasympathetic preganglionic) fibers in the intermediate nerve bring secretory signals to the **lacrimal gland** and the **submandibular** and the **sublingual salivary glands** (see Fig. 28.11 for the complicated route followed by the fibers). The **visceral afferent** fibers of the intermediate nerve come from **taste buds** in the anterior two-thirds of the tongue.

The Facial Nerve

The motor fibers of the facial nerve have their cell bodies in the **facial nucleus**, located in the lower pons. It belongs to the column of special somatic efferent nuclei (Figs. 27.2 and 27.3). The nucleus consists of several subdivisions, each supplying small groups of muscles. The root fibers of the facial nerve have a peculiar course before they leave the brain stem (Fig. 27.11). First, the fibers pass medially and lie dorsal to the abducens nucleus, forming the **genu of the facial nerve**, before they bend in the lateral and ventral direction. The facial fibers pass just beneath the floor of the fourth ventricle and form a

small elevation; the **facial colliculus** (see Fig. 6.19). Owing to the course of the nerve, symptoms of a peripheral facial paresis may occur in lesions that are located considerably more medial and dorsal than the nucleus itself. Figure 27.11 shows that damage to the abducens nucleus (affecting the lateral rectus muscle of the eye) is also likely to be accompanied by signs of pareses of the facial muscles of the same side.

The Mimetic Muscles

The facial or mimetic muscles originate from the facial skeleton and insert with elastic tendons in the dermis. There are many small muscles, with the majority located around the mouth and the eyes. Of particular practical value are the muscles responsible for blinking and closure of the eye (the **orbicularis oculi muscle**) and the muscles around the mouth (the **orbicularis oris** and several other muscles that move the lips). The **buccinator muscle** prevents the cheeks from being pressed out when the intraoral pressure is increased and, perhaps more importantly, prevents the cheeks from being sucked in between the teeth.

Central and Peripheral Facial Pareses

Signals from the facial nucleus evoke contractions of the mimetic muscles and are therefore responsible for our facial expressions. These muscles function also in conjunction with speech, eating, blinking, and so forth. The **pyramidal tract** (corticobulbar fibers) conveys signals for voluntary movements of the facial muscles. The fibers arise from the face region of the MI in the precentral gyrus (see Fig. 22.5).

The part of the facial nucleus supplying the muscles in the forehead and around the eyes receive both uncrossed and crossed pyramidal tract fibers, whereas the muscles in the lower part of the face receive purely crossed fibers. A **lesion of the pyramidal tract** (e.g., in the internal capsule) therefore produces clear-cut pareses only in the lower part of the face on the opposite side. Most obvious is the sagging corner of the mouth. The patient can still wrinkle the forehead and close the eyes voluntarily. A **peripheral lesion** (of the facial nucleus or the nerve), however, produces pareses of all the facial muscles on the same side as the lesion (Fig. 27.12). For example, the eye cannot be closed, so there is danger of drying and ulceration of the cornea (and permanent loss of vision).

Peripheral lesions of the facial nerve may be caused by hemorrhage, infarctions, or tumors in the pons, by infections of the middle ear (to which the nerve passes in close proximity), or by damage to the branches in the face. Most often, however, the cause of peripheral facial paresis is unknown (**Bell's palsy**). In such cases, the muscle power usually returns after some time.

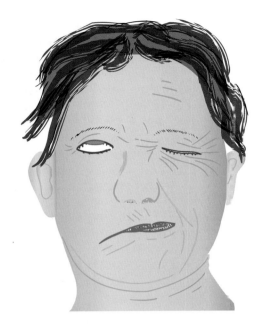

FIGURE 27.12 *Peripheral facial paralysis (right side).* The patient is asked to close her eyes and to retract the corners of the mouth. (Based on Monrad-Krohn 1954.)

Facial Expressions of Emotion Do Not Depend on the Pyramidal Tract

Whereas signals mediated by the pyramidal tract activate the motoneurons of the facial nucleus in voluntary movements (such as speech and eating), other descending pathways are responsible for facial expressions of emotions, such as sorrow and pleasure. As most of us know from personal experience, a genuine smile cannot be produced on command but arises independent of any conscious will. Indeed, our facial expressions often reveal emotions we would rather have concealed. A voluntary effort is required to suppress spontaneous facial expressions, which most likely are controlled by descending connections from the **hypothalamus** and possibly the **basal ganglia**. Thus, lesions of the pyramidal tract do not abolish spontaneous facial expressions. The patient smiles and laughs when told a good joke but cannot present a polite social smile. In **central pareses** (such as capsular hemiplegia) emotional facial expressions are in fact often exaggerated, and the patient cannot suppress a smile or prevent crying. Diseases of the basal ganglia, such as **Parkinson's disease,** present the opposite picture: the emotional, spontaneous expressions are lacking, whereas a voluntary, social smile is possible.

The Facial Nerve and Reflexes

The facial nucleus is also a link in some important reflex arcs. One is the **corneal** or **blink reflex.** It is elicited by touch or irritation of the cornea, and the sensory signals are conducted centrally in the trigeminal nerve to the spinal trigeminal nucleus (Fig. 27.13). From there the signals pass via interneurons in the reticular formation to the facial nucleus of both sides, and a contraction of the muscles of the eyelid is produced. The corneal reflex can be weakened or abolished by a lesion anywhere along the course of the afferent and efferent links or in the rather extensive reflex center.

Another reflex mediated by the facial nerve is the **stapedius reflex,** in which the response is contraction of the tiny **stapedius muscle** in the middle ear. The stimulus is an intense sound conducted centrally in the cochlear (acoustic) nerve to the cochlear nuclei. Most likely, interneurons in the reticular formation transfer the signals to the facial nucleus. The stapedius muscle pulls the stapes a little out of the oval window (see Fig. 17.7) and thereby dampens the transmission of sound waves to the cochlear duct. Accordingly, peripheral facial paresis can produce hypersensitivity to sounds, or **hyperacusis.**

Secretion of Tears and Saliva

The preganglionic parasympathetic fibers of the **intermediate nerve**—acting on the **lacrimal,** the **submandibular,** and the **sublingual glands**—have their cell bodies in the small **superior salivatory nucleus.** This nucleus belongs to the column of visceral efferent nuclei (Fig. 27.2). As mentioned, preganglionic parasympathetic fibers acting on the parotid gland have their cell bodies in the inferior salivatory nucleus and leave the brain stem in the glossopharyngeal nerve.

The **secretion of saliva** is brought about primarily by stimulation of the taste receptors but also by signals from higher levels of the brain (such as the thought of tasty food; it is especially effective to imagine that one

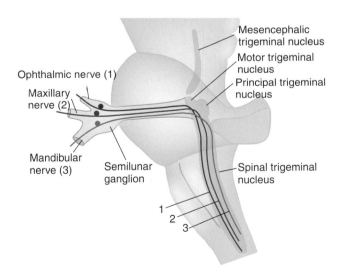

FIGURE 27.13 *The trigeminal nuclei.* In addition, the figure shows the topographic arrangement in the spinal trigeminal nucleus of the fibers from the three main trigeminal branches.

is eating a lemon). Strong emotions, for example, anxiety before a performance, can inhibit the secretion of saliva, as experienced by mouth dryness.

The **secretion of tears**, even more than the salivary secretion, is an example of how visceral functions can be influenced from higher levels of the brain. The continuous secretion of tears is of course primarily a physiological protection of the eyes and increases in response to any irritation of the cornea or the conjunctiva; nevertheless, the most profuse tear production occurs when we express strong emotions by crying. The signals to the superior salivatory nucleus producing the flow of tears when crying are not mediated by the pyramidal tract or other efferent cortical fibers descending in the internal capsule, in correspondence with the fact that tears cannot be produced voluntarily nor can the secretion of tears be suppressed. Most likely, fibers from the **hypothalamus** are responsible for the activation of the visceral efferent neurons during crying. Nevertheless, the hypothalamus is under the influence of higher levels, such as parts of the cerebral cortex and the limbic structures. Thus, the conscious experience of the emotions (such as sorrow or pity) starts the train of neural events leading to tear secretion.

The Intermediate Nerve

The small **geniculate ganglion**, containing the cell bodies of the sensory fibers of the intermediate nerve, is found where the facial nerve bends posteriorly in the temporal bone. Here a branch of the intermediate nerve, the **greater petrosal nerve**, leaves the main trunk of the facial nerve to course anteriorly. It contains **visceral efferent** (parasympathetic) fibers that end in the small parasympathetic **pterygopalatine ganglion** located behind the orbit. From there postganglionic fibers follow trigeminal branches to the **lacrimal gland** and **glands in the nasal cavity** (see Fig. 28.11). The rest of the intermediate nerve fibers leave the facial nerve as it passes downward posterior to the middle ear. This branch is called the **chorda tympani** because it passes through the middle ear (tympanic cavity) on its way forward to join the **lingual nerve** (a trigeminal branch) outside the skull. The chorda tympani contains **visceral afferent** fibers from **taste buds** in the anterior two-thirds of the tongue. These fibers have their cell bodies in the geniculate ganglion. In addition, the chorda tympani carries **visceral efferent** (parasympathetic) fibers that end in the small **submandibular ganglion**. From this ganglion, postganglionic parasympathetic fibers pass to the submandibular and the sublingual (salivary) glands.

THE TRIGEMINAL NERVE

The **fifth cranial nerve** is primarily the sensory nerve of the face, with mainly **somatic afferent fibers**. In addition,

it contains a small portion with **special somatic efferent** fibers to the masticatory muscles. The trigeminal nerve is the nerve of the **first branchial (visceral) arch** and innervates structures that are developed from this arch.

The nerve leaves the brain stem laterally on the pons (Fig. 27.1) with a small (medial) motor root and a large (lateral) sensory root. Shortly after leaving the pons, the nerve expands to form the large **semilunar ganglion**, which contains the cell bodies of the pseudounipolar (sensory) ganglion cells. Three large branches continue anteriorly from the ganglion: the **ophthalmic**, the **maxillary**, and the **mandibular** nerves (Fig. 27.13).

The **ophthalmic nerve** enters the orbit and supplies the eye bulb (including the cornea), the upper eyelid, the back of the nose, and the skin of the forehead with sensory fibers (Fig. 27.14). It also sends fibers to the mucous membranes of the anterior part of the nasal cavity. The **maxillary nerve** runs forward in a sulcus in the bottom of the orbit and sends fibers to the lower eyelid, the skin above the mouth, the upper teeth and the gingiva, and, finally, the hard palate and the posterior (major) part of the nasal cavity. The **mandibular nerve** innervates the lower teeth and gingiva, the tongue, and the skin of the lower jaw and upward, well into the temporal region (Fig. 27.14). The branch of the mandibular nerve supplying the tongue with somatic sensory afferent fibers is called the **lingual nerve**. This nerve receives visceral afferent (taste) fibers from the **chorda tympani**, destined for the anterior two-thirds of the tongue.

The **motor fibers** of the trigeminal nerve follow the mandibular nerve but leave this in several smaller twigs

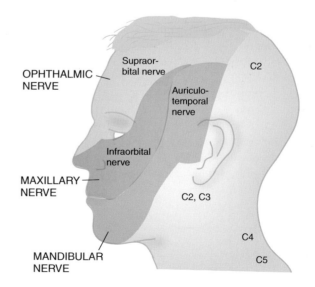

FIGURE 27.14 *Distribution in the facial skin of the three main trigeminal branches.* The names of some further branches and the segmental origins of sensory fibers to the rest of the head and the neck are indicated.

to the masticatory muscles (and some other muscles with relation to the lower jaw and the soft palate).

The Sensory Trigeminal Nucleus

With regard to function and fiber composition, the sensory part of the trigeminal nerve corresponds to the spinal dorsal roots. The trigeminal nerve, therefore, belongs to the somatosensory system and conducts signals from **low-threshold mechanoreceptors, thermoreceptors**, and **nociceptors** in the face and in the mucous membranes of the face. As with other spinal nerves, fibers leading from different kinds of receptors are intermingled in the nerve but are arranged by receptor type when entering the CNS. Then the fibers distribute to the three subdivisions of the long sensory trigeminal nucleus (Figs. 27.2 and 27.13). Fibers from proprioceptors (muscle spindles, joint receptors) end in the **mesencephalic nucleus**, fibers from low-threshold mechanoreceptors end in the main or **principal nucleus**, whereas signals from **nociceptors** end in the **spinal trigeminal nucleus**.[4]

Central Transmission of Signals from the Trigeminal Nucleus

Functionally, **the spinal trigeminal nucleus** (especially its caudal part) corresponds to the dorsalmost laminae of the cord, whereas the **principal sensory nucleus** corresponds to the dorsal column nuclei. These similarities are evident also in the central pathways. The secondary sensory fibers from the cells in the spinal nucleus join the **spinothalamic tract** (see Fig. 14.4) and end in the thalamus. Fibers from the main nucleus join the **medial lemniscus** (see Fig. 14.2). The somatotopic pattern within the thalamic terminal region is such that the fibers from the trigeminal nucleus—carrying signals from the face—end most medially, in the VPM (see Fig. 14.6). The ascending fibers from the trigeminal nucleus cross to the opposite side before they join the large sensory tracts. As discussed (under "Brain Stem Lesions Can Produce Symptoms from Several Cranial Nerves and Long Tracts"), a lesion affecting lateral parts of the medulla is likely to interrupt the spinothalamic tract and the spinal trigeminal nucleus. This will usually cause reduced or abolished pain and temperature sensation in the opposite body half but on the same side of the face (Fig. 27.6).[5] From the thalamus, the

signals are transmitted to the **face region** of the **SI** in the postcentral gyrus.

More about the Subdivisions of the Sensory Trigeminal Nucleus

The thinnest fibers of the trigeminal nerve (Aδ and C fibers)—conducting primarily from nociceptors and thermoreceptors—bend caudally after entering the pons (Fig. 27.13). They continue as a small bundle, the **spinal tract of the trigeminal nerve**, located just beneath the medullary surface. It is joined by somatic afferent fibers that have followed the glossopharyngeal and the vagus nerves peripherally. Just like the solitary tract, the spinal tract, strictly speaking, is not a tract, as it consists of the central process of the pseudounipolar ganglion cells. The spinal tract continues down into the upper cervical segments and corresponds to the zona terminalis (bundle of Lissauer) in the cord (see Fig. 13.16). The fibers enter the **spinal trigeminal nucleus** (nucleus of the spinal trigeminal tract), which corresponds largely to the dorsalmost laminae of the cord. For example, a layer very similar to the substantia gelatinosa is present. The spinal trigeminal nucleus can be further subdivided in a rostrocaudal sequence. The **caudal subnucleus** appears to be especially involved in pain mechanisms and corresponds most closely with the dorsal laminas of the cord. It also receives dorsal root fibers from the upper cervical segments. This may perhaps explain why a certain condition with paroxysms of facial pain of unknown origin—**trigeminal neuralgia**—may sometimes irradiate outside the area innervated by the trigeminal nerve. The spinal trigeminal nucleus furthermore shows a dorsoventral topographic localization. Thus the main trigeminal branches end sequentially, with the ophthalmic nerve ending most ventrally and the mandibular nerve most dorsally (Fig. 27.13).

Thick myelinated fibers (Aβ) in the trigeminal nerve from the skin end mostly in the principal sensory trigeminal nucleus (Fig. 27.13) with a precise somatotopic pattern.

The **mesencephalic trigeminal nucleus** stretches as a slender column from the upper part of the pons and into the mesencephalon. This is a very unusual nucleus, as its neurons look like pseudounipolar ganglion cells and, indeed, send one process peripherally into the trigeminal nerve. Afferent fibers from the **muscle spindles** of the **masticatory muscles** follow the mandibular nerve, whereas those from the **extraocular muscles** follow the ophthalmic and perhaps the oculomotor nerve. Signals from mechanoreceptors in the root sheaths of the **teeth** end in the mesencephalic nucleus.

Reflexes Involving the Trigeminal Nerve

Like the spinal dorsal root fibers, the trigeminal nerve constitutes the afferent link of several reflex arcs. The trigeminal nucleus, especially the spinal subdivision,

---

4 The separation of fibers of different types is not quite as sharp as this account may indicate. Many trigeminal fibers divide after entering the brain stem into an ascending and a descending branch (just like the sensory fibers entering the cord). In this manner, single ganglion cells may end in more than one nuclear subdivision.

5 If the lesion is situated high in the medulla or in the lower pons the ascending (secondary sensory) fibers from the spinal trigeminal nucleus have crossed and joined the spinothalamic tract. In such cases, loss of pain and temperature sensation in the face occurs on the opposite side of the lesion.

midline in the mesencephalon, ventral to the aqueduct (Figs. 27.2 and 27.5). The medial longitudinal fasciculus, with ascending fibers from the vestibular nuclei, lies close to the oculomotor nucleus (and to the abducens and trochlear nuclei as well). The **visceral efferent** (preganglionic parasympathetic) fibers come from the small **nucleus of Edinger-Westphal** located near the oculomotor nucleus. Often the term "oculomotor complex" is used for the somatic efferent and visceral efferent nuclei together.

The **oculomotor nerve** passes forward to the orbit through the **cavernous sinus** together with the other nerves to the eye (entering through the superior orbital fissure). The somatic efferent and parasympathetic fibers part in the orbit (Fig. 27.16). The somatic efferent fibers innervate the following extraocular muscles: the **superior** and **inferior rectus**, the **medial rectus**, and the **inferior oblique**. These muscles can move the eye medially, upward, and downward and rotate it around the sagittal axis (see Fig. 25.2). In addition, the oculomotor nerve supplies the **levator palpebrae** muscle, which serves to lift the upper eyelid.

The **visceral efferent** oculomotor fibers end in the small **ciliary ganglion** situated behind the eye (Fig. 27.16). Here the fibers establish synapses with the postganglionic neurons, which send their axons anteriorly in the wall of the eye to innervate the intrinsic (smooth) muscles of the eye: the **pupillary sphincter** and the **ciliary muscle** (see Fig. 16.2). Contraction of the ciliary muscle increases the lens curvature when looking at near objects (see Chapter 16, under "The Lens and the Far and Near Points of the Eye: Accommodation"). The sphincter constricts the pupil to reduce the amount of light reaching the retina.

A **lesion** of the **oculomotor nerve** produces, among other symptoms, an abnormal position of the eye, which is directed laterally (due to the unopposed pull of the lateral rectus) and downward (due to the superior oblique muscle). As in lesions of the abducens or the trochlear nerves, the patient will have double vision. In addition, the upper eyelid droops—ptosis—because of paralysis of the levator palpebrae (Fig. 27.18). The **interruption** of the **parasympathetic fibers** makes the pupil larger (due to loss of action of the pupillary sphincter), and the light reflex is absent (in an incomplete lesion of the nerve, the pupil may be slightly larger and the reaction to light more sluggish than on the normal side). **Accommodation** of the lens is abolished, making it impossible to see near objects sharply. The intracranial course of the oculomotor nerve makes it especially vulnerable in cases of temporal herniation caused by increased intracranial pressure (see Chapter 3). Thus, examination of the size of the pupils, and their reaction to light, is of great practical value in patients who are unconscious after **head trauma**.

The Light Reflex and the Accommodation Reflex

The oculomotor nerve is the efferent link of both of these reflexes, even though they are quite different in other respects. The **light reflex** is relatively simple, with its reflex center in the brain stem (Fig. 27.19). Increased amount of light hitting the retina elicits a contraction of the pupillary sphincter muscle. Both pupils constrict even when the light hits only one eye. The afferent link consists of fibers of the optic nerve that leave the optic tract before it reaches the lateral geniculate body. The fibers end in the pretectal nuclei on both sides. From these nuclei, the signals pass to the Edinger-Westphal nuclei on both sides, and by means of the ciliary ganglion, the signals reach the sphincter. The bilaterality of the connections explains why a unilateral stimulus produces a bilateral response.

Unilateral **interruption** of the **oculomotor nerve** abolishes the light reflex in the eye on the side of the lesion, but the reflex is present in the other eye. In case

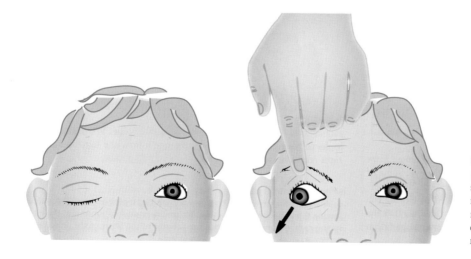

FIGURE 27.18 *Paresis of the oculomotor nerve (right side)*. **Left:** The upper eyelid droops (ptosis) due to paresis of the levator palpebrae muscle. **Right:** The examiner lifts the eyelid and reveals that the right eye is abducted and lowered due to the unopposed actions of the lateral rectus and the superior oblique muscles.

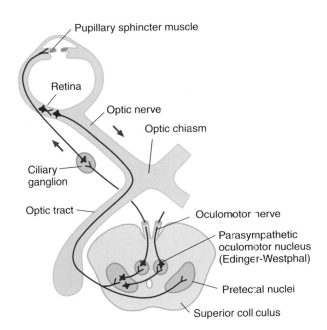

FIGURE 27.19 *The reflex arc for the light reflex.*

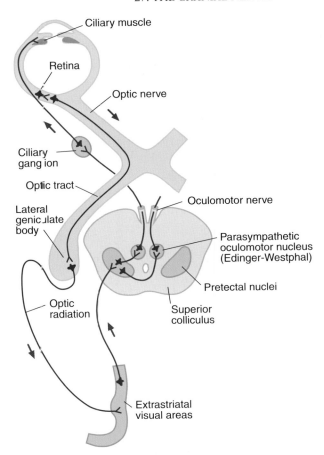

FIGURE 27.20 *The reflex arc for the accommodation reflex.*

of interruption of the **afferent link** on one side (damage to the retina or the optic nerve), the light reflex is absent in both eyes when light is shone into the eye on the lesioned side but is present in both sides when the other eye is illuminated. Thus, examination of the light reflex can provide valuable information with regard to the site of a lesion.

The **accommodation reflex** is a cortical reflex: the reflex arc passes through the cerebral cortex. The afferent link is fibers passing in the optic nerve from the retina, and the efferent link consists of parasympathetic fibers in the oculomotor nerve to the ciliary ganglion (Fig. 27.20). From there the postganglionic fibers pass to the ciliary muscle. The reflex center is not known in detail, but recent studies indicate that the cortical fibers pass to the superior colliculus (not the pretectal nuclei,

as shown in Fig. 27.18) and from there to the nearby reticular formation. Neurons in the reticular formation mediate the signals to the Edinger-Westphal nucleus. The accommodation reflex is elicited only when we fix the gaze on an object that is moving toward us. Together with the accommodation, a **pupillary constriction** occurs as the object comes closer.

VI | THE AUTONOMIC NERVOUS SYSTEM

THE autonomic nervous system (or visceral system) is not a term that can be defined precisely, either anatomically or functionally. The old belief that the somatic and the autonomic parts of the nervous system are completely independent is not tenable. The more we have learned about the nervous system, the clearer it has become that simplistic divisions like this are arbitrary. Some authors therefore maintain that the term "autonomic nervous system" should be abandoned and replaced by simply referring to **visceral neurons**—that is, the neurons that innervate visceral organs. For practical reasons, it is nevertheless helpful to use the term "autonomic nervous system" and to **define** it very broadly as the neuronal groups and fiber connections that control the activity of **visceral organs, vessels, and glands** (also the vessels and glands that are not parts of visceral organs). Visceral organs contain smooth-muscle cells and glandular cells. We can therefore also define the autonomic system as the parts of the nervous system that control the activity of **smooth muscles** and **glands**, regardless of their location in the body (in contrast to the somatic or cerebrospinal system, which controls striated skeletal muscles). Mostly, we are not aware of the processes going on in the organs controlled by the autonomic nervous system, and their activities are not subject to voluntary, conscious control.

The autonomic system can be subdivided in different ways. As with the somatic system, we distinguish **peripheral** and **central** parts. Whereas the peripheral parts of the autonomic and somatic systems can be separated fairly well, the division becomes much less clear within the central nervous system. The peripheral parts of the autonomic system are described in Chapters 28 and 29. Although the nerves to visceral organs contain both efferent (motor) and afferent (sensory) fibers, the anatomic differences between the autonomic and the somatic systems concern primarily the efferent side. Chapter 28 deals with the **visceral efferent neurons**, while Chapter 29 describes the characteristic features of **visceral afferent neurons**—that is, the sensory innervation of visceral organs. Even though visceral afferent neurons do not differ structurally from somatic afferent neurons, there are nevertheless physiological differences that are important in a clinical context—in particular, in relation to pain arising in the visceral organs. Although Chapter 29 contains discussion of some visceral reflexes and their central control, main topics concerning the central control of the autonomic system, notably the hypothalamus, are discussed in Chapter 30.

The autonomic system can also be divided into a **sympathetic** and a **parasympathetic** part, differing anatomically and functionally (again, the separation is most obvious in the peripheral nervous system). The actions of the two parts of the autonomic system are often antagonistic: where the sympathetic system activates, the parasympathetic reduces the activity, and vice versa. In addition, the **enteric nervous system** is now regarded as a distinct part of the autonomic nervous system. It consists of some million neurons and an extensive network in the wall of the digestive tract. The enteric system is influenced by both the sympathetic and the parasympathetic systems but functions independently as well.

In a superior perspective, a major function of the autonomic system is to contribute to **bodily homeostasis**, that is, the maintenance of a relatively constant internal milieu. The autonomic nervous system is not the only means by which the central nervous system can control homeostasis, however. In addition, the **endocrine system**, which is controlled from the central nervous system via the pituitary gland, serves this purpose. Further, homeostasis requires appropriate somatic motor activity to secure, for example, the supply of water and nutrients. The role of the **hypothalamus** is to organize the autonomic, endocrine, and somatic-motor processes into behavior that is appropriate for the immediate and long-term needs of the organism.

28 | Visceral Efferent Neurons: The Sympathetic and Parasympathetic Divisions

OVERVIEW

In general, the actions of the sympathetic system suggest that it is of special importance in situations of stress, requiring mobilization of bodily resources. The parasympathetic system, in contrast, contributes primarily to processes of maintenance, such as digestion and reproductive behavior. Such generalized statements are useful only as rules of thumb, however, because the actions of the two systems are much more varied than this. Table 28.1 gives an overview of the main actions of the two systems in various organs.

The sympathetic and parasympathetic system both consist of two consecutive neurons leading from the central nervous system (CNS) to the target organs. The **preganglionic neuron** has its cell body in the cord or in the brain stem and the axon terminates in a **ganglion**. **Postganglionic neurons** have their cell bodies in the ganglia while their axons terminate close to **smooth muscle cells** and **glandular cells**. The **preganglionic** sympathetic neurons are found in the **intermediolateral column** of the cord, stretching from T_1 to L_2, whereas the preganglionic parasympathetic cell bodies reside in the **brain stem** and in the **sacral cord**. All preganglionic neurons use **acetylcholine** as transmitter in the ganglia, where they act on **nicotinic** receptors. Most sympathetic neurons use **norepinephrine** (and various neuropeptides) as transmitter, while parasympathetic neurons use **acetylcholine** binding to **muscarinic** receptors.

Preganglionic sympathetic and parasympathetic fibers leave the cord and the brain stem through ventral roots and motor cranial nerves. Their further course differs, however. The parasympathetic fibers pass directly to ganglia that lie close to or in the wall of the target organ. The sympathetic fibers leave the spinal nerves just outside the intervertebral foramen and enter the **sympathetic trunk**, which stretches from the base of the skull to the lower end of the cord. The sympathetic trunk forms a chain of interconnected sympathetic ganglia. From these ganglia, sympathetic postganglionic fibers follow the spinal nerves to the extremities and somatic structures of the trunk. Preganglionic sympathetic fibers destined for visceral organs pass through the ganglia and leave the sympathetic trunk in separate **splanchnic nerves**. These end in **prevertebral ganglia**, and from there postganglionic fibers follow arteries to the target organs.

The **enteric system** consists of some million neurons in the wall of the gastrointestinal tract, controlling peristaltic movements, secretion, and absorption. While it operates to a large extent independently of the CNS, this "mini-brain of the gut" integrates local information from the gut with central commands through the sympathetic and parasympathetic systems.

GENERAL ORGANIZATION

Two Succeeding Neurons Constitute the Efferent Pathway

Despite their different actions, the sympathetic and the parasympathetic systems have certain features of peripheral organization in common that should be known before discussing the differences between them. In contrast to the somatic efferent fibers (leading from motoneurons to skeletal muscles), the visceral efferent fibers do not pass nonstop to the organs. The transmission of signals is synaptically interrupted in **autonomic ganglia** (Figs. 28.1 and 28.2). The multipolar neurons in the ganglia send their axons to the effectors (smooth-muscle cells and glands) in the visceral organs. The neurons conducting signals to the ganglia are called **preganglionic**, whereas the ganglion cells and their axons are called **postganglionic**. The cell bodies of the preganglionic neurons are located in the spinal cord and the brain stem. The **preganglionic neurons**, both the sympathetic and the parasympathetic ones, use **acetylcholine** as a neurotransmitter.

Another typical feature of the visceral efferent neurons is that, as a rule, the postganglionic fibers form extensive **plexuses** around the organs they innervate.

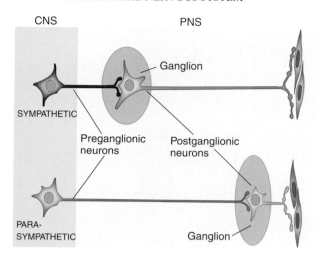

FIGURE 28.1 *Basic organization of the peripheral part of the autonomic system.* Two consecutive neurons conduct the signals from the central nervous system to the effectors. Note the difference in length between the pre- and postganglionic fibers in the sympathetic and the parasympathetic systems. Effectors may be glandular cells and not only smooth-muscle cells, as shown here.

Postganglionic Fibers Do Not Establish Typical Synapses

The thin, unmyelinated postganglionic fibers do not form typical synapses with the effector cells; in contrast to the somatic efferent fibers innervating skeletal muscle cells (see Fig. 21.5). When the postganglionic fibers reach the vicinity of the effector cells, they branch extensively, and there are small swellings—varicosities—along the branches (Fig. 28.1). In each varicosity, there are vesicles with neurotransmitters. The varicosities do not form synapses but can be located fairly close to the effector cells. In some places, the distance is only 50 nm, thus permitting very direct and precise control of the effector cell. Most often, however, the distance between the varicosities and the effectors is so great that the neurotransmitter, after being released, must diffuse over a considerable distance to reach its target. This means that the neurotransmitter acts on several effector cells within a certain distance. When the diffusion distance is great, the transmitter acts slowly, with a long latency and a prolonged action (compared with the fast action at the neuromuscular junction). Often, only a few of the smooth-muscle cells in the wall of a hollow organ (such as a vessel) are close enough to the varicosities to be directly influenced by the transmitter. In such cases, the action potential elicited in some smooth-muscle cells is propagated from cell to cell via **gap junctions** between them (electric coupling). In general, therefore, the actions of the autonomic nervous system are more **diffusely distributed**, both **spatially** and **temporally**, than is the case in the somatic system. The properties of the smooth-muscle cells contribute to increase this difference, because their action potentials last much longer

than those of skeletal muscle cells do. Further, smooth-muscle cells (e.g., in the wall of the gastrointestinal tract) can be made to contract by stimuli other than nervous ones, such as by stretching and by the actions of hormones. The autonomic system therefore contributes to the regulation of the contraction of smooth-muscle cells in the gastrointestinal tract and in the walls of the vessels, but it is not alone in this capacity (again in contrast to the control of skeletal muscle cells by the motoneurons).

Some Organs Are Subject to More Precise Autonomic Control than Others

There are, nevertheless, great differences between different organs with regard to the precision of their autonomic innervation. Some visceral organs require much faster and more accurate control than others. The smooth muscles of the **eye** (the ciliary muscle and the pupillary sphincter, regulating the curvature of the lens and the diameter of the pupil) must be subject to very precise control. The same holds for the muscles of the **ductus deferens**, in which the propulsive contractions must be fast and well coordinated. Such demands are not made of the smooth muscles of the gastrointestinal tract and the vessels. Corresponding to different functional requirements, the pattern of autonomic innervation varies in different organs. The intrinsic eye muscles, for example, receive a large number of nerve fibers so that all muscle cells come in close contact with varicosities of nerve fibers. This is called **multiunit arrangement**, because it is similar to the conditions in the somatic system with many precisely controlled motor units. In places with few nerve fibers to supply a large number of smooth-muscle cells, so that only a few cells are close to nerve varicosities, we use the term **single-unit arrangement**. Thus, numerous muscle cells behave as a unit when one or a few of them are activated.

Autonomic Ganglia and Plexuses

The autonomic ganglia contain **multipolar neurons** of various sizes (Fig. 28.3) with long, branching dendrites. The axons are mostly unmyelinated and very thin. The cell bodies of the ganglion cells are embedded in a meshwork of fibers consisting of afferent fibers, ganglion cell dendrites, and axons of the ganglion cells. At least some of the ganglia receive **sensory fibers** from visceral organs. There are also **interneurons** in the autonomic ganglia. Such features, and other data, indicate that the ganglia are not just simple synaptic interruptions of purely motor (efferent) pathways but can serve as **reflex centers** for some visceral reflexes.

When an organ is innervated by both sympathetic and parasympathetic fibers, these two components intermingle and form **autonomic plexuses** just outside

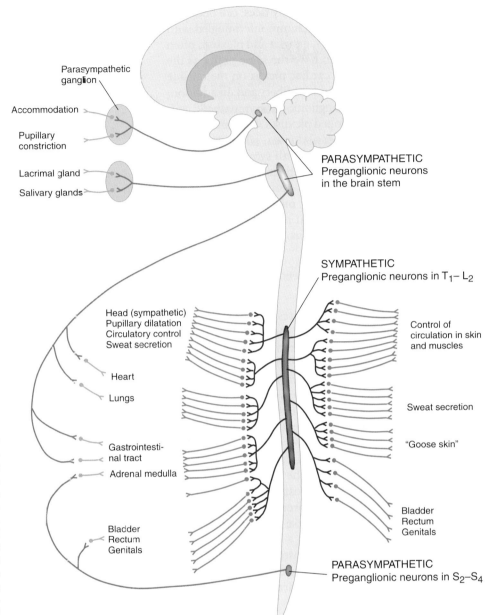

FIGURE 28.2 *Main anatomic features of the autonomic nervous system.* The preganglionic sympathetic neurons have their cell bodies in the intermediolateral column, whereas the corresponding parasympathetic neurons are located in the brain stem and the sacral cord. The cell bodies of sympathetic postganglionic neurons in ganglia lie close to the vertebral column (paravertebral and prevertebral ganglia), whereas those of parasympathetic postganglionic neurons lie in ganglia close to the organ. The sympathetic fibers reach all parts of the body, but the parasympathetic fibers have a more restricted distribution. (After Pick 1970.)

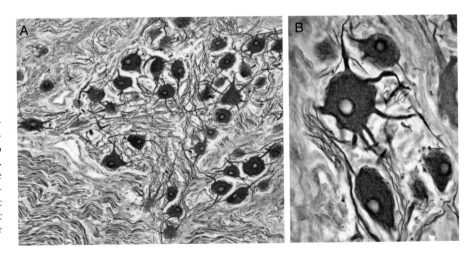

FIGURE 28.3 *Autonomic ganglion.* Photomicrograph of section through the celiac ganglion impregnated with heavy metals to show nerve fibers (black) and neurons (red). **A:** The multipolar postganglionic neurons lie in a wickerwork of preganglionic and postganglionic nerve fibers. Thus, the autonomic ganglia consist of groups of postganglionic neurons embedded in a plexus. **B:** Higher magnification of postganglionic neurons.

The difference in innervation precision between the sympathetic and the parasympathetic systems mentioned above have several **exceptions**, however. One example is the ductus deferens, in which the rhythmic contractions are elicited by sympathetic fibers. A multi-unit arrangement is required to ensure the necessary precision and speed of the contractile wave moving the sperm during ejaculation. Another example is that the parasympathetic innervation of the gastrointestinal tract is rather diffuse (single-unit arrangement).

PERIPHERAL PARTS OF THE SYMPATHETIC SYSTEM

Preganglionic Fibers and the Sympathetic Trunk

The peripheral parts of the sympathetic system consist of both neurons conveying signals to visceral organs and sensory fibers leading in the opposite direction. The efferent, preganglionic sympathetic neurons have their cell bodies in the **intermediolateral column** in the spinal cord (Fig. 28.4). The preganglionic fibers leave the cord (like other efferent fibers) through the ventral roots, but because the intermediolateral column is present

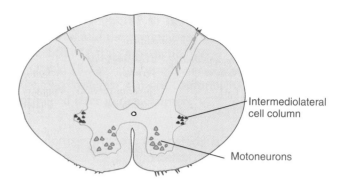

FIGURE 28.4 *The intermediolateral cell column contains the cell bodies of the preganglionic sympathetic neurons.* Cross section of the thoracic cord.

in only the T_1–L_2 segments, only the ventral roots of these segments contain preganglionic sympathetic fibers (the sympathetic system is also called the thoracolumbar system). The sympathetic fibers follow the somatic ones for a short distance, however. Just after the ventral and the dorsal roots fuse, the sympathetic preganglionic fibers leave the spinal nerve to end in a **sympathetic ganglion** (Fig. 28.5). In early embryonic life, one ganglion is

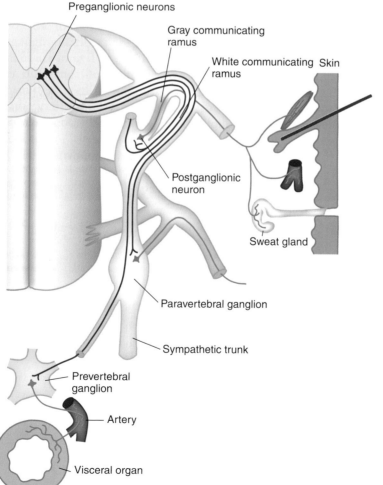

FIGURE 28.5 *The sympathetic system.* Postganglionic neurons are located in the ganglia of the sympathetic trunk and in the prevertebral ganglia. Sympathetic fibers to the trunk and the extremities follow the spinal nerves, whereas fibers to the visceral organs form separate nerves and follow the main vessels to the organs.

produced on each side for every spinal segment, but during further development, some ganglia fuse, so the final number is smaller than the number of segments. This reduction is most marked in the cervical region.

The ganglia are located just outside the intervertebral foramen, laterally on the vertebral column (Fig. 28.6). The row of such **paravertebral ganglia** extends from the base of the skull to the coccygeal bone in the pelvis minor. Because fiber bundles interconnect the ganglia, a continuous string called the **sympathetic trunk** is formed (Figs. 28.5 and 28.6). The ganglia form small swellings along the trunk. There is usually one ganglion for each pair of spinal nerves, except in the cervical region, where there are only three: the **superior, middle, and inferior cervical ganglia**. The middle ganglion can be missing, and the inferior cervical ganglion is usually fused with the uppermost thoracic ganglion to form the large **stellate ganglion** (Fig. 28.6). Some cross connections are present in the lumbar and sacral parts of the sympathetic trunks.

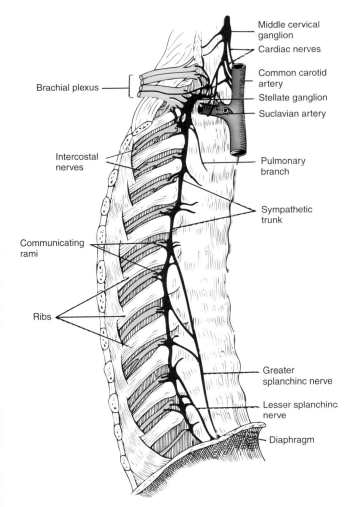

FIGURE 28.6 *The sympathetic trunk.* Part of the thoracic vertebral column and the ribs, as viewed from the right. Note the communicating rami and the splanchnic nerves. (Redrawn from Spalteholz 1933.)

The preganglionic sympathetic fibers leave the spinal nerve as a small bundle called the **white communicating ramus** (branch), which connects the nerve with the sympathetic trunk (Figs. 28.5 and 28.6). The whitish color arises because the preganglionic fibers are myelinated. Because of the restricted extension of the intermediolateral column, only the thoracic and the upper two lumbar spinal nerves give off white communicating rami.

When reaching the ganglia of the sympathetic trunk, some preganglionic fibers establish synapses with **postganglionic neurons** in that ganglion, whereas others continue uninterrupted through the ganglion (Fig. 28.5). In the upper part of the trunk, the fibers continue rostrally, in the lower part caudally, to establish synapses with ganglion cells in ganglia at levels above and below the intermediolateral column (Figs. 28.7, 28.8, and 28.9). This arrangement ensures that preganglionic fibers reach all the ganglia of the sympathetic trunk (the paravertebral ganglia).

Some of the preganglionic fibers pass directly through the ganglia and form separate nerves—**splanchnic nerves**—destined for **prevertebral sympathetic ganglia** (Figs. 28.5 and 28.7). We return to this point later in this chapter.

Postganglionic Sympathetic Fibers

The postganglionic fibers from the ganglia of the sympathetic trunk take different routes. From all of the ganglia, some fibers pass back to the spinal nerve as the thin **gray communicating ramus** (Figs. 28.5 and 28.6). This ramus is more grayish than the white ramus because most of the postganglionic fibers are unmyelinated.[1] All of the spinal nerves receive postganglionic fibers through the communicating rami (Fig. 28.6). The postganglionic fibers follow the spinal nerves out into all their branches (Figs. 28.8 and 28.9). Some postganglionic fibers leave the trunk, pass to larger arteries in the vicinity, and innervate the smooth-muscle cells of the artery. Many of the postganglionic sympathetic fibers that follow the spinal nerves leave them peripherally to innervate small vessels. Other fibers from the spinal nerves innervate the sweat glands and the smooth muscles attached to hair follicles (Fig. 28.5).

Sympathetic Innervation of the Head and Extremities

The head, neck, and upper extremity receive **preganglionic** sympathetic fibers from the **upper thoracic segments** (Table 28.2). The fibers enter the sympathetic trunk

---

1 White and gray rami often fuse into one, so that even at the levels T_1–L_2 there may be only one communicating ramus on each side. This contains, as will be understood, both the pre- and postganglionic fibers. In the case of two rami, the color difference between them is not very marked.

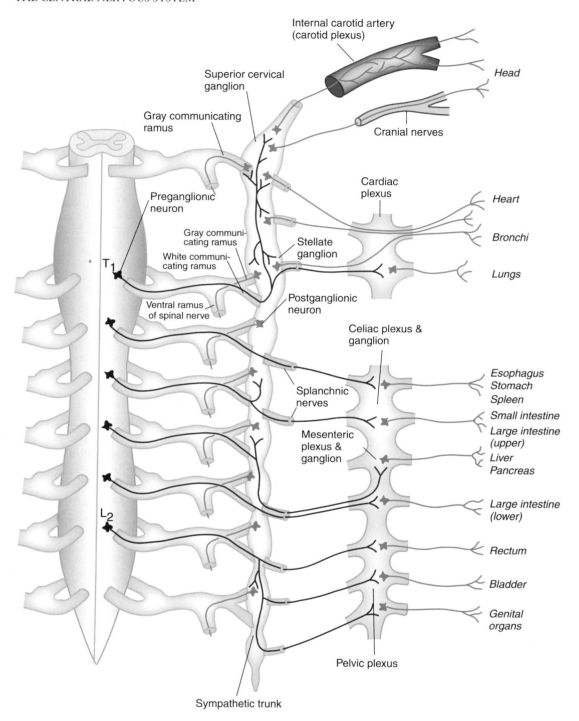

FIGURE 28.7 *The sympathetic system.* The sympathetic trunk with the paravertebral ganglia, and the prevertebral ganglia and plexuses are shown. The organs innervated from the various ganglia are also specified.

through the communicating rami. Some establish synaptic contacts with postganglionic neurons in the upper thoracic ganglia, whereas other fibers pass through these ganglia to end in the cervical ganglia (Figs. 28.7 and 28.8). From these ganglia, postganglionic fibers enter the spinal nerves to the neck (C_1–C_4) and the upper extremity (C_5–T_1).

The **head** receives **postganglionic** fibers from the **superior cervical ganglion**. From the ganglion, the fibers follow arteries and cranial nerves to the skin, the eye, the lacrimal gland, and the salivary glands (Table 28.2).

With regard to the **lower extremities**, the arrangement corresponds to that described for the upper extremity,

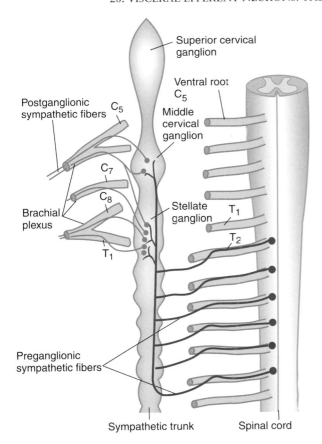

FIGURE 28.8 *Sympathetic innervation of the upper extremity.* The preganglionic fibers come from the upper thoracic segments of the cord and synapse in the ganglia of the sympathetic trunk up to the middle cervical ganglion. The postganglionic fibers follow the spinal nerves to the arm. (Redrawn from Haymaker and Woodhall 1945.)

with postganglionic fibers following the spinal the spinal nerves (Fig. 28.9).

Interruption of the Sympathetic Innervation of the Head: Horner's Syndrome

A lesion of the sympathetic trunk in the neck is the most common cause of sympathetic denervation of the head. Because all preganglionic fibers enter the trunk below the inferior cervical ganglion (Fig. 28.8), a lesion anywhere above the level of the thoracic outlet can interrupt the sympathetic innervation of the head. It may be caused, for example, by a tumor in the apex of the lung, in the thyroid gland, or in any of the numerous lymph nodes in the neck. The ensuing symptoms can be understood based on the effects of sympathetic fibers on the skin and the eye (Table 28.1). In the case of a unilateral lesion, the facial skin on the side of the lesion becomes redder (warmer) and drier than that on the other side (caused by vasodilatation and lack of sweat secretion). The pupil is miotic (smaller) on the side of the lesion (paralysis of the pupillary sphincter), and there is slight ptosis (the eyelid droops) owing to paralysis of the

smooth tarsal muscle. This constellation of symptoms—**red** and **dry** skin, **miosis**, and **ptosis**—affecting half of the face is called **Horner's syndrome** (Fig. 28.10).

Horner's syndrome can also be caused by lesions in the brain stem, interrupting the descending fibers to the intermediolateral column (cf. Chapter 27, under "Brain Stem Lesions Can Produce Symptoms from Several Cranial Nerves and Long Tracts" and "Lateral Pontine Infarctions").

Sympathetic Innervation of the Viscera

As mentioned, the postganglionic sympathetic fibers to the extremities and the body wall follow mainly the spinal nerves. The visceral organs of the thorax and the abdomen do not receive branches from the spinal nerves, however. Therefore, the sympathetic fibers destined for these organs have to form separate nerves. Such **splanchnic nerves** are thin twigs that leave the sympathetic trunk at various levels.

The sympathetic fibers to the **heart** follow the superior, middle, and inferior **cardiac nerves** leaving the corresponding cervical ganglia. The cell bodies of the postganglionic neurons lie in the cervical ganglia. In addition, some smaller branches to the heart take off from the upper thoracic sympathetic ganglia.

Most sympathetic fibers to the **abdominal viscera** form the **greater** and **lesser splanchnic nerves** (Fig. 28.6). These nerves consist mainly of preganglionic fibers from spinal segments T_6–T_{11}, which pass uninterrupted through the ganglia of the sympathetic trunk (Figs. 28.5 and 28.7). The nerves penetrate the diaphragm and end in ganglia located on the ventral side of the abdominal aorta in the upper abdomen. As mentioned, these are called **prevertebral ganglia**, to distinguish them from the paravertebral ganglia of the sympathetic trunk.

The largest among the prevertebral ganglia is the **celiac ganglion**, located where the celiac artery emerges from the aorta. Smaller prevertebral ganglia occur where the **superior** and **inferior mesenteric** arteries emerge. The postganglionic fibers follow the arteries to the various organs.

The greater and lesser splanchnic nerves and the corresponding prevertebral ganglia supply the visceral organs in the **upper** and **middle** part of the **abdomen**, such as the stomach, pancreas, gallbladder, small intestine, and the large intestine to the descending part. The **adrenal medulla**, which also receives preganglionic fibers from the splanchnic nerves, is special. The medullary endocrine cells (**chromaffin cells**)—which are transformed postganglionic neurons—release **epinephrine** (and small amounts of norepinephrine) into the bloodstream on sympathetic stimulation.

The visceral organs of the **lower abdomen** and the **pelvis** receive their sympathetic innervation from the intermediolateral column in the lower thoracic and upper two

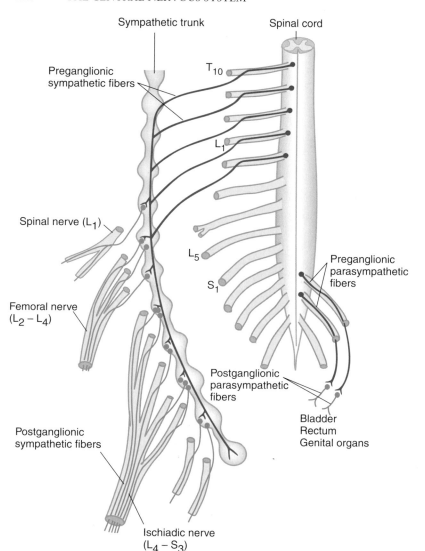

Symphathetic trunk

Spinal cord

Preganglionic
symphathetic fibers

T₁₀

L₁

Spinal nerve (L₁)

L₅

S₁

Preganglionic
parasympathetic
fibers

Femoral nerve
(L₂ – L₄)

Postganglionic
parasympathetic
fibers

Bladder
Rectum
Genital organs

Postganglionic
symphathetic fibers

Ischiadic nerve
(L₄ – S₃)

FIGURE 28.9 *Sympathetic innervation of the lower extremity*. On the right side, pre- and postganglionic parasympathetic fibers from the sacral cord are also shown. (Redrawn from Haymaker and Woodhall 1945.)

lumbar segments (Table 28.2). These fibers also leave the sympathetic trunk as separate nerves (lumbar splanchnic nerves) to reach prevertebral ganglia. The postganglionic fibers follow the arteries to the organs (Fig. 28.6).

The prevertebral ganglia are embedded in a meshwork of fibers, forming **prevertebral plexuses**, with names corresponding to those of the ganglia (Fig. 28.7). The plexuses formed mainly by sympathetic fibers continue

from the lower part of the abdominal aorta into the pelvis minor as the **hypogastric plexus**. In the pelvis, the hypogastric plexus mixes with parasympathetic fibers from the pelvic nerves and forms the **pelvic plexus** around the pelvic organs, as mentioned earlier.

PERIPHERAL PARTS OF THE PARASYMPATHETIC SYSTEM

As mentioned, the **preganglionic parasympathetic** (visceral efferent) neurons have their cell bodies in the brain stem and in the sacral cord. The neurons look like the sympathetic preganglionic neurons of the intermediolateral column.

The Cranial Nerves Contain Preganglionic Parasympathetic Fibers

The preganglionic fibers of the **cranial part** of the parasympathetic system follow the **oculomotor**, the **facial**

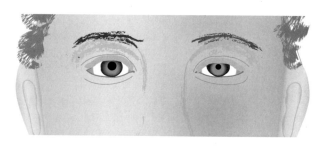

FIGURE 28.10 *Horner's syndrome*. The left half of the face shows the characteristic symptoms of loss of sympathetic innervation: red and dry skin, constricted pupil (miosis), and drooping of the upper eyelid (ptosis).

(intermediate), the **glossopharyngeal**, and the **vagus nerves**. The fibers come from the visceral efferent column of cranial nerve nuclei (see Figs. 27.2 and 27.3). The preganglionic fibers of the cranial nerves supplying structures in the head end in several parasympathetic **ganglia**, located outside the skull close to large cranial nerve trunks (Fig. 28.11). These are the **ciliary**, the

pterygopalatine, the **otic**, and the **submandibular ganglia**. From these ganglia, the postganglionic fibers pass to the effector organs (the intrinsic muscles of the eye, the lacrimal gland, and the salivary glands).

The preganglionic fibers of the **vagus nerve** do not end in well-defined ganglia but in more diffusely distributed collections of postganglionic neurons in the

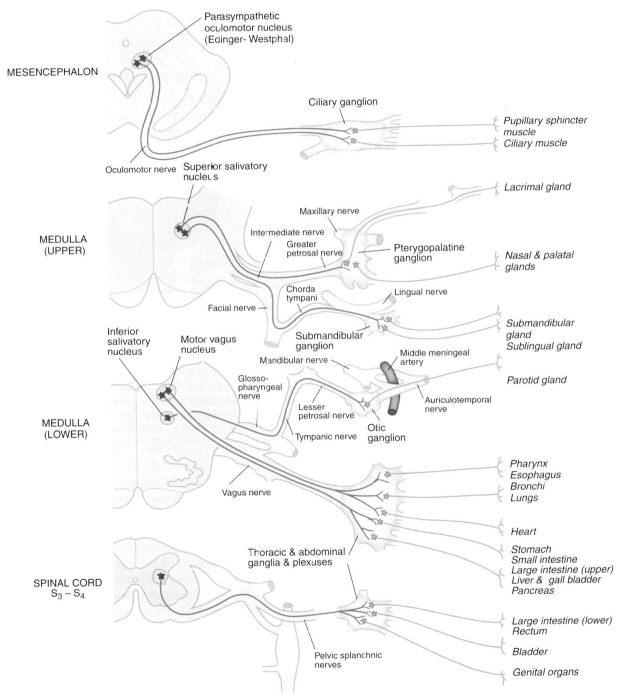

FIGURE 28.11 *The parasympathetic system.* The cell bodies of the preganglionic neurons are located in the brain stem and in the sacral cord. The peripheral course of the parasympathetic fibers is often quite complicated because they "jump" from one cranial nerve to another on their way to the target.

stroke volume increases. Cardiac muscle cells with a lower spontaneous firing frequency than the cells of the sinus node are activated by spread of the signal from the sinus node before the spontaneous depolarization has reached the threshold for an action potential. At rest, the heart is under a certain dominance of the parasympathetic system (the vagus nerve), which "restrains" the cardiac activity. Actions on the stroke volume by the autonomic system are mediated by fibers ending near the muscle cells of the ventricles.

Because the vascular smooth-muscle cells are arranged circularly, contraction reduces the diameter and increases the vascular resistance. Such vasoconstriction is most marked in the smallest arteries, the **arterioles**, which are especially concerned with the regulation of blood flow to the organs. Action potentials in the sympathetic fibers ending in the vessel walls produce vasoconstriction and, thus, reduced blood flow. By varying the signal frequency of the sympathetic nerves, the CNS can vary the diameter of the vessels.[2] When there are no signals in the sympathetic fibers innervating the vessel (and no other substances act to produce contraction), the arterioles are maximally widened by the internal blood pressure. This is called **vasodilatation** (vasodilation).

In many situations, the task of the sympathetic system is to ensure that there is a sufficient blood flow through **high-priority organs**, primarily the brain and the heart. When the blood flow through these organs diminishes, sympathetic neurons to vessels in other parts of the body increase their firing rate. Thus, the blood flow through skeletal muscles and the visceral organs is reduced. Sudden vasodilatation in large parts of the body leads to a fall in blood pressure and fainting, because the cerebral blood flow is reduced.

Sympathetic innervation of the **large veins** is also important for the maintenance of adequate blood pressure. Constriction of such capacity vessels distributes more of the blood volume to the arterial side—that is, the **effective blood volume** increases. This mechanism is important in case blood volume is reduced (on bleeding or dehydration).

Signals in sympathetic fibers to arterioles in **skeletal muscles** produce (as their main effect) vasoconstriction. Whether some sympathetic fibers may have the opposite effect in humans is not settled. Epinephrine—released from the adrenal medulla on sympathetic stimulation—may, however, inhibit the vascular smooth-muscle cells and thereby produce vasodilatation.

The vessels of the **lungs** receive sympathetic fibers producing vasodilatation. It is doubtful whether postganglionic sympathetic fibers act on the bronchial smooth musculature in humans, even though such innervation is present in several animal species. Thus, using histofluorescence techniques, which visualize catecholaminergic nerve fibers in tissue sections, studies in humans have shown the presence of such fibers around the vessels but not around the bronchi. **Epinephrine**, however, has a powerful inhibitory effect on the bronchial musculature; that is, it produces bronchial dilation. Most likely, therefore, the sympathetic system acts on the resistance of the airways by its stimulation of the adrenal medulla.

Control of Blood Pressure and Blood-Flow Distribution

Normally, the sympathetic neurons are activated reflexly, and many of them are links in arcs for so-called **vasomotor reflexes**, the reflexes in which the response is a change of vascular diameter (and thus resistance). The reflex arcs go through the cord or higher levels (the reticular formation or the hypothalamus). The superior aim of the control of **blood pressure** is to ensure that the brain (and the heart) always has a sufficient blood flow. **Baroreceptors** in the large arteries in the neck and the aortal arch record the slightest fall in blood pressure and produce an automatic increase of the signal frequency of sympathetic fibers. This is most marked for the skeletal muscles, but, if necessary, the heart rate is also increased. In this manner, vasoconstriction of the skeletal muscle arterioles is produced, thus increasing the vascular resistance and elevating the blood pressure, with the end result that the blood flow to the brain is increased to an adequate level.

Vasomotor reflexes have been studied with the **microneurographic technique**, enabling the recording of the activity of small groups of postganglionic sympathetic fibers in humans. This makes it possible to study the relationship between the sympathetic signal frequency and, for example, blood pressure. The postganglionic sympathetic fibers to muscle arterioles fire in bursts in pace with the pulse. The bursts are evoked by baroreceptor activation during the diastole of the heart. The overall firing frequency changes in association with changes of blood pressure. Considering the enormous blood flow that can pass through working muscles, we must obviously have central control of this part of the vascular system. Only if the heart increases its output and other vascular beds are constricted (e.g., in the abdominal organs) can the sympathetic "throttling" of the muscles be relieved without fall in the blood pressure.

Individual Differences in Sympathetic Activity

There are striking differences among persons with regard to the level of activity of sympathetic fibers under identical circumstances, as shown with the microneurographic technique. Postganglionic fibers to skeletal muscles,

2 The degree of vasoconstriction is influenced not only by the nervous system but also by circulating hormones, in particular, epinephrine. Further, substances produced by the local metabolism in the tissue influence the degree of contraction of the vascular smooth-muscle cells.

which constitute a large fraction of all postganglionic fibers in peripheral nerves, have been studied in particular. As mentioned, the activity of these fibers changes in close correlation with changes of the central blood pressure. Comparison of persons with normal blood pressure shows that the resting activity of sympathetic fibers varies by a factor of 10 from person to person. Thus, each person appears to have his own characteristic pattern, which is unchanged over a long time. From this "baseline" value, the signal frequency is up- or down-regulated in response to alterations in blood pressure caused by, for example, the change of body position from sitting to standing. No clear correlation has been found between the level of activity in sympathetic fibers to muscles and elevated blood pressure (hypertension).

Effects of Sympathetic Fibers in the Skin

The sympathetic innervation of the skin serves first and foremost the control of **body temperature**. The activity of the postganglionic sympathetic fibers to the skin appears not to be clearly related to the blood pressure, in contrast to the activity of fibers supplying vessels in skeletal muscles, but skin sympathetic fiber activity is closely correlated with the ambient temperature.

The **sweat glands** of the skin are innervated by sympathetic fibers, producing sweat secretion. Increased activity of fibers innervating the sweat glands occurs together with reduced activity of fibers to the small vessels. This produces **vasodilatation** and **sweat secretion** with increased loss of heat. A special feature of the innervation of sweat glands is that the neurotransmitter released from the postganglionic fibers is **acetylcholine** (and not norepinephrine).[3]

Sweat secretion may also occur in extreme situations with a large drop in blood pressure or with strong pain. In such situations, the skin vessels are maximally constricted and the skin is, consequently, pale and cold (**cold sweat**).

Signals in sympathetic fibers also activate the small smooth muscles attached to the **hair roots**, which make the hairs stand up. This is called **piloerection** (piloarrection). At the same time, the muscles compress the **sebaceous glands**, so that they empty their product into the hair follicle. In humans, the sympathetic control of hair position is of minor importance, whereas in animals it is of great significance for control of body temperature.

Irritation of Peripheral Nerves Can Produce Changes in the Skin

The effects of sympathetic fibers to the skin—that is, sweat secretion, vasoconstriction, and piloerection—can be reproduced by electrical stimulation of the ventral roots or the peripheral branches of the spinal nerves. The sympathetic fibers can be irritated by infections or by compression or traction of the nerves. In such cases, there is abnormal sweat secretion from pale and cold areas of the skin. Destruction of the sympathetic fibers (by, e.g., prolonged compression) leads to abolished sweat secretion and vasodilatation, resulting in areas of the skin that are abnormally warm and red and at the same time dry. Observations of such local changes of the skin can be helpful in the diagnosis of diseases that affect the peripheral nerves.

Effects of Sympathetic Fibers in the Gastrointestinal Tract, the Genital Organs, and the Eyes

In the **abdominal viscera**, signals in sympathetic fibers produce **vasoconstriction** and reduced contractile activity of the smooth muscles of the walls of hollow organs (i.e., reducing the amplitude and frequency of the peristaltic movements). At the same time, the secretion of the glands of the digestive tract is reduced. In sum, these effects result in a marked reduction of the digestive processes. The sympathetic system also inhibits the emptying of the **rectum**, both by inhibition of the smooth muscles of the wall and by activating the smooth muscles of the internal anal sphincter. The sympathetic system seems to play a minor role in the control of the bladder in humans (see later, "Normal Emptying of the Bladder").

The sympathetic innervation of the **genital organs** concerns vessels and the smooth musculature. The innervation of the **ductus deferens** is of particular importance because signals in sympathetic fibers are responsible for the rhythmic contractions during ejaculation. The **uterus** receives sympathetic fibers but their functional role is not clear. Thus, even after complete denervation, the uterus may function normally in pregnancy and in parturition.

The sympathetic fibers to the **eye** have their cell bodies in the **superior cervical ganglion**. They produce dilation of the pupil by activating the **pupillary dilatator muscle** and by causing contraction of the radially oriented vessels of the iris (the latter effect is probably most important for pupillary dilation). A small smooth muscle attached to the upper eyelid, the **tarsal muscle**, is also innervated by sympathetic fibers. The tonic activity of this muscle helps to keep the eyelid up while we are awake (the paresis of the tarsal muscle is responsible for the slight drooping of the eyelid occurring in Horner's syndrome).

---

3 Human hairy skin (but not glabrous skin) receives sympathetic fibers of two kinds: the ordinary noradrenergic vasoconstrictor fibers innervating vessels in all parts of the body, and cholinergic vasodilator fibers. The latter fibers mediate reflex responses to rise in core temperature (whole body heating) when the need to dissipate heat is great. The cholinergic vasodilator fibers co-release neuropeptides (e.g., VIP). In addition, local NO production contributes to vasodilatation.

Noncholinergic and Nonadrenergic Transmission in the Autonomic System

In addition to the classical neurotransmitters acetylcholine and norepinephrine, several other neuroactive substances have been demonstrated in the autonomic nervous system. As mentioned, many preganglionic and postganglionic neurons contain neuropeptides, as well as acetylcholine or norepinephrine. Further, some autonomic neurons—notably in the enteric system—contain neither acetylcholine nor norepinephrine. Such **noncholinergic** and **nonadrenergic** (NANC) autonomic fibers are also found in the respiratory tract, the gastrointestinal tract, the bladder, and the external genitals. Some of them release **ATP** or **NO** as a neurotransmitter; others contain neuropeptides such as **somatostatin, substance P, VIP,** and **CCK.**

The **coexistence** of norepinephrine and other transmitters was first suggested by the observation that blocking the receptors for norepinephrine did not prevent all effects of sympathetic nerve stimulation. In the **ductus deferens,** which receives a very dense sympathetic innervation, stimulation of the nerves produces, first, a fast contraction caused by release of ATP and, subsequently, a slow contraction produced by norepinephrine. In the **salivary glands,** the parasympathetic postganglionic fibers release both acetylcholine and VIP. The acetylcholine produces secretion from the glandular cells, whereas the VIP produces vasodilatation. Another example concerns the arteries of the **penis** and the **clitoris,** which dilate to cause erection. This vasodilatation is caused by parasympathetic postganglionic fibers that release NO (but not acetylcholine).

Some parasympathetic postganglionic fibers in the **heart** release somatostatin and probably VIP, thus increasing the heart rate. In the **stomach,** vagus stimulation can produce release of VIP in addition to acetylcholine. Stimulation of nerves to the human **airways** can produce bronchial dilatation, although not by release of norepinephrine or acetylcholine. The effect appears to be mediated by release of **VIP** from postganglionic nerve varicosities.

Presynaptic Receptors Modulate the Transmitter Release from Postganglionic Nerve Terminals

Neurotransmitters released from the postganglionic neurons bind not only to postsynaptic receptors in the membrane of smooth-muscle and glandular cells but also to presynaptic receptors in the membrane of the varicosities along the fibers (see Fig. 5.1). Thus, for example, norepinephrine that is released from sympathetic fibers can bind presynaptically and inhibit further release of norepinephrine or bind to parasympathetic cholinergic terminals in the vicinity. In the **heart,** sympathetic fibers inhibit the release of acetylcholine in this manner.

The sympathetic inhibiting effect on the peristaltic contractions of the gastrointestinal tract is mediated, at least partly, by binding of norepinephrine to α receptors on the parasympathetic, cholinergic terminals: that is, the release of acetylcholine is inhibited.

Sensitization

When the postganglionic autonomic fibers to an organ are interrupted, the sensitivity of the organ to the transmitter (which is no longer released) is increased. Epinephrine and norepinephrine in the bloodstream, for example, have a more powerful action after an organ has lost its sympathetic innervation, and the same holds for adrenergic drugs. This phenomenon, called **sensitization,** is not restricted to the autonomic system, however. It occurs, presumably, after denervation of any neuron. For example, skeletal muscle cells have increased sensitivity to acetylcholine after having lost their nerve supply. The underlying mechanism is probably increased postsynaptic density of receptors, as though the neuron attempts to maintain normal synaptic activity.

Drugs with Actions on the Autonomic Nervous System

Several drugs influence the synaptic transmission in the autonomic nervous system. **Atropine** blocks the action of acetylcholine (released from postganglionic parasympathetic fibers) on **muscarinic** receptors. Other drugs have similar **anticholinergic** effects, often as a side effect. This is the case for several psychopharmaceuticals. The peripheral actions of the parasympathetic system are inhibited, causing symptoms such as dilated pupils (mydriasis) and reduced accommodation of the lens (causing difficulties in seeing close objects clearly). The heart rate increases, and the secretory activity is reduced in several glands. The reduced salivary secretion causes dryness of the mouth, a very bothersome side effect of anticholinergic drugs. Atropine, for example, is used to reduce secretion of glands in the respiratory tract during surgical anesthesia. The peristaltic contractions of the bowel are reduced, causing constipation. The bladder contractility is reduced, with danger of incomplete emptying (especially in cases of prostatic enlargement causing increased urethral resistance, the danger of urinary retention should be kept in mind). Because the sweat glands receive a cholinergic innervation, their secretion may also be reduced (most antiperspirants contain substances with an anticholinergic action).

Pilocarpine is an example of a drug with a **parasympathicomimetic** action: that is, a cholinergic drug. Administration of pilocarpine causes increased salivation and tear flow, reduced heart rate, and increased secretion from, and peristaltic movements of, the gastrointestinal tract. The pupil is small (miotic), causing reduced vision in dim light.

Many drugs activate adrenergic receptors—that is, they have **sympathicomimetic** effects. Some act on both α and β receptors; others act preferentially on one or the other receptor type (or on subtypes). **Isoprenaline** (isoproterenol) acts selectively on β receptors and produces increased heart rate and bronchial dilatation. **Metaraminol** acts preferentially on α receptors and causes peripheral vasoconstriction and, thereby, increased blood pressure.

Drugs that **block α receptors** (such as phentolamine) produce peripheral vasodilatation and a fall in blood pressure, whereas drugs that **block β receptors** mainly cause reduced heart rate and stroke volume, and bronchial constriction. The development of more selective β blockers, acting selectively on β_1 receptors present in the heart, has made it possible to treat hypertension without unwanted bronchial constriction (β_2 receptors are found primarily in the lungs). In contrast, the development of adrenergic drugs acting selectively on β_2 receptors (and not on β_1 receptors) has made it possible to treat patients with bronchial obstruction (as asthmatics) without such side effects as increased cardiac activity and hypertension.

Drugs can also influence the signal transmission in the **autonomic ganglia**. As mentioned, acetylcholine is the main transmitter in both sympathetic and parasympathetic ganglia. The nicotinic receptors in the ganglia are nevertheless somewhat different from those present at the neuromuscular junction. This makes it possible to influence one of these targets without affecting the other.

All neurotransmitters present in the peripheral parts of the autonomic system are also found in the CNS, together with adrenergic and cholinergic receptors. Therefore, drugs designed to act on peripheral parts of the autonomic nervous system may produce side effects through actions in the **CNS**—that is, in case they pass the blood-brain barrier. **Beta (β) blockers**, for example, which are used extensively to treat hypertension, can give central side effects, such as dizziness, disturbed sleep, and depression.

effects of lesions. Nevertheless, there is evidence that signals in the dorsal columns can contribute to the experience of pain in humans. For example, a patient with intense pain due to cancer of the large bowel was made pain free by bilateral sectioning of the gracile fascicles at the T_{10} level (the effect lasted until his death three months later). Animal experiments confirm that nociceptive signals from the lower abdomen and the pelvis cease to activate the cerebral cortex after transection of the gracile fascicle. Finally, the convergence mediated by the dorsal columns may also contribute to **referred pain** (discussed later).

VISCERAL REFLEXES

Many of the visceral reflexes elicited by signals from visceral receptors and receptors in the walls of vessels have their **reflex centers** in the spinal cord. The more complex reflexes, however, requiring coordination of activity in several parts of the body, have reflex centers in the brain stem or in the hypothalamus. We return to this in Chapter 30. **Vasomotor reflexes** were discussed earlier in this chapter. Other important visceral reflexes are produced by stimulation of receptors in the **lungs** and the **airways**, such as coughing and respiratory adjustments (see later). The **vomiting reflex** can be elicited by irritation of the mucosa of the stomach but also in various other ways (see Chapter 27, under "The Vomiting Reflex"). The **emptying reflexes** of the rectum and the bladder are elicited by stimulation of stretch receptors in their walls and have reflex centers partly in spinal segments (S_2) S_3–S_4 and partly in the brain stem. These visceral reflexes are unusual because they can be suppressed voluntarily. The emptying reflex of the bladder is discussed further later.

Reflexes Elicited from Receptors of the Lungs

Signals from **stretch receptors** in the bronchial walls contribute to inhibition of inspiratory movements when the lungs have been inflated to a certain extent (the Hering-Breuer reflex). Receptors producing **coughing** are probably free endings between the epithelial cells of the airways, in part located very close to the epithelial surface (irritation receptors). Such free nerve endings contain **substance P** (as do many other sensory neurons), which is released by exposure to irritant gases.

A special kind of receptor—the **J**, or **juxtapulmonary**, **receptor**—is located close to the lung alveoli. It responds to increased pulmonary capillary pressure. Increased pressure in the left atrium (which receives the blood from the lungs) immediately leads to increased pulmonary capillary pressure, with the danger of developing lung edema. Thus, it seems reasonable that the capillary pressure must be monitored closely. Stimulation of the

J receptors produces rapid and shallow breathing but may probably also cause bronchial constriction (this is known to occur in patients with heart failure and increased pulmonary capillary pressure). It is furthermore believed that signals from the J receptors can reach consciousness and cause a feeling of shortness of breath, or **dyspnea**. J receptors are also believed to elicit the dry cough typical of lunge edema, as occurring in patients with congestive heart failure or persons suffering from altitude sickness.

The Emptying Reflex of the Bladder

As mentioned, the bladder emptying reflex is evoked by stimulation of **stretch receptors** in the wall of the bladder, which record filling. The signals are conducted in myelinated afferent fibers to the lumbosacral cord (Fig. 29.2; see Fig. 28.12). Many sensory units that lead from the bladder are slowly adapting with dynamic sensitivity; that is, they respond more upon rapid than upon slow distension of the bladder. No signals are sent when the bladder is empty, but when urine starts to accumulate the sensory units start firing. Normal adult **bladder capacity** is about 500 mL. The pressure in the human bladder during filling is typically between 5 and 15 mm Hg, whereas emptying is normally elicited at 25 to 30 mm Hg. At night (during sleep), the bladder fills to about the double of daytime volume before evoking an urge to void. This is a prerequisite for 8 hours uninterrupted sleep.[3] Urine does not leak out in the filling phase because the **intraurethral pressure** is kept higher than the **intravesical** pressure. The intraurethral pressure is maintained by several factors, among them smooth muscles and elastic tissue in the urethral wall. In the filling phase, the smooth muscle of the bladder wall—the **detrusor muscle**—is relaxed, while the striated external sphincter in the pelvic floor is tonically active. When the intravesical pressure reaches the critical level, brisk activity of parasympathetic neurons makes the detrusor muscle contract. In addition, the striated sphincter muscle and other muscles in the pelvic floor must relax. Normal emptying of the bladder thus requires **coordinated control** of parasympathetic preganglionic neurons in the S_3–S_4 segments and of α motoneurons in the S_1–S_3 segments.

The **parasympathetic** control of the detrusor muscle is mediated by **acetylcholine**. In addition, **vasoactive intestinal peptide (VIP)** released from parasympathetic fibers might contribute to inhibition of the smooth muscles surrounding the urethra.

---

3 One or more of the centers of the micturition reflex must therefore be inhibited during sleep. This inhibition develops between the ages of three and five. In children with **enuresis** (bedwetting), this inhibition seems to be lacking, as about the same bladder filling volume elicits emptying during night and during daytime.

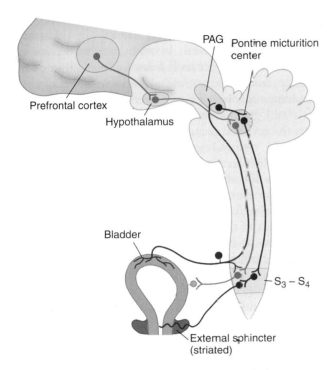

FIGURE 29.2 *Pathways and nuclei involved in control of micturition.* The reflex center for the emptying reflex is located in the sacral cord but is controlled by descending connections from the pontine micturition center. This is under control of higher centers, like the PAG, the hypothalamus, and the cerebral cortex.

The Role of the Sympathetic System in Bladder Control Is Not Clear

Evidence in experimental animals (cats and dogs) indicates that sympathetic activity increases during the filling phase, inhibiting the detrusor and activating smooth-muscle cells around the urethra in the bladder neck (internal sphincter). Few noradrenergic fibers are found in the human detrusor region (fundus), however, and sympathetic stimulation does not seem to inhibit the detrusor in the filling phase. (Because many noradrenergic fibers are found in the pelvic plexus and associated small parasympathetic ganglia, sympathetic inhibition of the detrusor muscle might theoretically occur by inhibition of the postganglionic parasympathetic neurons.) There is a richer noradrenergic innervation acting on α_1-adrenergic receptors to produce contraction of smooth-muscle cells in the bladder neck and trigonal area. These smooth muscles function as a "genital sphincter" that prevents backflow of semen to the bladder during ejaculation. The role of sympathetic innervation of the bladder neck for maintaining the urethral pressure during the bladder-filling phase is not equally clear, however. Nevertheless, drugs acting on α adrenergic receptors affect bladder emptying. Thus, α-adrenergic agonists may worsen urinary retention in patients with an enlarged prostatic gland and,

conversely, selective α antagonists are used to improve bladder outflow in such patients. Alpha (α)-adrenergic receptors are present at many levels of the reflex pathway—centrally in the cord and at higher levels, in the autonomic ganglia, and in the smooth-muscle cell membrane; further, they are located both pre- and postsynaptically and are activated by both norepinephrine released from postganglionic sympathetic fibers and by circulating epinephrine. Thus, deciding the site of action of a certain adrenergic drug is not straightforward.

Central Control of Micturition

Normal emptying of the bladder requires more than intact spinal reflex arches. This is evident in patients with **transsection of the cord** above the sacral level. If the lesion is complete, all descending connections acting on the sacral reflex centers are interrupted. The patients experience great difficulties with emptying the bladder because, among other problems, the activities of the detrusor muscle and the internal sphincter are not coordinated. This is called **dyssynergia**. (In addition, the bladder often becomes hyperactive—i.e., the emptying reflex is elicited at a lower pressure than before.) Patients with lesions of the brain stem above the pons do not have dyssynergia. Further observations show that the **dorsolateral pons** (near the locus coeruleus) contains a neuronal network that coordinate the spinal reflexes involved in micturition—the **pontine micturition center** (Fig. 29.2). Ascending spinoreticular fibers, which inform about the filling pressure, join the spinothalamic tract ventrolaterally in the cord. The fibers end in the **PAG**, which is assumed to send signals to the micturition center. The marked **emotional** influence on micturition, such as frequent urination in association with nervousness and fear, is probably mediated by connections from the **amygdala** to the PAG (see Fig. 31.6). Animal experiments indicate that the descending (reticulospinal) fibers from the pontine micturition center lie dispersed in the lateral funiculus, with the majority in its dorsal part. Clinical observations, however, indicate that in humans the fibers might lie more ventrally, close to the pyramidal tract in the lateral funicle. Thus, damage of the **pyramidal tract** in the spinal cord is often associated with **urge incontinence** (inability to inhibit the emptying reflex) as a sign of impaired central bladder control.

Although lesions above the pons do not disturb the normal emptying of the bladder, patients with such lesions may have problems with controlling of the initiation of micturition (inhibition in particular). The cell groups responsible for the voluntary control of micturition are not known in detail, although medial parts of the **frontal lobe** and the **hypothalamus** appear to be involved (Fig. 29.2). Clinical observations indicate that damage to the frontal lobes may cause **urge incontinence**.

Referred Pain

As mentioned, pain of visceral origin is often not felt where the organ is located but in some other place, often in the body wall or the extremities (Fig. 29.3). This phenomenon is called **referred pain**. The referred pain—for example, in the left arm in the case of angina, and under the right scapula in the case of a gallstone—can be localized fairly precisely by the patient. At the site of the diseased organ, however, there is usually only a diffuse pain, difficult both to localize and to describe. As mentioned, it typically takes some time for referred pain to develop.

The most widely accepted explanation of referred pain is based on the observed **convergence** of signals from somatic structures (especially the skin) and viscera.[5] Such convergence occurs in the dorsal horn, in the dorsal column nuclei, and in the thalamus, as discussed above and in Chapter 14 (under "Spinothalamic Neurons Receive Signals from Both Somatic and Visceral Structures"). As a rule, the diseased organ and the site of referred pain receive sensory innervation from the same **spinal segments**. Conceivably, the signals coming from the visceral organs are interpreted as arising in the skin and not in the visceral organ because signals from the visceral organs are never consciously perceived under normal circumstances (e.g., nociceptors of the heart are not normally stimulated). The referred pain usually takes some time to develop, and the occurrence of (referred) hyperesthesia and hyperalgesia is presumably explained by **sensitization** of central neurons receiving convergent inputs, leading to hyperexcitability and even spontaneous firing (i.e., independent of signals from the periphery). The importance of central sensitization is supported by the observation that the referred pain is felt even after blocking the sensory nerve fibers that lead from the area of referred pain. Further, the expansion of the painful area after some time is best explained by central sensitization of propriospinal neurons—transmitting signals to segments above and below those innervating the diseased organ. Indeed, animal experiments show that the receptive fields of dorsal horn neurons expand dramatically when the tissue from which they receive sensory signals is chronically inflamed.

Another peculiarity is that referred pain shows a tendency to localize to parts of the body that previously have been the site of a painful process. For example, a patient felt the pain of angina in a part of the spine that had been fractured many years ago. It seems as if a pain can be "remembered" as a persistent central sensitization (plasticity).

The peripheral axon of some **spinal ganglion cells** divides, with one branch going to the skin and another

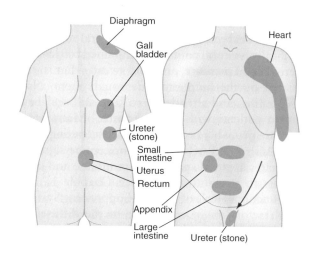

FIGURE 29.3 *Referred pain.* Examples of typical sites of pain in diseases affecting various visceral organs. (Based on Cope 1968.)

going to a visceral organ or a muscle. For example, one study found that about one-fifth of the fibers in the splanchnic nerve could be activated by electric stimulation of a somatic nerve. This may also contribute to the occurrence of referred pain. In such instances, an **axon reflex** (see later) may cause cutaneous hyperesthesia and vascular changes, as sensory signals from the visceral organ are conducted not only into the cord but also peripherally in the branch into the skin. There sensory fibers may release **neuropeptides** such as substance P and VIP, which cause changes of blood flow and sensitize sensory nerve endings (see Chapter 13, under "Primary Sensory Fibers and Neurotransmitters").

Examples of Referred Pain

The pain arising in the **heart** is usually referred to the ulnar aspect of the left arm or the upper part of the chest (Fig. 29.3). These regions of the skin and the heart both receive sensory innervation from the upper thoracic segments of the cord. The **gallbladder** and the skin in the region of the lower end of the scapula are both innervated from the eighth thoracic segment. The shoulder pain on irritation of the **diaphragm** is explained by the common innervation from the fourth and fifth cervical segments. Pain from the urinary **bladder** can be referred to two areas of the skin: one innervated by the spinal segments S_2-S_3 and one higher up on the back innervated by the lower thoracic and upper lumbar segments (see Fig. 13.15). This fits with the segments of the cord innervating the bladder (see Fig. 28.12).

Antidromic Signals and the Axonal Reflex

Electrical stimulation of dorsal roots can produce vasodilatation in the dermatome of the root concerned. This is caused by signals conducted in the peripheral direction by the sensory fibers. Signals conducted in the

---

5 That local anesthesia of the diseased organ prevents the development of referred pain proves that it depends on the nervous system.

direction opposite the normal direction are called **antidromic**. Of course, the action potentials are exactly the same as those conducted in the normal—**orthodromic**—direction. Antidromic signals in **C fibers** appear to release **substance P** from the peripheral branches. Substance P probably causes the release of **histamine** (presumably from mast cells). Histamine causes vasodilatation, especially of the capillaries, and at the same time the capillaries become leaky. Thus, a local edema is produced.

Various phenomena can probably be explained by this phenomenon. When the skin is stroked with a fairly sharp object, it reddens (vasodilatation) after a few seconds on both sides of the stripe. This can be explained as follows: the stroking of the skin stimulates C fiber nociceptors, and action potentials are conducted to the CNS (and we experience a sharp pain). At the same time, however, the action potential is also conducted peripherally in the branches of the C fiber that do not innervate the stimulated skin stripe. These branches end in the skin outside the stripe, where they liberate substance P and cause vasodilatation. The process is called a reflex, and because it uses only the peripheral process of a pseudounipolar ganglion cell, it is called an **axon reflex**. The reflex cannot be elicited in an area of the skin that has been deprived of its sensory innervation, proving that the phenomenon is mediated by nerve fibers.

Under normal conditions, the antidromic signals in sensory fibers hardly play any role, but they may help explain certain pathological phenomena. An example from the **airways** can be mentioned. In disposed individuals, irritating gases can produce a marked edema of the mucous membranes. The edema is caused apparently by histamine release, which, in turn, is caused by substance P released by an axon reflex from the sensory fibers that innervate the mucous membrane (partly coming close to the surface of the epithelium).

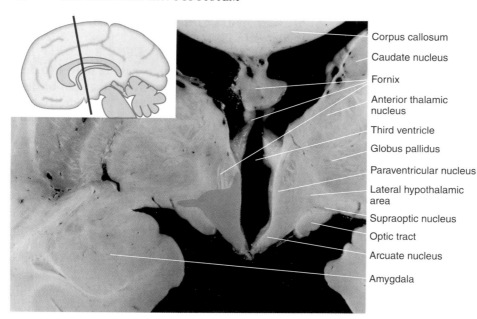

Corpus callosum
Caudate nucleus
Fornix
Anterior thalamic nucleus
Third ventricle
Globus pallidus
Paraventricular nucleus
Lateral hypothalamic area
Supraoptic nucleus
Optic tract
Arcuate nucleus
Amygdala

FIGURE 30.1 *The hypothalamus.* Frontal section through the hemisphere.

between the medial nuclei and the lateral area (nucleus) of the hypothalamus.

The Hypothalamus Contains Many Neurotransmitters

Numerous neurotransmitters are present in the hypothalamus, as demonstrated with immunocytochemical and biochemical methods. **Acetylcholine, norepinephrine, dopamine, serotonin, histamine,** and many **neuropeptides** occur with a differential distribution among the hypothalamic nuclei. Norepinephrine is among the neurotransmitters found in highest concentration (some of the norepinephrine is related to terminals of fibers from the locus coeruleus). Some of the neuropeptides are involved in the hypothalamic control of the pituitary gland or are released to the bloodstream in the pituitary. We return to some of the neuropeptides and

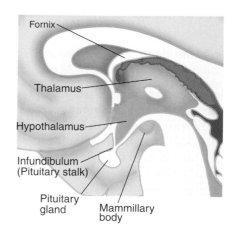

Fornix
Thalamus
Hypothalamus
Infundibulum (Pituitary stalk)
Pituitary gland
Mammillary body

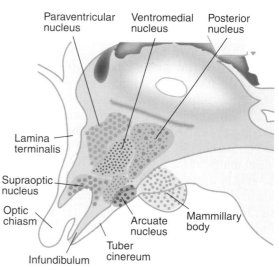

Paraventricular nucleus
Ventromedial nucleus
Posterior nucleus
Lamina terminalis
Supraoptic nucleus
Optic chiasm
Infundibulum
Tuber cinereum
Arcuate nucleus
Mammillary body

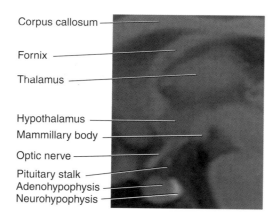

Corpus callosum
Fornix
Thalamus
Hypothalamus
Mammillary body
Optic nerve
Pituitary stalk
Adenohypophysis
Neurohypophysis

FIGURE 30.2 *The hypothalamus and the pituitary as seen in a midsagittal MRI scan.* (Courtesy of Dr. S.J. Bakke, Rikshospitalet University Hospital, Oslo, Norway.)

FIGURE 30.3 *The hypothalamus.* Median section through the third ventricle. Some of the major hypothalamic nuclei are shown with colored dots. The size of the dots indicates the relative size of the neurons of the various nuclei. (Redrawn after Le Gros Clark et al. 1936.)

their possible functions later in this chapter. Here we note that each neuropeptide takes part in different functional tasks, even though only one is mentioned in this discussion. The functional role of the various neurotransmitters in the hypothalamus is still incompletely known.

Afferent Connections and Other Kinds of Input to the Hypothalamus

Figure 30.4 shows diagrammatically the main afferent connections of the hypothalamus. It is immediately clear that many—perhaps most—parts of the brain are able to influence the hypothalamus! (The mammillary nucleus is in several aspects different from the other hypothalamic nuclei and is treated separately later in this chapter.) In addition, the hypothalamus is special because it receives information by **hormones** acting on specific receptors, and that it contains special **sensory neurons** that record blood temperature (**thermoreceptors**) and salt concentration (**osmoreceptors**). In addition, information about temperature and water balance is brought to the hypothalamus from peripheral receptors in the body. These features reflect the functions of the hypothalamus in homeostatic control.

Hypothalamic afferent nerve fibers bring signals from most kinds of **sense organ** and from higher levels of the brain, such as the **cerebral cortex** and the **limbic structures**. Thus, the hypothalamus receives information about **olfactory** and **taste** stimuli; the conditions in the **gastrointestinal tract**; the **blood pressure, noxious stimuli**, and **skin temperature**; and the intensity of **ambient light**. The afferent fibers from limbic structures, such as the amygdala, inform about **emotional** and **motivational** aspects.

The many groups of afferents end in at least partially different parts of the hypothalamus, which fits with physiological evidence that the hypothalamus consists of many functionally different parts (we discuss some of these later in this chapter). Nevertheless, both the many intrinsic connections and the properties of single cells show that the various afferent signals are considerably processed and integrated before commands are sent out to various targets.

The Connections and Functions of the Hypothalamic Nuclei Have Been Difficult to Clarify

Determining the exact connections and functional roles of the various nuclei has proved more difficult in the hypothalamus than in most other parts of the brain. This is partly because the nuclei are so small and are located in a part of the brain that is difficult to reach with experimental manipulations and partly because most of the afferent and efferent fibers are unmyelinated and mixed with fibers destined for other parts of the brain. In particular, lesions or stimulations of the lateral hypothalamic area are bound to affect the medial forebrain bundle and, thereby, fibers destined for other regions than the hypothalamus. Further, the rich network of intrahypothalamic connections means that a lesion of one nucleus will interfere with the functioning of several others as well. Modern methods using toxic agents that destroy the cell bodies without affecting fibers of passage have helped to settle some controversies, however. Finally, there are notable differences in both connections and neurotransmitters in various species, and most experimental data have been obtained in rats or cats.

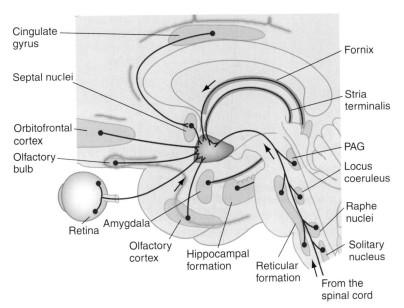

FIGURE 30.4 *Main afferent connections of the hypothalamus.* Arrows indicate direction of impulse conduction.

growth, and metabolism. The pituitary gland (the hypo-physis) consists of an **anterior lobe**, the **adenohypophy-sis**, which develops from the epithelium of the primitive foregut and consists of clusters of epithelial cells with a rich supply of wide capillaries (sinusoids). The **poste-rior lobe** of the pituitary, the **neurohypophysis**, devel-ops from the neural tube and consists of nerve terminals of fibers from the hypothalamus and a special kind of glial cell, the **pituicytes**.

Hypothalamic control concerns both the anterior and posterior parts of the pituitary (Fig. 30.7). Two different pathways exert the hypothalamo–pituitary interactions. The posterior pituitary receives a direct neural tract—often referred to as the supraopticohypo-physial or the **hypothalamohypophysial tract**—whereas the so-called **tuberoinfundibular tract** and a special **portal vascular system** reach the anterior pituitary (Fig. 30.6C). We return to this later.

The Anterior Pituitary Produces Several Hormones

The epithelial cells of he adenohypophysis produce and secrete the following hormones:

1. **Growth hormone** (GH) or **somatotropic** hormone, which stimulates body growth, particularly growth of long bones
2. **Thyroid-stimulating hormone** (TSH)
3. **Adrenocorticotropic hormone** (ACTH), which stim-ulates the production of steroid hormones, such as cor-tisol, in the adrenal cortex[2]
4. Two **gonadotropic hormones**—one **follicle-stimu-lating hormone** (FSH) that promotes the growth of the oocyte and its surrounding follicle cells and one **luteiniz-ing hormone** (LH) that is necessary for the ovulation and formation of the corpus luteum from the follicular cells
5. **Prolactin** (or lactogenic hormone), which stimu-lates growth of the mammary gland during pregnancy and maintains the milk production during the nursing period

Various observations indicate that, as a rule, a specific cell type produces each hormone. The cells are named for the hormone they produce, and are called **soma-totrophs** (GH), **thyrotrophs** (TSH), **mammotrophs** (pro-lactin), and so forth. In routine histological sections, however, only three kinds of epithelial cell can be recog-nized in the anterior pituitary: **acidophils**, **basophils**,

and **chromophobes**. The acidophils produce GH and prolactin, whereas the basophils probably produce the rest. The chromophobes may represent precursors to the acidophils and basophils. It follows that both the basophils and the acidophils are heterogeneous groups, as indeed has been shown with immunocytochemical techniques with antibodies raised against the various hormones.

Relationship between the Hypothalamus and the Posterior Pituitary

Two peptide hormones are released to the bloodstream in the posterior pituitary: **vasopressin** or **antidiuretic hormone** (ADH) and **oxytocin**. Both hormones consist of nine amino acids, are synthesized in the hypothalamus, and are brought to the pituitary by axonal transport. The thin, unmyelinated axons reaching the posterior lobe (in humans, about 100,000) come from two nuclei in the anterior part of the hypothalamus: the **supraoptic nucleus** and the **paraventricular nucleus** (Figs. 30.1, 30.3, and 30.7A). Most of the hormone-producing cells are large, with large vesicles in their cytoplasm that contain precursor molecules of the final hormones. The neurons are collectively termed the **magnocellular neuroendocrine system** (to distinguish them from the parvocellular neuroendocrine system that is discussed later). Even though vasopressin and oxytocin are pro-duced in both cell groups, vasopressin is produced predominantly in the supraoptic nucleus and oxytocin mainly in the paraventricular nucleus. The hormones can also be demonstrated within the axons, which end with large nerve terminals in close contact with the fenestrated capillaries of the posterior lobe (Fig. 30.7B). Action potentials invading the nerve terminals consti-tute the signal for release of the hormone (just as for the release of neurotransmitter in ordinary nerve cells). The cells of the supraoptic and the paraventricular nucleus are called **neurosecretory** because they have all the characteristic features of neurons but, at the same time, release their product to the bloodstream.

Vasopressin: Control of Osmolarity

Vasopressin (ADH) was extracted from the posterior lobe quite early, before the neural connection between the hypothalamus and the posterior lobe had been ascer-tained. The hormone acts by increasing the water reab-sorption in the kidneys by acting on **aquaporins** (water channels)—that is, it reduces the urine secretion (the hormone also elicits contraction of vascular smooth-muscle cells, which explains why it is also called vaso-pressin). It was known that destruction of the posterior lobe leads to a condition called **diabetes insipidus**, which is characterized by daily urine volume of 10 to 15 liters; diabetes insipidus also occurs as an inherited disease.

---

2 The hormone ACTH is synthesized from a large precursor protein called **pro-opiomelanocortin** or **pro-ACTH/endorphin**. This precursor molecule is cleaved into other peptides, notably β lipotropin (β-LPH) with a yet-unsettled function, and β **endorphin**, which is a potent opioid peptide with inhibitory actions on pain transmission. The functional role of the β endorphin secreted from the pitu-itary is not clear, however. Beta (β) endorphin is also found in a hypothalamic nucleus (the arcuate nucleus) with projections to brain stem nuclei of importance for pain transmission (see Chapter 15, under "Opiates and Endorphins").

Patients with this disease have pronounced cell loss in the supraoptic and paraventricular nuclei. Later it was discovered that the disease could also be produced by cutting the pituitary stalk. This was the beginning of a full understanding of the nature of the relationship between the hypothalamus and the pituitary. The production of ADH varies in accordance with the **osmolarity** of the blood.[3] Most likely, the cells of the supraoptic nucleus (and in some other nuclei) function as **osmoreceptors**. When the osmotic pressure of the blood increases because of extraordinary loss or reduced intake of fluid (e.g., by heavy sweating, diarrhea, or vomiting), the cells of the supraoptic nucleus are excited and increase the frequency of their action potentials, thus releasing more ADH into the bloodstream. This results in reduced urine volume (the urine becomes more concentrated). At the same time, the synthesis of the hormone is increased. Even a salty meal is enough to stimulate the osmoreceptors. Therefore, the hypothalamus is a control center for the body's "housekeeping" of water.

Oxytocin: Parturition and Milk Ejection

Oxytocin elicits contraction of the smooth-muscle cells in the wall of the **uterus** and thus has a role during parturition. It also produces contraction of the smooth-muscle cells (myoepithelial cells) of the mammary gland, thereby assisting in emptying the breast of milk. When the infant suckles, sensory impulses travel from the nipple (through the spinal nerves) to the cord and further to the hypothalamus, where the neurons of the paraventricular nucleus are influenced. Increased firing frequency leads to increased secretion of oxytocin to the bloodstream, and the hormone reaches the mammary gland in seconds. This is called the **milk ejection reflex**. It is special in that only the afferent link is neural; the efferent link is humoral. Although oxytocin is present in males, its function is so far unknown.

Vasopressin and Oxytocin Act in the Brain as Well as Peripherally

Although the peripheral actions of vasopressin and oxytocin have received most attention, both peptides exert effects on central neurons, influencing many aspects of behavior and cognition. For example, central infusion of oxytocin induces maternal behavior in rats, and oxytocin furthermore facilitates pair bonding (preference for a particular mate) in monogamous species. Central actions of vasopressin include sexual behavior, social

interactions, and anxiety reduction (and several other effects). These effects are produced by binding of vasopressin and oxytocin to specific receptors, modulating the activity of task-specific networks in several parts of the brain.

How the peptides reach their many central targets is less clear, however, because both peptides are mainly synthesized in the magnocellular neurons of the supraoptic and paraventricular nuclei that send their axons to the posterior lobe of the pituitary. However, some small (parvocellular) neurons in the paraventricular nucleus produce the peptides and send their axons to various central nuclei. Further, at least in some species, neurons in the suprachiasmatic nucleus, the amygdala, and in the basal forebrain also express vasopressin and oxytocin. Finally, the neurons of the magnocellular nuclei release peptides from the soma and the dendrites (Fig. 30.7B). Dendritic release probably enables vasopressin and oxytocin to act by volume transmission on neurons expressing the appropriate receptors near the paraventricular and supraoptic nuclei. While both peptides enter the cerebrospinal fluid (where their concentrations are usually higher than in the blood) it is not known whether this plays a functional role.

Influence of the Hypothalamus on the Anterior Pituitary: The Hypophyseal Portal System

It has long been known that altered growth, metabolism, and sexual functions—processes that are controlled by hormones produced in the anterior pituitary—can accompany diseases affecting the hypothalamus. There are no axonal connections from the thalamus to the anterior pituitary, however, and mechanisms other than those concerning the posterior lobe must be responsible for the influence of the hypothalamus on the anterior lobe. The discovery of a special vascular arrangement in the infundibulum (stalk) of the pituitary—the **hypophyseal portal system**—was a breakthrough in this respect (Fig. 30.7C). Most of the arteries reaching the anterior pituitary do not branch into capillaries among the epithelial cells but continue upward into the stalk (some arteries enter the stalk directly). In the upper part of the stalk, the vessels form wide capillaries (sinusoids) that finally collect into large veins. These hypophyseal **portal veins** course back to the anterior lobe, where they form a new set of sinusoids among the epithelial cells. From these sinusoids, the blood collects in veins that leave the pituitary. Because the blood in the sinusoids of the anterior lobe has first been through a capillary net in the stalk, substances can be transported from there to the anterior lobe. Numerous thin axons from the hypothalamus end in the uppermost part of the hypophyseal stalk, forming the **tuberoinfundibular tract**. This region is called the **median eminence** (Fig. 30.7C). The axons that end in contact with the capillaries in the median

3 The ADH secretion is also influenced by other factors, although in primates these appear to be much less potent than changes of osmolarity. For example, reduced blood volume leads to concentration of **angiotensin II** in the bloodstream, which, in turn, affects the supraoptic and paraventricular nuclei by means of the subfornical organ. **Ethanol** reduces the secretion of ADH, thereby increasing urine production.

the posterior parts contain neurons necessary for heat conservation. Together, these parts function as a **thermostat** that tries to keep the body temperature as close as possible to a **set point** of 37°C. If the temperature drops below the set point, the "heater" is turned on—that is, measures are initiated to conserve heat (skin vasoconstriction or putting on more clothes) and, if necessary, to increase heat production (shivering or voluntary muscular activity).

In humans, abnormal rise in the body temperature, **hyperthermia**, can occur in diseases that affect the hypothalamus or by an inadvertent lesion during surgery. The rise can also occur as a side effect of certain **drugs** acting on the brain (e.g., antipsychotics). Occasionally, hyperthermia occurs during **general anesthesia**.

Fever

Fever is part of the so-called **acute-phase response** elicited by immune system activation (see below, "Effects of the Immune System on the Nervous System"). Fever arises when the set point of the hypothalamic thermostat is altered. Especially neurons in the **preoptic area (POA)** in the anterior hypothalamus appear to be crucial, as judged from microinjections of fever-producing substances. If the set point is changed to, for example, 39°C, the normal body temperature is judged to be too low and measures to conserve and produce heat are started (skin vasoconstriction, shivering, curling up, putting on more clothes). The person feels cold while the temperature is below the new set point. Fever has most likely evolved as a defensive response, improving survival from infections (although fever is sometimes harmful).

Fever can be caused (indirectly) by lipopolysaccharides (called **pyrogens**) from bacterial membranes or by simple tissue injury that leads to inflammation (e.g., fever after severe sunburn). The pyrogens or other tissue changes make leukocytes release **cytokines**. The cytokines **interleukin 1β** (IL-1β), and **tumor-necrotic factor** (TNF) have been detected in the tissue fluid from the anterior hypothalamus in experimental animals with fever. IL-1β, which is the most potent fever-inducing substance, appears to act **via interleukin 6** (IL-6). Thus, IL-1β does not induce fever in knockout mice that lack the IL-6 gene. It is not quite clear, however, how the cytokines accumulate in the hypothalamus. Blood borne cytokines can bind specifically at sites without the blood–brain barrier—such as the **subfornical organ**—where the neurons express IL-1 and IL-6 receptors. In turn, these might induce synthesis of cytokines in the hypothalamus. It is also possible that cytokines are brought through the blood–brain barrier by specific transporters. Finally, there is evidence that sensory impulses in the **vagus nerve** may induce cytokine production in the hypothalamus. Thus, injections of IL–1β in the peritoneal cavity (mimicking a local inflammation) do not induce fever after cutting of the vagus nerve.

Whatever the cause of their presence, cytokines in the hypothalamus induce the synthesis of **prostaglandins** (among other substances), which increase the activity of cold-sensitive neurons and reduce the activity of heat-sensitive ones. That antipyretic (reduce fever) drugs, such as **aspirin**, inhibit the synthesis of prostaglandins supports a crucial role of prostaglandins in fever production.

Local adaptations in the hypothalamus ensure that the fever does not reach dangerous levels (**antipyresis**). Cytokines activate neurons in the paraventricular nucleus producing CRH and vasopressin. As discussed, CRH release leads to increased blood levels of cortisol. This would reduce the peripheral production of cytokines and, by that, reduce the fever. Further, fibers from the paraventricular nucleus release vasopressin in the **septal nuclei**. Experimental infusion of vasopressin in the septal nuclei suppresses almost completely the febrile response to intravenous injection of pyrogens. It appears most likely that the septal nuclei act back via septohypothalamic fibers to cancel the effect of cytokines on the thermostat.

The Hypothalamus, Sleep, and Hypocretins

Sleep disturbances often accompany lesions of the hypothalamus in experimental animals and in humans, sometimes as an abnormal amount of sleep and sometimes as insomnia or disturbed sleep rhythm. Animal experiments in the 1940s demonstrated that lesions in the **preoptic area** in the anterior hypothalamus caused insomnia, and later studies identified single neurons with their maximal activity during sleep in the same region. Later studies have identified two neuronal groups in the posterior hypothalamus of importance for wakefulness.[4]

The first is the **tuberomammillary nucleus** that contains histaminergic neurons with widespread axonal ramifications. Histamine binds to histamine receptors (H_1–H_3) in many brain regions. With regard to the histaminergic effect on wakefulness, the projections to the cerebral cortex, the locus coeruleus, and the raphe nuclei are probably most important (histamine has several additional actions, for example on learning and memory). GABAergic neurons in the preoptic area project to the (histaminergic) tuberomammillary nucleus, and may therefore contribute to sleep by inhibiting wake-active neurons.

The second group consists of diffusely spread neurons (about 7000 in humans) in the posterior and lateral

---

4 The epidemic in the early twentieth century of a presumed viral disease causing (among other complications) extreme somnolence—**encephalitis lethargica**—pointed to the posterior hypothalamus as important for waking.

hypothalamus that release two varieties of the neuro-peptide **hypocretin (orexin)**. The hypocretins bind to specific receptors and exert a wake-promoting effect when infused in animals. Further support for the impor-tance of hypocretins came from the observation that patients with **narcolepsy** have reduced levels of hypocre-tins in the cerebrospinal fluid and loss of hypocretiner-gic neurons (see Chapter 26, under "Narcolepsy"). The hypocretins exert effects several places but projections to the tuberomammillary nucleus may be of particular importance. Thus, hypocretins increase release of hista-mine and wakefulness but not in knockout mice lacking expression of the H$_1$ receptor. In addition, hypocretiner-gic fibers pass to the locus coeruleus and the raphe nuclei, both related to control of arousal (see Chapter 26, under "Multiple Pathways and Transmitters Are Responsible for Cortical Activation"). Interestingly, the **suprachias-matic nucleus**, which is responsible for the control of circadian rhythms, projects to regions with hypocretin-expressing neurons.[5]

The hypocretins are yet another example that each of the brain's many signal substances influences several different processes. Indeed, the hypocretins were dis-covered because of their ability to induce feeding behav-ior in experimental animals. Later, their importance for wakefulness was revealed, and now they are implicated in a number of other functions as well.

It should be emphasized that many more neuronal groups and neurotransmitters than those mentioned here are implicated in the control of wakefulness and sleep (see Chapter 26).

The Hypothalamus and Circadian Rhythms

The hypothalamus plays a role as a pacemaker for sev-eral functions showing a cyclic, diurnal variation. Such **circadian rhythms** are governed from the small **supra-chiasmatic nucleus** (SCN), situated just above the optic chiasm. γ-Aminobutyric acid (**GABA**) is the transmitter for most of the neurons in the SCN, colocalized with **neuropeptides** (either vasopressin or VIP). **Lesions** of the SCN disturb (but do not necessarily abolish) the cyclic variations of bodily functions Therefore, SCN is not alone in determining the circadian rhythms, even if it plays the leading part.

Several physiologic parameters—such as hormonal levels, blood pressure, body temperature, wakefulness, and sleep—are subject to circadian alterations. The same holds for several mental functions, such as reaction time and mood. The biologic significance of the cyclic varia-tions of bodily functions is presumably to adapt the level of activity to the most stable and predictable variations

in the environment. For example, in humans it seems appropriate that most bodily functions are at their low-est level during the night, whereas animals hunting at night would need a different activity profile. Persons staying in environments without any information about the time of the day develop a rhythm with cycles slightly longer than 24 hours. The capacity to produce circa-dian rhythms is inborn, and cyclic activity appears in the hypothalamus (rat) late in intrauterine life. The SCN functions as a **pacemaker** or **biologic clock**, pro-ducing a certain rhythm even in the absence of external inputs. Nevertheless, the exact rhythm—that is, at what time of the day the highest and lowest values occur—is modulated by sensory information. **Light stimuli** from the retina (Fig. 30.4), varying with length of the light/dark cycle, appear to be particularly important for the set of such circadian rhythms. Other factors also seem to contribute, however, such as activity level.

The **retinohypothalamic** fibers, which arise from retinal ganglion cells, end in the SCN. They inform only about the amount of light but do not provide specific information about patterns, movements, and so forth. In addition, the SCN receives afferents from a small part of the lateral geniculate nucleus and from the **raphe nuclei** (serotonin).

The SCN has **efferent** connections with several other parts of the hypothalamus, which enable it to synchro-nize the various functions mentioned above (and other functions as well). This concerns, for example, the **CRH**-containing neurons in the **paraventricular nucleus** that control the blood level of corticosteroids. Other connections reach the **thalamus** and cell groups in the **basal forebrain** (see Chapter 31, under "The Basal Forebrain"). Such connections might influence diurnal variations in motivation and memory. With regard to hypothalamic control of the **sleep–wake cycle**, newly dis-covered (polysynaptic) connections from the SCN to the **locus coeruleus** (norepinephrine) are of particular inter-est (see "The Hypothalamus, Sleep, and Hypocretins"). A special polysynaptic efferent pathway from the SCN to the **pineal gland** controls secretion of the hormone **melatonin**. Melatonin binds to high-affinity receptors in parts of the hypothalamus, among them the SCN, and modulates circadian rhythms. Light can influence the SCN pacemaker via variations in the melatonin level (in addition to by the retinohypothalamic fibers). Melatonin is secreted in response to low levels of light and can therefore be said to **signal darkness**.

Melatonin

The pineal body or gland (see Chapter 6, under "The Epithalamus and the Pineal Body") produces a number of neuroactive substances, among them several **neuropeptides** and large amounts of **serotonin**. The hor-mone **melatonin** has attracted most interest, however.

---

[5] Hypocretinergic connections to dopaminergic neurons in the mesencephalon (in the substantia nigra and the VTA) may explain why hypocretins also influ-ence motivation and "reward behavior."

Melatonin (*N*-acetylmethoxytryptamine) is synthesized from serotonin in two enzymatic steps. No nerve fibers leave the pineal body, which therefore is assumed to function only as an endocrine gland. The only known **afferent** nerve fibers arise in the **upper cervical sympathetic ganglion** (postganglionic fibers). Ambient **light** influences the secretion of melatonin; increased light (longer days) inhibits secretion. In humans, as in experimental animals, the level of melatonin varies with the light–darkness cycle, with the highest level occurring at night. The influence of light is mediated through a tortuous route: as mentioned, signals from the retina reach the SCN directly; neurons there forward signals directly or indirectly to the preganglionic sympathetic neurons in the upper thoracic cord, and their axons reach the upper cervical ganglion by means of the sympathetic trunk (see Fig. 28.7).

Melatonin acts by binding to G protein–coupled receptors, which occur with the highest concentrations in the SCN, the paraventricular nucleus, and parts of the anterior pituitary. The dominating effect of receptor activation seems to be reduced synthesis of cyclic AMP. Melatonin appears to inhibit the secretion of **gonadotropic hormones** (the effect seems to depend on the time of the day, however). In experimental animals, melatonin also have a number of other actions—for example, influencing **sleep**, **arousal**, body **temperature**, and blood level of **cortisol**. These effects are believed to be mediated mainly by the SCN.

Intake of melatonin in humans alters the phase of such rhythms, probably by setting the "circadian clock" in the SCN. Indeed, melatonin is now widely used to alleviate the unpleasant psychological and physiological effects of **jet lag** (even though its effect in this respect has not yet been convincingly documented). It has also been used to normalize sleep–wake patterns in blind people. The production of melatonin declines with age, and this has been taken to explain sleep disturbances in elderly people. Because melatonin counteracts the accumulation of cytotoxic free radicals, it has been suggested as a drug to halt the progression of degenerative brain diseases (Parkinson's disease, Alzheimer's disease, and others). The many reported beneficial effects of melatonin in humans lack documentation, however. It is fair to say that its normal role in humans is not yet clear, especially because most of what we know comes from experiments on rodents.

Control of Digestion and Feeding

The hypothalamus controls various metabolic processes. For example, lesions of certain parts can produce abnormal fat deposition, both in experimental animals and in humans. The gastrointestinal tract is influenced by the hypothalamus. Lesions can produce ulcers of the mucous membranes and bleeding in the stomach and the small intestine. Stimulation of the anterior hypothalamus, in particular, can elicit increased secretion of gastric juice and strengthening of peristaltic movements.

Not only the digestive processes but also **feeding behavior** is controlled from the hypothalamus. Early stimulation and lesion experiments indicated that the **lateral hypothalamic area** could induce increased eating (or behavior directed at acquiring food), whereas the **medial parts** (especially the ventromedial nucleus) reduce eating (induce satiety). Further studies have shown that, although essentially correct, this scheme is too simple. A complex network within the hypothalamus and between the hypothalamus and other parts of the brain controls food intake and body weight.

The inputs to the hypothalamic "feeding centers" are multifarious, as witnessed by data from animal experiments and by everyday experiences of the numerous factors that influence human feeding behavior. It is nevertheless remarkable how most people maintain their body weight over many years, although even the smallest daily surplus of food would cause a steady weight gain (a surplus of 10 calories a day would increase body weight by about 1 kg in a year). The hypothalamic centers governing food intake are thought to operate as a **homeostat** (a system maintaining a steady state by internal processes.) We also use the term **lipostat**, because the control of body fat is so central to maintaining constant body weight. **Feedback loops** ensure that the food intake oscillates around a set point. Reduced consumption automatically follows overeating.

The protein **leptin**, produced in fat cells, appears to be the single most important factor ensuring negative feedback from adipose tissue to the hypothalamus (**insulin** is another factor). The function of leptin is probably to inform about whether the energy reserves (fat) are sufficient. The so-called **ob** gene (ob for obesity) codes for leptin, while the **db** gene codes for the leptin receptor. Mice lacking either the ob or the db gene develop extreme obesity due to increased food intake and reduced metabolism (in addition, they develop diabetes and increased cortisol levels). Although leptin binds several places in the hypothalamus, a major effect is to inhibit the release of **neuropeptide Y** (NPY).[6] NPY reduces food intake, as shown by injections in certain parts of the hypothalamus in experimental animals.

Loss of Feeding Control

Of course, psychological factors—or, occasionally, hypothalamic disease—may disturb this finely tuned

6 NPY is involved in other hypothalamic tasks, such as control of circadian rhythms, and secretion of releasing hormones. It is often colocalized with catecholamines, GABA, or somatostatin. Finally, NPY is also found in the amygdala where it is involved in stress reactions (having an anxiolytic effect). Obviously, each of the numerous transmitters present in the hypothalamus may be expected to participate in quite diverse functions.

control mechanism. Studies of **obese people** indicate that they have normal leptin production.[7] A hypothalamic leptin resistance has been proposed, however, to account for the development of obesity (analogous to insulin resistance in some cases of diabetes). If so, the question remains how the resistance arises: is it due to a genetic abnormality, or is the lipostat altered by psychological and other factors? Only in about 25% of overweight people is there evidence of a genetic disposition.

Focusing on single actors like leptin, NPY, and hypothalamic nuclei should not make us forget that the hypothalamus does not operate in isolation. The many connections between the hypothalamus and the cerebral cortex, the amygdala, and other limbic structures tell us that the hypothalamus may be "overruled" by the higher parts of the brain engaged in cognitive and emotional processing. Thus, while the hypothalamus undoubtedly is the organizer for motivated behavior related to digestion and feeding, other regions than the hypothalamus determine whether such behavior occurs. Although we do not fully understand the causes of eating disorders such as **anorexia** and **bulimia**, it is unlikely that the primary cause is to be found in the hypothalamus.[8]

The Arcuate Nucleus, Neuropeptides, and Energy Metabolism

Several transmitters (especially many neuropeptides) are involved in the hypothalamic control of feeding behavior, although much remains before their mutual roles are clarified. Special interest attaches to **NPY**, which is found in high concentration in nerve terminals in the **paraventricular nucleus**. Most of the NPY-containing terminals come from the **arcuate nucleus**. Two groups of neurons in the arcuate nucleus have opposite effects: **NPY neurons** increase food intake while **POMC neurons** (pro-opiomelanocortin) reduce it. For example, injection of NPY near the paraventricular nucleus increases food intake in experimental animals. Further, it decreases the metabolism in **brown fat** and increases fat storage in ordinary (white) fat tissue. This leads to a larger weight gain than expected from the food intake. The NPY-containing connections to the paraventricular nucleus might therefore regulate the energy balance of the body by controlling both appetite and metabolism. How NPY release in the hypothalamus produces this is not known, although some effects may be mediated by

projections from the paraventricular nucleus to sympathetic preganglionic cell groups. In addition to **leptin**, the hormone **insulin** act as one of several **feedback signals** to the arcuate nucleus from the periphery, informing about the energy status of the body. Thus, hypothalamic injection of insulin reduces the food intake in normal rats (but not in rats with genetically determined obesity).

Several other factors contribute in the regulation of food intake. For example, **glucose-sensitive** hypothalamic neurons are likely to be involved in the control of appetite (for instance, the feeling of hunger when the blood glucose is low). The hormone **ghrelin**—produced in the stomach—may also contribute to regulation of hunger and food intake by acting on neurons in the arcuate nucleus. Indeed, ghrelin activates NPY neurons and inhibit POMC neurons, as one might expect from a signal informing about empty energy stores. (As other neuropeptides, ghrelin has diverse actions; it increases, for example, plasticity in the hippocampus.) Gut hormones, such as **cholecystokinin**, do not cross the blood–brain barrier, but can act on neurons in the **solitary nucleus** via the area postrema (lacking a blood–brain barrier). The **vagus nerve** provides the solitary nucleus with information about the filling of the stomach and probably about the levels of glucose and lipids in the liver. From the solitary nucleus, signals travel to the hypothalamus and notably the arcuate nucleus.

Hypothalamus, Sexual Functions, and Sex Differences

The efferent connections of the hypothalamus also enable it to influence sexual behavior—that is, to start and coordinate the autonomic, endocrine, and somatic motor components. This is verified by many animal experiments. For example, injection of the female sex hormone **estradiol** in the **ventromedial hypothalamic nucleus** in castrated male rats elicits copulatory behavior. Lesions of the ventromedial hypothalamic nucleus in female rats reduce their sexual activity. We have little precise knowledge of how the hypothalamus controls sexual functions, however. Neither do we understand fully the structural basis in the hypothalamus for behavioral sex differences, in spite of numerous findings of sex differences among hypothalamic nuclei.

In rodents a nucleus in the anterior hypothalamus— **the sexually dimorphic nucleus of the preoptic area, SDN-PO**—is three to eight times larger in males than in females. While several studies in humans have described sex differences in the corresponding region, it is remarkable that they do not agree on which one among three small nuclei that show such sexual dimorphism (neither is there agreement with regard to hypothalamic differences between heterosexual and homosexual men).

Several hypothalamic pathways are likely to be sexually dimorphic. One among many relevant pathways passes from the **paraventricular nucleus** directly to the

---

[7] A small minority of persons with extreme obesity have mutations of the ob or db genes. Such persons develop overweight very early. They also suffer from low levels of growth hormone and thyroid hormone, and they lack normal pubertal development.

[8] A review of 54 patients with eating disorders occurring in conjunction with a brain lesion showed that the majority had lesions in the right fronto-temporal region. Lesions of the hypothalamus were associated with reduced or increased appetite but not with more complex eating disorders (Uher and Treasure 2005).

themselves. Conceivably, the emotions are evoked by feedback connections from the hypothalamus to the limbic structures and the cerebral cortex—structures that are necessary for the experience of emotions (as distinct from emotional reactions). The higher regions presumably interpret the hypothalamic activity as evidence of external or internal stimuli that normally evoke strong emotions.

Emotions and Emotional Reactions

When discussing the relations between the hypothalamus and emotions, one must distinguish the emotions themselves from the emotional reactions—that is, the behavior expressing our emotions. We can experience the feelings or emotions only subjectively. Of course, we may learn that certain external stimuli or situations usually produce certain emotions in other people, but such correlations can only be tentative because so many psychological individual variations play a role. We cannot obtain information from animals about their emotions, but emotional reactions can be directly observed and are often more reliable in animals than in humans. Factors such as upbringing, social conventions, and conscious considerations determine to a large extent the emotional reactions in humans. That emotions in animals can only be inferred indirectly from their behavior explains why it is not quite clear how many basic emotions animals have. Commonly, however, only three basic emotions are identified (in cats, dogs, and monkeys): **rage, fear,** and **pleasure** (love). Even though the emotions of animals certainly are less schematic than this, there is no doubt that the emotions of humans have much more variation and nuances. This should be kept in mind when drawing conclusions with regard to emotions and psychosomatic interactions in humans on the basis of animal experiments. The anthropologist Paul Ekman (1984) identifies seven basic emotions in humans, based on their relation to culture-independent facial expressions: **happiness, sadness, anger, fear, disgust, surprise,** and **contempt.**

VII | LIMBIC STRUCTURES

THIS part of the book deals with parts of the fore-brain that are closely associated with the cerebral cortex with regard to development and connections. The cerebral cortex is divided into two parts (without definite delimitations) on the basis of phylogenetic development: the **neocortex**, which is the most recent part and comprises most of the cortex in higher mammals, and the **allocortex**, which is the oldest part. The neocortex is treated in Chapters 33 and 34, while this chapter deals with the allocortex and closely related subcortical nuclei. The nomenclature used for the oldest part of the cortex varies, but usually the term allocortex is used for the parts of the cortical mantle with a simple, often only three-layered structure instead of the six layers that are typical of the neocortex. In reptiles, the allocortex constitutes what little cortex there is. The allocortex receives afferents from adjacent subcortical nuclei (in contrast to the neocortex that is closely connected with the thalamus). Together, these subcortical nuclei and the allocortex are commonly said to comprise the so-called **limbic system** (gyrus limbicus is another name for the cingulate gyrus). The cell groups comprising the "limbic system" coincide in part with what was formerly called the **rhinencephalon**, although this term, strictly speaking, comprises only the parts of the brain that receive olfactory fibers. There are wide variations among authors, however, with regard to which neuronal groups are included in the "limbic system," indicating that the term lacks reasonable precision. Indeed, the term "system" becomes misleading when used to lump—rather arbitrarily—neuronal groups with major functional differences. In this book we therefore use the neutral term **limbic structures** to avoid giving a misleading impression of functional unity.

As witnessed by their numerous interconnections, all of these regions cooperate to exert an integrated influence on the peripheral somatic and autonomic effectors. What the American psychologist S.P. Grossman (1976, p. 361) said about the septal nuclei probably holds for the rest of the limbic structures, too: "Just about every behavior and/or psychological function which has been investigated to date has been shown to be affected in some way by septal lesions."

In **conclusion**, the "limbic system" does not represent a unity that can be defined with a reasonable degree of precision. As stated by the American neurologist Antonio Damasio (1995, p. 20), "the bizarre distinction between cognition and emotion, as if somehow one could have thoughts without emotion, a mind without affect . . . The rift between emotion and cognition acquired a neuroanatomical counterpart in the duality between limbic system and neocortex."

The Circuit of Papez

In 1937, Papez described what he considered a closed circuit of connections starting and ending in the hippocampus. From the hippocampus, the flow of signals was postulated to pass to the mammillary nucleus, from this nucleus to the anterior thalamic nucleus, from there to the cingulate gyrus, and then finally back to the hippocampus. This circuit of interconnected cell groups was hypothesized to form the anatomic basis of emotional reactions and expressions. These suggestions formed the basis for the concept of "the limbic system," which was introduced in the early 1950s by Paul MacLean.

THE AMYGDALA

Main Anatomic and Functional Subdivisions

The amygdala (the amygdaloid nucleus) is located in the temporal lobe, underneath the uncus (Figs. 31.1, 31.2, and 31.3; see Fig. 6.29). In humans, the amygdala is a complex of subnuclei, each with a distinctive internal structure, neurotransmitters, and connections.[2] Here we restrict ourselves to distinguishing between a small **corticomedial** (including a **central nucleus**) and a large **basolateral** nuclear group (including the **lateral nucleus**). The basolateral group increases in size from lower to higher mammals and is particularly well developed in humans. The corticomedial nuclear group lies close to

the olfactory cortex (see Fig. 19.3). To **simplify**, we may say that the corticomedial nuclei are connected primarily with the olfactory bulb, the hypothalamus, and the visceral nuclei of the brain stem, whereas the basolateral nuclei are mainly connected with the thalamus and prefrontal cortex. In addition, the basolateral nuclei send fibers to the ventral striatum and the basal nucleus. This would suggest that the corticomedial part of the amygdala is concerned primarily with autonomic functions, whereas the basolateral parts are more involved in conscious processes related to the frontal and temporal lobes. The many intrinsic connections among the various nuclei show that they must cooperate extensively, however.

The amygdala (or its many components) participates in several higher mental functions, each of which is highly complex. Its "functions" are correspondingly complex and hard to define. Nevertheless, some salient features are clear. Thus, a central task of the amygdala is the establishment of links between **stimuli** and their **emotional value** (put very simply, whether something is good or bad). Most of our memories have some—often quite strong—emotional coloring, which is crucial for our ability to react appropriately to a stimulus. Think of the importance of being able to judge the facial expressions of other people, the emotional aspects of their speech, and so forth. As we discuss in this chapter, damage to the amygdala in monkeys leads to, among other things, difficulties in **social interactions**.

Afferent Connections of the Amygdala

The **corticomedial** nuclei receive afferents from the **olfactory bulb**, the **hypothalamus**, the **intralaminar thalamic nuclei**, and the **septal nuclei** (Fig. 31.4). They also receive **dopaminergic** fibers from the ventral tegmental area in the mesencephalon, as well as fibers from

2 The amygdala as we describe it here is structurally and functionally heterogeneous, and we lump the various nuclei under one name purely for convenience. Indeed, in a critical review Larry Swanson and Gorica Petrovich (1998) concluded "...it is necessary to ask whether the concept of a structurally and functionally defined amygdala is indeed valid, or whether the concept is hindering attempts to understand general principles of telencephalic architecture by imposing an arbitrary classification on heterogeneous structures that belong to different functional systems."

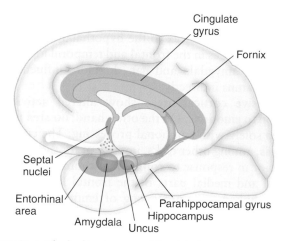

FIGURE 31.1 *The limbic structures.* The right hemisphere, as viewed from the medial aspect. The regions and cell groups indicated in red are usually included in the term "limbic system."

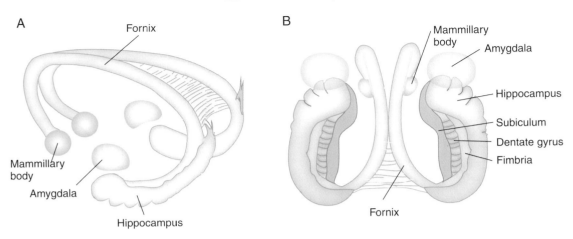

FIGURE 31.2 *The hippocampus, fornix, mammillary nucleus, and the amygdala.* **A:** Viewed obliquely from behind. **B:** Viewed from above.

the **parabrachial area** (in the dorsolateral pons). The latter projection may convey information about taste and, in addition, about painful stimuli. Thus, ascending fibers of spinal **lamina I** nociceptive neurons end in parts of the parabrachial area that project to the central amygdaloid nucleus (among other targets). The sensory units of this pathway have very large receptive fields and receive convergent inputs from the skin and viscera. It seems likely that this lamina I–parabrachial–amygdaloid pathway contributes to the **emotional aspects of pain**.

The **basolateral nuclei** receive fibers from several thalamic nuclei, the **prefrontal cortex**, parts of the temporal lobe, and the **cingulate gyrus** (Fig. 31.4). Together, the basolateral nuclei—the **lateral nucleus** in particular—receive all kinds of sensory information. This may be emotionally neutral information from cortical association areas and emotionally laden information about unpleasant and threatening stimuli from the reticular formation, the intralaminar thalamic nuclei, and perhaps parts of the cortex (the insula). Thus, the amygdala receives, for example, information about **fear-provoking stimuli** and their **context**. Efferents from the lateral nucleus reach other amygdaloid nuclei that may influence the cortex (conscious experience of emotions) and

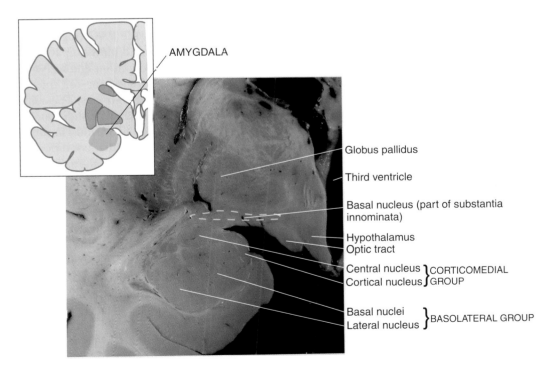

FIGURE 31.3 *The amygdala.* Frontal section through the left hemisphere (cf. Fig. 31.1). Some of the amygdaloid nuclei are marked with orange stippled lines. The basal nucleus is indicated with green stippled line. The amygdala and the cerebral cortex of the temporal lobe are closely connected. The section is placed more posteriorly than the one in Fig. 31.9.

Main Tasks of the Amygdala

The tasks performed by the amygdala have been clarified by lesion and stimulation experiments in animals, and recently by numerous functional magnetic resonance imaging (fMRI) studies in humans. Further, important information comes from examination of a few persons who lack the amygdala (usually after surgical treatment of epilepsy). While the connection between the amygdala and emotions is firmly established, much investigation remains before we understand its specific contributions to emotional processing and human behavior.

Animal experiments show that a central task for the amygdala is to establish **associations between sensory stimuli and their emotional coloring**. It is crucial that we can decide quickly—before slower conscious deliberations—whether a stimulus (or a situation) is threatening or safe (punishment or reward). Accordingly, fMRI studies in humans show activation of the amygdala when viewing pictures with an emotional content. Further, bilateral lesions of the amygdala in monkeys reduce behavior elicited by emotions. For example, the animals show no fear of snakes (monkeys have an inborn fear of snakes). This can probably be explained by the removal of amygdaloid effects on the hypothalamus and on the brain stem autonomic and somatic motor centers (among them the PAG; Fig. 31.6). Sensory stimuli (such as the sight of a snake), although reaching consciousness, would not be able to elicit the normal behavioral reactions.

The sight of **faces** expressing **anger** or **fear** causes a robust activation of the human amygdala, as shown via fMRI. Correspondingly, patients with amygdaloid lesions have difficulties with **recognizing facial expressions**. Interestingly, such patients do not show the normal tendency to remember events or stimuli that have an emotional coloring better than they remember neutral ones. This has been demonstrated, for example, by showing films containing emotionally neutral material and scenes that evoke strong emotions.

Selective lesions in adult monkeys produce a pattern of behavior characterized by **social disinhibition**.[3] For example, they initiate more physical contact, suggesting "...that heightened affiliative social interactions following amygdala lesions stems from a more general inability to properly perceive danger or threat in the environment and use such information to modulate social behavior adaptively" (Machado et al. 2008, p. 263). This would fit with the amygdala working as a sort of **alarm**—it

evaluates very rapidly a stimulus for its threatening value, and initiates appropriate behavior. However, selective lesions of the amygdala in monkeys produce fewer behavioral changes than reported in early experiments with lesions that included adjoining parts of the temporal lobe (see Chapter 34, under "Symptoms after Lesions of the Temporal Cortex"). For example, no signs of abnormal **social development** were observed the first 6 months after bilateral lesions of the amygdala in infant monkeys, in relationships with either the mother or other infants in the group. However, the infants did not exhibit the normal signs of distress to separation from the mother, presumably owing to a reduced ability to perceive danger and threatening situations.

Is the Amygdala Concerned Only with Negative Emotions?

Whereas most studies have focused on a correlation between amygdala activity and negative emotions such as fear and anger, recent studies suggest that the amygdala plays a role for the recognition of positive emotions as well. For example, a meta-analysis of human positron emission tomography (PET) and fMRI studies found that both negative and positive stimuli were associated with higher amygdala activity compared with neutral stimuli. Indeed, single-unit studies in monkeys identified distinct populations of amygdaloid neurons responding to positive and negative stimulus valence, respectively (the two kinds of neuron were not spatially segregated in the basolateral amygdala, however).

Electric Stimulation of the Human Amygdala

In humans, the amygdala has been stimulated in conjunction with brain surgery of the temporal lobe under local anesthesia. A wide spectrum of autonomic and emotional reactions has been produced in such cases, but most pronounced is a feeling of **anxiety**. Memory-like hallucinations and **déjà vu** experiences (the feeling of having experienced the same situation before) have also been reported. This is called a **dreamy state** and can occur in epileptic seizures that start in the temporal lobe. Similar effects—that is, fear and various kinds of hallucinations—have been produced by stimulation of the anterior portion of the hippocampus and the lateral cortex of the temporal lobe (in the superior temporal gyrus). This relationship can presumably be explained by the close connections between these regions and the amygdala, all being parts of a more widespread network for handling of emotions and memories.

Is Amygdala Necessary for the Experience of Emotions?

The finding that the amygdala is necessary for expression of emotions (at least some aspects) raises the question of

---

3 **Hypersexuality** was one of the behavioral changes reported in the early studies with large bilateral lesions of the amygdala in monkeys. However, this may be related to damage to allocortical areas near the amygdala rather than to the amygdala itself. Nevertheless, it is conspicuous that the amygdala is among the brain regions with the highest density of **receptors for sex hormones**. Conceivably, the level of sex hormones in the blood influences the activity of neurons in parts of the amygdala (the sex hormones are lipid-soluble and pass the blood–brain barrier easily).

whether the amygdala is necessary also for the subjective **experience** of emotions (such as fear or anger). A patient with bilateral destruction of the amygdala, described by the British psychiatrist R. Jacobson (1986), illustrates this point. She appeared calm and relaxed outwardly and had normal heart rate in situations in which she experienced great anxiety and wanted to run away. Presumably, the coupling between the emotions and the emotional reactions was disrupted in this patient (see Chapter 30, under "Emotions and Emotional Reactions"). Further, 20 patients with amygdaloid lesions after epilepsy surgery described their daily emotions—positive and negative—in the same manner as normal controls (Anderson and Phelps 2002).[4]

The Amygdala, Learning, and Unlearning

The conditioned-fear reaction discussed in the next subsection requires a learning process: the rat learns to associate an innocuous stimulus with something painful. Destruction of the amygdala prevents establishing the conditioned response. Indeed, induction of **LTP** occurs in certain parts of the amygdala in conjunction with development of a conditioned fear response. Thus, experiments with monkeys after a lesion restricted as far as possible to the amygdala show that they have difficulties in learning the association between objects and their meanings. They can recognize objects but cannot relate them to other kinds of information, such as whether the object was associated with a reward or something unpleasant. Many other observations support that the amygdala is necessary for the learning of associations between stimuli and their significance in terms of reward or punishment. We may say that the amygdala is crucial for the emotional coloring of experiences and sensations, and that associations are remembered. The amygdala is not alone in this respect, however. Both the amygdala and parts of the prefrontal cortex are necessary in monkeys for the learning and later retrieval of associations between visual stimuli and food rewards. The connections involved are partly direct fibers from the amygdala to the **ventromedial prefrontal cortex** and partly a pathway interrupted in the mediodorsal thalamic nucleus (MD). Experiments in rats suggest that connections between the basolateral amygdala and the **ventral striatum** are also necessary for establishing stimulus–reward associations.

Connections from medial parts of the prefrontal cortex appear to be necessary for unlearning—**extinction**—of the conditioned fear response. Extinction occurs when the conditioned stimulus regularly occurs without a subsequent unconditioned stimulus, but not in rats after removal of the medial prefrontal cortex. Other data also indicate that extinction depends on an active **inhibition** of the amygdala from the prefrontal cortex—not on the disappearance of the synaptic changes underlying the associations.

Amygdala, Anxiety, and Neurotransmitters

The amygdala contains many neurotransmitters, and to sort out the functional role of each is a formidable task. For practical reasons, therefore, scientists concentrate on studying one or a few at a time, with the danger of overlooking the contributions of other transmitters. We restrict ourselves here to the transmitters involved in **conditioned fear** and **psychic stress**. As mentioned, signals pass from the lateral to the central nucleus through both direct and indirect routes.

Electrical stimulation of the lateral nucleus evokes primarily γ-aminobutyric acid (**GABA**)-mediated inhibition in the central nucleus (acting at both $GABA_A$ and $GABA_B$ receptors). Some inhibition occurs presynaptically by reducing the release of **glutamate**. Drugs that reduce **anxiety** (anxiolytics) may function by interfering at this level. The **benzodiazepines** (Valium and others) bind to specific sites on the GABA receptor (benzodiazepine receptors) and potentiate the effect of GABA. The density of benzodiazepine receptors is high in the amygdala and particularly high in the lateral nucleus (and one other subnucleus of the basolateral complex). Local infusion of benzodiazepines in these nuclei reduces expressions of conditioned fear in experimental animals.

Corticotrophin-releasing hormone (CRH) may also be an important transmitter in the amygdala in relation to anxiety and stress. Besides containing CRH-positive cell bodies, the central nucleus receives many CRH-containing fibers (neurons in the parabrachial area and the locus coeruleus contain CRH, for example). Injection of CRH into the cerebral ventricles increases **stress reactions** and fear-related behavior, presumably by acting in the amygdala but also in other areas. For example, noradrenergic neurons in the locus coeruleus are activated, which may contribute to arousal as part of a stress reaction. Because acute and chronic stress increases CRH in the amygdala, microinjections of CRH antagonists in the central nucleus abolish some stress reactions.

The **expectation** of **pain** evokes an endocrine response, as one part of a stress reaction (see Chapter 30, under "Psychosomatic Disorders"). This may be mediated by neurons in the central nucleus, which project to the paraventricular hypothalamic nucleus. CRH-containing neurons in the paraventricular nucleus project to the

---

4 Not all patients with bilateral damage of the amygdala exhibit a dissociation of the experienced emotion and the emotional expressions, however. Indeed, there are surprisingly large individual variations in symptoms among patients with amygdaloid lesions. Conceivably, the age at which the lesion occurred plays a decisive part: with early lesions, other parts of the brain would be expected to at least partly take over the tasks of the amygdala. Further, prior experiences and subtle difference in context may strongly influence how different subjects with lesions of the amygdala experience and respond to identical stimuli.

median eminence. There CRH is released and reaches the anterior pituitary via the portal system (see Fig. 30.7). CRH increases the secretion of ACTH, thus increasing **cortisol** in the bloodstream.

Several transmitters other than CRH show changes in relation to anxiety and stress. **Neuropeptide Y** (NPY) has attracted much interest. Thus, microinjection of NPY in the amygdala evokes largely the opposite effects of CRH on stress and fear-related behavior. NPY is present in many neurons in the amygdala (colocalized with norepinephrine, GABA, or somatostatin) and in terminals of afferent axons. Animal experiments suggest that, whereas CRH is crucial in eliciting a stress reaction, NPY that is released after the reaction has started protects against overshooting.

The Amygdala and Depression

As mentioned, **CRH** is one likely transmitter (among several) for evoking fear-related behavior and stress reactions, and the amygdala is an important site of action. CRH also appears to be related to mood. Thus, the concentration of CRH in the cerebrospinal fluid is increased in many deeply depressed patients and victims of suicide. In the latter group, lowered density of the CRH receptor occurred in the frontal lobe (downregulation due to constantly increased CRH available?). A transgenic mouse strain overproducing CRH has increased levels of ACTH and cortisol in the blood as expected. In addition, mice from this strain show behavior indicative of anxiety (e.g., the way they behave in novel situations). This behavioral pattern is normalized by supply of CRH antagonists.

Measurement of **regional cerebral blood flow** supports the fact that the function of the amygdala is altered in seriously depressed patients. Thus, compared with a control group, depressed patients had increased blood flow in the left prefrontal cortex and amygdala. This observation does not tell us how the amygdala is involved in depression, however—for example, whether the blood flow changes are secondary to a change of mood, or whether changes in the amygdala come first.

SOME ASPECTS OF CORTICAL CONTROL OF AUTONOMIC FUNCTIONS AND EMOTIONS

Assigning specific functions to cortical regions builds on methods that can only provide indirect answers (functional deficits after lesions, blood flow changes associated with certain behaviors, EEG, single neurons recordings, and so forth). Because distributed networks—not single areas—are responsible for the execution of complex tasks, assigning functions to specific regions must be imprecise and simplistic. Although we need "pigeon holes" and labels to aid our thinking, we should bear in mind that our simplifying concepts have limited explanatory power. All cortical areas we mention here with focus on autonomic functions and emotions are also involved in other tasks (participate in other networks). For example, most of the cortical areas regulating autonomic functions also participate in processing of emotions. This is not unexpected, as the autonomic adjustments are an integral part of complex behavioral responses.

Autonomic Functions

Experimental and clinical data show that wide areas of the cerebral cortex influence the activity of structures innervated by the autonomic nervous system. This influence is mainly exerted via the amygdala, the hippocampal formation, and the septal nuclei, which in turn, influence the hypothalamus and brain stem nuclei. In addition, there are some direct connections from the **insula** and the **orbitofrontal cortex** to the hypothalamus. Further, neocortical areas in the frontal and temporal lobes project to the amygdala and can therefore influence the hypothalamus indirectly.

The **cingulate gyrus**—one of the limbic structures—appears to be involved in organization and initiation of various kinds of goal-directed behavior.[5] It projects to the hippocampal formation, to the septal nuclei, and to the amygdala—all of which have connections to various parts of the hypothalamus (Fig. 31.7). Electrical stimulation of the cingulate gyrus elicits a combination of autonomic (visceral) and somatic effects. Autonomic effects include, for example, alterations of **respiration** and **circulation** (reduced rate of breathing, heart rate, and blood pressure), of the **digestive tract** (altered peristaltic movements and secretory activity), and **pupillary dilatation**. Somatic effects are expressed mainly as changes of muscle tone and often inhibition of ongoing movements.

Alterations of functions controlled by the autonomic system can be produced by stimulation of parts of the cortex other than the cingulate gyrus. Stimulation of the **orbitofrontal cortex**, the **insula**, and the **pole of the temporal lobe** produces effects similar to those obtained from the cingulate gyrus—that is, combined behavioral, emotional, and autonomic responses. Stimulation of the aforementioned neocortical regions not only produces effects on autonomic functions; somatic functions are altered as well. In contrast, alterations of autonomic functions can occur after stimulation of cortical regions that one might believe to be purely somatic, such as the motor and the premotor cortical areas. Thus, stimulation

---

5 While minor parts of the cingulate gyrus belong to the allocortex, most of it probably belongs to the oldest parts of the neocortex. The terms **limbic** or **paralimbic cortex** are often used of cortical regions that have intimate connections with limbic structures, such as the amygdala and the hippocampus.

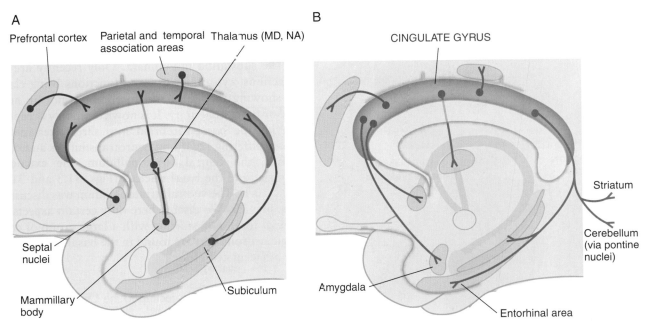

FIGURE 31.7 *Main connections of the cingulate gyrus.* **A:** Afferent connections **B:** Efferent connections. The cingulate gyrus has reciprocal connections with neocortical association areas and with limbic structures and may act as a mediator between them.

of the **motor cortex** produces **vasomotor changes** (i.e., changes of the blood vessel diameter and, therefore, of blood flow) of the opposite body half. On damage to these cortical areas (as seen in patients with a cerebral **stroke**), vasomotor changes often occur in the paralyzed parts of the body. Even alterations of the heart rate and blood pressure and of the digestive tract can occur. As a final example of combined somatic and autonomic effects, stimulation of the **frontal eye field** (see Fig. 25.7) produces pupillary dilatation in addition to the more obvious conjugated eye movements.

Emotions and the Neocortex

As mentioned, cortical areas that show altered activity (as measured with PET and fMRI) in relation to emotions are more extensive that those initially included in the "limbic system" (Fig. 31.8). On the other hand, no area is solely concerned with emotional processing. The **cingulate gyrus** is a pertinent example. Even if it consists of several smaller subdivisions that differ with regard to connections, they all seem to be involved in both cognitive and emotional processing, albeit to a varying degree. The anterior part of the cingulate gyrus (**anterior cingulate cortex [ACC]**) consists of rostral part that is more concerned with affect regulation and a caudal part more concerned with cognitive task. In general, the ACC appears to be important for the choice of behavior in response to **conflicting stimuli**. The ACC also seems to monitor mental and bodily processes with special focus on the detection of errors and conflicts.[6] For this monitoring, emotions provide important information about values of different signals. Parts of the cingulate gyrus (both anterior and posterior parts) and the anterior **insula** (Fig. 31.8) also alter their activity in relation to emotions such as admiration and **compassion**.

Several parts of the **prefrontal cortex** show altered activity in relation to emotions in humans, and accordingly, lesions often produce emotional disturbances (see Chapter 34, under "Symptoms after Prefrontal Lesions"). Especially the **orbitofrontal** and **ventromedial parts** seems important for emotional regulation (Fig. 31.8). As mentioned, these parts have reciprocal connections with the amygdala. The orbitofrontal cortex may integrate competing, emotionally colored signals to provide an appropriate response. For example, a study compared the behavior of normal and orbitofrontal-lesioned monkeys in a situation where a snake occurred between the monkey and a piece of food. Presumably, amygdala informs about the values of the signals (snake and food), whereas the orbitofrontal cortex is necessary for evaluation and appropriate action. Such studies strongly suggest that the orbitofrontal cortex is important for behavioral **flexibility**—that is, the ability to alter behavior when needed and to choose among conflicting choices.

---

6 Stimulation of the ACC in monkeys produces, for example, **aggressive reactions**, whereas bilateral removal makes the animals tamer. They may also become **socially indifferent**—that is, they appear to have lost interest in other members of their group and do not try to make contact.

basal forebrain show similarities with the basal ganglia (dorsal striatum and dorsal pallidum) regarding cyto-architectonics, cytochemistry, and connections (e.g., a dense dopaminergic innervation from the mesencepha-lon). In contrast to the dorsal striatum (the caudate nucleus and the putamen), which receives the main affer-ent input from the neocortex, the ventral striatum receives main inputs from the allocortex and the amygdala. A further characteristic of the ventral striatum is that it projects to the hypothalamus and brain stem nuclei, such as the periaqueductal gray (PAG) and the motor vagus nucleus. The ventral pallidum projects to the mediodorsal thalamic nucleus (MD) that sends fibers to the prefrontal cortex (cf. the projection of the dorsal pallidum to the VL/VA thalamic nuclei that project mainly to the premotor areas).

Another rather diffuse cell group in the basal fore-brain, continuous with the ventral pallidum, is called the **extended amygdala** because it forms a rostral exten-sion of the medial amygdala (Figs. 31.9 and 31.10). Most of it is made up of the **bed nucleus of the stria terminalis** (Figs. 31.6 and 36.9). The stria terminalis is a bundle of efferent fibers from the amygdala to the septal nuclei and the hypothalamus (Fig. 31.5). The bed nucleus lies medial to the pallidum at the same antero-posterior level and further anterior to the anterior com-missure (i.e., close to the septal nuclei). When this part of the basal forebrain is lumped with the amygdala, it is because they share many transmitters and connections. The anatomic distinction between the extended amygdala and the nucleus accumbens is not sharp, however, and both receive, for example, dopaminergic fibers from the mesencephalon.

The Medial Forebrain Bundle

Many fibers interconnecting the various limbic struc-tures are located in a diffusely delimited, parasagittal fiber mass in the basal part of the hemisphere. This ill-defined structure is called the **medial forebrain bundle** and passes through the lateral parts of the hypothala-mus. It extends from the region of the anterior commis-sure anteriorly and into the mesencephalon posteriorly. Most of the fibers are short, interconnecting nuclei found close to each other, such as the septal nuclei, other nuclei in the basal forebrain, various hypothalamic nuclei, and the PAG in the mesencephalon (see Fig. 31.4). Fibers from the **monoaminergic** cell groups of the brain stem pass through the medial forebrain bundle on their way to forebrain structures, such as the cortex (includ-ing the hippocampal formation). Functionally, the medial forebrain bundle is heterogeneous, and lesions of it cannot be expected to reveal the function of any particular cell group or fiber tract.

32 | The Hippocampal Formation: Learning and Memory

OVERVIEW

The hippocampus and nearby areas in the parahippocampal gyrus (the dentate gyrus and the entorhinal area) comprise the **hippocampal formation**, which plays a crucial role for certain kinds of learning and memory. The quantitatively dominating **afferent inputs** to the dentate gyrus and the hippocampus arise in the **entorhinal area**. The entorhinal area receives afferents from both nearby areas in the temporal lobe and cortical association areas. Thereby, it receives highly processed sensory information—that is, about all important events. The hippocampal projection neurons send signals via intermediaries to several areas, notably back to the entorhinal area and to the mammillary nucleus. Thus, the hippocampus acts largely back onto the areas from which it receives information.

Bilateral damage of the hippocampal formation leads to **amnesia**—impaired memory without intellectual reduction. Lesions restricted to the hippocampus proper produce amnesia, although it is much less severe than when the whole hippocampal formation has been damaged.

We can roughly distinguish two kinds of memory: one kind concerns the memory of events and facts and is called **declarative** or **explicit** memory; the other concerns skills and habits and is called **nondeclarative** or **implicit** memory. Only declarative memory depends critically on the integrity of medial parts of the temporal lobe. For nondeclarative memory, the basal ganglia, cerebellum, and parts of the neocortex appear to be most important.

Certainly, the hippocampal formation is not the only part of the brain that is important for memory. Parts of the parahippocampal gyrus outside the hippocampal formation appear to play an independent role in memory formation and retrieval. Further, amnesia has also been reported after lesions of the **medial thalamus**, and cholinergic cell groups of the basal forebrain also have a role (presumably by way of their connections with the hippocampus). Finally, **amygdala** is crucial for learning of associations between stimuli and their emotional value.

The hippocampal formation appears to be important for memory only for a certain time after an event. Thus, isolated damage of the hippocampal formation does not usually abolish recall of older memories, although it prevents the learning of new material. This is probably because, after a certain time, the memory traces are stored in many parts of the cerebral cortex.

THE HIPPOCAMPAL FORMATION

Macroscopic Appearance and Constituent Parts

The **hippocampal formation** consists of the **hippocampus** and nearby regions in the temporal lobe: the **dentate gyrus**, the **subiculum**, and the **entorhinal area** (located in the parahippocampal gyrus; Figs. 32.1 and 32.2). Whereas the interest formerly was directed mainly to the hippocampus itself, it is now realized that the function of the hippocampus can be understood only in conjunction with the nearby structures in the parahippocampal gyrus, which are closely interconnected with each other and with the hippocampus. Although hippocampus is included among the limbic structures (see Fig. 31.1), its functional role is distinct from that of the amygdala, the septal nuclei, and the cingulate gyrus. The amygdala and the hippocampal formation are, for example, both crucial for learning and memory, but for different kinds.

The **hippocampus** (Figs. 32.1 and 32.3; see Figs. 6.31 and 31.2) forms an elongated bulge medially in the temporal horn of the lateral ventricle, produced during early development by invagination of the ventricular wall by the hippocampal sulcus (see Fig. 9.12). The hippocampus is easily recognized in thionine-stained microscopic sections by its conspicuous layer of pyramidal cells (Fig. 32.2). Along the medial aspect of the hippocampus, the **dentate gyrus** forms a narrow, notched band (Fig. 32.1; see Fig. 31.2). Microscopically, the narrow, dark layer of small granule cells is characteristic (Fig. 32.2). The hippocampus and the dentate gyrus belong to the allocortex and have a simplified laminar pattern compared with the neocortex. Nevertheless, they are far from simply built, with several different cell types and precisely organized, complex patterns of connections. Figure 32.2 shows that the hippocampus (the CA1 field) continues into the **subiculum** but with a marked change in the thickness and organization of layers (both have three neuronal layers). The transition

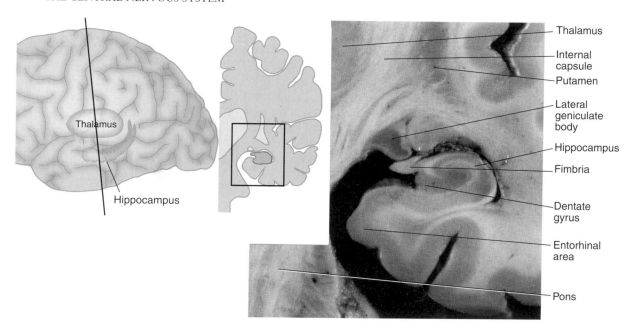

FIGURE 32.1 *The hippocampus*. Photograph of a frontal section through the left hemisphere. The hippocampus forms a continuation of the temporal cortex, as an invagination of the temporal horn of the lateral ventricle. Figure 22.2 shows the whole section. Compare Figs. 31.1 and 31.2.

between the subiculum and the **entorhinal cortex** is marked with the appearance of a six-layered cortex.

Two Main Sets of Connections

Two aspects of the connections of the hippocampal formation are, presumably, crucial for the understanding of its functional roles: first, the extensive, two-way connections with various cortical association areas and, second, the direct and indirect connections with the amygdala,

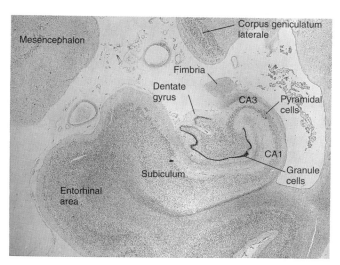

FIGURE 32.2 *The hippocampal formation*. Photomicrograph of thionine-stained frontal section through the human temporal lobe. The temporal horn of the lateral ventricle with some of the choroid plexus is seen above and to the right of the hippocampus. The mesencephalon with the crus and the substantia nigra is seen to the left. Compare with Fig. 32.1.

cingulate gyrus, and septal nuclei (Fig. 32.4). As for neocortical connections, the hippocampus obviously processes large amounts of information. The parallel increase in the size of the hippocampus and the neocortex during evolution furthermore indicates that its main functions are related to the neocortex. A large number of commissural fibers connect the hippocampus of the two sides, indicating a close cooperation between them.

Afferent Connections of the Hippocampal Formation

The main afferents to the **dentate gyrus** arise in the entorhinal area Figs. 32.4 and 32.5). Because the dentate gyrus sends its efferents to the hippocampus, the **entorhinal area** is the quantitatively dominating deliverer of information to the hippocampus. Smaller but functionally important contingents to the hippocampal formation come from the **septal nuclei** and **monoaminergic cell groups** in the brain stem (the locus coeruleus and the raphe nuclei). In addition, some fibers come from the **hypothalamus** and several **thalamic nuclei**. Finally, the **amygdala** projects to the subiculum and the entorhinal area. The latter connections most likely contribute to the well-known effect of emotions on learning, as discussed in Chapter 31 (see "Amygdala, Learning, and Unlearning").

To understand the nature of the information processed by the hippocampus, we must know the afferent connections of the **entorhinal area**. Recent studies with retrograde transport in monkeys have shown that most **association areas** of the neocortex are likely to influence the entorhinal area. Signals reach the entorhinal

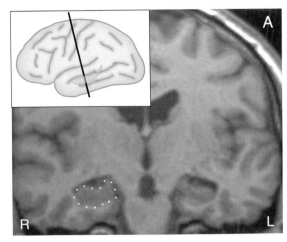
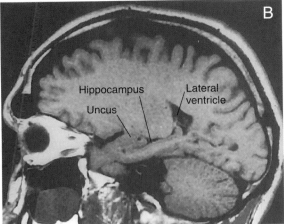

FIGURE 32.3 *Magnetic resonance images (MRIs) showing the hippocampus.* **A:** Frontal plane. The hippocampus is positioned medially in the temporal lobe (stippled outline on one side). Inset shows approximate position of the hippocampus in the temporal lobe and the plane of sectioning. **B:** Parasagittal plane through the medial part of the temporal lobe. (Courtesy of Dr. S. J. Bakke, Rikshospitalet University Hospital, Oslo, Norway.)

area directly, or indirectly by means of fibers to other areas in the parahippocampal gyrus, which, in turn, project to the entorhinal area. Thus, the majority of direct entorhinal afferents arise in adjacent parts of the **parahippocampal gyrus** (see Figs. 6.26 and 31.1) and in the **perirhinal cortex** (located around the rhinal sulcus; see Fig. 19.3). These areas form a continuous cortical region, although different parts are not identical regarding connections. Together, the region receives **visual** information from extrastriate areas in the inferior part of the temporal lobe, **auditory** information from the superior part of the temporal lobe, **somatosensory** information from the posterior parietal cortex, and

information from **polysensory** association areas—that is, areas that integrate several sensory modalities. Finally, afferents arrive from the **cingulate gyrus**, the **insula**, and the **prefrontal cortex**. Together, the entorhinal area receives highly processed sensory information. We assume, for example, that information about words comes to the hippocampus regardless of whether we see (read), hear, or read by touch (Braille writing).

The cortical areas that provide the entorhinal area (and thus the hippocampus) with its main inputs project to other areas as well. For example, both the **perirhinal cortex** and the **subiculum** project to the **mediodorsal thalamic nucleus** (MD), which projects to the prefrontal cortex and parts of the cingulate gyrus. This might explain why **amnesia** (memory loss) is more severe after damage of the perirhinal cortex and the areas neighboring the entorhinal area than after a lesion restricted to the entorhinal area and the hippocampus (we return to this point later).

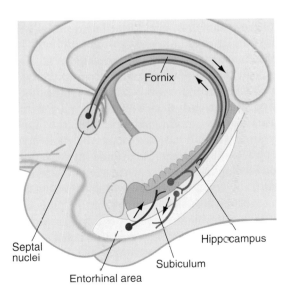

FIGURE 32.4 *Some main connections of the hippocampus.* The connections with the entorhinal area mediate specific, highly processed sensory information, whereas the connections with the septal nuclei are modulatory.

Modulatory Afferents Increase Hippocampal Plasticity

Although hippocampal afferents from the **septal nuclei** (Fig. 32.4) are not numerous, they have an important functional role. Many of the septohippocampal neurons release **acetylcholine** as a modulatory transmitter, increasing the excitability of the hippocampal pyramidal cells. The hippocampal afferents from the **raphe nuclei** (serotonin) and the **locus coeruleus** (norepinephrine) have modulatory effects on the hippocampal cells. Thus, there is evidence that hippocampal **long-term potentiation** (LTP; see later) is reduced after pharmacologic removal of monoamines from the hippocampus. These modulatory pathways may mediate the effects of attention and motivation, which we know have profound influences on both learning and memory.

amygdala (emotional coloring) and several parts of the cortex (Fig. 32.6). Common to declarative memories is that we as a rule must consciously "search our minds" to recall them. In contrast, **nondeclarative** memory is needed to learn and perform **skills** (riding a bicycle, dress, use a knife and fork, etc.). Habits and attitudes also largely fall in this category. The learning leads to altered behavior, but not so that the stored material can be subject to a conscious analysis. With skills like playing an instrument or arithmetic, the stored information becomes accessible only by performing the skill (memory of how). In ordinary teaching situations, much of the learning is implicit—for example, the acquisition of attitudes of which both the teacher and the student are unaware.

Relationship between Memory and Long-Term Potentiation

The cellular basis of brain plasticity is discussed in Chapter 4, under "Synaptic Plasticity"). Because the hippocampus is involved in learning and memory, it is of special interest that the synapses are plastic at several steps in the circuit shown in Figure 31.4. Thus, their efficacy can be increased for a long time after intensive stimulation. Indeed, **long-term potentiation** (LTP) was first discovered in the hippocampus, although it was later found in many other areas of the brain, among them the cerebral cortex and the amygdala. LTP is produced whenever the hippocampal pyramidal cells are subjected to excitatory inputs—for example, from the Schaffer collaterals—while they are in a depolarized state (i.e., caused by another excitatory input). Thus, simultaneous synaptic activation of the cell from two sources can make it "remember," in the sense that the next time the cell is activated by the same fibers the postsynaptic effects are stronger than earlier. To demonstrate a direct

relationship between LTP and learning is difficult, however. For example, only specific subsets of synapses in widely distributed networks are likely to show LTP in a natural learning situation. To look for such altered synapses would seem like looking for "a needle in a haystack." Nevertheless, much indirect evidence supports that hippocampal LTP is related to learning and memory. Increased synaptic efficacy has been found in the hippocampus in rats housed in an environment rich in stimuli and challenges (assuming that more learning takes place in this situation than in a standard cage). LTP-like phenomena have also been observed in the hippocampus after specific training situations. Another piece of evidence is that **N-methyl-D-aspartate** (**NMDA)-receptor** antagonists both prevent induction of LTP and reduce learning and memory in experimental animals. Gene-technological manipulations have produced strains of mice in which hippocampal LTP cannot be induced, and these animals also show reduced learning ability. Finally, structural synaptic changes have been observed in the hippocampus in conjunction with the induction of LTP. Even more compelling, structural synaptic changes (formation of new synapses and splitting of spines into two) have also been reported in the hippocampus in rats at the time they improve their performance in a learning situation.

Medial Parts of the Temporal Lobe Is Necessary for Declarative Memory

The belief that the hippocampus is of importance for memory goes back to the end of the nineteenth century and was based on careful examination of patients with amnesia (loss of memory) as a result of brain damage (Fig. 32.7). In particular, the importance of the medial temporal lobe for declarative memory was strikingly demonstrated in the 1950s by observations of the patient H.M. with bilateral removal of the hippocampus and surrounding regions. During the past few years, refined studies in monkeys with selective lesions, and observations with magnetic resonance imaging (MRI) and positron emission tomography (PET) in humans, have helped clarify the mutual roles of the hippocampus and other subregions of the medial temporal lobe.[3]

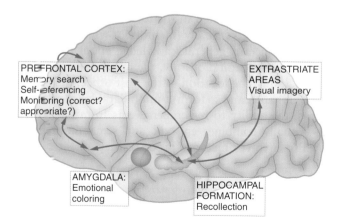

PREFRONTAL CORTEX:
Memory search
Self-referencing
Monitoring (correct?
appropriate?)

EXTRASTRIATE
AREAS
Visual imagery

AMYGDALA:
Emotional
coloring

HIPPOCAMPAL
FORMATION:
Recollection

FIGURE 32.5 *Network serving autobiographical memory.* Some of the regions showing increased activity in relation to retrieval of autobiographic memories, as revealed by fMRI. (Based on Cabeza and Jacques 2007.)

3 Various memory tests are used in experiments with monkeys to study the relationship between brain structures and memory. One common test is the so-called **delayed nonmatching-to-sample** test. The monkey is briefly shown an object. After a certain time, the same object is shown with a new one. To receive a reward (e.g., orange juice) the monkey must move the new object, thus showing that it remembers which one was seen before. The experiment goes on with continually new pairs of items. With a brief interval between the first and second presentation, the performance is independent of the integrity of medial temporal structures. With intervals above 10 sec, however, the frequency of errors increases in monkeys with such lesions as a sign of failing memory. With more than 2 min intervals, the performance is no better than chance, whereas normal monkeys reduce their performance to about 80% with intervals of 3 min.

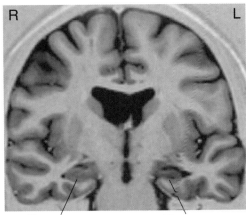

R   L

Hippocampus   Hippocampus
(normal)   (atrophic)

FIGURE 32.7 *MRI in the frontal plane showing hippocampal atrophy on the left side.* A nearby focus of epileptic activity is most likely the cause of hippocampal cell loss, causing so-called mesial temporal sclerosis. (Courtesy of Dr. S.J. Bakke, Rikshospitalet University Hospital, Oslo, Norway.)

Patients with severe **amnesia** that is not accompanied by intellectual reduction (dementia) typically have lesions that affect the medial parts of the temporal lobe (and often also the medial parts of the thalamus). Such lesions include the hippocampal formation as the most constant finding. Further, testing of patients with restricted lesions of the medial temporal lobe suggested that memory impairments concerned **long-term memory**, whereas **short-term memory** was virtually unimpaired (i.e., the ability to remember, e.g., numbers or words for up to a minute). Nevertheless, these conclusions may not be generally valid. Thus, conclusions were generally based on tests requiring the patients to retain simple motor sequences or short strings of digits or letters. Indeed, when using more natural test situations, requiring short-term memory of faces or locations, patients with restricted medial temporal lobe lesions show reduce performance.

The amnesia is **anterograde**—that is, the memory is lost for events that take place after the time of the brain damage. There are also varying degrees of **retrograde amnesia**—that is, the patient is unable to recall events that took place before the damage. Retrograde amnesia usually occurs together with anterograde amnesia (but some cases have been reported with relatively pure retrograde amnesia alone). Retrograde amnesia is usually graded, that is, is extends from the time of injury and a certain time backwards. Observations of patients with lesions restricted to medial temporal lobe indicate that the retrograde amnesia extends from about one year up to about 20 years. If the amnesia extends further back and include childhood memories, most studies suggest that there is damage also outside the medial temporal lobe. Not all researchers agree with this view, however, and maintain that lesions of the hippocampal formation

and surrounding areas can produce an amnesia that comprises all prior material without any gradation. Further, other evidence suggests the participation of the hippocampal formation in the retrieval of remote memories. For example, most functional MRI (fMRI) studies agree that the hippocampus increases its activity in relation to recollection of autobiographic memories, independent of how remote they are. As usually in science, the disagreements among authors may depend more on how questions are posed to nature (e.g., different tests and contexts) than on erroneous results.

The Contribution of the Perirhinal Cortex

The most pronounced memory loss occurs when the hippocampal formation, the perirhinal cortex, and areas outside the entorhinal area in the parahippocampal gyrus are destroyed on both sides. Especially, the inclusion of the **perirhinal cortex** appears to increase the severity of amnesia as compared with what occurs after lesions restricted to the hippocampal formation. Thus, the perirhinal cortex and the adjoining cortex of the parahippocampal gyrus appear to contribute to memory not only by their connections with the hippocampal formation but also by their connections to other parts of the brain. For example, the perirhinal cortex projects to the thalamus (MD), amygdala, mammillary body, and parts of the prefrontal cortex. The perirhinal cortex may be uniquely involved in **stimulus recognition memory.**

Amnesia: The Famous Case of H.M.

Patients with bilateral damage to medial aspects of the temporal lobe have pronounced anterograde (and often less severe retrograde) amnesia, as described previously. Scoville and Milner (1957) described the most famous case of this kind in the 1950s. This patient, called H.M. in the voluminous literature that deals with the results of tests to which he had been subjected, underwent surgery to remove bilaterally the medial aspects of his temporal lobes (the purpose was to cure his severe epilepsy). His lesion most likely comprised the hippocampal formation, additional parts of the parahippocampal gyrus, the uncus, and the amygdala. The epileptic seizures became less frequent, but, unfortunately, he acquired severe, permanent anterograde amnesia. Initially, he also had considerable retrograde amnesia that gradually improved to just 1 year before the operation. He remembered well the address of the place he lived before the operation, but he never learned the new address when moving afterward. He could easily recall songs he had learned before the operation but not those he heard for the first time afterward. He never learned where the lawn mower was kept in his new house. Shortly after eating dinner, he could start on a new meal without

One of the great challenges in understanding the hippocampus is to combine its role in spatial navigation and spatial memory with its undeniable importance for declarative memory. Recent animal experiments suggest that both tasks may be carried out simultaneously: neuronal populations may at the same time signal *where* something happens and *what* is going on. Such a double role might—loosely considered—fit with the everyday experience that recall depends strongly on **context**. For example, experiments with divers show that a series of numbers learned under water is better recalled under water than on dry land. Similarly, when unable to recall why we went into a room, it may help to go back to the place where we first got the idea to go into the room.

"Knowledge Systems of the Brain"

In a wide sense, memories represent our knowledge of the world and the actions that are necessary to relate successfully to it. Not all this knowledge is accessible for conscious "inspection" and analysis (nondeclarative or implicit memory, as described). Nevertheless, all memories presumably have as their substrate synaptic changes in specific parts of the central nervous system. Damasio and Tranel (1992) use the term "knowledge systems of the brain" about the widespread networks dedicated to specific tasks. Examples are knowledge systems dealing with social interactions, faces, objects, language, or ourselves. Although a part of the temporal lobe cortex is particularly important for recognition of faces, this does not necessarily mean that all information about faces is stored there. More likely, this part is unique because it has access to face-related information stored in many other areas. Presumably, the memory of faces fails after a stroke in the temporal lobe because there is "no one" to retrieve and process all the relevant information, not because the storehouse is empty.

VIII | THE CEREBRAL CORTEX

THE human cerebral cortex consists of about 20 billion neurons and constitutes more than half of all gray matter of the central nervous system. This gives a rough impression of its functional importance. In lower vertebrates, there are only very modest primordia of the cerebral cortex (allocortex), and it is first in mammals, particularly anthropoid apes and humans, that the cerebral cortex comes to dominate the rest of the nervous system quantitatively. This enormous increase in the volume of the cortex has necessitated a marked folding of the surface of the hemisphere. The outer layer of the human cerebral cortex is around 0.2 m^2, but only one-third of this is exposed on the surface. The **neocortex** constitutes most of the cerebral cortex in higher mammals, and this part deals only with the neocortex. In Chapter 33, we deal mainly with the structure and connections of the cerebral cortex from a functional perspective. In Chapter 34 we discuss the complex tasks attended to by the cortical association areas, which make up the bulk of the human cerebral cortex. In previous chapters we treated the role of the cerebral cortex in sensory processes (Chapters 14–19), control of body and eye movements (Chapters 22 and 25), autonomic functions and emotions (Chapter 31), and memory (Chapter 32). The role of the cerebral cortex in relation to sleep and consciousness is briefly discussed in Chapter 26.

33 | The Cerebral Cortex: Intrinsic Organization and Connections

OVERVIEW

In this chapter, we address two levels of organization. The first concerns information processing in a small volume of cortex; the second level concerns the interconnection of functionally different cortical units with long association and commissural fibers. These connections are essential parts of distributed, task-specific cortical networks.

The neurons of the neocortex are arranged in **six layers** parallel to the cortical surface. The layers differ with regard to afferent and efferent connections. In general, layers 2 and 4 are receiving, whereas layers 3 and 5 are mainly efferent. The bulk of afferents from the thalamus end in lamina 4, whereas layer 5 gives origin to subcortical tracts to the cord, brain stem, and basal ganglia. Layers 2 and 3 receive and send out most of the corticocortical fibers, interconnecting various parts of the cortex.

The cortex is divided into numerous **cytoarchitectonic** areas that differ with regard to connections and functional specializations. At a microstructural level, the cortical neurons are arranged in smaller **modules**, often in the form of **columns** perpendicular to the cortical surface. Each column, containing some thousand neurons, represents a computational unit. The neurons of the columns communicate with each other and with neurons in neighboring and distant columns.

There are two main kinds of cortical neuron: the **pyramidal cells** with long axons destined for other parts of the cortex or subcortical targets, and **interneurons** (with numerous subtypes) with short axons remaining in the cortical gray matter. The pyramidal cells are **glutamatergic**; whereas all interneurons are **GABAergic** (γ-aminobutyric acid [GABA] is colocalized with different combinations of neuropeptides). In addition, **modulatory transmitters**, such as dopamine and acetylcholine, regulate the cortical excitability level and the signal-to-noise ratio of cortical neurons.

Cortical connections fall into four groups. One group of afferents consists of precise, topographically organized connections from the **specific thalamic nuclei**; each thalamic nucleus supplies one particular part of the cortex. Another group consists of diffusely organized connections from the **intralaminar thalamic nuclei** and several other **subcortical nuclei** (releasing modulatory transmitters). The two final groups—making up the majority of all cortical connections—consist of corticocortical fibers; that is, **association fibers** and **commissural fibers**. Association fibers are precisely organized connections linking cortical areas within the same hemisphere, while commissural fibers pass in the corpus callosum and connect areas in the two hemispheres. The **efferent** connections of the cerebral cortex can also be divided into **subcortical** and **corticocortical** ones (association and commissural connections). The subcortical fibers are destined for the thalamus, the striatum, various brain stem nuclei (among them the pontine nuclei projecting to the cerebellum), and the spinal cord. The corticocortical connections are for the most part **reciprocal**—that is, an area receives fibers from the same areas to which it sends fibers.

STRUCTURE OF THE CEREBRAL CORTEX

Levels of Organization

To understand the relationship between the performance of the cerebral cortex and the underlying neural processes, we need to address two levels of organization. The first concerns information processing in a small volume of cortex; we may term this **intracortical synaptic organization**. The second level concerns the interconnection of functionally different cortical units with long association and commissural fibers, which we term **interareal synaptic organization**. How are signals arriving in a small bit of the cortex treated before "answers" are sent to other parts of the cortex or subcortical nuclei? How are the many different cortical areas interconnected to form networks designed for solving specific tasks? The enormous number of neurons and synaptic couplings in the human cerebral cortex explain why we do not have complete answers to such questions. For example, about 100,000 neurons reside below 1 mm^2 of cortical surface (rodent SI), and each neuron receives synaptic contacts from at least some hundred other neurons. Further, the tasks of the cerebral cortex are the most complex of all. To understand the relationship between the "machinery" of the

cortex (SI) with similar receptive fields and modalities are grouped together in columns with a diameter of some hundred micrometers. A similar columnar arrangement of neurons has been observed in the motor cortex (MI), but with respect to muscles rather than to receptors (neurons within one column act on one or a few synergistic muscles). Interestingly, a pyramidal cell with all its dendrites and recurrent collaterals is contained within a cortical tissue cylinder with a diameter of about 350 μm (Fig. 33.3A). Thousands of other neurons are present within the same cylinder.

Modular Organization of the Cerebral Cortex

Module is a more general term for columns and other assemblies of neurons that share salient properties (in the cortex and elsewhere; see Chapter 16, under "Modular Organization of the Visual Cortex"). It is striking how connections and cytochemical markers show a **patchy distribution** all over the cortex, strongly suggesting some kind of modular pattern as a basic principle in the organization of the cerebral cortex. For example, afferent projections—from the thalamus or from other parts of the cortex—end in many, regularly spaced patches in the cortex rather than continuously (Fig. 33.3B). This means that inputs from different sources may converge systematically on cortical neurons. Similarly, projection neurons with a common target tend to be lumped together. There is, furthermore, a striking correspondence between the diameters of cortical dendritic trees and of the terminal patches formed by afferent fibers.

It may not be feasible to find a definition that fits modules in all parts of the cortex, however. Indeed, different criteria are used to define modules in the cortex, and, depending on the criteria used, their shape and size vary greatly. Further, the distribution neurons with different properties is less schematic than the modular concept might imply. In the visual cortex, in which the segregation of functionally different neurons has been most thoroughly investigated, cells sharing functional properties are arranged in **bands** rather than in cylinders (see Fig. 16.23). Another problem with the columnar concept is that neurons in different layers—for example, of the striate area—are not functionally identical (e.g., cells that are color-specific and cells that are movement-specific are located in different layers). Thus, the modules may not always extend through the depth of the cortex but may be limited to one or a few layers (cf. color-specific "blobs" in the striate area; see Fig. 16.24). To apply the columnar concept to such cases confuses rather than clarifies.

The **biologic significance** of modular organization in the cortex and elsewhere (e.g., in the striatum and the cerebellum) is not fully understood. The modular pattern gives each cortical neuron a varied afferent

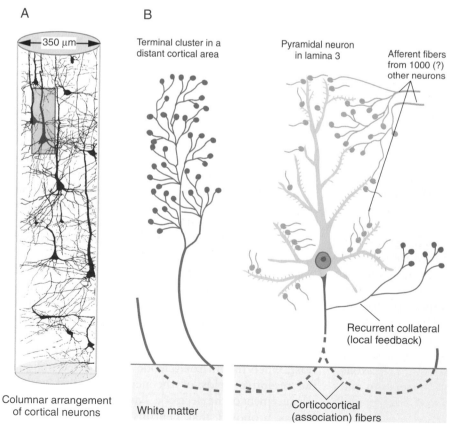

FIGURE 33.3 *Columnar arrangement of cortical neurons and clustering of cortico-cortical terminal areas.* **A:** A cylindrical volume of cortical tissue forms a functional unit (column), for example, in the somatosensory cortex. Golgi-impregnated neurons (from Conel 1939) show position of cell bodies and the main orientation of the dendrites. Note, however, that only a fraction of the total neuronal population within a column is shown in the figure. **B:** Schematic. A pyramidal neuron in cortical layer 3 (inset in A) and its main connections: recurrent collaterals and corticocortical fibers. A patch of termination in a distant cortical area is also shown. Each neuron forms many such patches in several areas. The number of neurons forming synapses on each layer 3 pyramidal neuron is indicated.

input, with each neuron receiving samples of information from several sources (several patches contact each neuron). In the motor cortex, for example, a neuron might need to integrate information from the thalamus (perhaps from different subgroups in the VL nucleus), from SI, and from the premotor cortex. Another advantage of modular organization may be that it permits shorter intracortical connections and thus saves nervous tissue. Further, modules may be advantageous during development by making it easier for growing axons to find their target. Some claim, however, that modular organization is merely a byproduct of how the nervous system develops and that it lacks an intrinsic functional meaning.

Afferents from Different Sources End in Different Cortical Layers

The cortical layers differ with regard to the origin of their extrinsic afferents. Thus, there is some degree of specialization among the laminae with regard to what kind of information they process. As we discuss later, however, connections between the laminae ensure integration of their outputs. Schematically, pathways that convey **precise sensory information** end primarily in **layer 4**. This includes thalamocortical fibers from the somatosensory relay nucleus, VPL, and from the relay nuclei of the visual and auditory pathways, the lateral and medial geniculate bodies. **Association fibers** (i.e., from other cortical areas) end preferentially in **layers 2 to 4**. Subcortical afferents with **modulatory effects** end in several layers but especially in **layer 1**. Such fibers arise in the intralaminar thalamic nuclei, in several brain stem nuclei (the raphe nuclei, nucleus locus coeruleus, and dopaminergic cell groups in the mesencephalon), and in the basal nucleus (acetylcholine).

The Cerebral Cortex Can Be Divided into Cytoarchitectonic Areas

Even though all parts of the neocortex consist of six cell layers, the thickness and structure of the various layers vary from one area to another. This is observed most easily in sections stained to visualize the cell bodies only (Figs. 33.1, 33.2; see Fig. 22.4). Such **cytoarchitectonic** differences form the basis of the subdivision of the entire cortex into cytoarchitectonic **areas**, as done around the turn of the century by Brodmann (1909) and others (Fig. 33.4). This is briefly described in Chapter 6, and several of the cytoarchitectonic areas are mentioned in previous chapters. The development of cytoarchitectonic areas is briefly discussed in Chapter 9 ("Specification of Cortical Cytoarchitectonic Areas").

The main importance of the division of the cortex into cytoarchitectonic areas is that these areas have proved in many instances to differ functionally, even though they were initially defined solely on the basis of the size, shape, and arrangement of the neuronal cell bodies. In many cases, a cytoarchitectonically defined area is unique with regard to its afferent and efferent connections and the physiological properties of its cells.

Although the borders between different cytoarchitectonic areas are sometimes easy to identify, as exemplified in the section of the visual cortex shown in Fig. 33.5, more often the differences are rather subtle. Thus, it should not come as a surprise that authors often disagree with regard to the parcellation of the cortex into areas. Today we try to define a cortical area not only based on cytoarchitectonics but also by additional criteria, such as fiber connections, cellular markers, recordings of single-cell activity, and the behavioral effects of stimulation or ablation of the area in question.

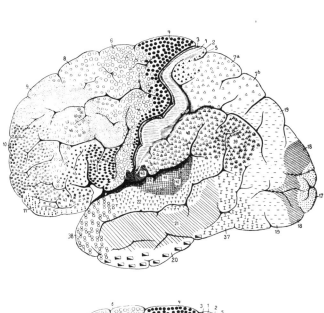

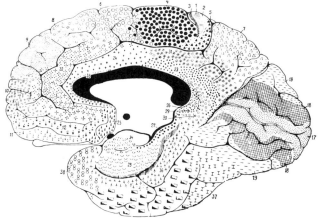

FIGURE 33.4 *Brodmann's cytoarchitectonic map of the human brain.* The various areas are labeled with different symbols and numbers. (From Brodmann 1909).

and GABA acting on **GABA**$_B$ receptors. In addition, **neuropeptides** colocalized with GABA exert modulatory effects, although we do not know their functional roles. Most studied, however, are modulatory actions mediated by diffusely organized fiber systems from several brain stem and basal forebrain cell groups. We mentioned such connections in Chapter 5 (under "Modulatory Transmitter 'Systems'") and in Chapter 26 (under "Pathways and Transmitters Responsible for Cortical Activation"). The following neurotransmitters are involved: **acetylcholine, norepinephrine, serotonin, dopamine,** and **histamine**. In general, they act to improve the precision of cortical signal transfer—for example, by improving the **signal-to-noise ratio**. Such effects are probably important in relation to **arousal,** focused **attention,** and **motivation**. Acetylcholine, for example, brings layer 5 pyramids in the motor cortex from a state with low-frequency burst firing to single-spike firing. In the latter state, the frequency of single spikes depends on the degree of depolarization: that is, the intensity of synaptic excitatory inputs to the neuron from, for example, the premotor cortex and the thalamus.

Intracortical Signal Traffic and Information Processing

Afferent fibers that end in a small volume of the cortex make excitatory synapses with a large number of projection neurons and interneurons. Thus, one afferent fiber from the thalamus has been estimated to contact about 5000 cortical neurons. The synaptic contacts are established in certain layers only, but the excitation is propagated to other layers by the pyramidal cell recurrent collaterals and **excitatory interneurons** (spiny stellate cells). At the same time, activation of numerous **inhibitory interneurons** serves to focus the excitatory signals and to limit the activity of the projection neurons. In addition, the inhibitory interneurons inhibit other inhibitory interneurons, with resulting **disinhibition**. **Horizontal** axonal collaterals propagate both inhibition and excitation laterally from the focus of cortical excitation. This does not occur at random but so that functionally related neurons are interconnected. Finally, the integrated signals are issued—especially from layer 3 and 5 pyramids—to other parts of the cortex and subcortical cell groups (among them, the motoneurons).

As we see, the activity of each cortical neuron (i.e., its firing frequency and firing pattern) depends on the activity of the numerous other neurons with which it is synaptically connected. Such connections reach a cortical neuron from subcortical nuclei and other parts of the cortex and from cells in its immediate vicinity (within a radius of a few millimeters in the horizontal direction). One cortical neuron, such as a pyramidal cell of the MI, integrates information from perhaps 600 nearby cortical cells and has been estimated to receive about 60,000 synapses (monkey).

The enormous number of neurons and their complex interconnections within even a small volume of cortical tissue explain why we still do not understand the basic rules underlying intracortical information processing. Promising advances have been made, however, especially in the visual cortex (see under "Intracortical Signal Traffic in the Visual Cortex").

Intracortical Signal Traffic in the Visual Cortex

Regarding intracortical signal traffic, detailed studies have been performed in the visual cortex with the use of methods enabling the recording of single-cell activity in relation to specific stimuli and subsequent intracellular injection of horseradish peroxidase. Thus, the dendritic and axonal patterns of individual, functionally characterized neurons can be determined. Successful attempts have also been made to abolish the activity of neurons in specific layers and then study how the properties of neurons in other layers are changed. As expected from the known terminal pattern of axons from the lateral geniculate body, neurons are first activated in **layer 4** after visual stimuli (in addition, neurons in other layers with dendrites extending into layer 4 can be influenced). From layer 4, the excitation is propagated to **layers 2** and **3,** and from there to **layers 5** and **6**. Some cells in layer 6 send axons upward to layer 4. Presumably, at every step in such a pathway through the cortex some processing of the sensory information takes place, such as integration by one neuron of the signals from other functionally different neurons. In accordance with this assumption, the functional properties of neurons in different layers vary, as shown with microelectrode recordings after natural stimulation of receptors. A projection neuron in layer 5 has quite different properties than a cell in layer 4; for example, the receptive fields of the layer 5 cells are larger (as a sign of convergence of signals from several neurons in layer 4). Other properties of layer 5 neuron also suggest that signals from functionally different layer 4 neurons converge on layer 5 cells (via processing in layers 2 and 3).

Cortical Neurons Are Coincidence Detectors

Many cortical neurons react primarily when information about two events reaches them simultaneously, like cells in the visual cortex that respond poorly to signals from one eye only but vigorously to simultaneous signals from both eyes (binocular cells). Like a good detective who has a special eye for **coincidences** (events occurring simultaneously) and disregards numerous trivial bits of information, the cortical neurons respond preferentially to certain coincidences of stimuli that have a survival value. This is the basis for association learning; that is, learning the relationship between cause and effect. We know that a novel or unexpected stimulus, or one occurring in an unusual context, causes arousal and improved retention of new material. Often, synaptic changes occur when a neuron receive simultaneous a specific input about a stimulus or the context and a modulatory input (e.g., acetylcholine from the basal nucleus) signaling the salience of the specific input (see Fig. 4.10). This characteristic property of cortical cells is probably built into the inborn wiring pattern ("hardware") of the brain, but it also needs proper use to be further developed and maintained (see later, "The Parietal Lobe and the Development of the Ability to Integrate Somatosensory and Visual Information").

Glutamatergic **thalamocortical fibers** appear to act through **AMPA** receptors on cortical neurons but not through NMDA receptors (the latter being related to induction of long-term potentiation [LTP]). The recurrent pyramidal cell collaterals, however, act also on **NMDA** receptors. Some experimental evidence shows that simultaneous activation of a cortical neuron from the thalamus (AMPA) and from other cortical neurons (NMDA) can induce **LTP**. In the monkey motor cortex, LTP has been established during the learning of new motor skills. Thus, not only are the cortical neurons especially sensitive to coincident inputs, they may also be the cellular basis of associative learning in the cortex.

Horizontal Integration and Cortical Plasticity

The extensive horizontal intracortical connections appear to be crucial for the working of the cortex. They help explain why the response of so many cortical neurons depends on the **context** of a stimulus (cf. Chapter 16, under "Color Constancy"). As mentioned, horizontal connections ensure that the **receptive fields** of cortical neurons are not static but subject to modification by inputs from their neighbors. For example, single cells in the visual cortex have smaller receptive fields and react more strongly when the **attention** of the animal is directed to the visual stimulus. Horizontal connections most likely also contribute to well-known **psychophysical phenomena**, such as the filling in of missing lines in otherwise meaningful visual images. When blocking GABA receptors (and thus inhibitory horizontal connections) the receptive fields of cortical neurons enlarge immediately. After blocking GABA transmission, stimulation of a small peripheral spot activates an area in the SI that is much larger than before. After **amputation** of a finger in monkeys, the area in SI activated from the neighboring fingers enlarges immediately. These examples show that there must exist excitatory connections in the cortex that are **suppressed** under ordinary conditions. Further, due to such modifiable connections there is a **dynamic balance** between the cortical representations of various body parts.

Training of a sensory task can alter the cortical representation of the trained part (e.g., training roughness discrimination with the index finger). It seems likely that such examples of **cortical plasticity** are due, at least partly, to changes in the synaptic efficacy of horizontal connections. The same mechanism probably operates during **recovery** after brain damage that affected the cerebral cortex or its connections.

CONNECTIONS OF THE CEREBRAL CORTEX

The connections of the cerebral cortex with subcortical structures are described in several of the previous chapters, where we deal with the terminal regions of the major sensory pathways and the areas that give origin to the descending pathways involved in motor control. Here we describe general aspects of connections between the **thalamus** and the cerebral cortex and of the **cortico-cortical connections** (association and commissural connections). Such knowledge is a necessary basis for the following treatment of the cortical association areas and their functional roles.

A Brief Survey of Cortical Connections

We can classify the **afferent** connections of the cerebral cortex as follows:

1. Precise, topographically organized connections from the "specific" thalamic nuclei; each thalamic nucleus supplies one particular part of the cortex
2. Diffusely organized connections from the **intralaminar thalamic nuclei** and several other **subcortical nuclei** (the raphe nuclei, the nucleus coeruleus, dopaminergic cell groups in the mesencephalon, and cholinergic cell groups in the basal forebrain); such connections do not respect the cytoarchitectonic borders in contrast to the connections from the specific thalamic nuclei
3. **Association fibers**—that is, precisely organized connections linking cortical areas within the same hemisphere
4. **Commissural fibers**—that is, precisely organized connections between areas in the two hemispheres

The **efferent** connections of the cerebral cortex can also be divided into **subcortical** and **corticocortical** ones (association and commissural connections). The subcortical fibers are destined for the thalamus, the striatum, various brain stem nuclei (among them the pontine nuclei projecting to the cerebellum), and the spinal cord. The corticocortical connections are for the most part **reciprocal**—that is, an area receives fibers from the same areas to which it sends fibers.

Specific Thalamocortical Connections

The thalamus has been mentioned in several contexts (see Chapters 6 and 14 for descriptions of its gross anatomy and main subdivisions). The thalamus supplies all parts of the neocortex with afferents. Each part of the cortex receives fibers primarily from one of the **specific thalamic nuclei**. The main features of this topographic arrangement of the thalamocortical projection are shown in Fig. 33.8 (as we believe it is organized in humans). Figures 14.6 and 24.16 show the projections from the ventral thalamic nucleus in more detail, based on experimental studies in monkeys with various axonal tracing methods. Figure 16.20 shows the projection from the lateral geniculate nucleus to the visual cortex.

Conditions are more complex than shown in the diagrams, however. In the first place, the topographic arrangement is much more fine-grained. Thus, the projection from one thalamic nucleus is precisely arranged, with subdivisions of the nucleus supplying minor parts only of the large fields shown in Fig. 33.8. As described in Chapters 14 and 16, the thalamocortical

connections from the (VPL) and the lateral geniculate body are somatotopically and retinotopically organized, respectively, with a precision that enables the cortex to extract information about minute spatial details. Further, each thalamic nucleus sends fibers to more than one cortical area. We can take the **mediodorsal nucleus** (MD) as an example. In the scheme, it is depicted as sending fibers to the prefrontal cortex (without any topographic arrangement). In reality, the MD sends fibers to other parts of the cortex, too, such as parts of the cingulate gyrus. The MD furthermore consists of several subdivisions, each supplying a different part of the prefrontal cortex. The main point emerging from such knowledge is that the MD is not a functional unit. A small lesion, for example, must be expected to produce quite different effects, depending on its exact location within the MD.

Some of the specific thalamic nuclei are relay stations in the pathways for signals from **sensory receptors** to specific cortical areas (vision, hearing, cutaneous sensation, etc.). The **ventral posterolateral nucleus** (VPL) receives afferents from the somatosensory pathways and projects to SI (areas 3, 1, and 2; see Figs. 14.2,

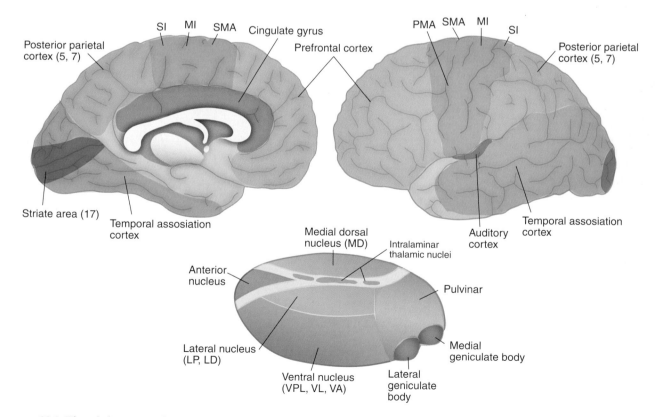

FIGURE 33.8 *The thalamocortical projection.* Highly simplified scheme showing the main features of its topographic organization. Overlap exists between the cortical terminal regions of different thalamic nuclei but is not shown in the figure.

14.4, and 14.6); the **lateral geniculate body** or nucleus receives afferents from the retina and projects to the striate area (see Figs. 16.14 and 16.20); the **medial geniculate body** is the last subcortical station in the auditory pathways and it sends efferents to AI (see Figs. 17.9 and 17.11). Other specific thalamic nuclei, the **ventrolateral nucleus** (VL) and the **ventral anterior nucleus** (VA), are relay stations in the pathways from the cerebellum and the basal ganglia to the motor and premotor cortical areas (see Fig. 24.16). Other thalamic nuclei relay signals from limbic structures: the **anterior thalamic nucleus** (A) receives afferents from the mammillary nucleus (which receives its main input from the hippocampal formation) and projects to the cingulate gyrus; and the **mediodorsal nucleus** (MD; Fig. 33.8) can relay signals from the amygdala to the frontal lobes. The posterior parietal cortex (areas 5 and 7) receives fibers from the posterior part of the thalamus, the **lateral posterior nucleus** (LP), and parts of the **pulvinar** (Fig. 33.8; see Figs. 6.21 and 6.22). Other parts of the pulvinar projects to the temporal lobe. The LP and the pulvinar receive afferents from nuclei related to vision and eye movements, such as the superior colliculus and the pretectal nuclei, and may relay such information to the posterior parietal cortex (see also Chapter 25, under "Cortical Control of Eye Movements"). However, the pulvinar is not primarily a relay nucleus but a link in a cortico–thalamic–cortical circuit, as we will return when discussing corticothalamic connections.

The Intralaminar Thalamic Nuclei

Modern tracer studies have shown that the cortical projections from each of the intralaminar nuclei end in certain parts of the cortex only; for example, the **contralateral nucleus** (CL) sends fibers predominantly to the parietal cortex. Nevertheless, the projections are considerably more widespread and diffuse than those from the specific thalamic nuclei and do not respect areal borders (the intralaminar nuclei were formerly termed the "unspecific thalamic nuclei"). Physiologic studies indicate that the intralaminar nuclei exert general effects on the **excitability** of cortical neurons. Thus, electrical stimulation produces a so-called **recruiting response** in extensive parts of the cortex, which resembles the **EEG** changes associated with **arousal** (desynchronization; see Chapter 26). The coactivation of cortical neurons by signals from the specific thalamic nuclei and the intralaminar nuclei may be important for the **binding** of specific stimuli with their salience—that is, a form of **coincidence detection** that perhaps may be necessary for awareness of the stimulus.

The tasks of the intralaminar nuclei are related not only to the cerebral cortex, because they have even stronger connections with the **striatum** (see Chapter 23,

under "Thalamostriatal Connections"). Such connections are precisely organized (another fact speaking against the use of the term "unspecific thalamic nuclei").

Extrathalamic, Modulatory Connections to the Cerebral Cortex

Apart from the major thalamocortical connections, several subcortical nuclei provide sparser cortical inputs without synaptic interruption in the thalamus (the raphe nuclei, the locus coeruleus, the mesencephalic ventral tegmental area [VTA], the basal nucleus, and the tuberomammillary nucleus in the hypothalamus). These nuclei supply most of the central nervous system with modulatory inputs and are in involved in a number of functions, as discussed in previous chapters. Briefly stated, the fibers from the aforementioned nuclei exert a modulatory control over the **excitability level** of cortical neurons, with relation to **wakefulness** and **phases of sleep**. In addition, they probably control more specifically selected cortical neuronal groups when our attention is focused on relevant, novel stimuli.

All of these transmitter-specific nuclei project to large parts of the cortex with no distinct topographic pattern. Nevertheless, recent studies in monkeys show that each nucleus (and thus fibers with a particular transmitter) projects with a higher density to some than to other parts of the cortex. For example, **dopaminergic fibers** from the VTA end with highest density in the prefrontal and temporal neocortex, whereas **noradrenergic** fibers from the locus coeruleus innervate especially the central region (MI, SI). Further, fibers from the various nuclei end in somewhat different cortical layers. A striking feature of the fibers is that, after having entered the cortex, they run **horizontally** for a considerable distance (in contrast to the vertical organization of the afferents from the specific thalamic nuclei). Further, their actions are partly mediated by **volume transmission**. (See Chapter 2, under "Modulatory Transmitter 'Systems'" and Chapter 16, under "Signal Pathways and Transmitters for the Activation of the Cerebral Cortex").

The Corticothalamic Connections

All of the thalamic nuclei receive massive **backprojections** from the cerebral cortex. In fact, the number of corticothalamic fibers is much higher than the number of thalamocortical ones; for example, the relationship for VPL has been estimated to 7:1. Yet, the corticothalamic connections have until recently received relatively little attention. The largest thalamic nuclei, with weak or no inputs from peripheral sense organs such, have reciprocal connections with association areas in the parietal, temporal, and frontal lobes

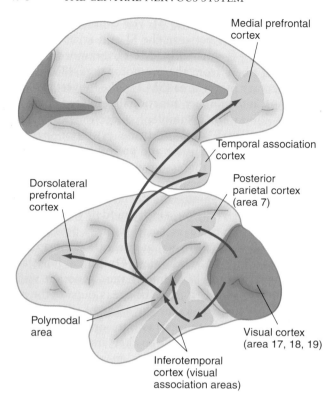

FIGURE 33.12 *Association connections of the visual cortex.* Compare with Figure 33.9 and note similarities with regard to the progression of information outward from the striate area. Only some connections are shown. (Based on Jones and Powell 1970.)

considerable **divergence** of information. At the same time, there is also considerable **convergence**, as each area receives afferents from several other areas (Figures 33.11 and 33.12 give very simplified accounts). Together, the many areas of the cortex are extensively interconnected, forming complex networks specialized for specific tasks. Complex functions—such as control of attention and speech—are carried out by many areas in conjunction with each other by way of their association connections. At the cellular level, the extensive association connections enable neurons to integrate many, different pieces of information and to act as coincidence detectors, as discussed in the preceding text.

Outward and Backward Corticocortical Connections

The discussion so far may give the impression that the flow of information between various cortical areas goes only in one direction, but this is not the case. Generally, the association connections are **reciprocal**, enabling areas to exert mutual influences. For example, there is not a one-way traffic outward from the striate area through successive stages of extrastriate areas, as at all levels areas send fibers back to each other and to the striate area. Differences exist, however, between the

connections going in opposite directions between two areas, notably with regard to laminar origin and destination. This has been most studied in visual cortical areas. Fibers going **outward**—also called **feedforward** connections—from the striate area to the extrastriate areas arise mainly in layer 3 and end primarily in layer 4. Fibers going **backward—feedback** connections—arise in deep layers (layer 6) and end mainly in the most superficial layers. The outward connections are precisely, topographically organized, whereas in general, the backward connections show a less fine-grained topography. Based on their anatomic characteristics, the outward connections from the sensory areas appear to be concerned with **segregation** and specific **convergence** of sensory information. For example, the striate area distributes different features of a visual image to extrastriate areas that are specialized for analysis of color, motion, form, and so forth. The backward connections are probably responsible for **context-dependent modifications** of sensory processing at the earlier stages—for example, the well-known effect of context on receptive fields of neurons in primary sensory areas. The backward connections may also provide a **prediction** of the sensory input expected to arise from a motor command, enabling the brain to compare the expected and actual results.

Commissural Connections of the Cerebral Cortex

Most commissural fibers pass in the **corpus callosum** (see Figs. 6.26 and 6.27). A small fraction courses in the **anterior commissure** (in humans, 1%–2%). The latter fibers are believed to belong primarily to the olfactory pathways. (In the monkey, the anterior commissure contains about 5% of all commissural fibers, mainly linking corresponding parts of the temporal lobes.)

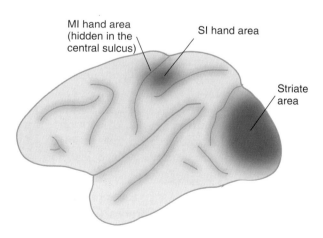

FIGURE 33.13 *Total distribution of commissural connections (monkey).* Almost all parts of the cerebral cortex send and receive commissural connections, except the representation of the central visual field in the striate area and the SI and MI hand regions (shown in red).

Generally, commissural fibers interconnect **corresponding areas** in the two hemispheres. The density of such fibers varies considerably among regions, however. Some regions are almost or totally devoid of commissural fibers (Fig. 33.13), especially the **striate area** and parts of the **MI** and **SI** that represent **distal parts of the extremities** (the regions representing the hands and feet). Thus, regions of the cortex dealing with parts of the body that usually work in a symmetrical fashion (such as the two halves of the back) are amply interconnected, whereas parts that usually work independently (such as the hands) have few commissural fibers. A corresponding organization is present in the somatosensory and the motor pathways; connections related to distal body parts are entirely crossed, whereas connections related to proximal parts are bilateral. It seems possible that commissural connections between, for example, the hand areas, would disturb the independent control of the hands (nevertheless, information about motor commands and sensory signals pertaining to the distal body parts of one side can reach the other hemisphere by other cortical areas and their commissural connections.

We return to the corpus callosum and the commissural connections in Chapter 34 when dealing with lateralization of functions—that is, tasks that are the division of tasks between the two hemispheres.

34 | Functions of the Neocortex

OVERVIEW

This chapter deals primarily with functional aspects of the cortical **association areas**, that is, parts of the cortex that neither receive direct sensory information through the major sensory pathways nor send direct fibers to subcortical motor nuclei. All of the cerebral lobes contain association areas, according to this definition. In Chapter 33, we discuss the connections of the association areas in general. Here we look at the main groups of association areas and their possible functions. It should be realized, however, that the functional roles of a group of association areas, for example, those of the frontal lobe, can be understood only if considered as part of distributed, task-specific networks involving other association areas and subcortical nuclei.

Typically, the association areas receive and **integrate** various kinds of information. Some are specialized for integration of two or more sensory modalities; others integrate highly processed sensory information with information about intentions and goals. The integrative capacity depends on proper use of sensory information, and must be learned in early childhood.

The **posterior parietal cortex** integrates visual and somatosensory information, and is responsible for, among other functions, the control of **visually guided behavior** and **spatial orientation**. From the parietal areas, signals pass to premotor and motor areas. The posterior parietal cortical areas also have reciprocal connections with the cingulate gyrus and the prefrontal cortex, mediating the influence of emotions, attention, and motivation on behavior produced by somatosensory and visual stimuli.

The **prefrontal cortex**, situated in front of the frontal lobe motor areas, receives information about all sensory modalities and also about the motivational and emotional state of the individual. It is of special importance for planning and initiation of **goal-directed behavior**. More specifically, the prefrontal cortex is important for attention, for selection of a specific behavior among several possible ones, and for suppression of unwanted behavior. These functions are of particular importance for social behavior.

The **temporal association areas** are particularly concerned with high-level processing of auditory and visual information. The cortex of the superior temporal gyrus is characterized by its connections with the auditory cortex, whereas the inferior part of the temporal lobe—the **inferotemporal cortex**—is dominated by processed visual information important for object recognition. The **medial parts** of the temporal lobe are of special importance for learning and declarative memory, as discussed in Chapter 32.

The **insula**, hidden in the lateral sulcus, receive all kinds of sensory information and is involved in pain perception, homeostasis, and bodily awareness.

Language and speech depends on a distributed network with two special hubs, one in the frontal lobe (**Broca's area**) and one at the temporoparietal junction (**Wernicke's area**). The anterior (frontal) area is particularly important for the expressive aspects of speech, while the posterior area is more concerned with the sensory aspects.

The left hemisphere is **dominant** for speech in 95% of the population. We also discuss further examples of hemispheric specialization (lateralization). The **corpus callosum** ensures that the two halves of the brain keep each other updated and cooperate to obtain common goals.

Finally, we discuss possible biologic bases of **cognitive sex differences**.

ASSOCIATION AREAS

For some of the cortical areas, functional aspects are discussed in previous chapters. Here we address primarily functions that can be ascribed to the so-called **association areas** of the cerebral cortex. This term is not precisely defined but is traditionally used for parts of the cortex that neither receive direct sensory information through the major sensory pathways nor send direct fibers to subcortical motor nuclei. All of the cerebral lobes contain association areas, according to this definition.

The connections of the association areas indicate that they are able to integrate information from sensory and "limbic" parts of the cortex (i.e., the cingulate gyrus, parts of the prefrontal cortex, and the hippocampal region) and thereafter issue commands to motor cortical areas and (indirectly) to the hypothalamus.

Comparison of the cerebral hemispheres of humans and monkeys shows that the association areas occupy a much larger fraction of the total in humans than in monkeys. Comparison of monkeys with other mammals, such as cats and dogs, shows again that the main difference between them with regard to the cerebral cortex is the relative size of the association areas. These parts of the cortex are of importance for what we may loosely call **higher mental functions**, as we discuss here. The association areas are not "centers" for specific mental faculties, however. First, several areas—often widely separated—participate in one task or function, and, further, one area participates in more than one function. This is witnessed by the high degree of divergence and convergence of the connections of the association areas, as discussed in the preceding text. Second, the operations of the association areas cannot be understood if considered in isolation; the intimate connections between the association areas and subcortical cell groups, such as the thalamus, the basal ganglia, the amygdala, and the hippocampus, are essential for their normal functioning.

Measurements of **regional cerebral blood flow** and metabolism during the performance of various **cognitive tasks** indicate that large parts of the cortex participate in all higher mental functions. When a person is asked to **imagine** that she is walking from one place to another in a city she knows, the activity increases in the extrastriate visual areas, in the posterior parietal cortex, in parts of the temporal lobe, and in several prefrontal areas. Solving a **mathematical** problem activates many of the same cortical areas but with certain differences, and a **verbal** task activates multiple areas that partly coincide with and partly differ from those activated in the spatial and the mathematical tasks.

In Chapter 16, we discussed the cortical substrate of visual imagery (under "Consciousness and Visual Experience").

Cognition and Cognitive Functions

The word **cognition** stems from the Latin word *cognitio*, meaning "acknowledge, come to know." According to the *Encyclopedia Britannica*, cognition "includes every mental process that can be described as an experience of knowing as distinguished from an experience of feeling or of willing. It includes, in short, all processes of consciousness by which knowledge is built up, including perceiving, recognizing, conceiving, and reasoning." Among neuroscientists today, the word is often used more broadly to include the **affective** aspects of higher mental functions. For example, the scholarly book *The New Cognitive Neurosciences* (2000) edited by Michael Gazzaniga deals not only with consciousness, language, memory, attention, and similar phenomena but also with emotions. This presumably reflects the realization that there is no sharp distinction between brain structures that govern rational thought and actions on the one hand and those that underlie emotions and subconscious drives on the other.

Integration of Different Sensory Modalities Depends on Learning

The ability to integrate somatosensory and visual information and to use visual information to guide voluntary movements is not inborn but learned in infancy and early childhood. Persons who were born blind but gained their vision back as young adults do not manage to coordinate the visual information with the other senses and therefore cannot use the "new" sense. They usually continue to use tactile sensation to "see" objects, and, in fact, the visual information can be more confusing than helpful (this is described by Oliver Sacks in *An Anthropologist on Mars* 1995).

Studies by Hyvärinen (1982) and coworkers exemplify how meaningful use of the systems is necessary for sensory integration to take place during early development. He studied how the properties of single cells in the parietal cortex change during the phase in which an infant monkey learns to combine **visual** and **somatosensory information**. Monkeys were prevented from seeing from birth (by suturing the eyelids) until they were between 6 months and 1 year old. At that time, few cells in area 7 responded to visual stimuli, in contrast to the normal situation at that age. An abnormally large fraction of the cells were activated by passive somatosensory stimuli and by active movements. Most striking was the almost total absence of cells that could be activated by both somatosensory and visual stimuli. Even 2 years after reestablishment of normal vision, the single-cell properties of area 7 remained virtually unaltered, with very few cells responding to visual stimuli. Properties of cells of the extrastriate cortex (area 19) were also altered in the visually deprived monkeys; for example, some cells were activated by somatosensory stimuli (which never occurred in normal monkeys), and there were fewer than normal visually driven cells. Behaviorally, the monkeys were blind after opening of the eyes, and no improvement occurred during the next month. They bumped into obstacles, fell off tables, and were unable to retrieve food by sight alone. Threatening faces did not frighten them, in contrast to normal monkeys at the same age. One monkey that was observed for 3 years improved to some extent, but it never regained the full use of vision. Brain-imaging studies of **humans born blind or deaf** also indicate that considerable reorganization takes place, as compared with normal persons. For example, in persons who have been blind since birth, the visual cortex is activated by somatosensory stimuli during Braille reading.

In conclusion, the data indicate that the functional properties of neurons in the association areas, and thus the capacity of the areas to contribute to certain tasks, are determined to a large extent in early childhood. Further, there is only a limited possibility of regaining the proper function of these regions at a later stage (see Chapter 9, under "Sensitive (Critical) Periods"). The experiments also show that when one kind of sensory information is lacking during an early stage of development, other sensory modalities take over parts of the cortex not normally used for processing that kind of sensory information. This has been shown also after early lesions of the auditory system.

Lesions of the Association Areas: Agnosia and Apraxia

Lesions of association areas typically disturb higher-level aspects of sensory and motor functions. **Agnosia** is usually defined as the lack of ability to recognize objects (when not due to reduced sensation or dementia). **Apraxia** is used similarly about the loss of the ability to do certain, formerly well-known skilled actions (such as dressing, using household tools, copy a drawing, etc.). There is no clear-cut distinction between these two categories of symptoms, however. Loss of the ability to copy a drawing—called **constructional apraxia**—for example, may be due to the patient not being able to perceive more than a small piece of the drawing at a time. Thus, she is not able mentally to put several pieces together.

Agnosia or apraxia seldom occurs as the only symptom, however, and even less frequent are cases with isolated subcategories. Such cases are nevertheless of great theoretical interest because they shed light on how the brain works to solve specific tasks. Depending on their site and size, cortical lesions can produce a wide specter of difficulties with perception. This concerns not only objects (strictly defined), but also all aspects of higher processing of sensory information. The word "agnosia" is therefore used more widely than the definition may suggest. For example, we use the term **visual agnosia** for loss of the ability to recognize objects and persons by sight, whereas **tactile agnosia** means loss of the ability to recognize objects by touch.

Visual agnosia is the most common kind and has been studied the most. It may appear in several varieties, each with a specific name. For example, **prosopagnosia** means inability to recognize familiar faces; **autotopagnosia** is inability to recognize one's own body parts; **simultanagnosia** is the inability to perceive more than one object at a time, and so forth. Inability to recognize letters, **alexia**, is regarded by some as a special kind of agnosia. To some extent, the different kinds of agnosia can be attributed to lesions of specific parts of the cortex. For example, several kinds of visual agnosia are associated with lesions of specific parts of extrastriate areas (see Chapter 16, under "Further Processing of Sensory Information outside the Striate Area"). **Tactile agnosia** has been described after lesions at the parieto-temporal junction (see Chapter 14, under "Lesions of the Somatosensory Areas"). Disturbances of the **body image** and **self-awareness** are typical of lesions in the posterior parietal cortex (see later).

There are numerous forms of apraxia (about 30 are listed by Petreska and coworkers in a comprehensive review). For example, **ideational apraxia** is used when it is not the execution of movements that is impaired (e.g., the use of a toothbrush) but the objects are used inappropriately (e.g., to eat with the toothbrush). **Ideomotor apraxia** is characterized by impaired execution of a movement rather than the conceptualization of its purpose. Basically, apraxia seems to ". . . result from a specific alteration in the ability to mentally evoke actions, or to use stored motor representations for forming mental images of actions" (Petreska et al. 2007, p. 64). Although apraxia is most frequently observed after parietal or frontal lesions, lesions in other parts of the cortex and even subcortical ones may produce apraxia too.

If in the term "agnosia" we include the inability to recognize **complex sounds** (like music, spoken words, and laughter), the distinction with speech disturbances after brain damage (aphasia) becomes blurred. Further, there are elements of apraxia in aphasia when it includes (as often happens) the inability to write (**agraphia**). Patients with lesions of the association areas often have symptoms belonging to several categories mentioned above—that is, elements of aphasia, agnosia, and apraxia. This can only partly be explained by the fact that many lesions are large and affect several specialized regions. It also reflects that, although they are anatomically separated, association areas are extensively interconnected and their normal functioning requires that they cooperate.

Parietal Association Areas

Usually **areas 5 and 7**—located in the upper and lower parietal lobules, respectively—are considered to constitute the parietal association cortex (Fig. 34.1; see Fig. 33.4). The term **posterior parietal cortex** is also used of this region. Both areas 5 and 7 can be further subdivided into parts differing in connections and functional properties.[1] These areas are intercalated between the visual cortical areas in the occipital lobe and the somatosensory cortex in the anterior parietal cortex. Functionally, as one might expect from this location, areas 5 and 7 process and integrate somatosensory and visual information. From these areas, signals are conveyed to premotor and motor areas (Fig. 34.1), explaining why a parietofrontal network is activated during

---

1 There is some disagreement in the literature with regard to the parcellation of the posterior parietal cortex in humans. Brodmann (Fig. 33.3) placed areas 5 and 7 in the superior parietal lobule, whereas the inferior lobule contained areas 39 and 40. Others, however, describe area 5 as located in the superior parietal lobule and area 7 in the inferior—that is, corresponding to the situation in monkeys.

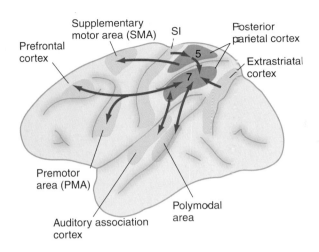

FIGURE 34.1 *Association connections of the posterior parietal cortex (monkey)*. Connections with the limbic cortical areas are not shown (see Fig. 33.11). Visual and somatosensory information converge in area 7. Connections are reciprocal.

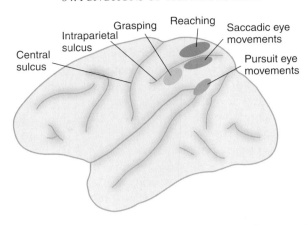

FIGURE 34.2 *Subregions within the posterior parietal cortex with relation to planning of specific kinds of movement.* (Based on Andersen and Buneo 2002.)

most voluntary movements. The posterior parietal cortical areas also have ample connections (both ways) with the **cingulate gyrus** and the **prefrontal cortex**. These connections are assumed to mediate the influence of emotions, attention, and motivation on behavior produced by somatosensory and visual stimuli.

Experiments with recording of **single-cell** activity in **area 5** of the monkey indicate that this area is essential for the proper use of somatosensory information, for goal-directed voluntary movements, and for the manipulation of objects. This fits well with the symptoms that arise in humans after damage to the posterior parietal cortex, as discussed next. Single-cell recordings indicate that **area 7** has an important role in the integration of visual and somatosensory stimuli, which is essential for the coordination of the eye and the hand—that is, for visual guidance of movements. Area 7 is also involved in the control of **eye movements**. Studies in monkeys suggest that certain subregions of the posterior parietal cortex are specialized for reaching movements, grasp, saccades, and smooth-pursuit eye movements (Fig. 34.2). It further appears that activity in these subregions is closely linked with the **intention** to move[2]—that is, the posterior parietal cortex contains a "map of intentions."

Lesions of the posterior parietal cortex in humans can cause different symptoms, depending on which

parts are most affected. Some of the symptoms can be summarized as difficulties with the transformation of sensory stimuli into adequate motor actions. This can probably be explained by lack of parietal influence on the premotor areas. The understanding of the meaning of sensory stimuli is seriously impaired (but usually not the mere recognition of a stimulus). This **agnosia** concerns especially the recognition of the form and spatial position of objects. A typical symptom after right-sided lesions is a tendency to **neglect** the opposite side of the body and the visual stimuli from the opposite side. Patients may suffer from **apraxia**—that is, they are unable to use well-known tools and objects. They may further have problems with **visually guided movements** (such as stretching out the arm to obtain an object).

Even though the symptoms mentioned here are most often seen after damage of the posterior parietal cortex, most of them have been described after lesions in other parts of the brain, too, especially of the prefrontal cortex, the thalamus, and the basal ganglia, all of which have connections with the parietal cortex. These structures take part in a **distributed network** responsible for, among other functions, the control of visually guided behavior and spatial orientation.

Properties of Single Neurons in the Posterior Parietal Cortex

Studies of monkeys with permanently implanted electrodes have demonstrated a wide repertoire of properties among neurons in areas 5 and 7. In general, a task-related increase in firing frequency occurs only when a stimulus is relevant and the **attention** of the animal is directed toward the stimulus. Thus, many neurons are virtually impossible to activate when the

---

2 Stimulation of parietal and premotor cortical areas in awake patients undergoing surgery corroborates the importance of the parietal cortex for movement intention and awareness of own movements. Stimulation of the Brodmann's areas 7, 39, and 40 (Fig. 34.4) provoked an intention to move, and with increasing stimulus strength, the patients reported that they had actually performed the movements (although no movement occurred). Stimulation of the premotor cortex, on the other hand, produced overt movements but the patients were not aware of them. Thus, "Conscious intention and motor awareness... arise from increased parietal activity before movement execution." (Desmurget et al. 2009).

animal is drowsy and inattentive. Some cells respond to stimulation of proprioceptors, but their response is much more vigorous when a movement (stimulating the proprioceptors) is **self-initiated** by the monkey than when the joint is passively manipulated by the examiner. In area 5, many neurons change their firing frequency in relation to manipulatory hand movements. Other neurons increase their firing in relation to reaching movements, but only when the hand is moved toward an object the monkey wants to obtain (such as an orange). The increase of firing in such neurons starts at the time the animal discovers the object—that is, before the arm movement starts—and is therefore not a result of proprioceptive stimulation. The American neurophysiologist Vernon B. Mountcastle, who first described such neurons, suggested that they might function as **command neurons** for the target-directed **exploration** of our immediate surrounding extrapersonal space. Such neurons appear to respond to the **coincidence** of two events: a sensory stimulus (e.g., the sight of an orange) and a signal that depends on motivation (whether the monkey is hungry and wants the orange; see Fig. 4.10).

More about Symptoms after Lesions of the Posterior Parietal Cortex

The most marked symptom produced by bilateral parietal lesions is the inability to **grasp** and to **manipulate** objects. Thus, the patient may be unable to move the hand toward an object that is clearly seen, even though there are no pareses and no visual defects. Movements that do not require visual guidance—such as buttoning, bringing an object to the mouth, and so forth—are performed normally. When the patient is asked to pour water from a bottle into a glass, he pours the water outside the glass over and over again, even though he can see clearly both the bottle and the glass. Such patients also have severe difficulties with the **appraisal** of **distances** and the **size** of objects. Further, to **fix the gaze** becomes difficult, especially to direct the gaze toward a point in the periphery of the visual field. The **identification of objects** is difficult, because of the inability to attend to more than one detail at a time (such as seeing a cigarette but not the person who smokes it). This may be a fundamental defect after parietal lobe lesions, perhaps also explaining the difficulties mentioned earlier with pouring water into a glass (the patient is unable to locate in space the bottle and the glass at the same time).

Patients with parietal lobe lesions typically have difficulties with **drawing** an object or a scene; again the inability to perceive more than one feature at a time is the probable basic defect. The parts of an object are drawn separately, without the proper spatial relations, or the drawing gives an extremely simplified representation.

This symptom occurs most often after damage to the right parietal cortex, in cases of unilateral lesions. The **use of tools** is also difficult or impossible: for example, the patient no longer knows how to use a hammer (**apraxia**).

Unilateral lesions of the right parietal lobe typically produce negligence—**neglect**—of the opposite body half and visual space. Such a patient behaves as if the left part of his body does not exist. He dresses only the right side, shaves only the right half of the face, and so forth. He may deny that the left leg belongs to him and claim that it belongs to the person in the adjacent bed, for example. A similar symptom is denial of the disease and the functional loss, called **anosognosia**. The patient may deny that the limb is paralytic or that he is blind. Thus, certain aspects of body knowledge no longer exist in the mind of the patient, but the loss is not consciously perceived. When drawing a face, for example, the right side is drawn normally, whereas the left side is vague or not included in the drawing.

A peculiar constellation of symptoms, the **Gerstmann syndrome**, can occur after lesions of the parietal lobe at the transition to the temporal lobe (usually of the left hemisphere). The symptoms are as follows: **finger agnosia** (the patient cannot recognize and distinguish the various fingers on her own or other people's hands), **agraphia** (inability to write), sometimes **alexia** (inability to read), **right–left confusion**, and, finally, **dyscalculia** (reduced ability to perform simple calculations, especially to distinguish categories of numbers such as tens, hundreds, and so forth). The most distinctive feature of the syndrome is the finger agnosia, which can occur in isolation. That finger agnosia can be the only symptom of a parietal lobe lesion indicates that a disproportionally large part of the human parietal cortex is devoted to the hand. Thus, the hand has a unique role as an exploratory sense organ and as a tool, and, further, it has a special place in our inner, mental, body image. The British neurologist M. Critchley (1953, p. 210) expressed it as follows: "The hand is largely the organ of the parietal lobe."

Frontal Association Areas

In this context we use the term "association cortex" only about the **prefrontal cortex**—that is, the parts of the frontal lobe in front of areas 6 (premotor area [PMA], supplementary motor area [SMA]) and 8 (the frontal eye field) (Fig. 34.3; see Fig. 33.4). The prefrontal cortex consists of several cytoarchitectonic areas, each with a specific set of connections. Together, the prefrontal areas receive strong **afferent** connections from areas in the occipital, parietal, and temporal lobes and, in addition, from the cingulate gyrus (Fig. 34.3). Thalamic afferents come from the **mediodorsal nucleus**, MD (see Fig. 33.8), which, in turn, receives afferents

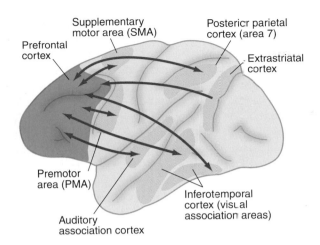

FIGURE 34.3 *Association connections of the prefrontal cortex (monkey).* Note the convergence of all kinds of processed sensory information and the connections with PMA and SMA. Connections with limbic cortical areas are not shown.

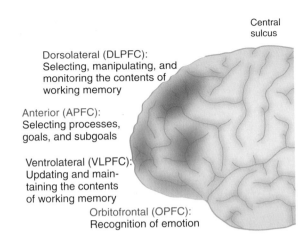

FIGURE 34.4 *Some functional specializations within the prefrontal cortex.* Regions that appear to be related to different aspects of memory, as judged from functional neuroimaging studies (PET and fMRI). The orbitofrontal cortex is activated in association with explicit identification of emotional facial expressions. (Based on Fletcher and Henson 2001, and Adolphs 2002.)

from the **amygdala** and the **ventral pallidum** (among other places). In sum, the prefrontal cortex appears to receive information about all sensory modalities and also about the motivational and emotional state of the individual.

The prefrontal cortex sends **efferents** back to most of the areas from which it receives afferents, among them the SMA and the PMA. In addition, many prefrontal efferents reach the caudate nucleus of the **striatum** (see Fig. 13.6). Finally, some efferents reach the **amygdala** and the **hypothalamus**.

Animal experiments, observations in brain-damaged humans, and brain imaging in normal persons all give a fairly consistent picture of the major tasks of the prefrontal cortex. Figure 34.4 shows some tasks associated with particular prefrontal subdivisions. The prefrontal cortex is obviously of crucial importance for **planning** and **initiation** of **goal-directed behavior**. More specifically, the prefrontal cortex is important for **attention**, for **selection** of a specific behavior among several possible, and for **suppression** of unwanted behavior. With regard to selection, the prefrontal cortex cooperates with the basal ganglia, as discussed in Chapter 23, under "Functions of the Basal Ganglia." Further, the prefrontal cortex is important for certain aspects of **memory**— both for working memory and for the long-term establishment of memory traces. Working memory enables us to retain a stimulus long enough for its evaluation and linking with ongoing processes and memory. We discussed in Chapter 32 that medial parts of the temporal lobe, including the hippocampus, are necessary for declarative memory. Functional magnetic resonance imaging (fMRI) studies indicate, however, that we remember words or pictures only if their presentation also activates the

prefrontal cortex. Probably, the prefrontal cortex tells the hippocampal region about the emotional coloring and the context of information that is transmitted to the hippocampus from sensory areas.

Learning of rules by association appears to be a central task of the prefrontal cortex. This may be performed by neurons that associate behaviorally relevant but otherwise dissimilar bits of information—such as that a red traffic light means stop. Appropriate behavior requires that we are able to learn such rules, but equally important is that we can replace them quickly with new ones. Both faculties suffer after damage to the prefrontal cortex.

In conclusion, the prefrontal cortex is of crucial importance for our ability to organize our own lives and to function socially. Indeed, the tasks mentioned previously, such as planning and choice of behavior, choosing between signals with different emotional coloring, suppression of unwanted behavior, and so forth, are indispensable for **social adaptation**. Another important factor in social functioning is **empathy**,[3] which also seems to depend on the integrity of the prefrontal cortex. However, the prefrontal cortex is not the only part of the cortex showing empathy-related activity. It appears that empathy activates the same network that is activated by the person experiencing the painful or

3 **Empathy** is used with somewhat different meanings. Hein and Singer (2008) refer to empathy as "...an affective state, caused by sharing the emotions and sensory states of another person." They distinguish empathy from **sympathy**, which they describe as emphatic concern or compassion. By emphasizing that empathy is an affective state, they also distinguish it from the understanding of other persons beliefs, intentions, and desires, which derives from reasoning (i.e., cognitively). Indeed, understanding another person's intentions is not the same as sharing them.

distressing situation. The exact distribution of activity would therefore vary with the specifics of the emotion experienced by the suffering person.

Symptoms after Prefrontal Lesions

The prefrontal cortex consists of several subregions, which differ with regard to their connections and functional properties. The symptoms of lesions that occur in this area in humans are correspondingly varied, and, further, the individual differences are fairly large even after seemingly identically placed lesions. In general, the symptoms are compatible with the functions discussed earlier.

Prefrontal lesions typically produce changes of **mood** and **personality**, distinguishing them from lesions of other parts of the cortex. Commonly, large lesions produce apathy, indifference, and emotional leveling-off. The patient appears to be uncritical compared with before the damage. For example, he may behave in a complacent and boastful manner, which he would never have done before. The ability to **alter** the **behavior** on the basis of experience from previous actions appears to be reduced. Clear-cut symptoms occur usually only after bilateral damage to the prefrontal cortex. Occasionally, however, the first signs of a **frontal-lobe tumor** are changes of behavior and personality.

More about Symptoms after Lesions of the Prefrontal Cortex

A striking defect after bilateral lesions of the **dorsolateral prefrontal cortex (DLPFC)** is the lack of the so-called **delayed response**. A monkey sees that food is put into one of two bowls. Then the sight of the bowls is blocked for up to 10 min before the monkey is allowed to choose one of the two. In contrast to normal monkeys, the lesioned ones do not remember which bowl contained the food (even though they do not show reduced performance in other more complicated memory tests). The dorsolateral parts of the prefrontal cortex thus appear to be necessary for the ability to form and retain an inner conception of the existence of an object in time and space when the object is no longer seen. Interestingly, humans manage a similar test first at the age of about 1 year. Before that age, everything that is not seen or felt is presumably nonexistent for the infant.

A characteristic symptom in humans with prefrontal lesions is the inability to **alter the response** when the stimulus changes; they continue to make the same response even though it is no longer adequate. This phenomenon is called **perseveration**. The **Wisconsin card sort test** is often used to reveal such a defect. The person is asked to sort cards in accordance with certain general rules, such as color, number, shape, and so forth. The correct rule to be applied is indicated by the response given by the examiner to the first attempts at sorting the cards. The rules can be changed without warning. Normal persons understand fairly quickly that the rule has been changed and alter their responses accordingly, whereas patients with prefrontal lesions continue sorting in accordance with the first rule, in spite of repeated warnings that they are making mistakes.

Emotional and **personality** changes after frontal lobe lesions are most common when the lesion includes the **orbitofrontal parts**. Such symptoms are difficult to evaluate, and the premorbid personality of the patients appears to play a decisive role. Nevertheless, a general tendency is to become less emotional and to show reduced emotional reactions to events. They also have difficulties in extracting the salient features from a complex situation, making their responses unpredictable and often inappropriate. A test designed for such symptoms uses drawings of complex situations, in part with a dramatic content, such as a man who has fallen through the ice on a lake and is in danger of drowning. Patients with frontal lesions usually attend only to details, saying, for example, "Since there is a sign saying 'Careful!' on the beach, there may be a high-voltage cable nearby." This kind of reduction results in inability to foresee the consequences of one's own actions and poor insight into other people's circumstances. This leads to poor **social adaptation**, with isolation as the final result.

The reduced capacity to retain inner conceptions is most likely the reason such patients have increased **distractibility**, with reduced ability to perform tasks that require continuous activity and attention. Motor hyperactivity, which can be a symptom, may perhaps result from the increased distractibility. Thus, in monkeys with prefrontal lesions, the hyperactivity disappears when they are placed in an environment with few stimuli.

In humans with frontal lobe tumors (e.g., a glioma or a metastasis from a malignant tumor elsewhere), a **depressive disorder** has been observed, but this may rather be a condition of de-emotionalization and social isolation.

The Temporal Association Cortex

A unitary functional role is even less evident for the temporal association areas than for those in the parietal and frontal lobes. Apart from the auditory cortex (areas 41 and 42) (see Fig. 17.11) and the phylogenetically old parts at the medial aspect (Fig. 31.1), the temporal lobe consists largely of Brodmann's areas 20, 21, and 22, which here are considered the association areas (Fig. 34.4).

The cortex of the **superior temporal gyrus** is characterized by its connections with the auditory cortex, whereas the inferior part of the temporal lobe—the **inferotemporal cortex**—is dominated by processed visual information from the extrastriate visual areas. In addition, there are strong connections with the **hippocampal formation** (through the entorhinal area) and the **amygdala**. Electrical **stimulation** of the temporal association cortex in humans evokes recall of memories of past events or the experience of dreamlike sequences of imagined events (such observations were first made by the Canadian neurosurgeon Wilder Penfield, who stimulated the temporal lobe and other parts of the cortex in patients in whom the cortex was exposed under local anesthesia for therapeutic reasons). Finally, long association fibers interconnect the temporal association areas with the prefrontal cortex (Fig. 34.3).

The **inferotemporal cortex** is important especially for the interpretation of **complex visual stimuli**, as judged from experiments in monkeys. Thus bilateral removal of these regions makes the monkeys unable to recognize and distinguish complex visual patterns.

These and other observations led to the conclusion that the inferotemporal cortex is of special importance for the **categorization** of visual stimuli. In monkeys, some neurons of the inferotemporal cortex respond only when the monkey sees, for example, a **face** or a **hand**. Some neurons respond preferentially to one particular face, whereas other neurons respond to any face. A neuron that responds briskly when the monkey is shown a drawing of a face may stop firing when important features are removed, such as the mouth or the eyes. Whether monkeys and humans—highly dependent on the ability to recognize faces and interpret facial expressions—have developed a separate system for face recognition is not settled. Selective loss of face recognition—**prosopagnosia**—sometimes occurs after lesions of the temporal lobe and would seem to suggest the existence of a separate "face" system. Further, fMRI studies show that activation in the **fusiform gyrus** in the inferotemporal cortex is associated with face recognition in humans (see Fig. 16.26). Other data, however, are more compatible with a general network for object identification that is used also for face recognition. Thus, objects other than faces can activate the fusiform gyrus, and, conversely, face recognition is associated with activation of several sites outside the fusiform gyrus. Because facial recognition is so important for social interactions and is used intensively from birth, presumably a larger proportion of neurons in temporal association areas become specialized for faces than for identification of other objects.

The **medial temporal lobe** and its importance for learning and declarative memory are discussed in Chapter 32. In addition, **lateral parts** of the temporal lobe is necessary for **semantic** memory—that is, knowledge about facts, meaning of words, objects, and so forth, which was acquired some time ago.

Symptoms after Lesions of the Temporal Cortex

Bilateral damage of the temporal lobes produces a syndrome dominated by pronounced **amnesia**.[4] The amnesia can be ascribed largely to the destruction of the hippocampal formation and neighboring areas in the parahippocampal gyrus. In addition, certain emotional changes are presumably caused by the concomitant destruction of the amygdala located in the tip of the temporal lobe. These aspects are discussed in Chapter 31. In addition, the patients become very **distractible**: they have difficulty maintaining their attention on a certain stimulus or task. Finally, psychic blindness or **visual agnosia** is a typical symptom of temporal lobe lesions that affect the **inferotemporal parts**. The patient is unable to recognize objects and persons she sees, even though her vision is normal. As for other association areas, it is the interpretation of sensory information that is deficient, not the sensory experience as such. Information about size and shape of objects may nevertheless be available to the posterior parietal cortex to be used in movement control, as discussed in Chapter 16, under "Consciousness and Visual Experience."

The Insula

The insula, sometimes called the fifth cerebral lobe, is mentioned in several chapters. This is because the insula, as evident from positron emission tomography (PET) and fMRI studies, participates in a wide range of cortical networks. Thus, activity changes in the insula occur in relation to somatic and visceral sensory processes, emotional regulation, and aspects of bodily awareness. This part of the neocortex is hidden at the bottom of the lateral fissure (see Figs. 6.29, 6.30, 14.9, and 31.9), and consists of several cytoarchitectonic subdivisions. Anatomically, the insula is characterized by receiving all kinds of sensory information and by its extensive corticocortical connections with major parts of the cortex. Further, there are ample connections among the subdivisions of the insula. It resides at the junction of the frontal, parietal and temporal lobes and has reciprocal connections with all three. This concerns, for example, the orbitofrontal cortex, the cingulate gyrus, the parahippocampal gyrus, the temporal pole, the superior temporal sulcus, premotor areas, SII, and the posterior parietal cortex—that is, regions involved in a wide specter of behaviors and mental processes.

4 The constellation of symptoms that occur after bilateral destruction of the temporal lobes is named after the two American neurosurgeons Klüver and Bucy (1937) who first described it in monkeys. Besides amnesia, the animals lack emotional responses and aggressive behavior (increased tameness), and they withdraw from social contact. Furthermore, the syndrome includes visual agnosia, a tendency to examine all objects by mouth, a tendency to pay attention to all visual stimuli, an irresistible urge to touch everything, and hypersexuality.

The insula receives afferents from several thalamic nuclei (Ventral anterior, Ventral posteromedial, Centromedian, VPM, CM, and some other nuclei). The insula also has reciprocal connections with the amygdala.

We discuss the insula in Chapter 14 because it is among the cortical regions activated by noxious stimuli and is an essential part of the network responsible for the experience of **pain**. Further, the anterior insula is activated in conjunction with strong **emotions** (especially disgust) and is presumably a part of a network for regulation of affect.

The insula receives not only sensory signals from somatic structures, but is consistently activated both by nonpainful and painful enteroceptive stimuli. For example, nonpainful distension of hollow organs such as the stomach and the esophagus activated the insula associated with the subjective feeling of fullness. Further, the awareness of one's own heartbeats is associated with activation of the insula. Indeed, the insula may thus play a particular role in our **awareness** of the state of our internal organs. However, its role does not seem to be limited to monitoring the internal organs and evoking subjective feelings referred to them. Thus, the awareness of voluntary movements, and especially the feeling of **body ownership**, involves a network that probably includes the insula (see Chapter 18). The contribution of the insula in this respect presumably depends on its integration of **proprioceptive, vestibular,** and **motor signals**.

Finally, the anterior part of the insula receives **olfactory** and **gustatory** signals and presumably contributes to the integration of these modalities, and their further integration with other enteroceptive signals.

Task-Specific Networks Integrate and Analyze Information

The brain receives innumerable pieces of information, which, to a large extent are treated in separate systems. For example, separate neuronal populations encode different features of objects, such as color, form, movement, surface texture, heaviness, and so forth. With regard to representation of space, the brain appears to possess several "maps." Yet, we experience ourselves and our surroundings as entities, not as isolated fragments. How can this paradox be explained? This **binding problem**—that is, how various bits of information represented in different parts of the cortex are integrated in the brain—is closely linked with the problem of consciousness (see also Chapter 16, under "Consciousness and Visual Experience," and Chapter 26, under "Neurobiological Basis of Consciousness"). The brain must possess the ability to integrate, almost instantaneously, the activity in numerous specialized neuronal groups, each representing different features of, for example, a visual scene. To be useful, the integrated

"picture" must furthermore be put into a meaningful context to form the basis for appropriate actions.[5] Imagine, for example, the continuous stream of changing information that must be evaluated and acted upon when driving a car in heavy traffic. No area appears to receive all necessary information. Rather, it seems likely that neuronal groups in many parts of the cerebral cortex are interconnected in task-specific networks. The vast number of association fibers must obviously be essential in this respect. There is now much evidence that **synchronization** of activity in large-scale networks may be the substrate for the binding together of related pieces of information—and thus for our conscious experience of our environment and ourselves. It should be emphasized that while the anatomic connectivity forms the "hardwiring" of the networks, their functioning depends on dynamic, moment-to-moment fluctuations in synchronized activity. Presumably, engagement of specific networks shifts in the time scale of milliseconds. For example, we know from everyday experience how our attention shifts instantaneously. Another example concerns viewing of ambiguous pictures; the experience (e.g., duck or rabbit) changes with no time delay in spite of unchanged sensory input.

The "Default-Mode Network"

Among the cortical networks so far identified, the so-called **default-mode network** seems to have a special position. It is characterized by consistently *decreased* activity during goal-directed tasks, while it is active when the person's attention is not directed to any specific task. The network comprises lateral parts of the parietal cortex and regions on the medial aspect of the hemisphere (posterior cingulate gyrus and adjoining posterior regions, and parts of the medial prefrontal cortex). The activity of the default-mode network is thought to be related to **introspection**. In support of this assumption, an fMRI study showed increased activity in the default-mode network when the subject contemplated a moral dilemma (requiring minimal cognitive engagement) whereas a color-word interference task produced deactivation (Harrison et al. 2008). Nevertheless, the moral dilemma situation produced a pattern of activity within the network that differed from the activity in an eyes-closed resting state.

Disturbances of the default-mode network-activity have been found in fMRI studies of several groups of patients (e.g., chronic pain, attention-deficit/hyperactivity disorder [ADHD], and mental diseases).

---

5 It takes several hundred milliseconds from the arrival of sensory signals at the cortical level to perception, as first shown by Libet (1991) with stimulation experiments in humans. This might perhaps reflect that in this situation it takes some time to bring the necessary networks in a state of synchronized activity.

For example, chronic pain patients show less than normal deactivation related to task performance.

The Cerebral Cortex and Mental Disease

It is to be expected that diseases affecting complex functions such as emotions, personality, sense of reality, and thought would involve alterations in many parts of the brain, as well as in many neurotransmitters. Indeed, attempts to explain mental illnesses by malfunction in a single brain "center" or of one transmitter have not been successful.

Evidence of changed structure, metabolism, or neurotransmitters has been found most consistently in **the prefrontal cortex** and several **limbic structures** in patients with mental disorders. However, altered neuronal activity in the prefrontal cortex (or any other structure) does not tell us that the primary pathology is there. Thus, the alterations in one area may be secondary to changed activity in other areas with which it is connected. Considering the many connections between the prefrontal cortex and the amygdala, ventral striatum, and hippocampal formation (among others), it seems likely that even if the primary pathology should arise in only one of these structures, the symptoms would be due to malfunctioning of the whole **network**. Interestingly, computational models of schizophrenia suggest that a basic problem may be that networks (especially prefrontal ones) are unstable due to a low signal-to-noise ratio. The latter may be due to faulty dopamine actions, as dopamine normally would stabilize networks by increasing signal-to-noise ratio (by acting on D_1 receptors). Presumably, the final symptomatology in a disease such as schizophrenia would reflect both the dysfunction caused by neuronal pathology and the attempts by the rest of the brain to cope with the disturbed functions. This would be so, regardless of whether schizophrenia turns out to be due to defective receptor genes, a prenatal disturbance of neuronal migration, or (most likely) a combination of many factors.

Ever since the first accurate description of schizophrenia, it has been postulated that the disease is caused by alteration of the frontal lobes. This assumption was partly based on similarities between the symptoms in schizophrenia and in cases of frontal lobe damage. Measurements of regional blood flow lend support to the theory that the prefrontal cortex may be involved in some manner. Thus, many schizophrenics have abnormally low blood flow in the prefrontal cortex at rest, and various tasks that give increased flow in normal people failed to do so in these patients. In homozygous twins discordant for schizophrenia, the affected twin was found to have slightly smaller volume of the cerebrum and of the hippocampus than the other, and significantly less activation of the dorsolateral prefrontal cortex during cognitive tasks. One may ask, however, whether the symptoms are caused by the abnormal prefrontal activity, or whether the low activity is due to other parts of the brain disturbing the execution of cognitive tasks in the prefrontal cortex? In contrast to some other studies, no signs of abnormal brain asymmetry or cortical structure were found in this twin study. The role of the ventral striatum—especially the nucleus accumbens—as a target for antipsychotic drugs was discussed in Chapter 23, under "The Ventral Striatum, Psychosis, and Drug Addiction." The fact that the drugs commonly used for the treatment of psychotic disorders are antidopaminergic (primarily D_2 antagonists) gave rise to the hypothesis that schizophrenia is caused by disturbances of dopamine actions pre- or postsynaptically. Recent studies have strengthened this theory—for example, by showing an increased level of dopamine receptors in the brains of schizophrenic patients. Other monoamines may be involved in schizophrenia as well, and PET studies suggest that untreated patients have reduced glutamate concentrations in the prefrontal cortex. Especially altered N-methyl-D-aspartate (NMDA)-receptor–mediated transmission has been reported in several studies. Needless to say, the interpretation of such findings is not straightforward.

Many questions remain about the etiology and pathophysiology of schizophrenia. Do defects of neurotransmitters and receptors produce structural abnormalities, or are abnormal brain networks the primary cause? There is evidence to suggest that the primary defect in schizophrenia is neurodevelopmental, but a hypothesis of neurodegeneration (based on evidence of slight but progressive loss of brain tissue) also has its proponents. We know that environmental factors must contribute, although we know little about their nature and how they interact with genetic predispositions.

LANGUAGE FUNCTIONS AND "SPEECH AREAS" OF THE CEREBRAL CORTEX

Clinical observations in the nineteenth century led to the identification of two so-called speech areas in the left hemisphere (Fig. 34.5). The anterior area is named after the French physician Paul Broca, who in 1861 described loss of speech—aphasia—caused by a lesion in the left frontal lobe just in front of the motor face area. The posterior speech area is named after the German neurologist Carl Wernicke, who discovered in 1874 that one of the clinically observed kinds of aphasia was associated with a lesion in the posterior part of the superior temporal gyrus. Aphasia is **defined** as loss (or disturbance) of speech due to a brain lesion. That speech depends almost entirely on only one hemisphere—in most people, the left—is the most marked and best-known example of **lateralization** (of function)

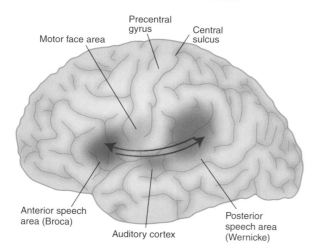

FIGURE 34.5 *Speech areas of the human brain*. Lesions of the anterior speech area (of Broca) produce predominantly motor aphasia, whereas lesions of the posterior speech area produce mainly sensory aphasia. The posterior speech area as shown here comprises parts of the inferior parietal lobule that were not included in the area described by Wernicke. Long association fibers interconnect the two areas, and these connections explain why a lesion between the two speech areas can produce aphasia (so-called conductance aphasia). Additional areas of the cerebral cortex are also involved in language processing, as shown with PET and fMRI.

or **hemispheric dominance**. We return to the topic of lateralization later.

What are termed "speech areas" should, more correctly, be termed "areas of aphasia," since we know that their destruction produces various disturbances of language functions (aphasia), but we know less of how these areas contribute to the normal production of language and speech. Further, what rather broadly is referred to as the "anterior" and "posterior" speech areas (Fig. 34.5) consist in reality of functionally different subregions.

fMRI and PET show that various tests of language functions activate regions corresponding roughly to the areas of Broca and Wernicke, but also that other parts of the cortex participate. This may not be surprising since language depends on several different processes, such as storage of words in short-term memory, phonologic (sound) and semantic (meaning) processing in relation to the "lexicon" in long-term memory, arranging words into sentences, and the issuing of commands to motor areas about sound production. Silent reading or repetition of words activates primarily the anterior region (Fig. 34.6). Specific tests for **semantic** analysis activate extensive areas in the temporal, prefrontal, and inferior parietal cortices, including Broca's and Wernicke's areas (primarily in the left hemisphere). Tests of **phonologic** analysis (like choosing matching words by sound similarity) activate partly the same and partly different areas than semantic tests. As for other complex mental functions, the main tendency is that extensive regions of the hemisphere participate in an extensive network for language and speech, and that different tasks activate overlapping regions.

Different parts of the **network** for language processing were suggested by Shalom and Poeppel (2008, p. 125) to specialize as follows: ". . . memorizing (learning new and retrieving stored primitives) in the temporal lobe, analyzing (accessing subparts of stored items) in the parietal lobe, and synthesizing (creating combinations of stored representations) in the frontal lobe." Further, there is evidence of a specialization within each region. For example, in Broca's area (or region), the superior part (closest to the ventral premotor area) appears to specialize in phonological processing, the midregion in syntactic processing, and the inferior part in semantic processing. A functional subdivision of Broca's area would agree with anatomic data, since it consists of several cytoarchitectonic areas with different connections.

Are There Brain Systems that Are Specific for Language?

A central question is whether language is produced by networks specialized for only this function, or by a

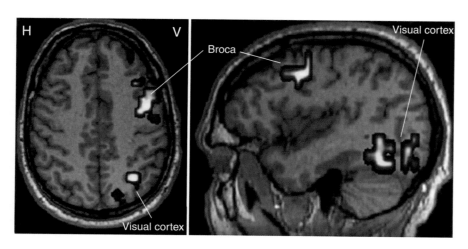

FIGURE 34.6 *Activation of Broca's area as demonstrated with fMRI.* An anatomic (T1-weighted) MRI is produced first, thereafter color-coded activity data are superimposed on the brain image. Activity in the visual cortex occurs because the test of language functions starts with reading of word. (Courtesy of Dr. S.J. Bakke, Rikshospitalet University Hospital, Oslo, Norway.)

more general system taking part also in other cognitive functions. Although rare, over the years many patients have been described with selective loss of language functions without other cognitive defects, and vice versa. Such observations have been taken to support the **specificity hypothesis**. Still, PET and fMRI data show considerable overlap among cerebral regions activated by language tasks and by other cognitive tasks. Further, connectionist-modeling (computer-based models of neural networks) shows that the **multipurpose hypothesis** is not incompatible with the evidence of selective defects from brain-damaged patients. Models can simulate language learning, such as learning to read words. Although such networks do not have segregated pathways for different functions, partial damage may produce selective visual or semantic defects (somewhat similar to a child with dyslexia). Such modeling experiments challenge "the commonly held assumption that the fractionation of behaviour reflects an underlying fractionation of the brain systems that control such behaviour" (Nobre and Plunkett 1997). Thus, a specific impairment after a brain damage does not mean that the brain possess a specific module responsible for the lost function.

Aphasia

There is an enormous literature dealing with the disturbances of speech and language, and there are numerous classifications of aphasias. Also, there is no lack of hypotheses for the cause, whereas understanding of the basic mechanisms underlying language and speech is still limited. This should come as no surprise, however, considering the complexity of the function in question.

Very schematically, there are two main types of aphasia. The simplest type is the so-called **motor aphasia**. This occurs most often after destruction of Broca's area (the anterior speech area). The patient more or less completely loses the ability to speak and typically produces only single words in a sort of telegraphic style. The few words used may also be applied wrongly. Other names used for this type are **nonfluent** aphasia (because the speech becomes stuttering) and **expressive** aphasia. The understanding of language is usually preserved, whereas the production of speech is deficient. Nevertheless, there are no signs of pareses of the muscles involved in speech production. Often, motor aphasia is combined with **agraphia**—the inability to express language in writing.

In patients with **sensory** or **receptive** aphasia, the lesion usually affects more posterior parts of the hemisphere at the junction between the parietal, temporal, and occipital lobes—that is, in or close to the Wernicke's or the posterior speech area (Fig. 33.5). Typically, the comprehension of language is most severely affected. The various elementary sounds are not properly put together to form meaningful words and sentences. Words that are heard cannot be repeated. In contrast to motor aphasia, spontaneous speech is fluent, but sounds are often put together into meaningless words, and proper words lack relation to each other ("word-salad"). Usually, sensory aphasia is combined with **alexia**—the inability to read.

In reality, the pure forms of aphasia are very seldom encountered; in most patients there is a mixture of motor and sensory symptoms, with one or the other dominating. Often there are other symptoms as well, since lesions of the hemispheres are rarely confined to the speech areas. Further, similarities between word blindness (alexia, dyslexia) and visual agnosia may be caused by lesions of the parietal lobe and the inferotemporal cortex. Alternatively, elementary symptoms of aphasia—such as agraphia or alexia—may sometimes occur in isolation or in combination with other kinds of symptoms (see Gerstmann's syndrome, described previously).

The relationship between specific aphasic symptoms and the anatomic location of a brain lesion is not absolute. Virtually all forms of aphasia have been described after lesions in unexpected parts of the brain. Thus, we can only say that the probability of speech disturbances is highest when the lesion affects one or both of the areas depicted in Fig. 33.5 (or the association fibers interconnecting the anterior and posterior speech areas).

THE DIVISION OF TASKS BETWEEN THE HEMISPHERES

The fact that the two hemispheres are connected by afferent and efferent fiber tracts with the opposite body half is proof that there *is* a division of tasks between the hemispheres. We have mentioned speech as a function that is largely taken care of by one hemisphere (the left), and here we discuss other examples of lateralization of functions. This does not mean, of course, that the two hemispheres are independent units: the **commissural connections** ensure that information reaching one hemisphere also reaches the other and that commands issued to lower parts of the brain also are known to both hemispheres. Complex functions are usually carried out by cooperation of the two hemispheres, and, as discussed, lesions of the association areas often have to be bilateral to produce clear-cut functional deficits.

Are the Two Hemispheres Anatomically Different?

Many differences have been reported but most of them are small and, further, based on small samples. This, together with the large individual variations in brain anatomy (e.g. with regard to size of cortical areas and total brain size) might explain why many reported

can understand concrete language. It understands both speech and writing of this kind but cannot express understanding through language—only through action. As mentioned, the right hemisphere can utter a few words especially when they are emotionally loaded, while it cannot manage abstract or rare words or grammatical analysis.

Not all aspects of language function are localized to the dominant hemisphere. The modulation and melody of the sounds of speech, **prosody**, appears to largely depend on the right hemisphere, as witnessed by several clinical reports. Thus, in some patients who suffered a right hemisphere stroke, prosody was changed or reduced without concomitant aphasia. Brain-imaging studies show activation in the right hemisphere in tests for perception of prosody, notably in the region corresponding to the Broca's area and in the superior temporal gyrus (but also some activation of the left hemisphere). Patients with loss of prosody may also be unable to judge the emotional aspects of the speech of other persons; for example, they cannot decide whether the person is sad or happy. Such an **intonational agnosia** may have serious effects on the social life of the patient. The importance of the prosody illustrates that much of what we regard as verbal communication is, in fact, nonverbal.

Lateralization of Music

With regard to the ability to appreciate and express **music**, there is no simple division of labor between the hemispheres, although it has been assumed that the right hemisphere is most important. Indeed, that the **perception of a melody** depends mainly on the right hemisphere was supported by a study using the Doppler technique to measure changes of total blood flow to the hemispheres during various tasks. The right-sided dominance was true only for nonmusicians, however: professional musicians showed left hemisphere dominance for the same task that was presented to the nonmusicians. Listening to **rhythm** activated the left hemisphere most strongly in both groups. Furthermore, left hemisphere activation was relatively larger when the person listened attentively, trying to discriminate musical elements, rather than having the music as a background. **Imagining** a familiar tune was found with PET to activate association areas around the right auditory cortex and frontal regions on both sides. The **supplementary motor area**—which is important for rhythmic and sequential movements—is activated when imagining tunes, perhaps because there is a motor element in music imagination.

Amusia most often occurs together with aphasia, but it has also been reported to occur in isolation. This suggests that language and music use largely separate parts of the cortex, although they appear to lie close together.

This is supported by PET studies of musicians practicing sight-reading (i.e., at the same time reading and playing an unfamiliar score).

Ear and Visual Field Dominance

A certain degree of "ear dominance" exists in most people, corresponding to speech lateralization—that is, the right ear is dominant for most people. This phenomenon can be studied by use of so-called **dichotic listening**. Two words are presented at the same time, one to each ear. Afterward, most people say that they heard the word presented to the right ear. **Visual field dominance** has been described in studies in which different visual stimuli are presented to the two hemispheres simultaneously. With regard to written words and letters, there is a tendency to prefer those presented in the right visual field (that is, those transferred to the left hemisphere). For **face recognition**, the reverse situation appears to exist for most people, as can be demonstrated by the presentation of so-called **chimeric portraits** composed of two left halves and two right halves, respectively. The person is asked which of the chimeric portraits most resembles the original (authentic) portrait. Most persons claim that the chimeric portrait consisting of two right facial halves most resembles the original. This is taken to suggest that the right hemisphere dominates in the analysis of faces and other complex visual patterns. Another indication of this is that when the **shape of letters** is made sufficiently ornate, the right hemisphere appears to become necessary for their interpretation.

Lateralization of Hand Function

With regard to lateralization of hand functions, the hemispheric differences are less clear-cut than for language. It is not a question of the ability to use the hand, but a matter of preference of one hand for most or all tasks. Even though hand preference is inheritable, there are also strong social factors that contribute to the final outcome of hand preference—for example, in writing. There is most likely a gradual transition with regard to the strength of hand preference, from those with a strong tendency to use the right hand for all tasks if possible (writing, drawing, use of tools, eating, and so forth) to those with an equally strong tendency to use the left hand. The latter group probably constitutes 2% to 3% of the total population. Hand preference starts to become expressed from the second year of life and is usually finally established at the age of 5 to 6.

Lateralization of Emotions

Early observations of split-brain patients suggest that the **right hemisphere** is dominant for the expression of emotions, but further studies show that the right hemisphere does not dominate all aspects of emotional behavior. Thus, the two hemispheres appear to be specialized for specific aspects of emotions. We mentioned **prosody** as an example of right hemisphere dominance. Overall, the right hemisphere appears to be the best at perceiving emotional expressions, whereas both hemispheres are involved in the experience and expression of emotions. The left hemisphere may be the best judge of certain kinds of emotional expressions, however. Some data have been interpreted to show that the right hemisphere is dominant as to the experience of strongly negative feelings (and the left as to positive feelings). Patients with **strokes** affecting the **left** hemisphere tend to have more depressive reactions than patients with corresponding right-sided lesions (the right hemisphere understands the agony of the left?). **Right** hemisphere lesions, especially when they affect the frontal lobe, appear to have a stronger tendency to produce a somewhat inadequate elevation of mood.

Further Examples of Hemispheric Specializations

Studies with detailed analyses of specific aspects of broader categories of cerebral functions reveal that the division of labor between right and left is more complicated than is apparent from the first split-brain observations. Sophisticated studies of visual perception show that the right hemisphere is superior to perceive and remember **specific characteristics** of objects (for example, the face of a person), whereas the left is better at **categories** (a face versus other kinds of objects). A different picture emerged in a study comparing patients with lesions in the superior temporal gyrus as to their ability to **identify letters**. Those with right-hemisphere lesions had difficulties with identification of a letter when it was composed of many small ones, but they easily perceive the small letters. Those with a left-hemisphere lesion had difficulties with identification of the small letters, but they easily identified the big one. Thus, the right hemisphere is good at identifying the **overall shape**, whereas the left is good at seeing the **details**. It may seem paradoxical that the left hemisphere is specialized both for identification of broad categories and details (and that the right hemisphere is specialized for identification of specific properties and the overall shape). Most likely, however, this reflects that different principles govern lateralization of visual and semantic memory. Another lateralization of a specific function does not fit with the usual right-left dichotomy of functions. Thus, the right hemisphere is best at **measuring distance** (e.g., the distance between a dot and a line), whereas the left hemisphere excels at judging **mutual positions** (whether the dot is above or below the line).

SEX DIFFERENCES AND THE CEREBRAL CORTEX

Gender and Cortical Structure

Many studies show that, on the average, men perform better than women on certain **spatial tasks** (shown most convincingly for imaginary rotation of a figure). Women, in contrast, excel on tasks that require **verbal fluency**, perceptual speed, and some fine-motor skills (many other cognitive differences have been proposed but few have been convincingly documented). Many speculative explanations have been offered. From an evolutionary point of view, it is now common to explain such sex differences by the living conditions during early human history, along with the different roles held by men and women. Although cognitive sex differences thus may have a genetic basis, environmental influences interact with genetic predispositions to produce the final cognitive make-up of the individual. Nevertheless, the average cognitive sex differences are small, and very much smaller than the variability among individuals of the same sex. As said by the Canadian psychologist Doreen Kimura (1996, 259): "In the larger comparative context, the similarities between human males and females far outweigh the differences."

With regard to neuroanatomic sex differences, the most obvious is the difference in **brain volume**: the brain is on average 10% heavier in men than in women. Most, but not all, of this difference can be accounted for by different body weights. The **temporal plane** (involved in language processing) has been reported to be larger in women than in men. Whether this is causally related to sex differences in verbal fluency is so far unknown, however. Studies at a more detailed level offer many data but, unfortunately, conflicting results make it difficult to draw conclusions. Yet, it seems fairly well documented that women have a slightly thicker cortex in parts of the parietal and temporal lobes (as studied with MRI). On the other hand, one study reported higher synaptic density in men than in women. A morphometric study found no difference in cortical thickness but that men had on average somewhat higher **cortical neuronal density** than women ($117,000 \pm 31,000$ and $101,000 \pm 26,000$ per mm^2, respectively). Even if this finding should be confirmed, the large individual variation within each sex makes any inferences about causal relationships doubtful. With PET and fMRI sex differences in brain activation patterns have been looked for. For example, one study found that men and women activated somewhat different parts of the brain when they were trying to find their way out of a (virtual) labyrinth. Apart from many regions activated in both sexes, men activated the left hippocampus, whereas women activated the right frontoparietal region. Other studies also point to gender differences in activation patterns but the interpretation

Literature

TEXTBOOKS AND REFERENCE WORKS

Blinkov, S.M., Glezer, I.I. *The human brain in figures and tables: a quantitative handbook.* New York: Plenum Press, 1968.

Brodal, A. *Neurological anatomy in relation to clinical medicine,* 3rd ed. Oxford: Oxford University Press, 1981.

Cooper, J.R., et al. *The biochemical basis of neuropharmacology,* 7th ed. New York: Oxford University Press, 1996.

Fain, G.L. *Molecular and cellular physiology of neurons.* Cambridge, MA: Harvard University Press, 1999.

Federative Committee on Anatomical Nomenclature. *Terminologia Anatomica. International anatomical terminology.* New York: Thieme, 1998.

Gazzaniga, M.S. *The new cognitive neurosciences.* Cambridge, MA: MIT Press, 2000.

Gazzaniga, M.S., et al. *Cognitive neuroscience: the biology of the mind.* 3rd ed. New York: W.W. Norton & Co. 2008.

Graham, D. (Ed.) *Greenfield's neuropathology,* 7th ed. London: Edward Arnold, 2002.

Kandel, E., et al. *Principles of neural science,* 4th ed. New York: McGraw-Hill, 1999.

Levitan, I.B., Kaczmarek, L.K. *The neuron: cell and molecular biology,* 3rd ed. New York: Oxford University Press, 2002.

Lockard, I. *Desk reference of neuroanatomy: a guide to essential terms.* New York: Springer-Verlag, 1977.

Martin, J.H. *Neuroanatomy: text and atlas.* Philadelphia: Elsevier, 1989.

Nicholls, J.G., et al. *From neuron to brain,* 4th ed. Sunderland, MA: Sinauer Associates, 2001.

Parent, A., Carpenter, M.B. *Carpenter's human neuroanatomy,* 9th ed. Philadelphia: Lippincott, Williams & Wilkins, 1995.

Paxinos, G. *The rat nervous system,* 3rd ed. Philadelphia: Elsevier, 2004.

Paxinos, G., Mai, J. *The human nervous system,* 2nd ed. Philadelphia: Elsevier Academic Press, 2004.

Rauber, A., Kopsch, F. *Anatomie des Menschen.* Vol. 3: *Nervensystem. Sinnesorgane.* Stuttgart: Georg Thieme Verlag, 1987.

Ropper, A., Samuels, M. *Adams and Victor's principles of neurology,* 9th ed. New York: McGraw, 2009.

Shepherd, G.M. *Neurobiology,* 3rd ed. New York: Oxford University Press, 1997.

Squire, L.R. (Editor in chief) *Encyclopedia of neuroscience,* 3rd ed. Philadelphia: Elsevier, 2009.

Squire, L.R., et al. *Fundamental neuroscience.* San Diego: Academic Press, 2002.

ATLASES

DeArmond, S.J., et al. *Structure of the human brain: a photographic atlas,* 3rd ed. Oxford: Oxford University Press, 1989.

Gouaze, A., Salomon, G. *Brain anatomy and magnetic resonance imaging.* New York: Springer-Verlag, 1988.

Haines, D.E. *Neuroanatomy: an atlas of structures, sections, and systems,* 7th ed. Philadelphia: Lippincott Williams & Wilkins, 2007.

Mai, J.K., et al. *Atlas of the human brain,* 3rd ed. Philadelphia: Academic Press, 2007.

Miller, R.A., Burack, E. *Atlas of the central nervous system in man,* 3rd ed. Baltimore: Williams & Wilkins, 1983.

Nieuwenhuys, R. *Chemoarchitecture of the brain.* New York: Springer-Verlag, 1985.

Nieuwenhuys, R., et al. *The human central nervous system: a synopsis and atlas,* 3rd ed. New York: Springer-Verlag, 1988.

Olszewski, J. *Cytoarchitecture of the human brain stem.* Basel: Karger, 1954.

O'Rahilly, R.R. *The embryonic human brain: an atlas of developmental stages,* 2nd ed. New York: John Wiley & Sons, 1999.

Roberts, M.P. *Atlas of the human brain in section.* Philadelphia: Lea & Febiger, 1987.

REVIEW JOURNALS

Annual Review of Neuroscience. Annual Reviews

Annual. Contains about twenty or more reviews by leading neuroscientists. Covers a wide range of topics. Requires background knowledge.

Clinical Neuroscience. Wiley-Liss

Quarterly. Issues focused on themes with a clinical origin, such as "Alzheimer's Disease," "Neuroscience of Depression," and "Pain: Mechanisms and Therapy." Aims at integrating basic neuroscience with clinical neurology, neurosurgery, and psychiatry.

Current Opinion in Neurobiology. Current Biology

Six issues annually. Concise reviews of the development the last few years within a special subfield. Contains comprehensive reference lists. Key references are supplied with brief, focused abstracts.

Nature Reviews Neuroscience. Nature Publishing Group

Monthly. Review articles by leading scientists, and neuroscience news in brief. The Web version features many useful links.

Neuron. Cell Press

Monthly. Each issue usually features one review article (basic neuroscience) and several mini-reviews of high standard, in addition to many research articles.

Scientific American. Scientific American Inc.

Monthly. Regularly one or more articles on various aspects of neuroscience. Requires less prior knowledge than the specialized neuroscience

Lehmann-Horn, F., Jurkat-Rott, K. Voltage-gated ion channels and hereditary disease. *Physiol. Rev.* 79:1317–1372, 1999.

Lisman, J.E. Bursts as a unit of neural information: making unreliable synapses reliable. *Trends Neurosci.* 20:38–43, 1997.

Madden, D.R. The structure and function of glutamate receptor ion channels. *Nat. Rev. Neurosci.* 3:91–101, 2002.

Mioshevsky, G.V., Jordan, P.C. Permeation of ion channels: the interplay of structure and theory. *Trends Neurosci.* 27:308–314, 2004.

Morisset, V., Nagy, F. Ionic basis for plateau potentials in deep dorsal horn neurons of the rat spinal cord. *J. Neurosci.* 19:7309–7316, 1999.

Novakovic, S.D., et al. Regulation of Na$^+$ channel distribution in the nervous system. *Trends Neurosci.* 24:473–478, 2001.

Wollmuth, L.P., Sobolevsky, A.I. Structure and gating of the glutamate receptor ion channel. *Trends Neurosci.* 27:308–214, 2004.

Zagotta, W.N., Siegelbaum, S.A. Structure and function of cyclic nucleotide-gated channels. *Annu. Rev. Neurosci.* 19:235–263, 1996.

Ziff, E.B. Enlightening the postsynaptic density. *Neuron* 19:1163–1174, 1997.

CHAPTER 4: SYNAPTIC FUNCTION

Alvarez, F.J. Anatomical basis for presynaptic inhibition of primary sensory fibers. In: Rudomin, P., et al. (Eds.), *Presynaptic inhibition and neural control* (pp. 13–49). New York: Oxford University Press, 1998.

Alvarez, V.A., Sabatini, B.L. Anatomical and physiological plasticity of dendritic spines. *Annu. Rev. Neurosci.* 30:79–97, 2007.

Bajjalieh, S.M. Synaptic vesicle docking and fusion. *Curr. Opin. Neurobiol.* 9:321–328, 1999.

Bialek, W., Rieke, F. Reliability and information transmission in spiking neurons. *Trends Neurosci.* 15:428–434, 1992.

Craig, A.M., Boudin, H. Molecular heterogeneity of central synapses: afferent and target regulation. *Nat. Neurosci.* 4:569–578, 2001.

De Camilli, P., Takei, K. Molecular mechanisms in synaptic vesicle endocytosis and recycling. *Neuron* 16:481–486, 1996.

Dermietzel, R., Spray, D.C. Gap junctions in the brain: where, what type, how many and why? *Trends Neurosci.* 16:186–192, 1993.

Eccles, J.C. *The physiology of synapses.* New York: Springer-Verlag, 1964.

Edwards, R.H. The neurotransmitter cycle and quantal size. *Neuron* 55:835–858, 2007.

Gaffield, M.A., Betz, W.J. Synaptic vesicle mobility in mouse motor nerve terminals with and without synapsin. *J. Neurosci.* 27:13691–13700, 2007.

Grillner, S. Bridging the gap: from ion channels to networks and behavior. *Curr. Opin. Neurobiol.* 9:663–669, 1999.

Guidolin, D., et al. On the role receptor-receptor interactions and volume transmission in learning and memory. *Brain Res. Rev.* 55:119–133, 2007.

Hall, Z.W., Sanes, J.R. Synaptic structure and development: the neuromuscular junction. *Neuron* 10 (Suppl.):99–121, 1993.

Kennedy, M.B., et al. Integration of biochemical signalling in spines. *Nat. Rev. Neurosci.* 6:423–434, 2005.

Kittel, R.J., et al. Bruchpilot promotes active zone assembly, Ca^{2+} channel clustering, and vesicle release. *Science* 312:1051–1054, 2006.

Koh, T.-W., Bellen, H.J. Synaptotagmin I, a Ca^{2+} sensor for neurotransmitter release. *Trends Neurosci.* 26:413–423, 2003.

Lisman, J.E., et al. The sequence of events that underlie quantal transmission at central glutamatergic synapses. *Nat. Rev. Neurosci.* 8:597–609, 2007.

MacDermott, A.B., et al. Presynaptic ionotropic receptors and the control of transmitter release. *Annu. Rev. Neurosci.* 22:443–485, 1999.

Magee, J.C., Cook, E.P. Somatic EPSP amplitude is independent of synapse location in hippocampal pyramid neurons. *Nat. Neurosci.* 3:895–903, 2000.

Malgaroli, A. Silent synapses: I can't hear you! Could you please speak aloud? *NatNeurosci.* 2:3–5, 1999.

Matthews, G. Neurotransmitter release. *Annu. Rev. Neurosci.* 19:219–233, 1996.

Monck, J.R., Fernandez, J.M. The exocytotic fusion pore and neurotransmitter release. *Neuron* 12:707–716, 1994.

Pietrobon, D. Function and dysfunction of synaptic calcium channels: insights from mouse models. *Curr. Opin. Neurobiol.* 15:257–265, 2005.

Rudomin, P., Schmidt, R.F. Presynaptic inhibition in the vertebrate spinal cord revisited. *Exp. Brain Res.* 129:1–37, 1999.

Schneggenburger, R., Neher, E. Presynaptic calcium and control of vesicle fusion. *Curr. Opin. Neurobiol.* 15:266–274, 2005.

Sjöström, P.J., Nelson, S.B. Spike timing, calcium signals and synaptic plasticity. *Curr. Opin. Neurobiol.* 12:305–314, 2002.

Sørensen, J.B. SNARE complexes prepare for membrane fusion. *Trends Neurosci.* 28:453–455, 2005.

Spruston, N. Pyramidal neurons: dendritic structure and synaptic integration. *Nat. Rev. Neurosci.* 9:206–221, 2008.

Stuart, G.J., Redman, S.J. The role of GABAA and GABAB receptors in presynaptic inhibition of Ia EPSPs in cat spinal motoneurons. *J. Physiol. (Lond.)* 447:675–692, 1992.

Unwin, N. Neurotransmitter action: opening of ligand-gated ion channels. *Neuron* 72 (Suppl. 10):31–41, 1993.

Ventura, R., Harris, K. Three-dimensional relationships between hippocampal synapses and astrocytes. *J. Neurosci.* 19:6897–6906, 1999.

Walmsey, B., et al. Diversity of structure and function at mammalian central synapses. *Trends Neurosci.* 21:81–88, 1998.

Yuste, R., Bonhoeffer, T. Morphological changes in dendritic spines associated with long-term synaptic plasticity. *Annu. Rev. Neurosci.* 24:1071–1089, 2001.

Yuste, R., Majewska, A. On the function of dendritic spines. *Neuroscientist* 7:387–395, 2001.

Synaptic Plasticity

Abraham, W.C. Metaplasticity: tuning synapses and networks for plasticity. *Nat. Rev. Neurosci.* 9:387–399, 2008.

Arshavsky, Y.I. "The seven sins" of the Hebbian synapse: Can the hypothesis of synaptic plasticity explain long-term memory consolidation? *Prog. Neurobiol.* 80:99–113, 2006.

Bailey, C.H., et al. The persistence of long-term memory: a molecular approach to self-sustaining changes in learning-induced synaptic growth. *Neuron* 44:49–57, 2004.

Barry, M.F., Ziff, E.B. Receptor trafficking and the plasticity of excitatory synapses. *Curr. Opin. Neurobiol.* 12:279–286, 2002.

Bastrikova, N., et al. Synapse elimination accompanies functional plasticity in hippocampal neurons. *Proc. Natl. Acad. Sci. USA* 105:3123–3127, 2008.

Bekinschtein, P., et al. BDNF is essential to promote persistence of long-term memory storage. *Proc. Natl. Acad. Sci. USA* 105:2711–2716, 2008.

Blitz, D.M., et al. Short-term synaptic plasticity: a comparison of two synapses. *Nat. Rev. Neurosci.* 5:630–640, 2004.

Bramham, C.R., Wells, D.G. Dendritic mRNA: transport, translation and function. *Nat. Rev. Neurosci.* 8:776–789, 2007.

Caporale, N., Dan, Y. Spike timing-dependent plasticity: a Hebbian learning rule. *Annu. Rev. Neurosci.* 31:25–46, 2008.

Cheng, Q., Augustine, G.J. Calcium channel modulation as an all-purpose mechanism for short-term plasticity. *Neuron* 57:171–172, 2008.

Costa-Mattioli, M., et al. Translational control of long-lasting synaptic plasticity and memory. *Neuron* 61:10–26, 2009.

DeRoo, M., et al. Spine dynamics and synapse remodeling during LTP and memory processes. *Prog. Brain Res.* 169:199–207, 2008.

Dudek, S.M., Fields, R.D. Gene expression in hippocampal long-term potentiation. *Neuroscientist* 5:275–279, 1999.

Flavell, S.W., Greenberg, M.E. Signaling mechanisms linking neuronal activity to gene expression and plasticity of the nervous system. *Annu. Rev. Neurosci.* 31:563–590, 2008.

Harvey, C.D., Svoboda, K. Locally dynamic synaptic learning rules in pyramidal neuron dendrites. *Nature* 450:1195–1200, 2007.

Hebb, D.O. The organization of behavior; a neuropsychological theory. New York: John Wiley & Sons, 1949.

Holtmaat, A., et al. Experience-dependent and cell-type-specific spine growth in the neocortex. *Nature* 441:979–983, 2006.

Kerchner, G.A., Nicholl, R.A. Silent synapses and the emergence of a postsynaptic mechanism for LTP. *Nat. Rev. Neurosci.* 9:813–825, 2008.

Levenson, J.M., Sweatt, J.D. Epigenetic mechanisms in memory formation. *Nat. Rev. Neurosci.* 6:108–118, 2005.

Linden, D.J., Connor, J.A. Long-term synaptic depression. *Annu. Rev. Neurosci.* 18:319–357, 1995.

Lynch, M.A. Long-term potentiation and memory. *Physiol. Rev.* 84:87–136, 2004.

Malinov, R., Malenka, R.C. AMPA receptor trafficking and synaptic plasticity. *Annu. Rev. Neurosci.* 25:103–126, 2002.

Martin, S.J., et al. Synaptic plasticity and memory: an evaluation of the hypothesis. *Annu. Rev. Neurosci.* 23:649–711, 2000.

Park, M., et al. Plasticity-induced growth of dendritic spines by exocytotic trafficking from recycling endosomes. *Neuron* 52:817–830, 2006.

Roo, M. De, et al. Spine dynamics and synapse remodeling during LTP and memory processes. *Prog. Brain Res.* 169:199–207, 2008.

Sanes, J.R., Lichtman J.W. Can molecules explain long-term potentiation? *Nat. Neurosci.* 2:597–604, 1999.

Segal, M.: Dendritic spines and long-term plasticity. *Nat. Rev. Neurosci.* 6:277–284, 2005.

Sossin, W.S. Molecular memory traces. *Prog. Brain Res.* 169:3–25, 2008.

Wang, Z., et al. Myosin Vb mobilizes recycling endosomes and AMPA receptors for postsynaptic plasticity. *Cell* 135:535–548, 2008.

Zucker, R.S. Calcium- and activity-dependent synaptic plasticity. *Curr. Opin. Neurobiol.* 9:305–313, 1999.

CHAPTER 5: NEUROTRANSMITTERS AND THEIR RECEPTORS

Neurotransmitters in General

Cooper, J.R., et al. *The biochemical basis of neuropharmacology.* 8th ed. New York: Oxford University Press, 2003.

Davletov, B., et al. Beyond BOTOX: advantages and limitations of individual botulinum neurotoxins. *Trends Neurosci.* 28:446–452, 2006.

DeFelice, L.J. Transporter structure and function. *Trends Neurosci.* 27:352–359, 2004.

Kelly, R.B. Storage and release of neurotransmitters. *Neuron* 10 (Suppl.):43–53, 1993.

Torrealba, F., Carrasco, M.A. A review of electron microscopy and neurotransmitter systems. *Brain Res. Rev.* 47:5–17, 2004.

Amino Acid Transmitters

Allen, T.G.J., et al. Simultaneous release of glutamate and acetylcholine from single magnocellular "cholinergic" basal forebrain neurons. *J. Neurosci.* 25:1588–1595, 2006.

Beart, P.M., O'Shea, R.D. Transporters for L-glutamate: an update on their molecular pharmacology and pathological involvement, *Br. J. Pharmacol.* 150:5–17, 2006.

Camacho, A., Massieu, L. Role of glutamate transporters in the clearance and release of glutamate during ischemia and its relation ot neuronal death. *Arch. Med. Res.* 37:11–18, 2006.

Chittajallu, R., et al. Kainate receptors: subunits, synaptic localization and function. *Trends Pharmacol. Sci.* 20:26–35, 1999.

Conti, F., et al. GABA-transporters in the mammalian cerebral cortex: localization, development and pathological implications. *Brain Res. Rev.* 45:196–212, 2004.

Danbolt, N.C. Glutamate uptake. *Prog. Neurobiol.* 63:1–105, 2001.

Dingledine, R., et al. The glutamate receptor ion channel. *Pharmacol. Rev.* 51:7–62, 1999.

Dzubay, J.A., Jahr, C.E. The concentration of synaptically released glutamate outside of the climbing fiber-Purkinje cell synaptic cleft. *J. Neurosci.* 19:5265–5274, 1999.

Erickson, J.D., et al. Activity-dependent regulation of vesicular glutamate and GABA transporters: a means to scale quantal size. *Neurochem. Int.* 48:643–649, 2006.

Farrant, M., Nusser, Z. Variations on an inhibitory theme: phasic and tonic activation of $GABA_A$ receptors. *Nat. Rev. Neurosci.* 6:215–229, 2005.

Featherstone, D.E., Shippy, S.A. Regulation of synaptic transmission by ambient extracellular glutamate. *Neuroscientist* 14:171–181, 2008.

Ferraguti, F., Shigemoto, R. Metabotropic glutamate receptors. *Cell Tissue Res.* 326:483–504, 2006.

Gaspary, H.L. AMPA receptors: players in calcium mediated neuronal injury? *Neuroscientist* 4:149–153, 1998.

Gundersen, V., et al. Synaptic vesicular localization and exocytosis of L-aspartate in excitatory nerve terminals: a quantitative immunogold analysis in rat hippocampus. *J. Neurosci.* 18:6059–6070, 1998.

Hanson, J.E., Smith, Y. Group I metabotropic glutamate receptors at GABAergic synapses in monkeys. *J. Neurosci.* 19:6488–6496, 1999.

Hentschke, H., et al. Neocortex is the major target of sedative concentrations of volatile anaesthetics: strong depression of firing rates and increase of $GABA_A$ receptor-mediated inhibition. *Eur. J. Neurosci.* 21:93–102, 2005.

Herz, L. Glutamate, a neurotransmitter—and so much more. A synopsis of Wierzba III. *Neurochem. Int.* 48:416–425, 2006.

Jacob, T.C., et al. $GABA_A$ receptor trafficking and its role in the dynamic modulation of neuronal inhibition. *Nat. Rev. Neurosci.* 9:331–343, 2008.

Lerma, J. Roles and rules of kainite receptors in synaptic transmission. *Nat. Rev. Neurosci.* 4:481–495, 2003.

Li, W.C., Roberts, A. Glutamate and acetylcholine corelease at developing synapses. *Proc. Natl. Acad. Sci. USA* 101:15488–15493, 2004.

Lüddens, H., Korpi, E.R. $GABA_A$ receptors: pharmacology, behavioral roles, and motor disorders. *Neuroscientist* 2:15–23, 1996.

Mayer, M.L. Glutamate receptor ion channels. *Curr. Opin. Neurobiol.* 15:282–288, 2005.

Misgeld, U., et al. A physiological role for $GABA_B$ receptors and the effects of baclofen in the mammalian central nervous system. *Prog. Neurobiol.* 46:423–462, 1995.

Owens, D.F,. et al. Changing properties of GABAA receptor-mediated signaling during early neocortical development. *J. Neurophysiol.* 82:570–583, 1999.

Ozawa, S., et al. Glutamate receptors in the mammalian central nervous system. *Prog. Neurobiol.* 54:581–618, 1998.

Pinheiro, P.S., Mulle, C. Presynaptic glutamate receptors: physiological functions and mechanisms of action. *Nat. Rev. Neurosci.* 9:423–436, 2008.

Represa, A., Ben-Ari, Y. Trophic actions of GABA on neuronal development. *Trends Neurosci.* 28:278–283, 2005.

Scremin, O.U. Cerebral Vascular System. In: Paxinos, G., Mai, J.K. (Eds.), *The human nervous system*, 2nd ed. (pp. 1325–1348). Philadelphia: Elsevier Academic Press, 2004.

Tatu, L., et al. Arterial territories of human brain: brainstem and cerebellum. *Neurology* 47:1125–1135, 1996.

Control of Cerebral Circulation

Cohen, Z., et al. Serotonin in the regulation of brain microcirculation. *Prog. Neurobiol.* 50:335–362, 1996.

Drake, T.C., Idadecola, C. The role of neuronal signaling in controlling cerebral blood flow. *Brain Lang.* 107:141–152, 2007.

Faraci, F.M., Heistad, D.D. Regulation of the cerebral circulation: role of endothelium and potassium channels. *Physiol. Rev.* 78:53–97, 1998.

Jakovcevic, D., Harder, D.R. Role of astrocytes in matching blood flow to neuronal activity. *Curr. Top. Dev. Biol.* 79:75–97, 2007.

Peppiatt, C.M., et al. Bidirectional control of CNS capillary diameter by pericytes. *Nature* 443:700–704, 2006.

Raichle, M.E., Mintum, M.A. Brain work and brain imaging. *Annu. Rev. Neurosci.* 29:449–476, 2006.

Schaller, B. Physiology of cerebral venous blood flow: from experimental data in animals to normal function in humans. *Brain Res. Rev.* 46:243–260, 2004.

Sirotin, Y.B., Das, A. Anticipatory haemodynamic signal in sensory cortex not predicted by local neuronal activity. *Nature* 457:475–480, 2009.

Stefanovic, B., et al. Functional reactivity of cerebral capillaries. *J. Cereb. Blood Flow Metab.* 28:961–972, 2008.

Takano, T., et al. Astrocyte-mediated control of cerebral blood flow. *Nat. Rev. Neurosci.* 9:260–267, 2006.

Unterberg, A.W., et al. Edema and brain trauma. *Neuroscience* 129:1019–1027, 2004.

Yang, G., Iadecola, C. Activation of cerebellar climbing fibers increases cerebellar blood flow: role of glutamate receptors, nitric oxide, and cGMP. *Stroke* 29:499–508, 1998.

Blood–Brain Barrier

Abbot, N.J., et al. Astrocyte-endothelial interactions at the blood-brain barrier. *Nat. Rev. Neurosci.* 7:41–53, 2006.

Banks, W.A., et al. Passage of cytokines across the blood–brain barrier. *Neuroimmunomodulation* 2:241–248, 1995.

Friedman, A., et al. Pyridostigmine in brain penetration under stress enhances neuronal excitability and induces early immediate transcriptional response. *Nat. Med.* 2:1382–1385, 1996.

Hawkins, B.T., Davis, T.P. The blood–brain barrier/neurovascular unit in health and disease. *Pharmacol.Rev.* 57:173–185, 2005.

Janzer, R.C., Raff, M.C. Astrocytes induce blood-brain barrier properties in endothelial cells. *Nature* 325:253–257, 1987.

Johansson, P.A., et al. The blood–CSF barrier explained: when development is not immaturity. *BioEssays* 30:237–248, 2008.

Lai, C.H., et al. Critical role of actin in modulating BBB permeability. *Brain Res. Rev.* 50:7–13, 2005.

Lammert, E. Brain Wnts for blood vessels. *Science* 322:1195–1196, 2008.

Rechthand, E., Rapoport, S.I. Regulation of the microenvironment of peripheral nerve: role of the blood–nerve barrier. *Prog. Neurobiol.* 28:303–343, 1987.

Saunders, N.R., et al. Barriers in the brain: a renaissance? *Trends Neurosci.* 31:279–286, 2008.

Weidenfeller, C., et al. Differentiating embryonic neural progenitor cells induce blood–brain barrier properties. *J. Neurochem.* 1001:555–565, 2008.

Wolburg, H., et al. Agrin, aquaporin-4, and astrocyte polarity as an important feature of the blood–brain barrier. *Neuroscientist* 15:180–193, 2009.

Zlokovic, B.V. The blood–brain barrier in health and chronic neurodegenerative disorders. *Neuron* 57:178–201, 2008.

CHAPTER 9: PRENATAL AND POSTNATAL DEVELOPMENT

Prenatal Development

Anderson, D.J. Stem cells and pattern formation in the nervous system: the possible versus the actual. *Neuron* 30:19–35, 2001.

Ang, S.B.C. Jr., et al. Four-dimensional migratory coordinates of GABAergic interneurons in the developing mouse cortex. *J. Neurosci.* 23:5805–5815, 2003.

Ashwell, K.W.S., Waite, P.M.E. Development of the peripheral nervous system. In: Paxinos, G., Mai, J.K. (Eds.), *The human nervous System*, 2nd ed. (pp. 95–110). Philadelphia: Elsevier Academic Press, 2004.

Bourgeois, J.-P. Rakic, P. Changes of synaptic density in the primary visual cortex of the macaque monkey from fetal to adult stage. *J. Neurosci.* 13:2801–2820, 1993.

Bystron, I., et al. Development of the human cerebral cortex: Boulder Committee revisited. *Nat. Rev. Neurosci.* 9:110–122, 2008.

Chan, S. Kilby, M.D. Thyroid hormone and central nervous development. *J. Endocrinol.* 165:1–8, 2000.

Cholfin, J.A., Rubenstein, J.R. Patterning of frontal cortex subdivisions by Fgf17. *Proc. Natl. Acad. Sci. USA* 104:7652–7657, 2007.

Colamarino, S.A., Tessier-Lavigne, M. The role of the floor plate in axon guidance. *Annu. Rev. Neurosci.* 18:497–529, 1995.

Cragg, B.G. The development of synapses in the cat visual cortex. *Invest. Ophthalmol.* 11:377–389, 1972.

Donoghue, M.J., Rakic, P. Molecular evidence for the early specification of presumptive functional domains in the embryonic primate cerebral cortex. *J. Neurosci.* 19:5967–5979, 1999.

Elias, L.A.B., et al. Gap junction adhesion is necessary for radial migration in the neocortex. *Nature* 448:901–906, 2007.

Finlay, B.L. Cell death and the creation of regional differences in neuronal numbers. *J. Neurobiol.* 23:1159–1171, 1992.

Fogarty, M., et al. Spatial genetic patterning of the embryonic neuroepithelium generates GABAergic interneuron diversity in the adult cortex. *J. Neurosci.* 27:10935–10946, 2007

Freeman, M.R. Sculpting the nervous system: glial control of neuronal development. *Curr. Opin. Neurobiol.* 16:119–125, 2006.

Geisen, M.J., et al. *Hox* Paralog group 2 genes control the migration of mouse pontine neurons through slit-robo signaling. *PLoS Biol.* 6:1178–1194, 2008.

Goldberg, D.J., Grabham P.W. Braking news: calcium and the growth cone. *Neuron* 22:423–425, 1999.

Goodrich, L.V., Scott, M.P. Hedgehog and Patched in neural development and disease. *Neuron* 21:1243–1257, 1998.

Hamilton, W.J., et al. *Human embryology. Prenatal development of form and function*, 4th ed. Baltimore: Williams & Wilkins, 1972.

Hatten, M.E. Central nervous system neuronal migration. *Annu. Rev. Neurosci.* 22:511–539, 1999.

Hennigan, A., et al. Neurotrophins and their receptors: roles in plasticity, neurodegeneration and neuroprotection. *Biochem. Soc. Trans.* 35 (2):424–427, 2007.

Huang, E.J., Reichardt, L.F. Neurotrophins: roles in neuronal development and function. *Annu. Rev. Neurosci.* 24:677–736, 2001.

Kalil, K., Dent, E.W. Touch and go: guidance signal to the growth cone cytoskeleton. *Curr. Opin. Neurobiol.* 15:521–526, 2005.

Keynes, R., Krumlauf R. Hox genes and regionalization of the nervous system. *Annu. Rev. Neurosci.* 17:109–132, 1994.

Kunes, S. Axonal signals in the assembly of neural circuitry. *Curr. Opin. Neurobiol.* 10:58–62, 2000.

Le Douarin, E., Dupin, E. Cell lineage analysis in neural crest ontogeny. *J. Neurobiol.* 24:146–161, 1993.

Levitt, P., et al. New evidence for neurotransmitter influences on brain development. *Trends Neurosci.* 20:269–274, 1997.

Lewin, G.R., Barde, Y.-A. Physiology of the neurotrophins. *Annu. Rev. Neurosci.* 19:289–317, 1996.

Mai, J.K, Ashwell, K.W.S. Fetal development of the central nervous system. In: Paxinos, G., Mai, J.K. (Eds.), *The human nervous system*, 2nd ed. (pp. 49–94). Philadelphia: Elsevier Academic Press, 2004.

McAllister, A.K., et al. Neurotrophins and synaptic plasticity. *Annu. Rev. Neurosci.* 22:295–318, 1999.

Meyer, G. Embryonic and early fetal development of the human neocortex. *J. Neurosci.* 20:1858–1868, 2000.

Momma, S., et al. Get to know your stem cells. *Curr. Opin. Neurobiol.* 10:45–49, 2000.

Müller, F., O'Rahilly, R. Embryonic development of the central nervous system. In: Paxinos, G., Mai, J.K. (Eds.), *The human nervous system*, 2nd ed. (pp. 22–48). Philadelphia: Elsevier Academic Press, 2004.

O'Leary, D.D.M., et al. Area patterning of the mammalian cortex. *Neuron* 56:252–269, 2007.

Parnevalas, J.G. The origin and migration of cortical neurones: new vistas. *Trends Neurosci.* 23:126–131, 2000.

Perris, R. The extracellular matrix in neural crest–cell migration. *Trends Neurosci.* 20:23–31, 1997.

Rubenstein, J.L.R., et al. Regionalization of the prosencephalic neural plate. *Annu. Rev. Neurosci.* 21:445–477, 1998.

Ruiz i Altaba, A. Pattern formation in the vertebrate neural plate. *Trends Neurosci.* 17:233–242, 1994.

Vyovodic, J.T. Cell death in cortical development: how much? why? so what? *Neuron* 16:693–696, 1996.

Wen, Z., Zheng J.Q. Directional guidance of nerve growth cones. *Curr. Opin. Neurobiol.* 16:52–58, 2006.

Wonders, C., Anderson, S.A. Cortical interneurons and their origins. *Neuroscientist* 11:199–205, 2005.

Development of Specific Neural Connections

Benson, D.L., et al. Molecules, maps and synapse specificity. *Nat. Rev. Neurosci.* 2:899–909, 2001.

Goodman, C.S., Shatz C.J. Developmental mechanisms that generate precise patterns of neuronal connectivity. *Neuron* 10 (Suppl.): 77–98, 1993.

Huberman, A.D., et al. Mechanisms underlying development of visual maps and receptive fields. *Annu. Rev. Neurosci.* 31 479–509, 2008.

Klein, R. Bidirectional modulation of synaptic functions by Eph/ephrin signaling. *Nat. Rev. Neurosci.* 12:15–20, 2009.

Kuang, R.Z., Kalil, K. Development of specificity in corticospinal connections by axon collaterals branching selectively into appropriate spinal targets. *J. Comp. Neurol.* 334:270–282, 1994.

Lambot, M-A., et al. Mapping labels in the human developing visual system and the evolution of binocular vision. *J. Neurosci.* 25:7232–7237, 2005.

Leergaard, T.B., et al. Topographical organization in the early postnatal corticopontine projection: a carbocyanine dye and 3-D computer reconstruction study in the rat. *J. Comp. Neurol.* 361:77–94, 1995.

Lemke, G., Reber, M. Retinotectal mapping: new insights from molecular genetics. *Annu. Rev. Cell. Dev. Biol.* 21:551–580, 2005.

Lichtman, J.W., Smith, S.J. Seeing circuits assemble. *Neuron* 60: 441–448, 2008.

McLaughlin, T., O'Leary, D.M. Molecular gradients and development of retinotopic maps. *Annu. Rev. Neurosci.* 28:327–355, 2005.

Petros, T.J., et al. Retinal axon growth at the optic chiasm: to cross or not to cross. *Annu. Rev. Neurosci.* 31:295–315, 2008.

Price, D.J., et al. The development of cortical connections. *Eur. J. Neurosci.* 23:910–920, 2006.

Sanes, J.R. Extracellular matrix molecules that influence neural development. *Annu. Rev. Neurosci.* 12:491–516, 1989.

Postnatal Development

Blakemore, S.-J., Frith U. *The learning brain. Lessons for education.* Oxford: Blackwell Publishing 2005.

Bredy, T.W., et al. Maternal care influences neuronal survival in the hippocampus of the rat. *Eur. J. Neurosci.* 18:2903–2909, 2003.

Bredy, T.W., et al. Peripubertal environmental enrichment reverses the effects of maternal care on hippocampal development and glutamate receptor subunit expression. *Eur. J. Neurosci.* 20: 1355–1362, 2004.

Brody, B.A., et al. Sequence of central nervous system myelination in human infancy. *J. Neuropathol. Exp. Neurol.* 46:283–301, 1987.

Chugani, H.T. Metabolic imaging: a window on brain development and plasticity. *Neuroscientist* 5:29–40, 1999.

Conel, J.L. *The postnatal development of the human cerebral cortex.* Vols. 1–6. Cambridge, MA: Harvard University Press, 1939–1959.

Dekaban, A.S., Sadowsky, D. Changes in brain weights during the span of human life: relation of brain weights to body heights and body weights. *Ann. Neurol.* 4:345–356, 1978.

Eriksson, P.S., et al. Neurogenesis in the adult human hippocampus. *Nat. Med.* 4:1313–1317, 1998.

Gogtay, N., et al. Three-dimensional brain growth abnormalities in childhood-onset schizophrenia visualized by using tensor-based morphometry. *Proc. Natl. Acad. Sci. USA* 105:15979–15984, 2008.

Helmeke, C., et al. Juvenile emotional experience alters synaptic inputs on pyramidal neurons in the anterior cingulated cortex. *Cereb. Cortex* 11:717–727, 2001.

Huttenlocher, P.R., Dabholkar, A.S. Regional differences in synaptogenesis in human cerebral cortex. *J. Comp. Neurol.* 387:167–178, 1997.

Matsuzawa, J. Age-related volumetric changes of brain gray and white matter in healthy infants and children. *Cereb. Cortex* 11:335–342, 2001.

McCue, M., Bouchard, T.J., Jr. Genetic and environmental influences on human behavioral differences. *Annu. Rev. Neurosci.* 21:1–24, 1998.

Rakic, P. Neurogenesis in adult primate neocortex: an evaluation of the evidence. *Nat. Rev. Neurosci.* 3:65–71, 2002.

Rampon, C., et al. Enrichment induces structural changes and recovery from nonspatial memory deficits in CA1 NMDAR1–knockout mice. *Nat. Neurosci.* 3:238–245, 2000.

Reiss, A.L., et al. Brain development, gender and IQ in children: a volumetric imaging study. *Brain* 119:1763–1774, 1996.

Sapolsky, R.M. Mothering style and methylation. *Nat. Neurosci.* 7:791–792, 2004.

Shaw, P., et al. Neurodevelopmental trajectories of the human cerebral cortex. *J. Neurosci.* 28:3586–3594, 2008.

Sowell, E.R., et al. In vivo evidence for post-adolescent brain maturation in frontal and striatal regions. *Nat. Neurosci.* 2:859–861, 1999.

Tsujimoto, S. The prefrontal cortex: functional neural development during early childhood. *Neuroscientist* 14:345–358, 2008.

Toga, A.W., et al. Mapping brain maturation. *Trends Neurosci.* 29:148–159, 2006.

Bertram, L., Tanzi, R.E. Thirty years of Alzheimer's disease genetics: the implications of systematic meta-analyses. *Nat. Rev. Neurosci.* 9:768–777, 2008.

Bruen, P.D., et al. Neuroanatomical correlates of neuropsychiatric symptoms in Alzheimer's disease. *Brain* 131:2455–2463, 2008.

Buckner, R.L., et al. Molecular, structural and functional characterization of Alzheimer's disease: evidence for a relationship between default activity, amyloid, and memory. *J. Neurosci.* 25:7709–7717, 2005.

Corey-Bloom, J., et al. Hippocampal sclerosis contributes to dementia in the elderly. *Neurology* 48:154–160, 1997.

Dickerson, B.C., et al. The cortical signature of Alzheimer's disease: regionally specific cortical thinning relates to symptom severity in very mild to mild AD dementia and is detectable in asymptomatic amyloid-positive individuals. *Cereb. Cortex* 19:497–510, 2009.

Finkbeiner, S., et al. Disease-modifying pathways in neurodegeneration. *J. Neurosci.* 26:10349–10357, 2006.

Giannakopoulos, P., et al. Cerebral cortex pathology in aging and Alzheimer's disease: a quantitative survey of large hospital–based geriatric and psychiatric cohorts. *Brain Res. Rev.* 25:217–245, 1997.

Gidalevitz, T., et al. Progressive disruption of cellular protein folding in models of polyglutamine diseases. *Science* 311:1471–1474, 2006.

Goedert, M., Spillantini, M.G., A century of Alzheimer's disease. *Science* 314:777–781, 2006.

Gomez-Isla, T., et al. Neuropathology of Alzheimer's disease. In: Duyckaerts, C., Litvan, I. (Eds.), *Handbook of clinical neurology.* Vol. 83, (pp. 233–243). Philadelphia: Elsevier, 2008.

Haas, C. Presenilins: genes for life and death. *Neuron* 18:687–690, 1997.

Hardy, J., et al. Genetic dissection of Alzheimer's disease and related dementias: amyloid and its relationship to tau. *Nat. Rev. Neurosci.* 1:355–358, 1998.

Jellinger, K.A. Morphological diagnosis of "vascular dementia" a critical update. *J. Neurol. Sci.* 270:1–12, 2008.

Kirik, D., et al. Localized striatal delivery of GDNF as a treatment for Parkinson disease. *Nat. Rev. Neurosci.* 7:105–110, 2004.

Lindvall, O., et al. Stem cell therapy for human neurodegenerative disorders Duyckaerts, C., Litvan, I. (Eds.), *Handbook of clinical neurology* how to make it work. *Nat. Med.* 10 Suppl. July: S42–S50, 2004.

Moorhouse, P., Rockwood, K. Vascular cognitive impairment: current concepts and clinical developments. *Lancet Neurol.* 7:246–255, 2008.

Parameshwaran, K., et al. Amyloid beta peptides and glutamatergic synaptic dysregulation. *Exp. Neurol.* 210:7–13, 2008.

Ross, C.A., Poirier, M.A. Protein aggregation and neurodegenerative disease. *Nat. Med.* 10 Suppl. July, S10–S17, 2004.

Wallace, W., et al. Amyloid precursor protein in the cerebral cortex is rapidly and persistently induced by loss of subcortical innervation. *Proc. Natl. Acad. Sci. USA* 90:8712–8716, 1993.

Wang, J.-Z., Liu, F. Microtubule-associated protein tau in development, degeneration and protection of neurons. *Prog. Neurobiol.* 85:148–175, 2008.

CHAPTER 11: RESTITUTION OF FUNCTION AFTER BRAIN DAMAGE

Cellular Mechanisms in Ischemia and in Restitution

Colbourne, F., et al. Electron microscopic evidence against apoptosis as the mechanism of neuronal death in global ischemia. *J. Neurosci.* 19:4200–4210, 1999.

Dirnagel, U., et al. Pathobiology of ischaemic stroke: an integrated view. *Trends Neurosci.* 22:391–397, 1999.

Emsley, J.G., et al. Adult neurogenesis and repair of the adult CNS with neural progenitors, precursors, and stem cells. *Prog. Neurobiol.* 75:321–41, 2005.

Farkas, O., Povlishock, J.T. Cellular and subcellular change evoked by diffuse traumatic brain injury: a complex web of change extending far beyond focal damage. *Prog. Brain Res.* 161:43–59, 2007.

Filbin, M.T. Myelin-associated inhibitors of axonal regeneration in the adult mammalian CNS. *Nat. Rev. Neurosci.* 4:703–713, 2003.

Fisher, M. Neuroprotection of acute ischemic stroke: where are we? *Neuroscientist* 5:392–401, 1999.

Gould, E., et al. Learning enhances adult neurogenesis in the hippocampal formation. *Nat. Neurosci.* 2:260–265, 1999.

Levin, B.E., et al. Widespread and lateralized effects of acute traumatic brain injury on norepinephrine turnover in the rat brain. *Brain Res.* 674:307–313, 1995.

Lindvall, O., et al. Neurotrophins and brain insults. *Trends Neurosci.* 17:490–496, 1994.

Lo, E.H. A new penumbra: transitioning from injury into repair after stroke. *Nat. Med.* 14:497–500, 2008.

Martinsson, L., Eksborg, S. Drugs for stroke recovery: the example of amphetamines. *Drugs Aging* 21:67–79, 2004.

Raisman, G., Li, Y. Repair of neural pathways by olfactory ensheathing cells. *Nat. Rev. Neurosci.* 8:312–319, 2007.

Samdani, A., et al. Nitric oxide synthase in models of focal ischemia. *Stroke* 28:1283–1288, 1997.

Sharp, F.R., et al. Molecular approaches to therapy of stroke. In: Martin, J.B. (Ed.), *Molecular neurobiology* (pp. 115–133). New York: Scientific American, Inc., 1998.

Wahlgren, N.G., Ahmed, N. Neuroprotection in cerebral ischaemia: facts and fancies the need for new approaches. *Cerebrovasc. Dis.* 17 (Suppl. 1):153–166, 2004.

Wictorin, K., et al. Reformation of long axon pathways in adult rat central nervous system by human forebrain neuroblasts. *Nature* 347:556–558, 1990.

Wieloch, T., Nikolich, K. Mechanisms of neural plasticity following brain injury. *Curr. Opin. Neurobiol.* 16:258–264, 2006.

Yepes, M., et al. Tissue-type plasminogen activator in the ischemic brain: more than a thrombolytic. *Trends Neurosci.* 32:48–55, 2008.

Neurogenesis and Axonal Regeneration

Aimone, J.B., et al. Computational influence of adult neurogenesis on memory encoding. *Neuron* 61:187–202, 2009.

Barnett, S.C., Riddell, J.S. Olfactory ensheathing cells (OECs) and the treatment of CNS injury: advantages and possible caveats. *J. Anat.* 204:57–67, 2004.

Dietz, V., Curt, A. Neurological aspects of spinal cord repair: promises and challenges. *Lancet Neurol.* 5:688–694, 2006.

Felling, R.J., Levison, S.W. Enhanced neurogenesis following stroke. *J. Neurosci. Res.* 73:277–283, 2003.

Ghashghaei, H.T., et al. Neuronal migration in the adult brain: are we there yet? *Nat. Rev. Neurosci.* 8:141–151, 2007.

Greenough, W.T., et al. New neurons in old brains: learning to survive? *Nat. Neurosci.* 2:203–205, 1999.

Ho, D.Y., Sapolsky, R.M. Gene therapy for the nervous system. *Sci. Am.* 276:96–100, 1997.

Li, Y., et al. TrkB regulates hippocampal neurogenesis and governs sensitivity to antidepressive treatment. *Neuron* 59:399–412, 2008.

Lledo, P.-M., et al. Adult neurogenesis and functional plasticity in neuronal circuits. *Nat. Rev. Neurosci.* 7:179–193, 2006.

Mackay-Sim, A., et al. Autologous olfactory ensheathing cell transplantation in human paraplegia: a 3 year clinical trial. *Brain* 131:2376–2386, 2008.

Olson, L. Regeneration in the adult central nervous system: experimental repair strategies. *Nat. Med.* 3:1329–1335, 1997.

Pettigrew, D.B., Crutcher K.A. White matter of the CNS support or inhibit neurite outgrowth *in vitro* depending on geometry. *J. Neurosci.* 19:8358–8366, 1999.

Svendsen, C.N., Smith A.G. New prospects for human stem-cell therapy in the nervous system. *Trends Neurosci.* 22:357–364, 1999.

Studies of Recovery in Humans and in Experimental Animals

Boyadjian, F.T., Devanne A.H. Motor cortex plasticity induced by extensive training revealed by transcranial magnetic stimulation. *Eur. J. Neurosci.* 21:259–266, 2005.

Bradbury, E.J., McMahon, S.B. Spinal cord repair strategies: why do they work? *Nat. Rev. Neurosci.* 7:744–753, 2006.

Brasted, P.J., et al. Associative plasticity in striatal transplants. *Proc. Natl. Acad. Sci. USA* 96:10524–10529, 1999.

Chouinard, P.A., et al. Changes in effective connectivity of the primary motor cortex in stroke patients after rehabilitative therapy. *Exp. Neurol.* 201:375–387, 2006.

Döbrössy, M.D., Dunnett, S.B. The influence of environment and experience on neural grafts. *Nat. Neurosci.* 2:871–879, 2001.

Doyon, J., Benali H. Reorganization and plasticity in the adult brain during learning of motor skills. *Curr. Opin. Neurobiol.* 15:161–167, 2005.

Edgerton, V.R., et al. Retraining the injured spinal cord. *J. Physiol.* 533:15–22, 2001.

Feeney, D.M., et al. Noradrenergic modulation of hemiplegia: facilitation and maintenance of recovery. *Restor. Neurol. Neurosci.* 22:175–190, 2004.

Fisher, C.M. Concerning the mechanism of recovery in stroke hemiplegia. *Can. J. Neurol. Sci.* 19:57–63, 1992.

Fries, W., et al. Motor recovery following capsular stroke: role of descending pathways from multiple motor areas. *Brain* 116:369–382, 1993.

Gauthier, L.V., et al. Remodeling the brain Plastic structural brain changes produced by different motor therapies after stroke. *Stroke* 39:1520–1525, 2009.

Gerloff, C., et al. Multimodal imaging of brain reorganization in motor areas of the contralesional hemisphere of well recovered patients after capsular stroke. *Brain* 129:791–808, 2006.

Goldberger, M.E., Murray, M. Recovery of movement and axonal sprouting may obey some of the same laws. In: Cotman, C.W. (Ed.), *Neuronal plasticity* (pp. 73–96). New York: Raven Press, 1978.

Johansen-Berg, H., et al. The role of the ipsilateral premotor cortex in hand movement after stroke. *Proc. Natl. Acad. Sci. USA* 99:14518–14523, 2002.

Jones, T.A., et al. Motor skills training enhances lesion-induced structural plasticity in the motor cortex of adult rats. *J. Neurosci.* 19:10153–10163, 1999.

Keller, A., et al. Formation of new synapses in the cat motor cortex following lesions of the deep cerebellar nuclei. *Exp. Brain Res.* 80:23–33, 1990.

Kolb, B., Whishaw I.Q. Brain plasticity and behavior. *Annu. Rev. Psychol.* 49:43–64, 1998.

Krakauer, J.W. Avoiding performance and task confounds: multimodal investigation of brain reorganization after stroke rehabilitation. *Exp. Neurol.* 204:491–495, 2007.

Lo, E.H., et al. Mechanisms, challenges and opportunities in stroke. *Nat. Rev. Neurosci.* 4:399–415, 2003.

Mackel, R. The role of the monkey sensory cortex in the recovery from cerebellar injury. *Exp. Brain Res.* 66:638–652, 1987.

Maier, I.C., et al. Constraint-induced movement therapy in the adult rat after unilateral corticospinal tract injury. *J. Neurosci.* 28:9386–9403, 2008.

Musso, M., et al. Training-induced brain plasticity in aphasia. *Brain* 122:1781–1790, 1999.

Nudo, R.J., et al. Role of adaptive plasticity in recovery of function after damage to motor cortex. *Muscle Nerve* 24:1000–1019, 2001.

Platz, T., et al. Motor learning after recovery from hemiparesis. *Neuropsychologia* 32:1209–1233, 1994.

Qureshi, A.I., et al. No evidence for an ischaemic penumbra in massive experimental intracerebral hemorrhage. *Neurology* 52:266–272, 1999.

Raineteau, O., Schwab, M.E. Plasticity of motor systems after incomplete spinal injury. *Nat. Rev. Neurosci.* 2:263–273, 2001.

Rijntjes, M. Mechanisms of recovery in stroke patients with hemiparesis or aphasia: new insights, old questions and the meaning of therapies. *Curr. Opin. Neurol.* 19:76–83, 2006.

Sanes, J.N., Donoghue, J.P. Plasticity and primary motor cortex. *Annu. Rev. Neurosci.* 23:393–415, 2000.

Schallert, T., Jones T.A. "Exuberant" neuronal growth after brain damage in adult rats: the essential role of behavioral experience. *J. Neural Transplant. Plast.* 4:193–198, 1993.

Schwab, J.M., et al. Experimental strategies to promote spinal cord regenerationan integrative perspective. *Prog. Neurobiol.* 78:91–116, 2006.

Stein, D.G. Brain injury and theories of recovery. In: Armonk, G.L. (Ed.): *Restorative neurology: advances in pharmacology for recovery after stroke* (pp. 1–34). Elmsford, NY: Futura, 1998.

Taub, E., et al. New treatments in neurorehabilitation founded on basis research. *Nat. Rev. Neurosci.* 3:228–236, 2002.

Taub, E., et al. Constraint-induced movement therapy: answers and questions after two decades of research. *NeuroRehab.* 21:93–95, 2006.

Vidal, P.P., et al. Vestibular compensation revisited. *Otolaryngol. Head Neck Surg.* 119:34–42, 1998.

Weiller, C., et al. Individual patterns of functional reorganization in the human cerebral cortex after capsular infarction. *Ann. Neurol.* 33:181–189, 1993.

Whitall, J. Stroke rehabilitation: time to answer more specific questions? *Neurorehabil. Neural Repair* 18:3–8, 2004.

Zeki, S. *A vision of the brain.* Oxford: Blackwell, 1993.

Restitution after Early Brain Damage

Bachevalier, J., Vargha-Khadem, F. The primate hippocampus: ontogeny, early insult and memory. *Curr. Opin. Neurobiol.* 15:168–174, 2005.

Balantyne, A.O., et al. Plasticity in the developing brain: intellectual, language and academic functions in children with ischaemic perinatal stroke. *Brain* 131:2975–2985, 2008.

Büchel, C., et al. Different activation patterns in the visual cortex of late and congenitally blind subjects. *Brain* 121:409–441, 1998.

Collignon, O., et al. Cross-modal plasticity for the spatial processing of sounds in visually deprived subjects. *Exp. Brain Res.* 192:343–358, 2009.

Eyre, J.A. Corticospinal tract development and its plasticity after perinatal injury. *Neurosci. Biobehav. Rev.* 31:1136–1149, 2007.

Friel, K.M., Martin, J.H. Bilateral activity-dependent interactions in the developing corticospinal system. *J. Neurosci.* 27:11083–11090, 2007.

Johnston, M.V. Clinical disorders of brain plasticity. *Brain Dev.* 26:73–80. 2004.

Martin, J.H., et al. Corticospinal development. In: Squire, L. (Ed.), *Encyclopedia of neuroscience* (pp. 203–214). Philadelphia: Elsevier, 2009.

Salimi, I., et al. Pyramidal tract stimulation restores normal corticospinal tract connections and visuomotor skill after early postnatal motor cortex activity blockade. *J. Neurosci.* 28:7426–7434, 2008.

Staudt, M., et al. Reorganization in congenital hemiparesis acquired at different gestational ages. *Ann. Neurol.* 56:854–863, 2004.

Stiles, J., et al. Cognitive development following early brain injury: evidence for neural adaptation. *Trends Cogn. Sci.* 9:136–143, 2005.

Trauner, D.A., et al. Behavioural profiles of children and adolescents after pre- or perinatal unilateral brain damage. *Brain* 124: 995–1002, 2001.

Vharga-Kadem. F., et al. Onset of speech after left hemispherectomy in a nine-year-old boy. *Brain* 120:159–182, 1997.

Villablanca, J.R., Hovda D.A. Developmental neuroplasticity in a model of cerebral hemispherectomy and stroke. *Neuroscience* 95:625–637, 2000.

CHAPTER 12: SENSORY RECEPTORS IN GENERAL

Anderson, D.J. Lineages and transcription factors in the specification of vertebrate primary sensory neurons. *Curr. Opin. Neurobiol.* 9:517–524, 1999.

Cahusac, P.M.B., Noyce, R. A pharmacological study of slowly adapting mechanoreceptors responsive to cold thermal stimulation. *Neuroscience* 148:489–500, 2007.

Cesare, P., et al. Ion channels gated by heat. *Proc. Natl. Acad. Sci. USA* 96:7658–7663, 1999.

Christensen, A.P., Corey, D.P. TRP channels in mechanosensation: direct or indirect activation? *Nat. Rev. Neurosci.* 8:510–521, 2007.

de Lafuente, Romo, V.R.: Neuronal correlates of subjective sensory experience. *Nat. Rev. Neurosci.* 8:1698–1703, 2005.

Gilbert, C.D. Plasticity in visual perception and physiology. *Curr. Opin. Neurobiol.* 6:269–274, 1996.

Gray, J. How are qualia coupled to functions? *Trends Cogn. Sci.* 7:192–194, 2003.

Hamill, O.P., McBride, D.W., Jr. The cloning of a mechano-gated membrane ion channel. *Trends Neurosci.* 17:439–443, 1994.

Koutalos, Y., Yau, K.-W. A rich complexity emerges in phototransduction. *Curr. Opin. Neurobiol.* 3:513–519, 1993.

Nielsen, K.J., Callaway, E.M. More than a feeling: sensation from cortical stimulation. *Nat. Rev. Neurosci.* 11:10–12, 2008.

Nilius, B., et al. Transient receptor potential cation channels in disease. *Physiol. Rev.* 165–217, 2007.

Parker, A.J., Newsome, W.T. Sense and the single neuron: probing the physiology of perception. *Annu. Rev. Neurosci.* 21:227–277, 1998.

Pedersen, S.F., et al. TRP channels: an overview. *Cell Calcium* 38:233–252, 2005.

Stock, J., et al. Chemosensing and signal transduction in bacteria. *Curr. Opin. Neurobiol.* 4:474–480, 1994.

Talavera, K., et al. Neuronal TRP channels: thermometers, pathfinders and life-savers. *Trends Neurosci.* 31:287–295, 2008.

CHAPTER 13: PERIPHERAL PARTS OF THE SOMATOSENSORY SYSTEM

Nociceptors and Thermoreceptors

Aley, K.O., et al. Nitric oxide signaling in pain and nociceptor sensitization in the rat. *J. Neurosci.* 18:7008–7014, 1998.

Bandel, M., et al. From chills to chilis: mechanisms for thermosensation and chemosthesis via thermo TRPs. *Curr. Opin. Neurobiol.* 17:490–497, 2007.

Belmonte, C., Viana, F. Nociceptor responses. In: Squire, L. (Ed.), *Encyclopedia of neuroscience* (pp. 1191–1198). Philadelphia: Elsevier, 2009.

Benarroch, E.E. Sodium channels and pain. *Neurology* 68:233–236, 2007.

Bjurholm, A., et al. Noradrenergic and peptidergic nerves in the synovial membrane of the Sprague-Dawley rat. *Arthritis Rheum.* 33:859–865, 1990.

Bove, G.M., Light A.L. Unmyelinated nociceptors of rat paraspinal tissue. *J. Neurosphysiol.* 73:1752–1762, 1995.

Caterina, M.J., Julius, D. Sense and specificity: a molecular identity for nociceptors. *Curr. Opin. Neurobiol.* 9:525–530, 1999.

Catteral, W.A., Yu, F.H. Painful channels. *Neuron* 52:743–749, 2006.

Cox, J.J., et al. An *SCN9A* channelopathy causes congenital inability to experience pain. *Nature* 444:894–898, 2006.

Cummins, T.R., et al. The roles of sodium channels in nociception: Implications for mechanisms of pain. *Pain* 131:243–257, 2007.

Gibson, W., et al. Referred pain and hyperalgesia in human tendon and muscle belly tissue. *Pain* 120:113–123, 2006.

Giles, L.G.F., Harvey, A.R. Immunohistochemical demonstration of nociceptors in the capsule and synovial folds of human zygoapophyseal joints. *Br. J. Rheumatol.* 26:362–364, 1987.

Graven-Nielsen, T., Mense, S. The peripheral apparatus of muscle pain: evidence from animal and human studies. *Clin. J. Pain* 17:2–10, 2001.

Guieu, R., Serratrice, G. Identifying the afferents involved in movement-induced pain alleviation in man. *Brain* 115:1073–1079, 1992.

Julius, D., Basbaum, A.I. Molecular mechanisms of nociception. *Nature* 413:203–10, 2001.

Lewin, G.R., et al. A plethora of painful molecules. *Curr. Opin. Neurobiol.* 14:443–449, 2004.

Light, A.R., et al. Dorsal root ganglion neurons innervating skeletal muscle respond to physiological combinations of protons, ATP, and lactate mediated by ASIC, P2X, and TRPV1. *J. Neurophysiol.* 100:1184–1201, 2008.

Momin, A., Wood, J.N. Sensory neuron voltage-gated sodium channels as analgesic drug targets. *Curr. Opin. Neurobiol.* 18:283–388, 2008.

Patapoutian, A., et al. ThermoTRP channels of temperature sensation. *Nat. Rev. Neurosci.* 4:529–539, 2003.

Paus, R., et al. Frontiers in pruritus research: scratching the brain for more effective itch therapy. *J. Clin. Invest.* 116:1174–1185, 2006.

Pethö, G., et al. Bradykinin-induced nociceptor sensitization to heat is mediated by cyclooxygenase products in isolated rat skin. *Eur. J. Neurosci.* 14:210–218, 2001.

Schmidt, R., et al. Novel classes of responsive and unresponsive C nociceptors in human skin. *J. Neurosci.* 15:333–341, 1995.

Schmidt, R., et al. Innervation territories of mechanically activated C nociceptors units in human skin. *J. Neuropshysiol.* 78:2641–2648, 1997.

Simone, D.A., et al. Identification of muscle afferents subserving sensation of deep pain in humans. *J. Neurophysiol.* 72:883–889, 1994.

Snider, W.D., McMahon, S.B. Tackling pain at the source: new ideas about nociceptors. *Neuron* 20:629–632, 1998.

Steen, K.H., et al. A dominant role of acid pH in inflammatory excitation and sensitization of nociceptors in rat skin, *in vitro*. *J. Neurosci.* 15:3982–3989, 1995.

Tai, C., et al. TRPA1: The central molecule for chemical sensing in pain pathway? *J. Neurosci.* 28:1019–1021, 2008.

Wong, G.F., Gavva, N.R. Therapeutic potential of vanilloid receptor TRPV1 agonists and antagonists as analgesics: recent advances and setbacks. *Brain Res. Rev.* doi:10.1016, 2009.

Woolf, C.J., Ma, Q. Nociceptors—noxious stimulus detectors. *Neuron* 55:353–364, 2007.

Low-Threshold Cutaneous Receptors

Birznieks, I., et al. Encoding of direction of fingertip forces by human tactile afferents. *J. Neurosci.* 21:8222–8237, 2001.

Macefield, G., et al. Perceptual responses to microstimulation of single afferents innervating joints, muscle and skin of the human hand. *J. Physiol.* 429:113–129, 1990.

Olausson, H., et al. Unmyelinated tactile afferents signal touch and project to insular cortex. *Nat. Rev. Neurosci.* 5:900–904, 2002.

Olausson, H., et al. Functional role of unmyelinated tactile afferents in human hairy skin: sympathetic response and perceptual localization. *Exp. Brain Res.* 184:135–140, 2008.

Torebjörk, H.E., et al. Intraneural microstimulation in man: its relation to specificity of tactile sensations. *Brain* 110:1509–1529, 1987.

Vallbo, Å.B., Johansson, R.S. The tactile sensory innervation of the glabrous skin of the human hand. In: Gordon, G. (Ed.), *Active touch. A multi-disciplinary approach* (pp. 29–54). Oxford: Pergamon Press, 1978.

Vallbo, Å.B., et al. Somatosensory, proprioceptive and autonomic activity in human peripheral nerves. *Physiol. Rev.* 59:919–957, 1979.

Witney, A.G., et al. The cutaneous contribution to adaptive precision grip. *Trends Neurosci.* 27:637–643, 2004.

Zelena, J. *Nerves and mechanoreceptors.* New York: Chapman & Hall, 1994.

Proprioceptors

Banks, R.W. An allometric analysis of the number of muscle spindles in mammalian skeletal muscles. *J. Anat.* 203:753–768, 2006.

Bloem, B.R., et al. Triggering of balance corrections and compensatory strategies in a patient with total leg proprioceptive poss. *Exp. Brain Res.* 142:91–107, 2002.

Cao, D.-Y., et al. Position sensitivity of feline paraspinal muscle spindles to vertebral movement in the lumbar spine. *J. Neurophysiol.* 101:1722–1729, 2009.

Cooper, S. Muscle spindles and motor units. In: Andrew B.L. (Ed.), *Control and innervation of skeletal muscle* (pp. 9–15). New York: Churchill Livingstone, 1966.

Gandevia, S.C. Kinaesthesia: roles of afferent signals and motor commands. In: Rowell, A.L. (Ed.), *Integration of motor, circulatory, respiratory and metabolic control during exercise* (pp. 128–172). Australian Physiological Society, 1996.

Hasan, Z., Stuart, D.G. Animal solutions to problems of movement control: the role of proprioceptors. *Annu. Rev. Neurosci.* 11:199–223, 1988.

Illert, M., et al. Beta innervation and recurrent inhibition: a hypothesis for manipulatory and postural control. *Eur. J. Physiol.* 432:R61–67, 1996.

Kellgren, J.H., Samuel E.P. The sensitivity and innervation of the articular capsule. *J. Bone Joint Surg.* 32:84–92, 1950.

Kokkorogiannis, T. Somatic and intramuscular distribution of muscle spindles and their relation to muscular angiotypes. *J. Theor. Biol.* 229:263–280, 2004.

Matthews, P.B.C. Evolving views on the internal operation and functional role of the muscle spindle. *J. Physiol.* 320:1–30, 1964.

Matthews, P.B.C. Muscle spindles and their motor control. *Physiol. Rev.* 44:219–288, 1981.

McCloskey, I., et al. Sensory effects of pulling or vibrating tendons in man. *Brain* 106:21–37, 1983.

Proske, U. Kinesthesia: the role of muscle receptors. *Muscle Nerve* 34:545–558, 2006.

Proske, U., et al. The role of muscle receptors in the detection of movements. *Prog. Neurobiol.* 60:85–96, 2000.

Refshauge, K.M., et al. Movement detection at the distal joint of the human thumb and fingers. *Exp. Brain Res.* 122:85–92, 1998.

Rothwell, J.C., et al. Manual motor performance in a deafferented man. *Brain* 105:515–542, 1982.

Sacks, O. The man who mistook his wife for a hat. New York: Picador, 1986.

Sanes, J.N., Shadmehr, R. Sense of muscular effort and somesthetic afferent information in humans. *Can. J. Physiol. Pharmacol.* 73:223–233, 1995.

Voss, H. Tabelle der absoluten und relativen Muskelspindelzahlen der menschlichen Skelettmuskulatur. *Anat. Anz.* 129:562–572, 1971.

Primary Sensory Neurons and the Dorsal Roots

Amaya, F., et al. Periganglionic inflammation elicits a distally radiating pain hypersensitivity by promoting COX-2 induction in the dorsal root ganglion. *Pain* 142:59–67, 2009.

Brain, S.D. Sensory neuropeptides: their role in inflammation and wound healing. *Immunopharmacology* 37:133–152, 1997.

Broman, J. Neurotransmitters in subcortical sensory pathways. *Anat. Embryol.* 189:181–214, 1994.

Brown, A.G. Organization in the spinal cord: the anatomy and physiology of identified neurones. New York: Springer-Verlag, 1981.

Coggeshall, R.E., Carlton, S.M. Receptor localization in the mammalian dorsal horn and primary afferent neurons. *Brain Res. Rev.* 24:28–66, 1997.

Foerster, O. The dermatomes in man. *Brain* 56:1–40, 1933.

Head, H. *Studies in neurology.* 2 vols. New York: Oxford University Press, 1920.

Honor, P., et al. Spinal substance P receptor expression and internalization in acute, short-term, and long-term inflammatory pain states. *J. Neurosci.* 19:7670–7678, 1999.

Howe, J.F., et al. Mechanosensitivity of dorsal root ganglia and chronically injured axons: a physiological basis for the radicular pain of nerve root compression. *Pain* 3:25–41, 1977.

Keegan, J.J., Garret F.D. The segmental distribution of cutaneous nerves in the limbs of man. *Anat. Rec.* 102:409–437, 1948.

Kraneveld, A.D., et al. Airway hyperresponsiveness: first eosinophils and then neuropeptides. *Int. J. Immunopharmacol.* 19:517–527, 1997.

Levine, J.D., et al. Peptides and the primary afferent nociceptor. *J. Neurosci.* 13:2273–2286, 1993.

Liguori, R., et al. Determination of the segmental sensory and motor innervation of the lumbosacral spinal nerves: an electrophysiological study. *Brain* 115:915–934, 1992.

Nakatsuka, T., Gu, J.G. P2X purinoceptors and sensory transmission. *Pflügers Arch. Eur. J. Physiol. (Lond.)* 452:598–607, 2006.

Sherrington, C.S. Experiments in examination of the peripheral distribution of the fibres of the posterior roots of some spinal nerves. Part II. *Philos. Trans. Roy. Soc., Lond. B* 190:45–186, 1898.

Waxman, S.G. Sodium channels, excitability of primary sensory neurons, and the molecular basis of pain. *Muscle Nerve* 22:1177–1187, 1999.

Wiesenfeld-Hallin, Z., Xu, X.J. Galanin in somatosensory function. *Ann. NY Acad. Sci.* 863:383–389, 1998.

Zhang, X., Bao L. The development and modulation of nociceptive circuitry. *Curr. Opin. Neurobiol.* 16:460–466, 2006.

CHAPTER 14: CENTRAL PARTS OF THE SOMATOSENSORY SYSTEM

The Spinal Cord and Sensory Pathways

Al-Chaer, E.D., et al. Comparative study of viscerosomatic input onto postsynaptic dorsal column and spinothalamic tract neurons in the primate. *J. Neurophysiol.* 82:1876–1882, 1999.

Andrew, D., Craig, A.D. Spinothalamic lamina I neurons selectively sensitive to histamine: a central neural pathway for itch. *Nat. Rev. Neurosci.* 4:72–77, 2001.

Apkarian, A.V., Hodges, C.J. Primate spinothalamic pathways: I. A quantitative study of the cells of origin of the spinothalamic pathway. *J. Comp.Neurol.* 288:447–473, 1989.

Apkarian, A.V., Hodges, C.J. Primate spinothalamic pathways: III. Thalamic terminations of the dorsolateral and ventral spinothalamic pathways. *J. Comp. Neurol.* 288:493–511, 1989.

Bagley, C.A., et al. Psychophysics of CNS pain-related activity: binary and analog channels and memory encoding. *Neuroscientist* 12:29–42, 2006.

Berkley, K., Hubscher, C.H. Are there separate central nervous system pathways for touch and pain? *Nat. Med.* 1:766–773, 1995.

Bester, H., et al. Physiological properties of the lamina I spinoparabrachial neurons in the rat. *J. Neurophysiol.* 83:2239–2259, 2000.

Blomqvist, A., et al. Cytoarchitectonic and immunohistochemical characterization of a specific pain and temperature relay, the posterior portion of the ventral medial nucleus, in the human thalamus. *Brain* 123:601–619, 2000.

Bourgeais, L., et al. Projections from the nociceptive area of the central nucleus of the amygdala to the forebrain: a PHA-L study in the rat. *Eur. J. Neurosci.* 14:229–255, 2001.

Cohen, L.G., Starr, A. Localization, timing and specificity of gating of somatosensory evoked potentials during active movement in man. *Brain* 110:451–467, 1987.

Cooper, B.Y., et al. Finger movement deficits in the stumptail macaque following lesions if the fasciculus cuneatus. *Somatosens. Mot. Res.* 10:17–29, 1993.

Craig, A.D., et al. A thalamic nucleus specific for pain and temperature sensation. *Nature* 372:770–773, 1994.

Cullen, K.E. Sensory signals during active versus passive movement. *Curr. Opin. Neurobiol.* 14:698–706, 2004.

Danziger, N., et al. A clinical and neurophysiological study of a patient with an extensive transection of the spinal cord sparing only a part of the anterolateral quadrant. *Brain* 119:1835–1848, 1996.

Dougherty, P.M., et al. Combined application of excitatory amino acids and substance P produces long-lasting changes in responses of primate spinothalamic tract neurons. *Brain Res. Rev.* 18: 227–246, 1993.

Fanselow, E.A., Nicolelis, M.A.L. Behavioral modulation of tactile responses in the rat somatosensory system. *J. Neurosci.* 19:7603–7616, 1999.

Giesler, G.J., et al. Direct spinal pathways to the limbic system for nociceptive information. *Trends Neurosci.* 17:244–250, 1994.

Glendenning, D.S., Vierck, C.J., Jr. Lack of proprioceptive deficit after dorsal column lesions in monkeys. *Neurology* 43:363–366, 1993.

Gordon, G. Active touch: the mechanism of recognition of objects by manipulation—a multi-disciplinary approach. Oxford: Pergamon Press, 1978.

Graziano, A., Jones, E.G. Widespread thalamic terminations of fibers arising in the superficial medullary dorsal horn of monkeys and their relation to calbindin immunoreactivity. *J. Neurosci.* 24:248–256, 2004.

Groenewegen, H.J., Berendse, H.W. The specificity of the "nonspecific" midline and intralaminar thalamic nuclei. *Trends Neurosci.* 17:52–57, 1994.

Han, Z.-S., et al. Nociceptive and thermoceptive lamina I neurons are anatomically distinct. *Nat. Rev. Neurosci.* 1:218–224, 1998.

Klop, E.M., et al. In cat four times as many lamina I neurons project to the parabrachial nuclei and twice as many to the periaqueductal gray as to the thalamus. *Neuroscience* 134:189–197, 2005.

Kohama, I., et al. Synaptic reorganization in the substantia gelatinosa after peripheral nerve neuroma formation: aberrant innervation of lamina II neurons by A*b* afferents. *J. Neurosci.* 20:1538–1539, 2000.

Lenz, F.A., et al. Stimulation in the human somatosensory thalamus can reproduce both the affective and sensory dimensions of previously experienced pain. *Nat. Med.* 1:910–913, 1995.

Macchi, G., et al. *Somatosensory integration in the thalamus.* Philadelphia: Elsevier, 1990.

Marple-Horvath, D.E., Armstrong D.M. Central regulation of motor cortex neuronal responses to forelimb nerve inputs during precision walking in the cat. *J. Physiol.* 519:279–299, 1999.

Mayer, D.J., et al. Neurophysiological characterization of the anterolateral spinal cord neurons contributing to pain perception in man. *Pain* 1:51–58, 1975.

Monconduit, L., et al. Convergence of cutaneous, muscular and visceral noxious inputs onto ventromedial thalamic neurons in the rat. *Pain* 103:83–91, 2003.

Nathan, P.W., et al. Sensory effects in man of lesions of the posterior columns and of some other afferent pathways. *Brain* 109:1003–1041, 1986.

Ralston, H.J., Ralston, D.D. Medial lemniscal and spinal projections to the macaque thalamus: an electron microscopic study of differing GABAergic circuitry serving thalamic somatosensory mechanisms. *J. Neurosci.* 14:2485–2502, 1994.

Seki, K., et al. Sensory input to primate spinal cord is presynaptically inhibited during voluntary movement. *Nat. Rev. Neurosci.* 6: 1309–1316, 2003.

Todd, A.J., Spike, R.C. The localization of classical transmitters and neuropeptides within neurons in laminae I–III of the mammalian spinal dorsal horn. *Prog. Neurobiol.* 41:609–645, 1993.

Urban, L., et al. Modulation of spinal excitability: co-operation between neurokinin and excitatory amino acid neurotransmitters. *Trends Neurosci.* 17:432–438, 1994.

Vierck, C.J., Jr., Cooper, B.Y. Cutaneous texture discrimination following transection of the dorsal spinal column in monkeys. *Somatosens. Mot. Res.* 15:309–315, 1998.

Voss, M., et al. Sensorimotor attenuation by central motor command signals in the absence of movement. *Nat. Rev. Neurosci.* 9: 26–227, 2006.

Willis, W.D., et al. A visceral pain pathway in the dorsal column of the spinal cord. *Proc. Natl. Acad. Sci. USA* 96:7675–7679, 1999.

Windhorst, U. Muscle proprioceptive feedback and spinal networks. *Brain Res. Bull.* 73:155–202, 2007.

Somatosensory Cortical Areas

Afif, A., et al. Middle short gyrus of the insula implicated in pain processing. *Pain* 138:546–555, 2008.

Blakemore, S.-J., et al. Central cancellation of self-produced tickle sensation. *Nat. Rev. Neurosci.* 1:635–640, 1998.

Bourgeais, L., et al. Parabrachial internal lateral neurons convey nociceptive messages from the deep laminas of the dorsal horn to the intralaminar thalamus. *J. Neurosci.* 21:2159–2165, 2001.

Burton, H., et al. Cortical areas within the lateral sulcus connected to cutaneous representations in areas 3b and 1: a revised interpretation of the second somatosensory area in macaque monkeys. *J. Comp. Neurol.* 355:539–562, 1995.

Bushnell, M.C., et al. Pain perception: is there a role for primary somatosensory cortex? *Proc. Natl. Acad. Sci. USA* 96:7705–7709, 1999.

Caselli, R. Ventrolateral and dorsomedial somatosensory association cortex damage produces distinct somesthetic syndromes in humans. *Neurology* 43:762–771, 1993.

Craig, A.D. How do you feel? Interoception: the sense of the physiological condition of the body. *Nat. Rev. Neurosci.* 3:655–666, 2002.

Darian-Smith, D., et al. Ipsilateral cortical projections to area 3a, 3b, and 4 in the macaque monkey. *J. Comp. Neurol.* 335:200–213, 1993.

Gehring, W.J., Taylor, S.F. When the going gets tough, the cingulated gets going. *Nat. Rev. Neurosci.* 7:1285–1287, 2004.

Hari, R., et al. Functional organization of the human first and second somatosensory cortices: a neuromagnetic study. *Eur. J. Neurosci.* 5:724–734, 1993.

Henderson, L.A., et al. Somatotopic organization of processing of muscle and cutaneous pain in the left right insula cortex: a single-trial fMRI study. *Pain* 128:20–30, 2007.

Kell, C.A., et al. The sensory cortical prepresentation of the human penis: revisiting somatotopy in the male homunculus. *J. Neurosci.* 25:5984–5987, 2005.

Lee, S.-H., et al. Motor modulation of afferent somatosensory circuits. *Nat. Rev. Neurosci.* 11:1430–1438, 2008.

Nicolelis, M.A.L., et al. Simultaneous encoding of tactile information by three primate cortical areas. *Nat. Med.* 1:621–630, 1998.

Pavlides, C., et al. Projection from the sensory to the motor cortex is important in learning motor skills in the monkey. *J. Neurophysiol.* 70:733–741, 1993.

Penfield, W., Rasmussen, T. *The cerebral cortex of man.* New York: Macmillan, 1950.

Ploner, M., et al. Differential organization of touch and pain in human primary somatosensory cortex. *J. Neurophysiol.* 83:1770–1776, 2000.

Ploner, M., et al. Cortical representation of first and second pain sensations in humans. *Proc. Natl. Acad. Sci. USA* 99:12444–12448, 2002.

Rainville, P., et al. Pain affect encoded in human anterior cingulate but not somatosensory cortex. *Science* 277 968–971, 1997.

Reed, J.L., et al. Widespread spatial integration in primary somatosensory cortex. *Proc. NY Acad. Sci.* 105 10233–10237, 2008.

Rosetti, Y., et al. Visually guided reaching: bilateral posterior parietal lesions cause a switch from fast visuomotor to slow cognitive control. *Neuropsychologia* 43:162–173, 2005.

Schneider, R.J. A modality-specific somatosensory area within the insula of the rhesus monkey. *Brain Res.* 621:116–120, 1993.

Tracey, I., Mantyh, P.W. The cerebral signature for pain perception and its modulation. *Neuron* 55:377–391, 2007.

Van Buren, J.M. Sensory responses from stimulation of the inferior Rolandic and Sylvian regions in man. *J. Neurosurg.* 59:119–130, 1983.

Woolsey, C.N. Organization of somatic sensory and motor areas of the cerebral cortex. In: Harlow, H.F. Woolsey, C.N. (Eds.), *Biological and biochemical bases of behavior* (pp. 63–81). Madison, WI: University of Wisconsin Press, 1958.

CHAPTER 15: PAIN

Apkarian, A.V. Pain perception in relation to emotional learning. *Curr. Opin. Neurobiol.* 18:464–468, 2008.

Baranauskus, G., Nistri, A. Sensitization of pain pathways in the spinal cord: cellular mechanisms. *Prog. Neurobiol.* 54:349–365, 1998.

Behbehani, M.M. Functional characteristics of the midbrain periaqueductal gray. *Prog. Neurobiol.* 46:575–605, 1995.

Brand, P., Yancey, P. *Pain: the gift nobody wants.* New York: Harper-Collins, 1993.

Brownstein, M.J. A brief history of opiates, opioid peptides, and opioid receptors. *Proc. Natl. Acad. Sci. USA* 90:5391–5393, 1993.

Carlsson, K., et al. Predictability modulates the affective and sensory-discriminative neural processing of pain. *NeuroImage* 32:1804–1814, 2006.

Carrive, P. The periaqueductal gray and defensive behavior: functional representation and neuronal organization. *Behav. Brain Res.* 58:27–47, 1993.

Casey, K.L. Forebrain mechanisms of nociception and pain: analysis through imaging. *Proc. Natl. Acad. Sci. USA* 96:7668–7674, 1999.

Cerevero, F., Laird, J.M.A. Mechanisms of touch-evoked pain (allodynia): a new model. *Pain* 68:13–23, 1996.

Coderre, T.J., Katz, J. Peripheral and central hyperexcitability: differential signs and symptoms in persistent pain. *Behav. Brain Sci.* 20:404–419, 1997.

Danziger, N., et al. Can we share a pain we never felt? Neural correlates of empathy in patients with congenital insensitivity to pain. *Neuron* 61:203–212, 2009.

Eisenberg, N.I., Lieberman, M.D. Why rejection hurts: a common neural alarm system for physical and social pain. *Trends Cogn. Sci.* 8:294–300, 2004.

Fields, H. State-dependent opioid control of pain. *Nat. Rev. Neurosci.* 5:565–575, 2004.

Gamsa, A. The role of psychological factors in chronic pain. II. A critical appraisal. *Pain* 57:17–29, 1994.

Gear, R.W., et al. Pain-induced analgesia mediated by mesolimbic reward circuits. *J. Neurosci.* 19:7175–7181, 1999.

Guieu, R., et al. Nociceptive threshold and physical activity. *Can. J. Neurol. Sci.* 19:69–71, 1992.

Gybels, J.M., Sweet, W.H. Neurosurgical treatment of persistent pain: physiological and pathological mechanisms of human pain. Basel: Karger, 1989.

Hardcastle, V.G. *The myth of pain.* Cambridge, MA: MIT Press, 1999.

Harris, J. Cortical origin of pathological pain. *Lancet* 354:1464–1466, 1999.

Iadarola, M.J., et al. Neural activation during acute capsaicin-evoked pain and allodynia assessed with PET. *Brain* 121:931–947, 1998.

Keltner, J.R. Isolating the modulatory effects of expectation on pain transmission: a functional magnetic resonance study. *J. Neurosci.* 26:4437–4443, 2006.

Kieffer, B.L. Opioids: first lessons from knockout mice. *Trends Pharmacol. Sci.* 20:19–26, 1999.

Lai, J., et al. The role of voltage-gated sodium channels in neuropathic pain. *Curr. Opin. Neurobiol.* 13:291–297, 2003.

Leknes, S., Tracey, I. A common neurobiology for pain and pleasure. *Nat. Rev. Neurosci.* 9:314–320, 2008.

Mason, P. Central mechanisms of pain modulation. *Curr. Opin. Neurobiol.* 9:436–441, 1999.

McCabe, C., et al. Don't look now! Pain and attention. *Clin. Med.* 5:482–486, 2005.

McCabe, C., et al. Simulating sensory-motor incongruence in healthy volunteers: implications for a cortical model of pain. *Rheumatology* 44:509–516, 2005.

Melzack, R., Wall, P.D. Pain mechanisms: a new theory. *Science* 150:971–979, 1965.

Melzack, R., Wall, P.D. Acute pain in an emergency clinic: latency of onset and descriptor patterns related to different injuries. *Pain* 14:33–43, 1982.

Mense, S. Nociception from skeletal muscle in relation to clinical muscle pain. *Pain* 54:241–289, 1993.

Mogil, J.S., et al. Pain genes? Natural variation and transgenic mutants. *Annu. Rev. Neurosci.* 23:777–811, 2000.

Moseley, G.L., Arntz, A. The context of a noxious stimulus affects the pain it evokes. *Pain* 133:64–71, 2007.

Padawer, W.J., Levine, F.M. Exercise-induced analgesia: fact or artifact? *Pain* 48:131–135, 1992.

Porro, C.A., et al. Temporal intensity coding of pain in human cortex. *J. Neurophysiol.* 80:3312–3320, 1998.

Ramachandran, V.S., Blakeslee, S. *Phantoms in the brain. Probing the mysteries of the human mind.* New York: William Morrow, 1998.

Reynolds, D.V. Surgery in the rat during electrical analgesia induced by focal brain stimulation. *Science* 164:444–445, 1969.

Sacks, O. *A leg to stand on.* New York; Picador, 1994.

Schaible, H.-G., Grubb, B.D. Afferent and spinal mechanisms of joint pain. *Pain* 55:5–54, 1993.

Stux, G., Pomeranz, B. *Basics of acupuncture*, 3rd ed. New York: Springer-Verlag, 1995.

Urban, M.O., Gebhart, G.F. Supraspinal contributions to hyperalgesia. *Proc. Natl. Acad. Sci. USA* 96:7687–7692, 1999.

Vanegas, H., Schaible H.-G. Descending control of persistent pain: inhibitory or facilitatory? *Brain Res. Rev.* 46:295–309, 2004.

Vogt, B.A. Pain and emotion interactions in subregions of the cingulate gyrus. *Nat. Rev. Neurosci.* 6:533–544, 2005.

Wang, S.-M., et al. Acupuncture analgesia: I. The scientific basis. *Pain Med.* 106:602–610, 2008.

Wolf, C.J., et al. Towards a mechanism-based classification of pain? *Pain* 77:227–229, 1998.

Chronic Pain Conditions (CRPS and Others)

Apkarian, A.V., et al. Towards a theory of chronic pain. *Prog. Neurobiol.* 87:81–97, 2009.

Baliki, M.N., et al. Beyond feeling: chronic pain hurts the brain, disrupting the default mode network dynamics. *J. Neurosci.* 28:1398–1403, 2008.

Baron, R., et al. Causalgia and reflex sympathetic dystrophy: does the sympathetic nervous system contribute to the generation of pain? *Muscle Nerve* 22:678–695, 1999.

Blumberg, H., et al. Sympathetic nervous system and pain: a clinical reappraisal. *Behav. Brain Sci.* 20:426–434, 1997.

Fields, H.L., et al. Postherpetic neuralgia: irritable nociceptors and deafferentation. *Neurobiol. Dis.* 5:209–227, 1998.

Flor, H., et al. Extensive reorganization of primary somatosensory cortex in chronic back pain patients. *Neurosci. Lett.* 224:5–8, 1997.

Geha, P.Y., et al. The brain in chronic CRPS pain: abnormal gray-white matter interactions in emotional and autonomic regions. *Neuron* 60:570–581, 2008.

Giummarra, M.J., et al. Central mechanisms in phantom limb perception: the past, present and future. *Brain Res. Rev.* 54:219–232, 2007.

Jänig, W., Baron, R. Complex regional pain syndrome: mystery explained? *Lancet Neurology* 2:687–697, 2003.

Jänig, W., Baron, R. Is CRPS I a neuropathic pain syndrome? *Pain* 120:227–229, 2006.

Lewis, J.S., et al. Body perception disturbance: a contribution to pain in complex regional pain syndrome (CRPS). *Pain* 133:111–119, 2007.

Loeser, J.D., Treede, R.-D. The Kyoto protocol of IASP basic pain terminology. *Pain* 137:437–477, 2008.

Maihöfner, C., et al. Cortical reorganization during recovery from complex regional pain syndrome. *Neurology* 63:693–701, 2004.

May, A. Chronic pain may change the structure of the brain. *Pain* 137:7–15, 2008.

Moisset, X., Bouhassira, D. Brain imaging of neuropathic pain. *NeuroImage* 27:S80–S88, 2007.

Perl, E.R. Causalgia, pathological pain, and adrenergic receptors. *Proc. Natl. Acad. Sci. USA* 96:7664–7667, 1999.

Peyron, R., et al. Parietal and cingulate processes in central pain: a combined positron emission tomography (PET) and functional magnetic resonance imaging (fMRI) study of an unusual case. *Pain* 84:77–87, 2000.

Schott, G.D. Complex? Regional? Pain? Syndrome? *Pract. Neurol.* 7:145–157, 2007.

Schweinhardt, P., et al. Fibromyalgia: a disorder of the brain? *Neuroscientist* 14:415–421, 2008.

Stanton-Hicks, M., et al. Reflex sympathetic dystrophy: changing concepts and taxonomy. *Pain* 63: 127–133, 1995.

Tsao, H., et al. Reorganization of the motor cortex is associated with postural control deficits in recurrent low back pain. *Brain* 131:2161–2171, 2008.

Yezierski, R.P. Pain following spinal cord injury: the clinical problem and experimental studies. *Pain* 68:185–194, 1996.

Placebo and Nocebo

Amanzio, M., Benedetti, F. Neuropharmacological dissection of placebo analgesia: expectation-activated opioid systems versus conditioning-activated specific subsystems. *J. Neurosci.* 19:484–494, 1999.

Beauregard, M. Mind does relally matter: evidence from neuroimaging studies of emotional self-regulation, psychotherapy, and placebo effect. *Prog. Neurobiol.* 81:218–236, 2007.

Benedetti, F., et al. Somatotopic activation of opioid systems by target-directed expectations of analgesia. *J. Neurosci.* 19: 3639–3648, 1999.

Benedetti, F., et al. When words are painful: unraveling the mechanisms of the nocebo effect. *Neuroscience* 147:260–271, 2007.

Colloca, L., et al. Learning potentiates neurophysiological and behavioral placebo analgesic responses. *Pain* 139:306–314, 2009.

Colloca, L., Benedetti, F. Placebo analgesia induced by social observational learning. *Pain* doi:10.1016/j.pain.2009.01.033.

Enck, P., et al. New insight into the placebo and nocebo responses. *Neuron* 59:195–206, 2008.

Kong, J., et al. A functional magnetic resonance imaging study on the neural mechanisms of hyperalgesic nocebo effect. *J. Neurosci.* 28:13354–13362, 2008.

Petrovic, P., et al. Placebo and opioid analgesia: imaging a shared neuronal network. *Science* 106:71–76, 2002.

Petrovic, P., et al. Placebo in emotional processing-induced expectations of anxiety relief activate a generalized modulatory network. *Neuron* 46:957–969, 2005.

Porro, C.A., et al. Does anticipation of pain affect cortical nociceptive systems? *J. Neurosci.* 22:3206–3214, 2002.

Price, D.D., et al. A comprehensive review of the placebo effect: recent advances and current thoughts. *Annu. Rev. Psychol.* 59: 565–590, 2008.

Scott, D.J., et al. Placebo and nocebo effects are defined by opposite opioid and dopaminergic responses. *Arch. Gen. Psychiatry* 65:220–231, 2008.

Turner, J.A., et al. The importance of placebo effects in pain treatment and research. *JAMA* 271:1609–1614, 1994.

Wager, T., et al. Placebo-induced changes in fMRI in the anticipation and experienceec of pain. *Science* 303:1162–1167, 2004.

Wager, T.D., et al. Placebo effects on human μ-opioid activity during pain. *Proc. Natl. Acad. Sci. USA* 104:11056–11061, 2007.

Wall, P.D. Pain and the placebo response. *Ciba Found. Symp.* 174:187–211, 1993.

CHAPTER 16: THE VISUAL SYSTEM

Retina

Bair, W. Spike timing in the mammalian visual system. *Curr. Opin. Neurobiol.* 9:447–453, 1999.

Demb, J.B. Functional circuitry of visual adapatation in the retina. *J. Physiol.* 586:4377–4384, 2008.

DeVries, S.H., Baylor, D.A. Synaptic circuitry of the retina and olfactory bulb. *Neuron* 10(Suppl.):139–149, 1993.

Dowling, J. *The retina: an approachable part of the brain.* Cambridge, MA: Harvard University Press, 1987.

Kuffler, S.W., et al. From neuron to brain. A cellular approach to the function of the nervous system, 2nd. ed. Sunderland, MA: Sinauer Associates, 1984.

Lee, B.B. Paths to color in the retina. *Clin. Exp. Optom.* 87:239–248, 2004.

Masland, R.H. The fundamental plan of the retina. *Nat. Rev. Neurosci.* 4:877–886, 2001.

Meister, M., Berry, M.J. II. The neural code of the retina. *Neuron* 22:435–450, 1999.

Nickle, B., Robinson, P.R. The opsins of the vertebrate retina: insights from structural, biochemical, and evolutionary studies. *Cell Mol. Life Sci.* 64:2917–2932, 2007.

Nierenberg, S., Latham, P.E. Population coding in the retina. *Curr. Opin. Neurobiol.* 8:488–493, 1998.

Schiller, P.H. The on and off channels of the visual system. *Trends Neurosci.* 15:86–92, 1992.

Schulte, D., Bumsted-O'Brien, K.M. Molecular mechanisms of vertebrate retina development: implications for ganglion cell and photoreceptor patterning. *Brain Res.* 1192:151–164, 2008.

Shapley, R., Perry, V.H. Cat and monkey retinal ganglion cells and their visual functional roles. *Trends Neurosc.* 9:229–235, 1986.

Vanleeuwen, M.T., et al. The contribution of the outer retina to color constancy: a general model for color constancy synthesized from primate and fish data. *Vis. Neurosci.* 24:277–290, 2007.

Zhou, Z.J., Lee, S. Synaptic physiology of direction selectivity in the retina. *J. Physiol.* 586:4371–4376, 2008.

Zrenner, E. Will retinal implants restore vision? *Science* 295:1022–1025, 2002.

Visual Pathways and Visual Cortex

Aine, C.J., et al. Retinotopic organization of human visual cortex: departures from the classical model. *Cereb. Cortex* 6:354–361, 1996.

Allison, T., et al. Face recognition in human extrastriate cortex. *J. Neurophysiol.* 71:821–825, 1994.

Bar, M. Visual objects in context. *Nat. Rev Neurosci.* 5:617–628, 2004.

Barbur, J.L., et al. Insights into the different exploits of colour in the visual cortex. *Proc. R. Soc. Lond. B Biol. Sci.* 258:327–334, 1994.

Barnes, G.R., et al. The cortical deficit in humans with strabismic amblyopia. *J. Physiol.* 533:281–297, 2001.

Berman, R.A., Wurtz, R.H. Exploring the pulvinar path to visual cortex. *Prog. Brain Res.* 171:467–473, 2008.

Blasdel, G., Campbell, D. Functional retinotopy of monkey visual cortex. *J. Neurosci.* 21:8286–8301, 2001.

Boussaoud, D., et al. Pathways for motion analysis: cortical connections of the medial superior temporal and fundus of the superior temporal visual areas in the macaque. *J. Comp. Neurol.* 296:462–495, 1990.

Bridge, H., Cumming, B.G. Representation of binocular surfaces by cortical neurons. *Curr. Opin. Neurobiol.* 18:425–430, 2008.

Buchtel, H., et al. Behavioural and electrophysiological analysis of strabismus in cats: modern context. *Exp. Brain Res.* 192:359–367, 2009.

Callaway, E.M. Local circuits in primary visual cortex of the macaque monkey. *Annu. Rev. Neurosci.* 21:47–74, 1998.

Cant, J., et al. fMR-adaptation reveals separate processing regions for the perception of form and texture in the human ventral stream. *Exp. Brain Res.* 192:391–405, 2009.

Cohen, M.R., Newsome, W.T. Context-dependent changes in functional circuitry in visual area MT. *Neuron* 60:162–173, 2008.

Courtney, S.M., Ungerleider, L.G. What fMRI has taught us about human vision. *Curr. Opin. Neurobiol.* 7:554–561, 1997.

Cumming, B.G., DeAngelis, G.C. The physiology of stereopsis. *Annu. Rev. Neurosci.* 24:203–208, 2001.

Das, A. Orientation in visual cortex: a simple mechanism emerges. *Neuron* 16:477–480, 1996.

DeAngelis, G.C. Seeing in three dimensions: the neurophysiology of stereopsis. *Trends Cogn. Sci.* 4:80–90, 2000.

Deco, G., Rolls, E.T. Attention, short-term memory, and action selection: a unifying theory. *Prog. Neurobiol.* 76:236–256, 2005.

Desimone, R., Duncan, J. Neural mechanisms of selective visual attention. *Annu. Rev. Neurosci.* 18:193–222, 1995.

Downing, P.E., et al. A cortical area selective for visual processing of the human body. *Science* 293:2470–2473, 2001.

Dupont, P. et al. The kinetic occipital region in human visual cortex. *Cereb. Cortex* 7:283–292, 1997.

Eagleman, D.M. Visual illusions and neurobiology. *Nat. Rev. Neurosci.* 2:920–926, 2002.

Fang, F., He, S. Cortical responsens to invisible objects in the human dorsal and ventral pathways. *Nat. Rev. Neurosci.* 8:1380–1385, 2005.

Gonzales, F., Perez, R. Neural mechanisms underlying stereoscopic vision. *Prog. Neurobiol.* 55:191–224, 1998.

Goodale, M.A., Milner, A.D. Separate visual pathways for perception and action. *Trends Neurosci.* 15:20–25, 1992.

Gulyás, B., Roland, P.E. Processing and analysis of form, colour and binocular disparity in the human brain: functional anatomy by positron emission tomography. *Eur. J. Neurosci.* 6:1811–1828, 1994.

Haxby, J.V., et al. Distributed and overlapping representations of faces and objects in ventral temporal cortex. *Science* 293:2425–2430, 2001.

Holmes, G. Disturbances of vision by cerebral lesions. In: Phillips, C.G. (Ed.), *Selected papers of Gordon Holmes* (pp. 337–367). Oxford: Oxford University Press, 1979.

Hubel, D., Wiesel, T. Receptive fields, binocular interaction and functional architecture in the cat's visual cortex. *J. Physiol.* 160:106–154, 1962.

Kaas, J.H. Why does the brain have so many visual areas? *J. Cogn. Neurosci.* 1:121–135, 1989.

Komatsu, H. The neural mechanism of perceptual filling-in. *Nat. Rev. Neurosci.* 7:220–231, 2006.

Kreiman, G. Single unit approaches to human vision and memory. *Curr. Opin. Neurobiol.* 17:471–475, 2007.

Lamme, V.A.F., Roelfsema, P.R. The distinct modes of vision offered by feedforward and recurrent processing. *Trends Neurosci.* 23:571–579, 2000.

Livingston, M.S., Hubel, D.H. Psychophysical evidence for separate channels for the perception of form, color, movement, and depth. *J. Neurosci.* 7:3416–3468, 1987.

Logothetis, N.K., Sheinberg, D.L. Visual object recognition. *Annu. Rev. Neurosci.* 19:577–621, 1996.

Löwel, S. Ocular dominance column development: strabismus changes the spacing of adjacent columns in cat visual cortex. *J. Neurosci.* 14:7451–7468, 1994.

Malach, R., et al. Relationship between intrinsic connections and functional architecture revealed by optical imaging and *in vivo* targeted biocytin injections in primate striate cortex. *Proc. Natl. Acad. Sci. USA* 90:10469–10473, 1993.

Menon, R.S. Ocular dominance in human V1 demonstrated by functional magnetic resonance imaging. *J. Neurophysiol.* 77:2780–2787, 1997.

Moutoussis, K., Zeki, S. Motion processing, directional selectivity, and conscious visual perception in the human brain. *Proc. Natl. Acad. Sci. USA* 105:16362–16367, 2008.

Nealey, T.A., Maunsell, J.H.R. Magnocellular and parvocellular contributions to the responses of neurons in macaque striate cortex. *J. Neurosci.* 14:2069–2079, 1994.

Parker, A.J. Binocular depth perception and the cerebral cortex. *Nat. Rev. Neurosci.* 8:379–391, 2007.

Pasupathy, A. Neural basis of shape representation in the primate brain. *Prog. Brain Res.* 154:293–313, 2006.

Poghosyan, V., et al. Effects of attention and arousal on early responses in striate cortex. *Eur. J. Neurosci.* 22:225–234, 2005.

Pollen, D.A. On the neural correlates of visual perception. *Cereb. Cortex* 9:4–19, 1999.

Reddy, L., Kanwisher, N. Coding of visual objects in the ventral stream. *Curr. Opin. Neurobiol.* 16:408–414, 2006.

Roland, P.E., Gulyás, B. Visual imagery and visual representation. *Trends Neurosci.* 17:281–287, 1994.

Schwarzlose, R.F., et al. Separate face and body selectivity on the fusiform gyrus. *J. Neurosci.* 23:11055–11059, 2005.

Self, M.W., Zeki, S. The integration of colour and motion by the human visual brain. *Cereb. Cortex* 15:1270–1279, 2005.

True, S., Maunsell, J.H. Effects of attention on the processing of motion in macaque middle temporal and medial superior temporal visual cortical areas. *J. Neurosci.* 19:7591–7602, 1999.

Vaina, L.M., et al. Functional neuroanatomy of biological motion perception in humans. *Proc. Natl. Acad. Sci. USA* 98:11656–11661, 2001.

Van Essen, D.C., Gallant, J.L. Neural mechanisms of form and motion processing in the primate visual system. *Neuron* 13:1–10, 1994.

Zeki, S. *A vision of the brain.* Oxford: Blackwell Scientific, 1993.

Zeman, A. Theories of visual awareness. *Prog. Brain Res.* 144: 321–329, 2004.

Color Vision

Barbur, J.L., et al. Insights into the different exploits of colour in the visual cortex. *Proc. Roy. Soc. Lond. B* 258:327–334, 1994.

Conway, B.R. Color vision, cones, and color-coding in the cortex. *Neuroscientist* 15:274–290, 2009.

Foster, D.H. Does color constancy exist? *Trends Cogn. Sci.* 7: 439–443, 2003.

Gegenfurtner, K.R. Cortical mechanisms of colour vision. *Nat. Rev. Neurosci.* 4:563–572, 2003.

Gulyás, B., Roland, P.E. Processing and analysis of form, colour and binocular disparity in the human brain: functional anatomy by positron emission tomography. *Eur. J. Neurosci.* 6:1811–1828, 1994.

Heywood, C., Cowey, A. With color in mind. *Nat. Rev. Neurosci.* 1:171–173, 1998.

Hofer, H., et al. Organization of the human trichromatic cone mosaic. *J. Neurosci.* 25:9669–9679, 2005.

Komatsu, H. Mechanisms of central color vision. *Curr. Opin. Neurobiol.* 8:503–408, 1998.

Solomon, S.G., Lennie P. The machinery of colour vision. *Nat. Rev. Neurosci.* 8:276–286, 2007.

CHAPTER 17: THE AUDITORY SYSTEM

Moore, J.K., Linthicum, F.H. Jr. Auditory system. In: Paxinos, G., Mai, J.K. (Eds.), *The human nervous system*, 2nd ed. (pp. 1241–1279). Philadelphia: Elsevier Academic Press, 2004.

Cochlea

Ashmore, J.F., Kolston, P.J. Hair cell based amplification in the cochlea. *Curr. Opin. Neurobiol.* 4:503–508, 1994.

Dallos, P. Cochlear amplification, outer hair cells and prestin. *Curr. Opin. Neurobiol.* 18:370–376, 2008.

Eatock, R.A. Adaptation in hair cells. *Annu. Rev. Neurosci.* 23: 285–314, 2000.

Fettiplace, R., Hackney C.M. The sensory and motor roles of auditory hair cells. *Nat. Rev. Neurosci.* 7:19–29, 2006.

Flock, Å., et al. Supporting cells contribute to control of hearing sensitivity. *J. Neurosci.* 19:4498–4507, 1999.

Gillespie, P.G., et al. Have we found the tip link, transduction channel and gating spring of the hair cell? *Curr. Opin. Neurobiol.* 15: 389–396, 2005.

Glowatzki, E., et al. Hair cell afferent synapses. *Curr. Opin. Neurobiol.* 18:389–395, 2008.

Hudspeth, A.J. Mechanical amplification by hair cells. *Curr. Opin. Neurobiol.* 7:480–486, 1997.

Kozlov, A.S., et al. Coherent motion of stereocilia assures the concerted gating of hair-cell transduction channels. *Nat. Neurosci.* 10:87–92, 2007.

Legan, P.K., et al. A deafness mutation isolates a second role for the tectorial membrane in hearing. *Nat. Neurosci.* 8:1035–1042, 2005.

Manley, G.A., Köppl, C. Phylogenetic development of the cochlea and its innervation. *Curr. Opin. Neurobiol.* 8:468–474, 1998.

Middlebrooks, J.C., et al. Cochlear implants: the view from the brain. *Curr. Opin. Neurobiol.* 15:488–493, 2005.

Nelson, E.G., Hinojosa, R. Presbyacusis: a human temporal bone study of individuals with downward sloping audiometric patterns of hearing loss and review of the literature. *Laryngoscope* 116:1–12, 2006.

Nilsen, K.E., Russel, I.J. Timing of cochlear feedback: spatial and temporal representation of a tone across the basilar membrane. *Nat. Neurosci.* 2:642–647, 1999.

Nobili, R., et al. How well do we understand the cochlea? *Trends Neurosci.* 21:159–167, 1998.

Ohlemiller, K.K., et al. Strial microvascular pathology and age-associated endocochlear potential decline in NOD congenic mice. *Hear. Res.* 244:85–97, 2008.

Pauler, M., et al. Atrophy of the stria vascularis as a cause of sensorineural hearing loss. *Laryngoscope* 98:754–759, 1988.

Prakash, R., Ricci, A.J. Hair bundles teaming up to tune the mammalian cochlea. *Proc. Natl. Acad. Sci. USA* 105:18651–18652, 2008.

Ren, T., Gillespie, P.G. A mechanism for active hearing. *Curr. Opin. Neurobiol.* 17:498–503, 2007.

Rubinstein, J.T., Miller, C.A. How do cochlear prosthesis work? *Curr. Opin. Neurobiol.* 9:399–404, 1999.

Sainz, M., et al. Assessment of auditory skills in 140 cochlear implant children using the EARS protocol. *J. Otorhinolaryngol. Relat. Spec.* 65:91–96, 2003.

Takeuchi, S., et al. Mechanism generating endocochlear potential: role played by intermediate cells in the stria vascularis. *Biophys. J.* 79:2572–2582, 2000.

Auditory Pathways and Auditory Cortex

Ahveninen, J., et al. Task modulated "what" and "where" pathways in human auditory cortex. *Proc. Natl. Acad. Sci. USA* 103:14608–14613, 2006.

Alain, C., et al. A distributed network for auditory sensory memory in humans. *Brain Res.* 812:23–37, 1998.

Arnott, S.E., et al. Assessing the auditory dual-pathway model in humans. *NeuroImage* 22:401–408, 2004.

Bamiou, D.E., et al. The insula (Island of Reil) and its role in auditory processing. *Brain Res. Rev.* 42:143–154, 2003.

Bavelier, D., et al. Do deaf individuals see better? *Trends Cogn. Sci.* 10:512–518, 2006.

Bisiach, E., et al. Disorders of perceived auditory lateralization after lesions of the right hemisphere. *Brain* 107:37–52, 1984.

Brainard, M.S. Neural substrates of sound localization. *Curr. Opin. Neurobiol.* 4:557–562, 1994.

Carlyon, R.P. How the brain separates sounds. *Trends Cogn. Sci.* 8:465–471, 2004.

Carney, L.H. Temporal response properties of neurons in the auditory pathway. *Curr. Opin. Neurobiol.* 9:442–446, 1999.

Creutzfeldt, O., et al. Neuronal activity in the human temporal lobe. II. Responses to the subject's own voice. *Exp. Brain Res.* 77: 476–489, 1989.

Dahmen, J.C., King, A.J. Learning to hear: plasticity of auditory cortex processing. *Curr. Opin. Neurobiol.* 17:456–464, 2007.

Edelman, G.M., et al. *Auditory function: neurobiological bases of hearing.* New York: John Wiley & Sons, 1988.

Ehret, G., Romand, R. *The central auditory system.* New York: Oxford University Press, 1997.

Galuske, R.A.W., et al. Interhemispheric asymmetries of the modular structure in human temporal cortex. *Science* 289:1946–1949, 2000.

Giraud, A.L., et al. Functional plasticity of language-related brain areas after cochlear implantation. *Brain* 124:1307–1316, 2001.

Howard, M.A., et al. Auditory cortex on the human posterior superior temporal gyrus. *J. Comp. Neurol.* 416:79–92, 2000.

Knudsen, E.I., Brainard M.S. Creating a unified representation of visual and auditory space in the brain. *Annu. Rev. Neurosci.* 18: 19–43, 1995.

Lewald, J., et al. Processing of sound location in human cortex. *Eur. J. Neurosci.* 27:1261–1270, 2008.

Lomber, S., Malhorta, S. Double dissociation of "what" and "where" processing in auditory cortex. *Nat. Neurosci.* 11:609–616, 2008.

Magnusson, A.K., et al. Retrograde GABA signaling adjusts sound localization by balancing excitation and inhibition in the brainstem. *Neuron* 59:125–137, 2008.

Masterton, R.B. Role of the central auditory system in hearing: the new direction. *Trends Neurosci.* 15:280–285, 1992.

Nelken, I., Bar-Yosef, O. Neurons and objects: the case of auditory cortex. *Front. Neurosci.* 2:107–113, 2008.

Oertel, D. Encoding of timing in the brain stem auditory nuclei of vertebrates. *Neuron* 19:959–962, 1997.

Penfield, W., Perot, P. The brain's record of auditory and visual experience. *Brain* 86:596–696, 1963.

Peretz, I., et al. Functional dissociations following bilateral lesions of auditory cortex. *Brain* 117:1283–1301, 1994.

Pickles, J.O., Corey, D.P. Mechanoelectrical transduction by hair cells. *Trends Neurosci.* 15:254–259, 1992.

Poulet, J.F.A., Hedwig, B. A corollary discharge maintains auditory sensitivity during sound production. *Nature* 418:872–876, 2002.

Rauschecker, J.P., Shannon, R.V. Sending sound to the brain. *Science* 295:1025–1029, 2002.

Romanski, L.M., et al. Dual streams of auditory afferents target multiple domains in the primate prefrontal cortex. *Nat. Neurosci.* 2:1131–1136, 1999.

Rutkowski, R.G., Weinberger, N.M. Encoding of learned importance of sound by magnitude of representational area in primary auditory cortex. *Proc. Natl. Acad. Sci. USA* 102:13664–13669, 2005.

Schneider, P., et al. Morphology of Heschl's gyrus reflects enhanced activation in the auditory cortex of musicians. *Nat. Neurosci.* 5:688–694, 2002.

Schreiner, C.E., et al. Modular organization of frequency integration in primary auditory cortex. *Annu. Rev. Neurosci.* 23:501–529, 2000.

Scott, S.K. Auditory processing—speech, space and auditory objects. *Curr. Opin. Neurobiol.* 15:197–201, 2005.

Syka, J. Plastic changes in the central auditory system after hearing loss, restoration of function, and during learning. *Physiol. Rev.* 82:601–636, 2002.

Tanaka, Y., et al. "So-called" cortical deafness. *Brain* 114:2385–2401, 1991.

Warren, J.E., et al. Sounds do-able: auditory-motor transformations and the posterior temporal plane. *Trends Neurosci.* 28:636–643, 2005.

Winer, J.A., et al. Auditory thalamocortical transformation: structure and function. *Trends Neurosci.* 28:255–263, 2005.

Winkler, I., et al. Object representation in the human auditory system. *Eur. J. Neurosci.* 24:625–634, 2006.

Zahorik, P., Wightman, F.L. Loudness constancy with varying sound distance. *Nat. Rev.Neurosci.* 4:78–83, 2001.

Zatorre, R.J., et al. Structure and function of auditory cortex: music and speech. *Trends Cogn. Sci.* 6:37–45, 2002.

CHAPTER 18: THE SENSE OF EQUILIBRIUM

Vestibular Apparatus and Vestibular Nuclei

Büttner-Ennever, J.A. *Neuroanatomy of the oculomotor system.* Philadelphia: Elsevier, 1988.

Büttner-Ennever, J.A. A review of otolith pathways to brainstem and cerebellum. *Ann. NY Acad. Sci.* 871:51–64, 1999.

Büttner-Ennever, J.A, Gerrits, N.M. Vestibular system. In: Paxinos, G., Mai, J.K. (Eds.), *The human nervous system*, 2nd ed. (pp. 1212–1240). Philadelphia: Elsevier Academic Press, 2004.

de Waele, C., et al. Vestibular projections in the human cortex. *Exp. Brain Res.* 141:541–551, 2001.

Lindeman, H.H. Anatomy of the otolith organs. *Adv. Oto-Rhino-Laryngol.* 20:405–433, 1973.

Manzoni, D. The cerebellum may implement the appropriate coupling of sensory inputs and motor responses: evidence from vestibular physiology. *Cerebellum* 4:178–188, 2005.

Meng, H., et al. Vestibular signals in primate thalamus: properties and origin. *J. Neurosci.* 27:13590–13602, 2007.

Nathan, P.W., et al. Vestibulospinal, reticulospinal and descending propriospinal nerve fibres in man. *Brain* 119:1809–1833, 1996.

Parker, D.E. The relative roles of the otolith organs and semicircular canals in producing space motion sickness. *J. Vestib. Res.* 8:57–59, 1998.

Rinne, T., et al. Bilateral loss of vestibular function. *Acta Otolaryngol. (Stockh)* Suppl. 520:247–250, 1997.

Sadeghi, S.G., et al. Efferent mediated responses in vestibular nerve afferents of the alert macaque, *J. Neurophysiol.* 101:988–1001, 2009.

Uchino, Y., et al. Otolith and canal integration on single vestibular neurons in cats. *Exp. Brain Res.* 164:271–285, 2005.

Wersäll, J. Studies on the structure and innervation of the sensory epithelium of the cristae ampullaris of the guinea pig. A light and electron microscopic investigation. *Acta Otolaryng. (Stockh.)* Suppl. 126:1–85, 1956.

Wilson, V.J., Melvill Jones, G. *Mammalian vestibular physiology.* New York: Plenum Press, 1979.

Wilson, V.J., et al. Cortical influences on the vestibular nuclei of the cat. *Exp. Brain Res.* 125:1–13, 1999.

Zwergal, A., et al. An ipsilateral vestibulothalamic tract adjacent to the medial lemniscus in humans- *Brain* 131:2928–2935, 2008.

Vestibular Reflexes and Postural Control

Allum, J.H.J., Honegger, F. Interactions between vestibular and proprioceptive inputs triggering and modulating human balance-correcting responses differ across muscles. *Exp. Brain Res.* 121:478–494, 1998.

Balaban, C.D. Vestibular autonomic regulation (including motion sickness and the mechanism of vomiting). *Curr. Opin. Neurol.* 12:29–33, 1999.

Balasubramaniam, R., Wing, A.M. The dynamics of standing balance. *Trends Cogn. Sci.* 6:531–536, 2002.

Barbieri, G., et al. Does proprioception contribute to the sense of verticality? *Exp. Brain. Res.* 185:545–552, 2008.

Bles, W., et al. Motion sickness: one provocative conflict? *Brain Res. Bull.* 15:481–487, 1998.

Bloem, B.R., et al. Is lower leg proprioception essential for triggering human automatic postural responses? *Exp. Brain Res.* 130: 375–391, 2000.

Boulinguez, P., Rouhana, J.I. Flexibility and individual differences in visuo-proprioceptive integration: evidence from a morphokinetic control task. *Exp. Brain Res.* 185:137–149, 2008.

Bronstein, A.M., Hood, D. The cervico-ocular reflex in normal subjects and patients with absent vestibular function. *Brain Res.* 373:399–408, 1986.

Deliagini, T.G., et al. Spinal and supraspinal postural networks. *Brain Res. Rev.* 57:212–221, 2008.

Denise, P., Darlot, C. The cerebellum as a predictor of neural messages. II. Role in motor control and motion sickness. *Neuroscience* 56:647–655, 1993.

Kaufmann, H., et al. Vestibular control of sympathetic activity. An otolith-sympathetic reflex in humans. *Exp. Brain Res.* 143:463–469, 2002.

Lackner, J.R. Motion sickness. In: Squire, L. (Ed.), *Encyclopedia of neuroscience* (pp. 989–993). Philadelphia: Elsevier, 2009.

Labuguen, R.H. Initial evaluation of vertigo. *Am. Family Phys.* 73:244–251, 2006.

Lekhel, H., et al. Postural responses to vibration of neck muscles in patients with idiopathic torticollis. *Brain* 120:583–591, 1997.

Lisberger, S.G. Physiologic basis for motor learning in the vestibulo-ocular reflex. *Otolaryngol. Head Neck Surg.* 119:43–48, 1998.

Nashner, L.M. Balance and posture control. In: Squire, L. (Ed.), *Encyclopedia of neuroscience* (pp. 21–29). Philadelphia: Elsevier, 2009.

Shelhamer, M.J. Nystagmus. In: Squire, L. (Ed.), *Encyclopedia of neuroscience* (pp. 1313–1317). Philadelphia: Elsevier, 2009.

Strupp, M., et al. Perceptual and oculomotor effects of neck muscle vibration in vestibular neuritis. Ipsilateral somatosensory substitution of vestibular function. *Brain* 121:677–685, 1998.

Weerdesteyn, V., et al. Automated postural responses are modified in a functional manner by instruction. *Exp. Brain Res.* 186:571–580, 2008.

Wilson, V.J., Schor R.H. The neural substrate of the vestibulocollic reflex: what needs to be learned. *Exp. Brain Res.* 129:483–493, 1999.

Wu, G., Chiang J.-H. The significance of somatosensory stimulations to the human foot in the control of postural reflexes. *Exp. Brain Res.* 114:163–169, 1997.

Yates, B.J., et al. Physiological basis and pharmacology of motion sickness: an update. *Brain Res. Bull.* 15:395–406, 1998.

Yates, B.J., Wilson, T.D. Vestibulo-autonomic responses. In: Squire, L. (Ed.), *Encyclopedia of neuroscience* (pp. 133–138). Philadelphia: Elsevier, 2009.

Cortical Level

Anastasopoulos, D., et al. The role of somatosensory input for the perception of verticality. *Ann. NY Acad. Sci.* 871:379–383, 1999.

Angelaki, D.E., Cullen, K.E. Vestibular system: the many facets of a multimodal system. *Annu. Rev. Neurosci.* 31:125–150, 2008.

Astafiev, S.V., et al. Extrastriate body area in human occipital cortex responds to the performance of motor actions. *Nat. Neurosci.* 7:542–548, 2004.

Berlucchi, G., Aglioti, S. The body in the brain: neural bases of corporeal awareness. *Trends Neurosci.* 20:560–564, 1997.

Berthoz, A., Viaud-Delmond, I. Multisensory integration in spatial orientation. *Curr. Opin. Neurobiol.* 9:708–712, 1999.

Blake, R., Shiffrar, M. Perception of human motion. *Annu. Rev. Psychol.* 58:47–73, 2007.

Blanke, O., Mohr, C. Out-of-body experience, heautoscopy, and autoscopic hallucination of neurological origin. Implications for neurocognitive mechanisms of corporeal awareness and self consciousness. *Brain Res. Rev.* 50:184–199, 2005.

Bos, E., van den, M. Jeannerod. Sense of body and sense of action both contribute to self-recognition. *Cognition* 85:177–188, 2002.

Bosbach, S., et al. Inferring another's expectation from action: the role of peripheral sensation. *Nat. Neurosci.* 8:1295–1297, 2005.

Bottini, G., et al. Cerebral representations for egocentric space. Functional-anatomical evidence from caloric vestibular stimulation and neck vibration. *Brain* 124:1182–1196, 2001.

Brandt, T., Dieterich, M. The vestibular cortex: its location, functions, and disorders. *Ann. NY Acad. Sci.* 871:293–312, 1999.

Carpenter, M.G., et al. The influence of postural threat on the control of upright stance. *Exp. Brain Res.* 138:210–218, 2001.

Dieterich, M., Brandt, T. Functional brain imaging of peripheral and central vestibular disorders. *Brain* 131:2538–2552, 2008.

Jeannerod, M. Being oneself. *J. Physiol. Paris* 101:161–168, 2007.

Kalueff, A.V., et al. Anxiety and otovestibular disorders: linking behavioral phenotypes in men and mice. *Behav. Brain. Res.* 186: 1–11, 2008.

Kavounoudias, A., et al. From balance regulation to body orientation: two goals for muscle proprioceptive information processing? *Exp. Brain Res.* 124:80–88, 1999.

Kerber, K.A., et al. Disequilibrium in older people: a prospective study. *Neurology* 51:574–580, 1998.

Lackner, J.R., DiZio, P.A. Aspects of body self-calibration. *Trends Cogn. Sci.* 4:279–289, 2000.

Lopez, C., et al. Body ownership and embodiment: vestibular and multisensory mechanisms. *Clin. Neurophysiol.* 38:148–161, 2008.

Moro, V., et al. The neural basis of body form and body action agnosia. *Neuron* 60:235–246, 2008.

Pérennou, D.A., et al. The polymodal sensory cortex is crucial for controlling lateral postural stability. Evidence from stroke patients. *Brain Res. Bull.* 53:359–365, 2000.

Reschke, M.F., et al. Posture, locomotion, spatial orientation, and motion sickness as a function of space flight. *Brain Res. Rev.* 28:102–117, 1998.

Schwoebel, J., Coslett, H.B. Evidence for multiple, distinct representations of the human body. *J. Cogn. Neurosci.* 17:543–553, 2005.

Shenton, J.T., et al. Mental motor imagery and the body schema: evidence for proprioceptive dominance. *Neurosci. Lett.* 370: 19–24, 2004.

Strupp, M., et al. Perceptual and oculomotor effects of neck muscle vibration in vestibular neuritis: ipsilateral somatosensory substitution of vestibular function. *Brain* 121:677–685, 1998.

Sundermier, L., et al. The development of balance control in children: comparisons of EMG and kinetic variables and chronological and developmental groupings. *Exp. Brain Res.* 136:340–350, 2001.

Tsakiris, M., et al. On agency and body-ownership: phenomenological and neurocognitive reflections. *Conscious. Cogn.* 16:645–660, 2007.

Tsakiris, M., et al. The role of the right temporo-parietal junction in maintaining a coherent sense of one's body. *Neuropsychologia* 46:3014–3018, 2008.

Urgesi, C., et al. Representation of body identity and body actions in extrastriate body area and ventral premotor cortex. *Nat. Neurosci.* 10:30–31, 2007.

Warren, W.H. Perception of heading is a brain in the neck. *Nat. Neurosci.* 1:647–649, 1998.

CHAPTER 19: OLFACTION AND TASTE

Barbas, H. Organization of cortical afferent input to orbitofrontal areas in the rhesus monkey. *Neuroscience* 56:841–864, 1993.

Finger, T.E., et al. (Eds.) *The neurobiology of taste and smell*. New York: John Wiley & Sons, 2001.

Olfaction

Ache, B.W., Young J.M. Olfaction: diverse species, conserved principles. *Neuron* 48:417–430, 2005.

Buck, L.B. Information coding in the vertebrate olfactory system. *Annu. Rev. Neurosci.* 19:517–544, 1996.

Firestein, S. How the olfactory system makes sense of scents. *Nature* 413:211–218, 2001.

Haberly, L.B., Bower, J.M. Olfactory cortex: model circuit for study of associative memory. *Trends Neurosci.* 12:258–264, 1989.

Hudson, R. Olfactory imprinting. *Curr. Opin. Neurobiol.* 3:548–552, 1993.

Jones-Gotman, M., et al. Contribution of medial versus lateral temporal-lobe structures to human odour identification. *Brain* 120:1845–1856, 1997.

Kay, L.M., Sherman, S.M. An argument for an olfactory thalamus. *Trends Neurosci.* 30:47–53, 2007

Laurent, G. Odor images and tunes. *Neuron* 16:473–476, 1996.

Laurent, G. Olfactory processing: maps, time and codes. *Curr. Opin. Neurobiol.* 7:547–553, 1997.

Laurent, G., et al. Odor encoding as an active dynamical process. *Annu. Rev. Neurosci.* 24:263–297, 2001.

Leopold, D.A., et al. Anterior distribution of human olfactory epithelium. *Laryngoscope* 110:417–421, 2000.

Mainland, J., Sobel, N. The sniff is part of the olfactory percept. *Chem. Sens.* 31:181–196, 2006.

Mombaerts, P. Targeting olfaction. *Curr. Opin. Neurobiol.* 6:481–486, 1996.

Mombaerts, P. Molecular biology of odorant receptors in vertebrates. *Annu. Rev. Neurosci.* 22:487–509, 1999.

Nakashima, T., et al. Structure of human fetal and adult olfactory neuroepithelium. *Arch. Otolaryngol.* 110:641–646, 1984.

Paik, S.I., et al. Human olfactory biopsy. The influence of age and receptor distribution. *Arch. Otolaryngol. Head Neck Surg.* 118:731–738, 1992.

Price, J.L. Olfaction. In: Paxinos, G., Mai, J.K. (Eds.), *The human nervous system*, 2nd ed. (pp. 1197–1211). Philadelphia: Elsevier Academic Press, 2004.

Ressler, K.J., et al. A molecular dissection of spatial patterning in the olfactory system. *Curr. Opin. Neurobiol.* 4:588–596, 1994.

Richardson, J.T.E., Zucco, G.M. Cognition and olfaction: a review. *Psychol. Bull.* 105:352–360, 1989.

Sanchez-Andrade, G., Kendrick, K.M. The main olfactory system and social learning in mammals. *Behav. Brain Res.* 200:323–335, 2009.

Shepherd, G.M. Discrimination of molecular signals by the olfactory receptor neuron. *Neuron* 13:771–790, 1994.

Trombley, P.Q., Shepherd, G.M. Synaptic transmission and modulation in the olfactory bulb. *Curr. Opin. Neurobiol.* 3:540–547, 1993.

Wilson, R.I., Mainen, Z.F. Early events in olfactory processing. *Annu. Rev. Neurosci.* 29:163–201, 2006.

Zatorre, R.J., et al. Functional localization and lateralization of human olfactory cortex. *Nature* 360:339–340, 1992.

Zelano, C., Sobel N. Humans as an animal model for systems-level organization of olfaction. *Neuron* 48:431–454, 2005.

Zou, D.J., et al. Postnatal refinement of peripheral olfactory projections. *Science* 304:1976–1979, 2004.

Zozulya, S., et al. The human olfactory receptor repertoire. *Genome Biol.* 2:1–12, 2001.

Zufall, F., Leinders-Zufall, T. Calcium imaging in the olfactory system: new tools for visualizing odor recognition. *Neuroscientist* 5:4–7, 1999.

Pheromones

Baxi, K.N., et al. Is the vomeronasal system really specialized for detecting pheromones? *Trends Neurosci.* 29:1–7, 2006.

Brennan, P.A., Zufall, F. Pheromonal communication in vertebrates. *Nature* 444:308–315, 2006.

Dulac, C., Torello, A.T. Molecular detection of pheromone signals in mammals: from genes to behaviour. *Nat. Rev. Neurosci.* 4:551–562, 2003.

Karlson, P., Lüscher M. "Pheromones": a new term for a class of biologically active substances. *Nature* 183:55–56, 1959.

Keller, M., et al. The main and the accessory olfactory systems interact in the control of mate recognition and sexual behavior. *Behav. Brain Res.* 200:268–276, 2009.

Swaney, W.T., Keverne, E.B. The evolution of pheromonal communication. *Behav. Brain Res.* 200:239–247, 2009.

Wysocki, C.J., Preti G. Facts, fallacies, fears, and frustrations with human pheromones. *Anat. Rec. A* 281A:1201–1211, 2004.

Zufall, F., Leinders-Zufall, T. Mammalian pheromone sensing. *Curr. Opin. Neurobiol.* 17:483–489, 2007.

Taste

Acolla, R., Carleton, A. Internal body state influences topographical plasticity of sensory representations in the rat gustatory cortex. *Proc. Natl. Acad. Sci. USA* 105:4010–4015, 2008.

Acolla, R., et al. Differential spatial representation of taste modalities in the rat gustatory cortex. *J. Neurosci.* 27:1396–1404, 2007.

Bermúdez-Rattoni, F. Molecular mechanisms of taste-recognition memory. *Nat. Rev. Neurosci.* 5:209–217, 2004.

Boughter, J.D., Gilbertson, T.A. From channels to behavior: an integrative model of NaCl taste. *Neuron* 22:213–215, 1999.

Finger, T.E., et al. ATP signaling is crucial for communication from taste buds to gustatory nerves. *Science* 310:1495–1499, 2005.

Frank, M.E., et al. Cracking taste codes by tapping into sensory neuron impulse traffic. *Prog. Neurobiol.* 86:245–263, 2008.

Gilbertson, T.A. Gustatory mechanisms for the detection of fat. *Curr. Opin. Neurobiol.* 8:447–452, 1998.

Heath, T.P., et al. Human taste thresholds are modulated by serotonin and noradrenaline. *J. Neurosci.* 26:12664–12671, 2006.

Huang, Y. J. et al.: Mouse taste buds use serotonin as a neurotransmitter. *J. Neurosci.* 25:843–847, 2005.

Hoon, M.A., et al. Putative mammalian taste receptors: a class of taste-specific GCPRs with distinct topographic sensitvity. *Cell* 96:541–551, 1999.

Kinnamon, S.C. Taste transduction: a diversity of mechanisms. *Trends Neurosci.* 11:491–496, 1988.

Margolskee, R.F. The biochemistry and molecular biology of taste transduction. *Curr. Opin. Neurobiol.* 3:526–531, 1993.

McCormack, D.N., et al. Detection of free fatty acids following a conditioned taste aversion in rats. *Physiol. Behav.* 87:582–594, 2006.

Mizushige, T., et al. Why is fat so tasty? Chemical reception of fatty acid on the tongue. *J. Nutr. Sci. Vitaminol.* 53:1–4, 2007.

Nelson, G., et al. An amino-acid taste receptor. *Nature* 416:199–202, 2002.

Pritchard, T.C., Norgren, R. Gustatory system. In: Paxinos, G., Mai, J.K. (Eds.), *The human nervous system*, 2nd ed. (pp. 1171–1196). Philadelphia: Elsevier Academic Press, 2004.

Reilly, S. The role of the gustatory thalamus in taste-guided behavior. *Neurosci. Biobehav. Rev.* 22:883–901, 1998.

Roper, S.D. Cell communication in taste buds. *Cell. Mol. Life. Sci.* 63:1494–1500, 2006.

Schoenfeld, M.A., et al. Functional magnetic resonance tomography correlates of taste perception in the human primary taste cortex. *Neuroscience* 127:347–353, 2004.

Scott, K. Taste recognition: food for thought. *Neuron* 48:455–464, 2005.

Shepherd, G.M. Smell images and the flavour system in the brain. *Nature* 444:316–321, 2006.

Simon, S.A., et al. The neural mechanisms of gustation: a distributed processing code. *Nat. Rev. Neurosci.* 7:890–901, 2006.

Small, D.M., Prescott, J. Odor/taste integration and the perception of flavor. *Exp. Brain Res.* 166:345–357, 2005.

Smith, D.V., St. John, S.J. Neural coding of gustatory information. *Curr. Opin. Neurobiol.* 9:427–435, 1999.

Spector, A.C., Travers, S.P. The representation of taste quality in the mammalian nervous system. *Behav. Cogn. Neurosci. Rev.* 4: 143–191, 2005.

Sugita, M., Shiba, Y. Genetic tracing shows segregation of taste neuronal circuitries for bitter and sweet. *Science* 309:781–785, 2005.

CHAPTER 20: MOTOR SYSTEMS AND MOVEMENTS IN GENERAL

Ahissar, E. And motion changes it all. *Nat. Neurosci.* 11:1369–1370, 2008.

d'Avella, A., Bizzi, E. Shared and specific muscle synergies in natural motor behaviors. *Proc. Natl. Acad. Sci. USA* 3076–3081, 2005.

Johansson, R.S., Flanagan, J.R. Coding and use of tactile signals from the fingertips in object manipulation tasks. *Nat. Rev. Neurosci.* 10:345–259, 2009.

Schütz-Bosbach, S., et al. Self and other in the human motor system. *Curr. Biol.* 16:1830–1834, 2006.

Synofzik, M., et al. I move, therefore I am: a new theoretical framework to investigate agency and ownership. *Conscious. Cogn.* 17:411–424, 2008.

Wolpert, D.M., et al. An internal model for sensorimotor integration. *Science* 269:1880–1882, 1995.

CHAPTER 21: THE PERIPHERAL MOTOR NEURONS AND REFLEXES

Muscles, Motoneurons, and Motor Units

Basmajian, J.V., De Luca, C. *Muscles alive: their functions revealed by electromyography*, 5th ed. Baltimore: Williams & Wilkins, 1985.

Bawa, P., Jones, K.E. Do lengthening contractions represent a case of reversal in recruitment order? *Prog. Brain Res.* 123:215–220, 1999.

Bigland-Ritchie, B., et al. Contractile properties of human motor units: is man a cat? *Neuroscientist* 4:240–249, 1998.

Bizzi, E., et al. Combining modules for movement. *Brain Res. Rev.* 57:125–133, 2008.

Burke, R.E. Revisiting the notion of "motor unit types." *Prog. Brain Res.* 123:167–175, 1999.

Carson, S., Riek, S. Changes in muscle recruitment patterns during skill acquisition. *Exp. Brain Res.* 138:71–87, 2001.

Collins, D.F., et al. Sustained contractions produced by plateau-like behavior in human motoneurons. *J. Physiol.* 538:289–301, 2002.

Dasen. J.S., et al. Hox repertoires for motor neuron diversity and connectivity gated by a single accessory factor, FoxP1. *Cell* 134:304–316, 2008.

Dong, M., et al. SV2 is the protein receptor for botulinum neurotoxin A. *Science* 312:592–596, 2006.

Enoka, R.M., Fuglevand, A.J. Motor unit physiology: some unresolved issues. *Muscle Nerve* 24:4–17, 2001.

Fallentin, N., et al. Motor unit recruitment during prolonged isometric contractions. *Eur. J. Appl. Physiol.* 67:335–341, 1993.

Gardiner, P., et al. Motoneurones "learn" and "forget" physical activity. *Can. J. Appl. Physiol.* 30:352–370, 2005.

Granit, R. The basis of motor control: integrating the activity of muscles, α and γ motoneurons and their leading control systems. New York: Academic Press, 1970.

Henneman, E., et al. Rank order of motoneurons within a pool: law of combination. *J. Neurophysiol.* 37:1338–1349, 1974.

Horowits, R. Passive force generation and titin isoforms in mammalian skeletal muscle. *Biophys. J.* 61:392–398, 1992.

Howell, J.N., et al. Motor unit activity during isometric and concentric-eccentric contractions of the human first dorsal interosseus muscle. *J. Neurophysiol.* 74:901–904, 1995.

Hultborn, H. Plateau potentials and their role in regulating motoneuronal firing. *Prog. Brain Res.* 123:39–48, 1999.

Jenny, A.B., Inukai, J. Principles of motor organization of the monkey cervical spinal cord. *J. Neurosci.* 3:567–575, 1983.

Johnson, M.A., et al. Data on the distribution of fibre types in thirty-six human muscles: an autopsy study. *J. Neurol. Sci.* 18:111–129, 1973.

Kandel, E., Schwartz, J.H. *Principles of neural science*. Philadelphia: Elsevier, 1985.

Khan, S.I., Burne, J.A. Reflex inhibition of normal cramp following electrical stimulation of the muscle tendon. *J. Neurosphysiol.* 98:1102–1107, 2007.

Kiehn, O., Eken, T. Functional role of plateau potentials in vertebrate motor neurons. *Curr. Opin. Neurobiol.* 8:746–752, 1998.

Löscher, W.N., et al. Excitatory drive to the α-motoneuron pool during fatiguing submaximal contraction in man. *J. Physiol.* 491:271–280, 1996.

Magnusson, S.P., et al. A mechanism for altered flexibility in human skeletal muscle. *J. Physiol.* 497:291–298, 1996.

McComas, A.J. Motor unit estimation: anxieties and achievements. *Muscle Nerve* 18:369–379, 1995.

Miller, K.J., et al. Motor-unit behavior in humans during fatiguing arm movements. *J. Neurophysiol.* 75:1629–1636, 1996.

Monti, R.J., et al. Role of motor unit structure in defining function. *Muscle Nerve* 24:848–866, 2001.

Navarrete, R., Vrbová, G. Activity-dependent interactions between motoneurones and muscles: their role in the development of the motor unit. *Progr. Neurobiol.* 41:93–124, 1993.

Piehl, F., et al. Calcitonin gene-related peptide-like immunoreactivity in motoneuron pools innervating different hind limb muscles in the rat. *Exp. Brain Res.* 96:291–303, 1993.

Taylor, J.L., Gandevia, S.C. Transcranial magnetic stimulation and human muscle fatigue. *Muscle Nerve* 24:18–29, 2001.

Wang, Y., et al. Motor learning changes GABAergic terminals on spinal motoneurons in normal rats. *Eur. J. Neurosci.* 23:141–150, 2006.

Reflexes and Spinal Interneurons

Aminoff, M.J., Goodin, D.S. Studies of the human stretch reflex. *Muscle Nerve* Suppl. 9:S3–S6, 2000.

Andersen, O.K., et al. Interaction between cutaneous and muscle afferent activity in polysynaptic reflex pathways: a human experimental study. *Pain* 84:29–36, 2000.

Bennett, D.J. Stretch reflex responses in the human elbow joint during a voluntary movement. *J. Physiol.* 474:339–351, 1994.

Brown, D.A., Kukulka, C.G. Human flexor reflex modulation during cycling. *J. Neurophysiol.* 69:1212–1224, 1993.

Capaday, C., et al. A re-examination of the effects of instruction on the long-latency stretch reflex response of the flexor pollicis longus muscle. *Exp. Brain Res.* 100:515–521, 1994.

Cody, F.J.W., et al. Observations on the genesis of the stretch reflex in Parkinson's disease. *Brain* 109:229–249, 1986.

Cody, F.J.W., et al. Stretch and vibration reflexes of wrist flexor muscles in spasticity. *Brain* 110:433–450, 1987

Dietz, V., et al. Task-dependent modulation of short- and long-latency electromyographic responses in upper limb muscles. *Electroencephalogr. Clin. Neurophysiol.* 93:49–56, 1994.

Edgerton, R., et al. Does motor learning occur in the spinal cord? *Neuroscientist* 3:287–294, 1997.

Fellows, S.J., et al. Changes in the short- and long-latency stretch reflex components of the triceps surae muscle during ischaemia in man. *J. Physiol.* 472:737–748, 1993.

Glendenning, D.S. The effect of fasciculus cuneatus lesions on finger positioning and long-latency reflexes in monkeys. *Exp. Brain Res.* 93:104–116, 1993.

Hultborn, H. State-dependent modulation of sensory feedback. *J. Physiol.* 533:5–13, 2001.

Iles, J.F. Evidence for cutaneous and corticospinal modulation of presynaptic inhibition of Ia afferents from the human lower limb. *J. Physiol.* 481:197–207, 1996.

Katz, R., Pierrot-Deseilligny, E. Recurrent inhibition in humans. *Prog. Neurobiol.* 57:325–355, 1999.

Lacquaniti, F., et al. Transient reversal of the stretch reflex in human arm muscles. *J. Neurophysiol.* 66:939–954, 1991.

Liddell, E.G.T. *The discovery of reflexes.* New York: Oxford University Press, 1960.

Marsden, C.D., et al. Stretch reflex and servo action in a variety of human muscles. *J. Physiol. (Lond.)* 259:531–560, 1976.

Matthews, P.B.C. The human stretch reflex and the motor cortex. *Trends Neurosci.* 14:87–91, 1991.

Mazzocchio, R., et al. Depression of Renshaw recurrent inhibition by activation of corticospinal fibres in human upper and lower limb. *J. Physiol.* 481:487–498, 1994.

McCrea, D.A. Can sense be made of spinal interneuron circuits? *Behav. Brain Sci.* 15:633–643, 1992.

Nakazawa, K., et al. Short- and long-latency reflex responses during different motor tasks in elbow flexor muscles. *Exp. Brain Res.* 116:20–28, 1997.

Prochazka, A., et al. What do *reflex* and *voluntary* mean? Modern views on an ancient debate. *Exp. Brain Res.* 130:417–432, 2000.

Rossi, A., Decchi, B. Flexibility of lower limb reflex responses to painful cutaneous stimulation in standing humans: evidence of load-dependent modulation. *J. Physiol.* 481:521–532, 1994.

Sherrington, C.S. *The integrative action of the brain.* Cambridge, UK: Cambridge University Press, 1947.

Wolpaw, J.R. The complex structure of a simple memory. *Trends Neurosci.* 20:588–594, 1997.

Zehr, E.P., Stein R.B. Interaction of the Jendrássik maneuver with segmental presynaptic inhibition. *Exp. Brain Res.* 124:474–480, 1999.

Muscle Tone and Injury of Motoneurons

Baldissera, F., et al. Motor neuron "bistability": a pathogenetic mechanism for cramps and myokymia. *Brain* 117:929–939, 1994.

Brushart, T.M.E. Motor axons preferentially reinnervate motor pathways. *J. Neurosci.* 13:2730–2738, 1993.

Chen, Z.-L., et al. Peripheral regeneration. *Annu. Rev. Neurosci.* 30:209–233, 2007.

Chleboun, G.S., et al. Relationship between muscle swelling and stiffness after eccentric exercise. *Med. Sci. Sports Exerc.* 30:529–535, 1998.

Cope, T.C., Clark, B.D. Motor-unit recruitment in self-reinnervated muscle. *J. Neurophysiol.* 70:1787–1796, 1993.

Futagi, Y., et al. Primitive reflex profiles in infants: differences based on categories of neurological abnormality. *Brain Dev.* 14:294–298, 1992.

Gerrits, H.L., et al. Contractile properties of the quadriceps muscle in individuals with spinal cord injury. *Muscle Nerve* 22:1249–1256, 1999.

Hallin, R.G., et al. Spinal cord implantation of avulsed ventral roots in primates: correlation between restored motor function and morphology. *Exp. Brain Res.* 124:304–310, 1999.

Pisano, F., et al. Quantitative evaluation of normal muscle tone. *J. Neurol. Sci.* 135:168–172, 1996.

Rafuse, V.F., et al. Proportional enlargement of motor units after partial denervation of cat triceps surae muscles. *J. Neurophysiol.* 68:1261–1276, 1992.

Sakai, F., et al. Pericranial muscle hardness in tension-type headache: a non-invasive measurement method and its clinical application. *Brain* 118:523–531, 1995.

Simons, D., Mense, S. Understanding and measurement of muscle tone as related to clinical muscle pain. *Pain* 75:1–17, 1998.

Swash, M., et al. Focal loss of anterior horn cells in the cervical cord in motor neuron disease. *Brain* 109:939–952, 1986.

Van der Meché, F.G.A., Van Gijn, J. Hypotonia: an erroneous clinical concept? *Brain* 109:1169–1178, 1986.

CHAPTER 22: THE MOTOR CORTICAL AREAS AND DESCENDING PATHWAYS

Descending Motor Tracts

Biber, M.P., et al. Cortical neurons projecting to the cervical and lumbar enlargements of the spinal cord in young and adult Rhesus monkeys. *Exp. Neurol.* 59:492–508, 1978.

Bortoff, G.A., Strick, P.L. Corticospinal terminations in two new-world primates: further evidence that corticomotoneuronal connections provide part of the neural substrate for manual dexterity. *J. Neurosci.* 13:5105–5118, 1993.

Capaday, C., et al. Studies on the corticospinal control of human walking. I. Responses to focal transcranial magnetic stimulation of the motor cortex. *J. Neurophysiol.* 81:129–139, 1999.

Danek, A., et al. Tracing of neuronal connections in the human brain by magnetic resonance imaging *in vivo*. *Eur. J. Neurosci.* 2:112–115, 1990.

Dum, R.P., Strick, P.L. The origin of corticospinal projections from the premotor areas in the frontal lobe. *J. Neurosci.* 11:667–689, 1990.

Englander, R.N., et al. The location of human pyramidal tract in the internal capsule: anatomic evidence. *Neurology* 25:823–826, 1975.

Eyre, J.A. Corticospinal tract development and its plasticity after perinatal injury. *Neurosci. Biobehav. Rev.* 31:1136–1149, 2007.

Foerster, O. *Motorische Felder und Bahnen* In: *Hdb. d. Neurol.* Vol. 6. Heidelberg: Springer Verlag, 1936.

He, S.-Q., et al. Topographic organization of corticospinal projections from the frontal lobe: motor areas on the lateral surface of the hemisphere. *J. Neurosci.* 13:952–980, 1993.

Holstege, J.C. The ventro-medial medullary projections to spinal motoneurons: ultrastructure, transmitters and functional aspects. *Prog. Brain Res.* 107:160–181, 1996.

Jacobs, B.L., Fornal, C.A. Serotonin and motor activity. *Curr. Opin. Neurobiol.* 7:820–825, 1997.

Luppino, G., et al. Corticospinal projections from mesial frontal and cingulate areas in the monkey. *NeuroReport* 5:2545–2548, 1994.

Maier, M.A., et al. Differences in corticospinal projection from primary motor cortex and supplementary motor area to Macaque upper limb motoneurons: an anatomical and electrophysiological study. *Cereb. Cortex* 12:281–296, 2002.

Matsuyama, K., et al. Multi-segmental innervation of single pontine reticulospinal axons in the cervico-thoracic region of the cat: anterograde PHA-L tracing study. *J. Comp. Neurol.* 377:234–250, 1997.

Nathan, P.W., Smith, M.C. The rubrospinal and central tegmental tracts in man. *Brain* 105:223–269, 1982.

Nathan, P.W., et al. The corticospinal tracts in man: course and location of fibres at different segmental levels. *Brain* 113:303–324, 1990.

Nathan, P.W., et al. Vestibulospinal, reticulospinal and descending propriospinal nerve fibres in man. *Brain* 119:1809–1833, 1996.

Nudo, R.J., Masterton, R.B. Descending pathways to the spinal cord. III: Sites of origin of the corticospinal tract. *J. Comp. Neurol.* 296:559–583, 1990.

Ralston, D.D., Ralston, H.J. III. The terminations of corticospinal tract axons in the macaque monkey. *J. Comp. Neurol.* 242: 325–337, 1985.

Strutton, P.H., et al. Corticospinal activation of internal oblique muscles has a strong ipsilateral component and can be lateralised in man. *Exp. Brain Res.* 158:474–479, 2004.

Turton, A., Lemon, R. The contribution of fast corticospinal input to the voluntary activation of proximal muscles in normal subjects and in stroke patients. *Exp. Brain Res.* 129:559–572, 1999.

Control of Posture and Automatic Movements

Allum, J.H.J., Honegger, F. Interactions between vestibular and proprioceptive inputs triggering and modulating human balance-correcting responses differ across muscles. *Exp. Brain Res.* 121:478–494, 1998.

Armstrong, D.M. The supraspinal control of mammalian locomotion. *J. Physiol.* 405:1–37, 1988.

Berger, W. Characteristics of locomotor control in children with cerebral palsy. *Neurosci. Biobehav. Rev.* 22:579–582, 1998.

Bloem, B.R., et al. Is lower leg proprioception essential for triggering human automatic postural responses? *Exp. Brain Res.* 130:375–391, 2000.

Brenière, Y., Bril, B. Development of postural control of gravity forces in children during the first 5 years of walking. *Exp. Brain Res.* 121:255–262, 1998.

Buccino, G., et al. Action observation activates premotor and parietal areas in a somatotopic manner: an fMRI study. *Eur. J. Neurosci.* 13:400–404, 2001.

Calancie, B., et al. Involuntary stepping after chronic spinal cord injury: evidence for a central rhythm generator for locomotion in man. *Brain* 117:1143–1159, 1994.

Capaday, C. The special nature of human walking and its neural control. *Trends Neurosci.* 25:370–376, 2002.

Caronni, A., Cavallari, P. Anticipatory postural adjustments stabilise the whole upper-limb prior to a gentle index finger tap. *Exp. Brain Res.* 194:59–66, 2009.

Cordo, P.J., Gurfinkel, V.S. Motor coordination can be fully understood only by studying complex movements. *Prog. Brain Res.* 143:29–38, 2004.

Deliagina, T.G., et al. Spinal and supraspinal postural networks. *Brain Res. Rev.* 57:212–221, 2008.

Dietz, V. Evidence for a load receptor contribution to the control of posture and locomotion. *Neurosci. Biobehav. Rev.* 22:495–499, 1998.

Dietz, V., et al. Level of spinal cord lesion determines locomotor activity in spinal man. *Exp. Brain Res.* 128:405–409, 1999.

Fitzpatrick, R.C., et al. Ankle stiffness of standing humans in response to imperceptible perturbation: reflex and task-dependent components. *J. Physiol.* 454:533–547, 1992.

Forssberg, H. Neural control of human motor development. *Curr. Opin. Neurobiol.* 9:676–682, 1999.

Grasso, R., et al. Development of anticipatory orienting strategies during locomotor tasks in children. *Neurosci. Biobehav. Rev.* 22:533–539, 1998.

Grillner, S., Wallén, P. Innate versus learned movements—a false dichotomy? *Brain Res.* 143:297–309, 2004.

Grillner, S., et al. Neural bases of goal-directed locomotion in vertebrates—an overview. *Brain Res. Rev.* 57:2–12, 2008.

Hultborn, H. Plateau potentials and their role in regulating motoneuronal firing. *Prog. Brain Res.* 123:39–48, 1999.

Ito, Y., et al. The functional effectiveness of neck muscle reflexes for head-righting in response to sudden fall. *Exp. Brain Res.* 117:266–272, 1997.

Ivanenko, Y.P., et al. Distributed neural networks for controlling human locomotion. Lessons from normal and SCI subjects. *Brain Res. Bull.* 78:13–21, 2009.

Kavounoudias, A., et al. From balance regulation to body orientation: two goals for muscle proprioceptive information processing? *Exp. Brain Res.* 124:80–88, 1999.

Kuo, A.D., et al. Effect of altered sensory conditions on multivariate descriptions of human postural sway. *Exp. Brain Res.* 122:185–195, 1998.

Lackner, J.R., DiZio, P.A. Aspects of body self-calibration. *Trends Cogn. Sci.* 4:279–288, 2000.

Lacour, M., et al. Sensory strategies in human postural control before and after unilateral vestibular neurotomy. *Exp. Brain Res.* 115:300–310, 1997.

Lacquaniti, F., et al. Posture and movement: coordination and control. *Arch. Ital. Biol.* 135:353–367, 1997.

Lemon, R.N., et al. Direct and indirect pathways for corticospinal control of upper limb motoneurons in the primate. *Prog. Brain Res.* 143:263–279, 2004.

Massion, J., et al. Why and how are posture and movement coordinated? *Prog. Brain Res.* 143:13–27, 2004.

McCrea, D.A., Rybak, I.A. Organization of mammalian locomotor rhythm and pattern generation. *Brain Res. Rev.* 57:134–146, 2008.

Mergner, T., Rosemeier, T. Interaction of vestibular, somatosensory and visual signals for postural control and motion perception under terrestrial and microgravity conditions: a conceptual model. *Brain Res. Rev.* 28:118–135, 1998.

Muir, G.D., Stevens J.D. Sensorimotor stimulation to improve locomotor recovery after spinal cord injury. *Trends Neurosci.* 20:72–77, 1997.

Pearson, K.G. Generating the walking gait: role of sensory feedback. *Prog. Brain Res.* 143:123–129, 2004.

Perennou, D.A., et al. The polymodal sensory cortex is crucial for controlling lateral postural stability: evidence from stroke patients. *Brain Res. Bull.* 53:359–365, 2000.

Pettersen, T.H., et al. Cortical involvement in anticipatory postural reactions in man. *Exp. Brain Res.* 193:161–171, 2009.

Runge, C.F., et al. Role of vestibular information in initiation of rapid postural responses. *Exp. Brain Res.* 122:403–412, 1998.

Schiepatti, M., Nardone, A. Group II spindle afferent fibers in humans: their possible role in reflex control of stance. *Prog. Brain Res.* 123:461–472, 1999.

Schmitz, C., et al. Building of anticipatory postural adjustment during childhood: a kinematic and electromyographic analysis of unloading in children from 4 to 8 years of age. *Exp. Brain Res.* 142:354–364, 2002.

Stapley, P., et al. Investigating centre of mass stabilisation as the goal of posture and movement coordination during human whole body reaching. *Biol. Cybern.* 82:161–172, 2000.

Wu, A.M., et al. Anticipatory postural adjustments in stance and grip. *Exp. Brain Res.* 116:122–130, 1997.

Wu, G., Chiang J.-H. The significance of somatosensory stimulations to the human foot in the control of postural reflexes. *Exp. Brain Res.* 114:163–169, 1997.

Cortical Motor Areas and Voluntary Movements

Abe, M., Hanakawa, T. Functional coupling underlying motor and cognitive functions of the dorsal premotor cortex. *Behav. Brain Res.* 198:13–23, 2009.

Ansuini, C., et al. Bresaking the flow of action. *Exp. Brain Res.* 192:287–292, 2009.

Ashe, J., et al. Cortical control of motor sequences. *Curr. Opin. Neurobiol.* 16:213–221, 2006.

Bizzi, E., Mussa-Ivaldi, F.A. Neural basis of motor control and its cognitive implication. *Trends Cogn. Sci.* 2:97–102, 1998.

Boecker, H., et al. Role of human rostral supplementary motor area and the basal ganglia in motor sequence control: investigations with H$_2$ ^{15}O PET. *J. Neurophysiol.* 79:1070–1080, 1998.

Bush, G., et al. Dorsal anterior cingulate cortex: a role in reward-based decision making. *Proc. Natl. Acad. Sci. USA* 99:523–528, 2002.

Castiello, U. The neuroscience of grasping. *Nat. Rev. Neurosci.* 6:726–736, 2005.

Chouinard, P.A., Paus T. Ther primary motor and premotor areas of the human cerebral cortex. *Neuroscientist* 12 143–152, 2006.

Culham, J.C., Valyear K.F. Human parietal cortex in action. *Curr. Opin. Neurobiol.* 16:205–212, 2006.

Deiber, M.-P., et al. Cerebral structures participating in motor preparation in humans: a positron emission tomography study. *J. Neurophysiol.* 75:233–247, 1996.

Fadiga, L., et al. Human motor cortex excitability during the perception of other's action. *Curr. Opin. Neurobiol.* 15:213–218, 2005.

Flanders, M. Functional somatotopy in sensorimotor cortex. *NeuroReport* 16:313–316, 2005.

Fogassi, L., et al. Parietal lobe: from action organization to intention understanding *Science* 308:662–667, 2005.

Georgopoulos, A.P. New concepts in generation of movement. *Neuron* 13:257–268, 1994.

Grafton, S.T., et al. Functional anatomy of pointing and grasping in humans. *Cereb. Cortex* 6:226–237, 1996.

Graziano, M.S., et al. Complex movements evoked by microstimulation of precentral cortex. *Neuron* 34:841–851, 2002.

Graziano, M. The organization of behavioral repertoire in motor cortex. *Annu. Rev. Neurosci.* 29:105–134, 2006.

Halsband, U., et al. The role of the premotor cortex and the supplementary motor area in the temporal control of movement in man. *Brain* 116:243–266, 1993.

Hikosaka, O., et al. Differential roles of the frontal cortex, basal ganglia, and cerebellum in visuomotor sequence learning. *Neurobiol. Learn. Mem.* 70:137–149, 1998.

Hoshi, E., Tanji J. Distinctions between dorsal and ventral premotor areas: anatomical connectivity and functional properties. *Curr. Opin. Neurobiol.* 17:234–242, 2007.

Kawato, M. Internal models for motor control and trajectory planning. *Curr. Opin. Neurobiol.* 9:718–727, 1999.

Keller, A. Intrinsic synaptic organization of the motor cortex. *Cereb. Cortex* 3:430–441, 1993.

Lacquaniti, F., Carminiti, R. Visuo-motor transformations for arm reaching. *Eur. J. Neurosci.* 10:195–203, 1998.

Loeb, G.E. What might the brain know about muscles, limbs and spinal circuits? *Prog. Brain Res.* 123:405–409, 1999.

Luria, A.R. *Higher cortical functions in man.* 2nd ed. New York: Consultants Bureau, 1980.

Macchi, G., Jones, E.G. Toward an agreement on terminology of nuclear and subnuclear subdivisions of the motor thalamus. *J. Neurosurg.* 86:670–685, 1997.

Marsden, J.F., et al. Organization of cortical activities related to movements in humans. *J. Neurosci.* 15:2307–2314, 2000.

Mountcastle, V.B. et al. Posterior parietal association cortex of the monkey: command functions for operations within extrapersonal space. *J. Neurophysiol.* 38:871–908, 1975.

Nachev, P., et al. Functional role of the supplementary motor areas. *Nat. Rev. Neurosci.* 9:856–869, 2008.

Orban de Xivry, J.J., Ethier, V. Neural correlates of internal models. *J. Neurosci.* 28:7931–7932, 2008.

Paus, T., et al. Role of the human anterior cingulate cortex in the control of oculomotor, manual, and speech responses: a positron emission tomography study. *J. Neurophysiol.* 70:453–469, 1993.

Pearce, A.J., et al. Functional reorganisation of the corticomotor projection to the hand in skilled racquet players. *Exp. Brain Res.* 130:238–243, 2000.

Penfield, W., Rasmussen, T. *The cerebral cortex of man.* New York: Macmillan, 1950.

Phillips, C.G. *Movements of the hand.* Liverpool: Liverpool University Press, 1986.

Phillips, C.G., Porter, R. *Corticospinal neurones: their role in movement.* New York: Academic Press, 1977.

Picard, N., Strick, P.L. Motor areas of the medial wall: a review of their location and functional activation. *Cereb. Cortex* 6: 342–353, 1996.

Prochazka, A. Sensorimotor gain control: a basic strategy of motor systems? *Prog. Neurobiol.* 33:281–307, 1989.

Rademacher, J., et al. Variability and asymmetry in the human precentral motor system: a cytoarchitectonic and myeloarchitectonic brain mapping study. *Brain* 124:2232–2258, 2001.

Rao, S.M., et al. Somatotopic mapping of the human motor cortex with functional magnetic resonance imaging. *Neurology* 45: 919–924, 1995.

Rathelot, J.-A., Strick, P.L. Subdivisions of primary motor cortex based on cortico-motoneuronal cells. *Proc. Natl. Acad. Sci. USA* 106:918–923, 2009.

Rioult-Pedotti, M.-S., et al. Strengthening of horizontal cortical connections following skill learning. *Nat. Rev. Neurosci.* 1:230–234, 1998.

Rizzolatti, G., et al. Motor and cognitive functions of the ventral premotor cortex. *Curr. Opin. Neurobiol.* 12:149–154, 2002.

Rowe, J.B., Frackowiak, R.S.J. The impact of brain imaging technology on our understanding of motor function and dysfunction. *Curr. Opin. Neurobiol.* 9:728–734, 1999.

Rushworth, M.F.S., et al. Parietal cortex and movement. I. Movement selection and reaching. *Exp. Brain Res.* 117:292–310, 1997.

Sanes, J.N., Donoghue, J.P. Plasticity and primary motor cortex. *Annu. Rev. Neurosci.* 23:393–415, 2000.

Schieber, M.H. How might the motor cortex individuate movements? *Trends Neurosci.* 13:440–445, 1990.

Schluter, N.D., et al. Temporary interference in human lateral premotor cortex suggests dominance for the selection of movements: a study using transcranial magnetic stimulation. *Brain* 121: 785–799, 1998.

Serrien, D.J., et al. The missing link between action and cognition. *Prog. Neurobiol.* 82:95–107, 2007.

Sessle, B.J., Wiesendanger, M. Structural and functional definition of the motor cortex in the monkey (*Macaca fascicularis*). *J. Physiol.* 323:245–265, 1982.

Shima, K., Tanji, J. Both supplementary and presupplementary motor areas are crucial for the temporal organization of multiple movements. *J. Neurophysiol.* 80:3247–3260, 1998.

Shindo, K., et al. Spatial distribution of thalamic projections to the supplementary motor area and the primary motor cortex: a multiple retrograde labeling study in the macaque monkey. *J. Comp. Neurol.* 357:98–116, 1995.

Stephan, K.M., et al. The role of ventral medial wall motor areas in bimanual co-ordination: a combined lesion and activation study. *Brain* 122:351–368, 1999.

Sumner, P., Husain, M. At the edge of consciousness: automatic motor activation and voluntary control. *Neuroscientist* 14:474–486, 2008.

Tanji, J., Hoshi, E. Premotor areas: medial. In: Squire, L. (Ed.), *Encyclopedia of neuroscience* (pp. 925–933). Philadelphia: Elsevier, 2009.

Todorov, E. Direct cortical control of muscle activation in voluntary arm movements: a model. *Nat. Rev. Neurosci.* 3:391–398, 2000.

Tokuno, H., et al. Reevaluation of ipsilateral corticocortical inputs to the orofacial region of the primary motor cortex in the macaque monkey. *J. Comp. Neurol.* 389:34–48, 1997.

Wilson, S.A., et al. Transcranial magnetic stimulation mapping of the motor cortex in normal subjects: the representation of two intrinsic hand muscles. *J. Neurol. Sci.* 118:134–144, 1993.

Woolsey, C.N. Organization of somatic sensory and motor areas of the cerebral cortex. In: Harlow, H.F., Woolsey, C.N. (Eds.), *Biological and biochemical bases of behavior.* Madison, WI: University of Wisconsin Press, 1958.

Xiao, J. Premotor neuronal plasticity in monkeys adapting to a new dynamic environment. *Eur. J. Neurosci.* 22:3266–3280, 2005.

Yue, G.H., et al. Brain activation during finger extension and flexion movements. *Brain Res.* 856:291–300, 2000.

Motor Learning, Imagery, and Mirror Neurons

Berger, S.E., Adolph, K.E. Learning and development in infant locomotion. *Prog. Brain Res.* 164:237–255, 2007.

Catmur, C., et al. Through the looking glass: countermirror activation following incomparable sensorimotor learning. *Eur. J. Neurosci.* 28:1208–1215, 2008.

Gazzola, V., et al. The anthropomorphic brain: the mirror neuron system responds to human and robotic actions. *NeuroImage* 25:1674–1684, 2007.

Gentili, R., et al. Improvement and generalization of arm motor performance through motor imagery practice. *Neuroscience* 137:761–772, 2005.

Jacob, P., Jeannerod, M. The motor theory of social cognition. *Trends Cogn. Sci.* 9:21–25, 2005.

Jeannerod, M., Frak, V. Mental imaging of motor activity in humans. *Curr. Opin. Neurobiol.* 9:735–739, 1999

Decety, J., Grezes J. The power of simulation: imaging one's own and other's behavior. *Brain Res.* 1079:4–14, 2006.

Laforce, R., Doyon, J. Distinct contribution of the striatum and cerebellum in motor learning. *Brain Cogn.* 45:189–211, 2001.

Lalazar, H., Vaadia, E. Neural basis of sensorimotor learning: modifying internal models. *Curr. Opin. Neurobiol.* 18:573–581, 2008.

Li, S., et al. The effect of motor imagery on spinal segmental excitability. *J. Neurosci.* 24:9624–9680, 2004.

Naito, E., et al. Internally simulated sensations during motor imagery activate cortical motor areas and the cerebellum. *J. Neurosci.* 22:3683–3691, 2002.

Oztop, E., et al. Mirror neurons and imitation: a computationally guided review. *Neural Netw.* 19:254–271, 2006.

Pascual-Leone, A., et al. Modulation of muscle responses evoked by transcranial magnetic stimulation during the acquisition of new fine motor skills. *J. Neurophysiol.* 74:1037–1045, 1995.

Shmuelof, L., Zohary, E. Mirror-image representation of action in the anterior parietal cortex. *Nat. Rev. Neurosci.* 11:1267–1269, 2008.

Solodkin, A., et al. Fine modulation in network activation during motor execution and motor imagery. *Cereb. Cortex* 14:146–1255, 2004.

Stoeckel, M.C., et al. Congenitally altered motor experience alters somatotopic organization of human primary motor cortex. *Proc. Natl. Acad. Sci. USA* 106:2395–2400, 2009.

Wolpert, D.M., et al. Perspectives and problems in motor learning. *Trends Cogn. Sci.* 5:487–494, 2001.

Injury of Central Motor Pathways (Upper Motor Neurons)

Adams, M.M., Hicks, A.L. Spasticity after spinal cord injury. *Spinal Cord* 43:577–586, 2005.

Beer, R., et al. Disturbances of voluntary movement coordination in stroke: problems of planning or execution? *Prog. Brain Res.* 123:455–460, 1999.

Bennett, D.J., et al. Evidence for plateau potentials in tail motoneurons of awake chronic spinal rats with spasticity. *J. Neurophysiol.* 86:1972–1982, 2002.

Burne, J.A., et al. The spasticity paradox: movement disorder or disorder of resting limbs? *J. Neurol. Neurosurg. Psychiatry* 76:47–54, 2005.

Classen, J., et al. The motor syndrome associated with exaggerated inhibition within the primary motor cortex of patients with hemiparetic stroke. *Brain* 120:605–619, 1997.

Cleland, C.L., et al. Neural mechanisms underlying the clasp-knife reflex in the cat: stretch-sensitive muscular-free nerve endings. *J. Neurophysiol.* 64:1319–1330, 1990.

Dietz, V., Sinkjaer, T. Spastic movement disorder: impaired reflex function and altered muscle mechanics. *Lancet Neurol.* 6: 725–733, 2007.

Faist, M., et al. Impaired modulation of quadriceps tendon jerk reflex during spastic gait: differences between spinal and cerebral lesions. *Brain* 117:1449–1455, 1994.

Freund, H.-J., Hummelsheim, H. Lesions of premotor cortex in man. *Brain* 108:697–733, 1985.

Grey, M., et al. Post-activation depression of soleus stretch reflexes in healthy and spastic humans. *Exp. Brain Res.* 185:189–197, 200

Lance, J.W. The Babinski sign. *J. Neurol. Neurosurg. Psychiatry* 73:360–362, 2202.

Landau, W.M. Muscle tone: hypertonus, spasticity, rigidity. In: Adelman, G. (Ed.), *Encyclopedia of neuroscience* (pp. 721–723). Boston: Birkhauser, 1987.

Latash, M.L., Anson, J.G. What are "normal movements" in atypical populations? *Behav. Brain Sci.* 19:55–106, 1996.

Leon, F.E., Dimitrijyevic, M.R. Recent concepts in the pathophysiology and evaluation of spasticity. *Invest. Clin.* 38:155–162, 1997.

Levin, M.F. Interjoint coordination during pointing movements is disrupted in spastic hemiparesis. *Brain* 119:281–293, 1996.

Mayer, N.H. Clinicophysiologic concepts of spasticity and motor dysfunction in adults with an upper motoneuron lesion. *Muscle Nerve* 20(Suppl. 6):S1–S13, 1997.

Monrad-Krohn, G.H. *The clinical examination of the nervous system,* 10th. ed. London: H.K. Lewis, 1954.

Nathan, P.W. Effects on movement of surgical incisions into the human spinal cord. *Brain* 117:337–346, 1994.

Nielsen, J.B., et al. The spinal pathophysiology of spasticity—from a basic science point of view. *Acta Physiol.* 189:171–180, 2007.

Nudo, R.J. Recovery after damage to motor cortical areas. *Curr. Opin. Neurobiol.* 9:740–747, 1999.

Ropper, A.H., et al. Pyramidal infarction in the medulla: a cause of pure motor hemiplegia sparing the face. *Neurology* 29:91–95, 1979.

Sharma, N., et al. Motor imagery: a backdoor to the motor system after stroke? *Stroke* 37:1941–1952, 2006.

Sinkjær, T., et al. Non-reflex and reflex mediated ankle joint stiffness in multiple sclerosis patients with spasticity. *Muscle Nerve* 16:69–76, 1993.

Turton, A., Lemon R.N. The contribution of fast corticospinal input to the voluntary activation of proximal muscles in normal subjects and in stroke patients. *Exp. Brain Res.* 129:559–572, 1999.

Wilson, L.R., et al. Muscle spindle activity in the affected upper limb after a unilateral stroke. *Brain* 122:2079–2088, 1999.

Wirth, B., et al. Ankle dexterity remains intact in patients with incomplete spinal cord injury in contrast to stroke patients. *Exp. Brain Res.* 191:353–361, 2008.

Woallacott, A., Burne, J. The tonic stretch reflex and spastic hypertonia after spinal cord injury. *Exp. Brain Res.* 174:386–396, 2006.

Zadikoff, C., Lang, A.E. Apraxia in movement disorders. *Brain* 128:1480–1497, 2005.

CHAPTER 23: THE BASAL GANGLIA

Structure, Connections, and Physiology

Alexander, G.E., et al. Parallel organization of functionally segregated circuits linking basal ganglia and cortex. *Annu. Rev. Neurosci.* 9:357–381, 1986.

Chevalier, G., Deniau, J.M. Disinhibition as a basic process in the expression of striatal functions. *Trends Neurosci.* 13:277–280, 1990.

Draganski, B., et al. Evidence of segregated and integrative connectivity patterns in the human basal ganglia. *J. Neurosci.* 28:7143–7152, 2008.

Flaherty, A.W., Graybiel A.M. Input–output organization of the sensorimotor striatum in the squirrel monkey. *J. Neurosci.* 14:599–610, 1994.

Gerfen, C.R. The neostriatal mosaic: multiple levels of compartmental organization. *Trends Neurosci.* 15:133–138, 1992.

Gerfen, C.R. Basal ganglia. In: Paxinos, G. (Ed.), *The rat nervous system*, 3rd ed. (pp. 455–508). Philadelphia: Elsevier Academic Press, 2004.

Groenewegen, H.J., et al. Organization of the output of the ventral striatopallidal system in the rat: ventral pallidal afferents. *Neuroscience* 57:113–142, 1993.

Haber, S., Calzavara, R. The cortico-basal ganglia integrative network: the role of the thalamus. *Brain Res. Bull.* 78:69–74, 2009.

Haber, S., Gdowski, M.J. The basal ganglia. In: Paxinos, G., Mai, J.K. (Eds.), *The human nervous system*. 2nd ed. (pp. 676–738). Philadelphia: Elsevier Academic Press, 2004.

Lavoie, B., Parent, A. Pedunculopontine nucleus in the squirrel monkey: projections to the basal ganglia as revealed by anterograde tract-tracing methods. *J. Comp. Neurol.* 344:210–231, 1994.

Levesque, M., Parent, A. The striatofugal fiber system in primates: a reevaluation of its organization based on single-axon tracing studies. *PNAS* 102:11888–11893, 2005.

McFarland, N.R., Haber, S.N. Convergent inputs from thalamic motor nuclei and frontal cortical areas to the dorsal striatum in the primate. *J. Neurosci.* 20:3798–3813, 2000.

Meck, W.H., et al. Cortico-striatal representation of time in animals and humans. *Curr. Opin. Neurobiol.* 18:145–152, 2008.

Mena-Segovia, J., et al. Pedunculopontine nucleus and basal ganglia: distant relatives or part of the same family? *Trends Neurosci.* 27:585–589, 2004.

Middleton, F.A., Strick, P.L. Basal ganglia and cerebellar loops: motor and cognitive circuits. *Brain Res. Rev.* 31:236–250, 2000.

Munro-Davies, L.E., et al. The role of the pedunculopontine region in basal-ganglia mechanisms of akinesia. *Exp. Brain Res.* 129:511–517, 1999.

Obeso, J. A., et al. Functional organization of the basal ganglia: therapeutic implications for Parkinson's disease. *Mov. Disord.* 23 (Suppl. 3):S548–S549, 2008.

Postuma, R.B. Dagher, A. Basal ganglia functional connectivity based on a meta-analysis of 126 positron emission tomography and functional magnetic resonance imaging publications. *Cereb. Cortex* 16:1508–1521, 2006.

Romanelli, P., et al. Somatotopy in the basal ganglia: experimental and clinical evidence for segregated sensorimotor channels. *Brain Res. Rev.* 48:112–128, 2005.

Shink, E., et al. Efferent connections of the internal globus pallidus in the squirrel monkey. II. Topography and synaptic organization of pallidal efferents to the pedunculopontine nucleus. *J. Comp. Neurol.* 382:348–363, 1997.

Sidibé, M., et al. Efferent connections of the internal globus pallidus in the squirrel monkey. I. Topographic and synaptic organization of the pallidothalamic projection. *J. Comp. Neurol.* 382:323–347, 1997.

Smith, Y., et al. The thalamostriatal systems: anatomical and functional organization in normal and parkinsonian states. *Brain Res. Bull.* 78:60–68, 2009.

Tepper, J.M., et al. Feedforward and feedback inhibition in neostriatal GABAergic spiny neurons. *Brain Res. Rev.* 58:272–281, 2008.

Voorn, P., et al. Putting a spin on the dorsal-ventral divide of the striatum. *Trends Neurosci.* 27:468–474, 2005.

Wichmann, T., et al. The primate subthalamic nucleus. I. Functional properties in intact animals. *J. Neurophysiol.* 72:494–506, 1994.

Wilson, C.J. Striatum: Internal physiology. In: Squire, L. (Ed.), *Encyclopedia of neuroscience* (pp. 563–572). Philadelphia: Elsevier, 2009.

Neurotransmitters and Receptors

Aizman, O., et al. Anatomical and physiological evidence for D1 and D2 dopamine receptor colocalization in neostriatal neurons. *Nat. Rev. Neurosci.* 3:226–230, 2000.

Alcaro, A., et al. Behavioral functions of the mesolimbic dopaminergic system: an affective neuroethological perspective. *Brain Res. Rev.* 56:283–321, 2007.

Aubert, I., et al. Phenotypical characterization of the neurons expressing the D1 and D2 dopamine receptors in the monkey striatum. *J. Comp. Neurol.* 418:22–32, 2000.

Calabresi, P., et al. Acetylcholine-mediated modulation of striatal function. *Trends Neurosci.* 23:120–126, 2000.

Georges, F., Aston-Jones, G. Activation of ventral tegmental area cells by the bed nucleus of the stria terminalis: a novel excitatory amino acid input to midbrain dopaminergic neurons. *J. Neurosci.* 22:5173–5187, 2002.

Horvitz, J.C. Mesolimbocortical and nigrostriatal dopamine response to salient non-reward events. *Neuroscience* 96:651–656, 2000.

Joel, D., Weiner I. The connections of the dopaminergic system with the striatum in rats and primates: an analysis with respect to the functional and compartmental organization of the striatum. *Neuroscience* 96:451–474, 2000.

Kitai, S.T., et al. Afferent modulation of dopamine neuron firing patterns. *Curr. Opin. Neurobiol.* 9:690–697, 1999.

McNab, F., et al. Changes in cortical dopamine D1 receptor binding associated with cognitive training. *Science* 323:800–802, 2009.

Nicola, S.M., et al. Dopaminergic modulation of neuronal excitability in the striatum and nucleus accumbens. *Annu. Rev. Neurosci.* 23:185–215, 2000.

Redgrave, P., et al. What is reinforced by phasic dopamine signals? *Brain Res. Rev.* 58:322–339, 2008.

Schultz, W. Behavioral dopamine signals. *Trends Neurosci.* 30:203–210, 2007.

Soiza-Reilly, M., et al. Different D1 and D2 receptors expression after motor activity in the striatal critical period. *Brain Res.* 1004:217–221, 2004.

Tepper, J.M., et al. GABAergic microcircuits in the neostriatum. *Trends Neurosci.* 27:662–669, 2004.

Wise, RA. Dopamine, learning and motivation. *Nat. Rev. Neurosci.* 5:483–494, 2004.

Functions

Bhatia, K.P., Marsden C.D. The behavioral and motor consequences of focal lesions of the basal ganglia in man. *Brain* 117:859–876, 1994.

Calabresi, P., et al. The neostriatum beyond the motor function: experimental and clinical evidence. *Neuroscience* 78:39–60, 2002.

Desmurget, M., Turner, R.S. Testing basal ganglia motor functions through reversible inactivations in the posterior internal globus pallidus. *J. Neurophysiol.* 99:1057–1076, 2007.

Doya, K. Complementary roles of basal ganglia and cerebellum in learning and motor control. *Curr. Opin. Neurobiol.* 10:732–739, 2000.

Grahn, J.A., et al. The cognitive functions of the caudate nucleus. *Prog. Neurobiol.* 86:141–155, 2008.

Grahn, J.A., et al. The role of the basal ganglia in learning and memory: neuropsychological studies. *Behav. Brain Res.* 199:53–60, 2009.

Graybiel, A.M. The basal ganglia: learning new tricks and loving it. *Curr. Opin. Neurobiol.* 15:638–644, 2005.

Grillner, S., et al. Mechanisms for selection of basic motor programs—roles for the striatum and pallidum. *Trends Neurosci.* 28: 364–370, 2005.

Jog, M.S., et al. Building neural representations of habits. *Science* 286:1745–1748, 1999.

Marsden, C.D., Obeso J.A. The functions of the basal ganglia and the paradox of stereotaxic surgery in Parkinson's disease. *Brain* 117:877–897, 1994.

Meck, W.H., et al. Cortico-striatal representation of time in animals and humans. *Curr. Opin. Neurobiol.* 18:145–152, 2008.

Nambu, A. Seven problems on the basal ganglia. *Curr. Opin. Neurobiol.* 18:595–604, 2008.

Packard, M.G., Knowlton, B.J. Learning and memory functions of the basal ganglia. *Annu. Rev. Neurosci.* 25:563–593, 2002.

Redgrave, P., et al. The basal ganglia: a vertebrate solution to the selection problem? *Neuroscience* 89:1009–1023, 1999.

Stevens, M.C., et al. Functional neural circuits for timekeeping. *Hum. Brain Map.* 28:394–408, 2007.

Takakusaki, K., et al. Role of basal ganglia-brainstem systems in the control of postural muscle tone and locomotion. *Prog. Brain Res.* 143:231–237, 2004.

Temel, Y., et al. The functional role of the subthalamic nucleus in cognitive and limbic circuits. *Prog. Neurobiol.* 76:393–413, 2005.

Zweifel, L.S., et al. Disruption of NMDAR-dependent burst firing by dopamine neurons provides selective assessment of phasic dopamine-dependent bahvior. *Proc. Natl. Acad. Sci. USA* 106:7281–7288, 2009.

Ventral Striatum

Breiter, H.C., Rosen B.R. Functional magnetic resonance imaging of brain reward circuitry in the human. *Ann. NY Acad. Sci.* 877:523–547, 1999.

Cannon, C.M., Palmiter R.D. Reward without dopamine. *J. Neurosci.* 23:10827–10831, 2003.

de Olmos, J.S., Heimer L. The concepts of the ventral striatopallidal system and extended amygdala. *Ann. NY Acad. Sci.* 877:1–32, 1999.

Ellison, G. Stimulant-induced psychosis, the dopamine theory of schizophrenia, and the habenula. *Brain Res. Rev.* 19:223–239, 1994.

Floresco, S.B., et al. Dissociable roles for the nucleus accumbens core and shell in regulating set shift. *J. Neurosci.* 26:2449–2457, 2006.

Geisler, S. The lateral habenula: no longer neglected. *CNS Spectr.* 13:484–489. 2008.

Goto, Y., Grace, A.A. Limbic and cortical information processing in the nucleus accumbens. *Trends Neurosci.* 31:552–558, 2008.

Groenewegen, H.J., et al. Convergence and segregation of ventral striatal inputs and outputs. *Ann. NY Acad. Sci.* 877:49–63, 1999.

Hikosaka, O. New insights on the subcortical representation of reward. *Curr. Opin. Neurobiol.* 18:203–208, 2008.

Kelley, A.E. Nicotinic receptors: addiction's smoking gun? *Nat. Med.* 8:447–449, 2002.

Koob, G.F. The neurocircuitry of addiction: implications for treatment. *Clin. Neurosci. Res.* 5:89–101, 2005.

Koob, G.F., et al. Neuroscience of addiction. *Neuron* 21:467–476, 1998.

McCann, U.D., et al. Long-lasting effects of recreational drugs of abuse on the central nervous system. *Neuroscientist* 3:399–411, 1997.

Nestler, E.J., et al. Drug addiction: a model for the molecular basis of neural plasticity. *Neuron* 11:995–1006, 1993.

O'Doherty, J., et al. Dissociable roles of ventral and dorsal striatum in instrumental conditioning. *Science* 304:452–454, 2004.

Okun, M.S., et al. Deep brain stimulation in the internal capsule and nucleus accumbens region: responses observed during active and sham programming. *J. Neurol. Neurosurg. Psychiatry* 78:310–314, 2007.

Parkinson, J.A., et al. Dissociation in effects of lesions of the nucleus accumbens core and shell on appetitive pavlovian approach behavior and the potentiation of conditioned reinforcement and locomotor behavior by D-amphetamine. *J. Neurosci.* 19:2401–2411, 1999.

Sartorius, A., Henn, F.A. Deep brain stimulation of the lateral habenula in treatment resistant major depression. *Med. Hypotheses* 69:1305–1308, 2007.

Spanagel, R., Weiss F. The dopamine hypothesis of reward: past and current status. *Trends Neurosci.* 22:521–527, 1999.

Volkov, N., Li, T.K. The neuroscience of addiction. *Nat. Neurosci.* 8:1429–1430, 2005.

Weiss, F., Porrino, L.J. Behavioral neurobiology of alcohol addiction: recent advances and challenges. *J. Neurosci.* 22:3332–3337, 2002.

Diseases of the Basal Ganglia

Ackermans, L., et al. Deep brain stimulation in Tourette's syndrome. *Neurotherapeutics* 5:339–344, 2008.

Albin, R.L., Mink, J.W. Recent advances in Tourette syndrome research. *Trends Neurosci.* 29:175–182, 2006.

Antonini, A., et al. The metabolic anatomy of tremor in Parkinson's disease. *Neurology* 51:803–810, 1998.

Barker, R.A., Dunnett, S.B. Functional integration of neural grafts in Parkinson's disease. *Nat. Rev. Neurosci.* 2:1047–1048, 1999.

Baron, M.S., et al. Effects of transient focal inactivation of the basal ganglia in parkinsonian primates. *J. Neurosci.* 22:592–599, 2002.

Bezard, E., Gross, C.E. Compensatory mechanisms in experimental and human parkinsonism: towards a dynamic approach. *Prog. Neurobiol.* 55:1–24, 1998.

Björklund, A., Lindvall, G. Cell replacement therapies for central nervous system disorders. *Nat. Rev. Neurosci.* 3:537–544, 2000.

Brandt, J., Butters, N. The neuropsychology of Huntington's disease. *Trends Neurosci.* 9:118–120, 1986.

Breakfield, X.O., et al. The pathophysiological basis of dystonias. *Nat. Rev. Neurosci.* 9:222–234, 2208.

Brown, P. Abnormal oscillatory synchronization in the motor system leads to impaired movement. *Curr. Opin. Neurobiol.* 17:656–664, 2007.

Brown, R.G., Marsden C.D. Cognitive function in Parkinson's disease: from description to theory. *Trends Neurosci.* 13:21–29, 1990.

Cattaneo, E., et al. Normal huntingtin function: an alternative approach to Huntington's disease. *Nat. Rev. Neurosci.* 6:919–930, 2005.

Centonze, D., et al. Subthalamic nucleus lesion reverses motor abnormalities and striatal glutamatergic overactivity in experimental parkinsonism. *Neuroscience* 133:831–840, 2005.

Cody, F.W.J. Observations on the genesis of the stretch reflex in Parkinson's disease. *Brain* 109:229–249, 1986.

Edwards, R.H. Molecular analysis of Parkinson's disease. In: Martin, J.B. (Ed.), *Molecular neurology* (pp. 155–174). New York: Scientific American, Inc., 1998.

Gil, J.A., Rego, A.C. Mechanisms of neurodegeneration in Huntington's disease. *Eur. J. Neurosci.* 27:2803–2820, 2008.

Gray, J.M., et al. Impaired recognition of disgust in Huntington's disease gene carriers. *Brain* 120:2029–2038, 1997.

Hutchison, W.D., et al. Neuronal oscillations in the basal ganglia and movement disorders: evidence from whole animal and human recordings. *J. Neurosci.* 24:9240–9243, 2004.

Jankovic, J. Parkinson's disease: clinical features and diagnosis. *J. Neurol. Neurosurg. Psychiatry* 79:368–376, 2008.

Jellinger, K.A. Pathology of Parkinson's disease: changes other than the nigrostriatal pathway. *Mol. Chem. Neuropathol.* 14:153–197, 1991.

Levy, R., et al. Re-evaluation of the functional anatomy of the basal ganglia in normal and parkinsonian states. *Neuroscience* 76:335–343, 1997.

Levy, R., et al. Dependence of subthalamic nucleus oscillations on movement and dopamine in Parkinson's disease. *Brain* 125:1196–1209, 2002.

Lindvall, O., et al. Stem cell therapy for human neurodegenerative disorders—how to make it work. *Nat. Med.* 10:S42–S50, 2004.

Lozano, A.M., Kalia, S.K. New movements in Parkinsons's. *Sci. Am.* 293:68–75, 2005.

Magnin, M., et al. Single-unit analysis of the pallidum, thalamus and subthalamic nucleus in parkinsonian patients. *Neuroscience* 96:549–564, 2000.

Moore, D.J., et al. Molecular pathophysiology of Parkinson's disease. *Annu. Rev. Neurosci.* 28:57–87, 2005.

Obeso, J.A., et al. Basal ganglia pathophysiology: a critical review. In: *The basal ganglia and new surgical approaches for Parkinson's disease* (pp. 3–18). Advances in Neurology. Vol. 74. New York: Lippincott-Raven, 1997.

Obeso, J.A., et al. The globus pallidus pars externa and Parkinson's disease. Ready for prime time? *Exp. Neurol.* 202:1–7, 2006.

Pahapill, P.A., Lozano, A.M. The pedunculopontine nucleus and Parkinson's disease. *Brain* 123:1767–1783, 2000.

Pfann, K.D., et al. Pallidotomy and bradykinesia: implications for basal ganglia function. *Neurology* 51:796–803, 1998.

Reddy, P.H., et al. Recent advances in understanding the pathogenesis of Huntington's disease. *Trends Neurosci.* 22:248–255, 1999.

Riaz, S.S., Bradford, H.F. Factors involved in the determination of the neurotransmitter phenotype of developing neurons of the CNS: Applications in cell replacement treatment for Parkinson's disease. *Prog. Neurobiol.* 76:257–273, 2005.

Robertson, M.M. Tourette syndrome, associated conditions and the complexity of treatment. *Brain* 123:425–462, 2000.

Rodriguez-Oroz, M.C., et al. The subthalamic nucleus in Parkinson's disease: somatotopic organization and physiological characteristics. *Brain* 124:1777–1790, 2001.

Rodriguez-Oroz, M.C., et al. Bilateral deep brain stimulation in Parkinson's disease: a multicentre study with 4 years follow-up. *Brain* 128:2240–2249, 2005.

Sacks, O. *The man who mistook his wife for a hat* (pp. 87–97). New York: Picador, 1986.

Sheppard, D.M., et al. Tourette's and comorbid syndromes: obsessive compulsive and attention deficit hyperactivity disorder. A common etiology? *Clin. Psychol. Rev.* 19:531–532, 1999.

Singer, H.S. Tourette's syndrome: from behaviour to biology. *Lancet Neurology* 4:149–159, 2005.

Stephens, B. Evidence of a breakdown of corticostriatal connections in Parkinson's disease. *Neuroscience* 132:741–754, 2005.

York, M.K. Cognitive declines following bilateral subthalamic nucleus deep brain stimulation for the treatment of Parkinson's disease. *J. Neurol. Neurosurg. Psychiatry* 79:789–795, 2008.

Young, A.B. Huntington's disease and other trinucleotide repeat disorders. In: Martin, J.B. (Ed.), *Molecular neurology* (pp. 35–54). New York: Scientific American, Inc., 1998.

CHAPTER 24: THE CEREBELLUM

Structure, Connections, and Physiology

Andersen, B.B., et al. A quantitative study of the human cerebellum with unbiased stereological techniques. *J. Comp. Neurol.* 326:549–560, 1992.

Apps, R. Movement-related gating of climbing fibre input to cerebellar cortical zones. *Prog. Neurobiol.* 57:537–562, 1999.

Apps, R., Garwicz M. Anatomical and physiological foundations of cerebellar information processing. *Nat. Rev. Neurosci.* 6:297–311, 2005.

Bengtsson, F., Hesslow G. Cerebellar control of the inferior olive. *Cerebellum* 5:7–14, 2006.

Bloedel, J.R., Bracha, V. Current concepts of climbing fiber function. *Anat. Rec. (New Anat.)* 253:118–126, 1998.

Bosco, G., Poppele, R.E. Representation of multiple kinematic parameters of the cat hindlimb in spinocerebellar activity. *J. Neurophysiol.* 78:1421–1432, 1997.

Brodal, P., Bjaalie, J.G. Salient anatomic features of the cortico-ponto-cerebellar pathway. *Prog. Brain Res.* 114:227–249, 1997.

Cerminara, N.I., et al. An internal model of a moving target in the lateral cerebellum. *J. Physiol.* 587:429–442, 2009.

Dow, R.S., Moruzzi, G. *The physiology and pathology of the cerebellum.* Minneapolis, MN: University of Minnesota Press, 1958.

Eccles, J.C., et al. *The cerebellum as a neuronal machine.* New York: Springer-Verlag, 1967.

Garwicz, M., et al. Organizational principles of cerebellar neuronal circuitry. *News Physiol. Sci.* 13:26–32, 1998.

Gauck, V., Jaeger, D. The control of rate and timing of spikes in the deep cerebellar nuclei by inhibition. *J. Neurosci.* 20:3006–3016, 2000.

Grodd, W., et al. Sensorimotor mapping of the human cerebellum: fMRI evidence of somatotopic organization. *Hum. Brain Map.* 13:55–73, 2001.

Hawkes, R., Mascher, C. The development of molecular compartmentation in the cerebellar cortex. *Acta Anat.* 151:139–149, 1994.

Hoshi, E., et al. The cerebellum communicates with the basal ganglia. *Nat. Rev. Neurosci.* 8:1491–1493, 2005.

Ito, M. *The cerebellum and neural control.* New York: Raven Press, 1984.

Jacobsen, G.A., et al. A model of the of lignendeivo-cerebellar system as a temporal pattern generator. *Trends Neurosci.* 31:617–625, 2008.

Jahnsen, H. Electrophysiological characteristics of neurones in the guinea-pig deep cerebellar nuclei *in vitro. J. Physiol.* 372:129–147, 1986.

Jankowska, E., Puczynska, A. Interneuron activity in reflex pathways from group II muscle afferents is monitored by dorsal spinocerebellar tract neurons in the cat. *J. Neurosci.* 28:3615–3622, 2008.

King, J.S. *New concepts in cerebellar neurobiology.* New York: Alan R. Liss, 1987.

Lang, E.J., et al. Patterns of spontaneous Purkinje cell complex spike activity in the awake rat. *J. Neurosci.* 19:2728–2739, 1999.

Larouche, M., Hawkes, R. From clusters to stripes: the developmental origins of adult cerebellar compartmentation. *Cerebellum* 5:77–88, 2006.

Llinás, R., Sugimori, M. The electrophysiology of the cerebellar Purkinje cell revisited. In: Llinás, R., Sotelo, C. (Eds.), *The cerebellum revisited* (pp. 167–181). New York: Springer-Verlag, 1992.

Macchi, G., Jones, E.G. Toward an agreement on terminology of nuclear and subnuclear divisions of the motor thalamus. *J. Neurosurg.* 86:670–685, 1997.

Manni, E., Petrosini, L. A century of cerebellar somatotopy: a debated representation. *Nat. Rev. Neurosci.* 5:241–249, 2004.

Nietschke, M.F., et al. The cerebellum in the cerebro-cerebellar network for the control of eye and hand movements—an fMRI study. *Progr. Brain Res.* 148:151–164, 2005.

Odeh, F. et al. Pontine maps linking somatosensory and cerebellar cortices are in register with climbing fiber somatotopy. *J. Neurosci.* 15:5680–5690, 2005.

Ramnani, N. The primate cortico-cerebellar system: anatomy and function. *Nat. Rev. Neurosci.* 7:511–522, 2006.

Sakai, K., et al. Separate cerebellar areas for motor control. *NeuroReport* 9:2359–2363, 1998.

Sakai, S.T., et al. Comparison of cerebellothalamic and pallidothalamic projections in the monkey (*Macaca fuscata*): a double anterograde labeling study. *J. Comp. Neurol.* 368:215–228, 1996.

Thach, W.T., et al. Cerebellar output: multiple maps and modes of control in movement coordination. In: Llinas, R., Sotelo, C. (Eds.), *The cerebellum revisited* (pp. 283–300). New York: Springer-Verlag, 1992.

Their, P., Möck M. The oculomotor role of the pontine nuclei and the nucleus reticularis tegmenti pontis. *Prog. Brain Res.* 151: 293–2320, 2006.

Valle, M., et al. Cerebellar cortical activity in the cat anterior lobe during hindlimb stepping. *Exp. Brain Res.* 187:359–372, 2008.

Voogd, J., Ruigrok T.J.H. Transverse and longitudinal pattern in the mammalian cerebellum. *Prog. Brain Res.* 114:21–37, 1997.

Welker, W. Spatial organization of somatosensory projections to granule cell cerebellar cortex: functional and connectional implications of fractured somatotopy. In: King, J.S. (Ed.), *New concepts in cerebellar neurobiology* (pp. 239–280). New York: Alan R. Liss, 1987.

Wiesendanger, R., Wiesendanger, M. Cerebello-cortical linkage in the monkey as revealed by transcellular labeling with the lectin wheat germ agglutinin conjugated to the marker horseradish peroxidase. *Exp. Brain Res.* 59:105–117, 1985.

Cerebellum and Learning

Anderson, B.J., et al. Motor-skill learning: changes in synaptic organization of the rat cerebellar cortex. *Neurobiol. Learn. Mem.* 66:221–229, 1996.

Asanuma, H., Pavlides, C. Neurobiological basis of motor learning in mammals. *NeuroReport* 8:i–vi, 1997.

Bracha, V., et al. The human cerebellum and associative learning: dissociation between the acquisition, retention and extinction of conditioned eyeblinks. *Brain Res.* 860:87–94, 2000.

Catz, N., et al. Cerebellar-dependent motor learning is based on pruning of a Purkinje cell population response. *Proc. Natl. Acad. Sci. USA* 105:7309–7314, 2008.

D'Angelo, E., De Zeeuw, C.I. Timing and plasticity in the cerebellum: focus on the granular layer. *Trends Neurosci.* 32:30–40, 2008.

De Zeeuw, C.I., et al. Causes and consequences of oscillations in the cerebellar cortex. *Neuron* 58:655–658, 2008.

Hesslow, G., et al. Learned movements elicited by direct stimulation of cerebellar mossy fiber afferents. *Neuron* 24:179–185, 1999.

Ilg, W., et al. The influence of focal cerebellar lesions on the control and adaptation of gait. *Brain* 131:2913–2927, 2008.

Ioffe, M.E., et al. Role of cerebellum in learning postural tasks. *Cerebellum* 6:87–94, 2007.

Ito, M. Bases and implications of learning in the cerebellum—adaptive control and internal model mechanisms. *Prog. Brain Res.* 148: 95–107, 2005.

Jirenhed, D.-A., et al. Acquisition, extinction and reacquisition of a cerebellar cortical memory trace. *J. Neurosci.* 27:2493–2502, 2007.

Kassardjian, C.D., et al. The site of a motor memory shifts with consolidation. *J. Neurosci.* 25:7979–7985, 2005.

Kleim, J.A., et al. Structural stability within the lateral cerebellar nucleus of the rat following complex motor learning. *Neurobiol. Learn. Mem.* 69:290–306, 1998.

Lisberger, S.G. Cerebellar LTD: a molecular mechanism of behavioral learning? *Cell* 92:701–704, 1998.

Llinás, R., Welsh, J.P. On the cerebellum and motor learning. *Curr. Opin. Neurobiol.* 3:958–965, 1993.

Medina, J.F., Lisberger, S.G. Links from complex spikes to local plasticity and motor learning in the cerebellum of awake-behaving monkeys. *Nat. Rev. Neurosci.* 11:1185–1192, 2008.

Molinari, M., et al. Cerebellum and procedural learning: evidence from focal cerebellar lesions. *Brain* 120:1753–1762, 1997.

Nixon, P.D., Passingham, R.E. Predicting sensory events: the role of the cerebellum in motor learning. *Exp. Brain Res.* 138:251–257, 2001.

Optican, L.M., Robinson, D.A. Cerebellar-dependent adaptive control of primate saccadic system. *J. Neurophysiol.* 44:1058–1076, 1978.

Pascual-Leone, A., et al. Procedural learning in Parkinson's disease and cerebellar degeneration. *Ann. Neurol.* 34:594–602, 1993.

Raymond, J.L., et al. The cerebellum: a neuronal learning machine? *Science* 272:1126–1131, 1996.

Sacchetti, B., et al. Cerebellar role in fear-conditioning consolidation. *Proc. Natl. Acad. Sci. USA* 99:8406–8411, 2002.

Thach, W.T. On the specific role of the cerebellum in motor learning and cognition: clues from PET activation and lesion studies in man. *Behav. Brain Sci.* 19:411–431, 1996.

Thompson, R.F., et al. The nature of reinforcement in cerebellar learning. *Neurobiol. Learn. Mem.* 70:150–176, 1998.

Welsh, J.P., Harvey J.A. Acute inactivation of the inferior olive blocks associative learning. *Eur. J. Neurosci.* 10:3321–3332, 1998.

Werner, S., et al. The effect of cerebellar cortical degeneration on adaptive plasticity and movement control. *Exp. Brain Res.* 193:189–196, 2009.

Cerebellum and Cognitive Functions

Ackermann, H., et al. Does the cerebellum contribute to cognitive aspects of speech production? A functional magnetic resonance imaging (fMRI) study in humans. *Neurosci. Lett.* 247:187–190, 1998.

Andreasen, N.C., et al. "Cognitive dysmetria" as an integrative theory of schizophrenia: a dysfunction in cortical-subcortical-cerebellar circuitry? *Schizophr. Bull.* 24:203–218, 1998.

Copeland, D.R., et al. Neurocognitive development of children after a cerebellar tumor in infancy: a longitudinal study. *J. Clin. Oncol.* 17:3476–3486, 1999.

Frank, B., et al. Aphasia, neglect and extinction are no prominent clinical signs in children and adolescents with acute surgical cerebellar lesions. *Exp. Brain Res.* 184:511–519, 2008.

Gottwald, B., et al. Evidence for distinct cognitive deficits after focal cerebellar lesions. *J. Neurol. Neursosurg. Psychiatry* 75:1524–1531, 2004.

Hoppenbrouwers, S.S., et al. The role of the cerebellum in the pathophysiology and treatment of neuropsychiatric disorders. *Brain Res. Rev.* 59:185–200, 2008.

Ioannides, A.A., Fenwick, P.B.C. Imaging cerebellum activity in real time with magnetoencephalographic data. *Prog. Brain Res.* 148:139–150, 2005.

Ito, M. Control of mental activities by internal models in the cerebellum. *Nat. Rev. Neurosci.* 9:304–313, 2008.

Ivry, R.B., Schlerf, J.E. Dedicated and intrinsic models of time perception. *Trends Cogn. Sci.* 12:273–280, 2008.

Kim, S.-G., et al. Activation of a cerebellar output nucleus during cognitive processing. *Science* 265:949–951, 1994.

Le, T.H., et al. 4T-fMRI study of nonspatial shifting of selective attention: cerebellar and parietal contributions. *J. Neurophysiol.* 79:1535–1548, 1998.

Mangels, J.A., et al. Dissociable contributions of the prefrontal and neocerebellar cortex to time perception. *Cogn. Brain Res.* 7:15–39, 1998.

Mukhopadhyay, P., et al. Identification of neuroanatomical substrates of set-shifting ability: evidence from patients with focal brain lesions. *Prog. Brain Res.* 168:95–104, 2008.

Nixon, P.D., Passingham, R.E. The cerebellum and cognition: cerebellar lesions do not impair spatial working memory or visual associative learning in the monkey. *Eur. J. Neurosci.* 11:4070–4080, 1999.

O'Reilly, J.X., et al. The cerebellum predicts the timing of perceptual events. *J. Neurosci.* 28:2252–2260, 2008.

Ravizza, S.M., et al. Cerebellar damage produces selective deficits in verbal working memory. *Brain* 129:306–320, 2006.

Schmahmann, J.D., Sherman, J.C. The cerebellar cognitive affective syndrome. *Brain* 121:561–579, 1998.

Townsend, J., et al. Spatial attention deficits in patients with acquired or developmental cerebellar abnormality. *J. Neurosci.* 19:5632–5643, 1999.

Cerebellar Function and Symptoms in Disease

Bastian, A.J. Learning to predict the future: the cerebellum adapts feedforward movement control. *Curr. Opin. Neurobiol.* 16:645–649, 2006

Blakemore, S.J., et al. The cerebellum is involved in predicting the sensory consequences of action. *NeuroReport* 12:1879–1885, 2001.

Bower, J.M. Is the cerebellum sensory for motor's sake, or motor for sensory's sake: the view from the whiskers of a rat? *Prog. Brain Res.* 114:463–497, 1997.

Braitenberg, V., et al. The detection and generation of sequences as a key to cerebellar function. *Behav. Brain Sci.* 20:229–277, 1997.

Cerri, G., et al. Coupling hand and foot voluntary oscillations in patients suffering cerebellar ataxia: different effect of lateral and medial lesions on coordination. *Prog. Brain Res.* 148:227–241, 2005.

Ghelarducci, B., Sebastiani, L. Contributions of the cerebellar vermis to cardiovascular control. *J. Auton. Nerv. Syst.* 56:149–156, 1996.

Glickstein, M., et al. Cerebellum and finger use. *Cerebellum* 4:189–197, 2005.

Gorassani, M., et al. Cerebellar ataxia and muscle spindle sensitivity. *J. Neurophysiol.* 70:1853–1862, 1993.

Holmes, G. The cerebellum. In: Phillips, C.G. (Ed.), *Selected papers of Gordon Holmes* (pp. 186–247). Oxford: Oxford University Press, 1979.

Imamizu, H., et al. Human cerebellar activity reflecting an acquired internal model of a new tool. *Nature* 403:192–195, 2000.

Kawato, M. Internal models for motor control and trajectory planning. *Curr. Opin. Neurobiol.* 9:718–727, 1999.

Keele, S.W., Ivry, R. Does the cerebellum provide a common computation for diverse tasks? *Ann. NY Acad. Sci.* 608:179–207, 1990.

Luft, A.R., et al. Comparing motion- and imagery-related activation in the human cerebellum: a functional MRI study. *Hum. Brain Map.* 6:105–113, 1998.

Marti, S., et al. A model-based theory on the origin of downbeat nystagmus. *Exp. Brain Res.* 188:613–631, 2008.

Morton, S.M., Bastian, A.J. Cerebellar control of balance and locomotion. *Neuroscientist* 10:247–259, 2004.

Müller, F., Dichgans, J. Dyscoordination of pinch and lift forces during grasp in patients with cerebellar lesions. *Exp. Brain Res.* 101:485–492, 1994.

Ohyama, T., et al. What the cerebellum computes. *Trends Neurosci.* 26:222–227, 2003.

Palliyath, S., et al. Gait in patients with cerebellar ataxia. *Mov. Disord.* 13:958–964, 1998.

Paulin, M.G. The role of the cerebellum in motor control and perception. *Brain Behav. Evol.* 41:39–50, 1993.

Pekhletski, R., et al. Impaired cerebellar synaptic plasticity and motor performance in mice lacking the mGluR4 subtype of metabotropic glutamate receptor. *J. Neurosci.* 16:6364–6373, 1996.

Robinson, F.R., Fuchs, A.F. The role of the cerebellum in voluntary eye movements. *Annu. Rev. Neurosci.* 24:981–1004, 2001.

Straube, A., et al. Unilateral cerebellar lesions affect initiation of ipsilateral smooth pursuit eye movements in humans. *Ann. Neurol.* 42:891–898, 1997.

Takagi, M., et al. Effects of lesions of the oculomotor cerebellar vermis on eye movements in primate: smooth pursuit. *J. Neurophysiol.* 83:2047–2062, 2000.

Timmann, D., et al. Classically conditioned withdrawal reflex in cerebellar patients. 1. Impaired conditioned responses. *Exp. Brain Res.* 130:453–470, 2000.

Walker, M.F., Zee D.S. Directional abnormalities of vestibular and optokinetic responses in cerebellar disease. *Ann. NY Acad. Sci.* 871:205–220, 1999.

Welsh, J.P., Harvey J.A. The role of the cerebellum in voluntary and reflexive movements: history and current status. In: Llinás, R., Sotelo, C. (Eds.), *The cerebellum revisited* (pp. 301–334). New York: Springer-Verlag, 1992.

Werner, S., et al. The effect of cerebellar cortical degeneration on adaptive plasticity and movement control. *Exp. Brain Res.* 193:189–196, 2009.

Wolpert, D.M., et al. Internal models in the cerebellum. *Trends Cogn. Sci.* 2:338–347, 1998.

CHAPTER 25: CONTROL OF EYE MOVEMENTS

Eye Muscles and Eye Movements

Büttner-Ennever, J.A., et al. Sensory control of extraocular muscles. *Prog. Brain Res.* 151:81–93, 2006.

Donaldson, I.M. The functions of proprioceptors of the eye muscles. *Philos. Trans. R. Soc. Lond. B Biol. Sci.* 355:1685–1754, 2000.

Gilchrist, I.D. Saccades without eye movements. *Nature* 390:130–131, 1997.

Goldberg, S.J., Shall M.S. Motor units of extraocular muscles: recent findings. *Prog. Brain Res.* 123:221–232, 1999.

Hayhoe, M., Ballard, D. Eye movements in natural behavior. *Trends Cogn. Sci.* 9:188–194, 2005.

Jampel, R.S. The function of the extraocular muscles, the theory of the coplanarity of fixation planes. *J. Neurol. Sci.* 280:1–9, 2009.

Lewis, R.F., et al. Oculomotor function in the rhesus monkey after deafferentation of the extraocular muscles. *J. Exp. Brain Res.* 141:349–358, 2001.

Ruff, R.L. More than meets the eye: extraocular muscle is very distinct from extremity skeletal muscles. *Muscle Nerve* 25:311–313, 2002.

Spencer, R.F., Porter J.D. Biological organization of the extraocular muscles. *Prog. Brain Res.* 151:43–80, 2006.

Brain Stem and Cerebellum

Büttner-Ennever, J.A. Mapping the oculomotor system. *Prog. Brain Res.* 171:3–11, 2008.

Büttner, U., Büttner-Ennever, J.A. Present concepts of oculomotor organization. *Prog. Brain Res.* 151:1–42, 2006.

Curthoys, I.S. Generation of the quick phase of horizontal vestibular nystagmus. *Exp. Brain Res.* 143:397–405, 2002.

Dean, P., et al. Event or emergency? Two systems in the mammalian superior colliculus. *Trends Neurosci.* 12:137–147, 1989.

duLac, S., et al. Learning and memory in the vestibulo-ocular reflex. *Annu. Rev. Neurosci.* 18:409–441, 1995.

Gaymard, B., et al. Smooth pursuit eye movement deficits after pontine nuclei lesions in humans. *J. Neurol. Neurosurg. Psychiatry* 56:799–807, 1993.

Grosbras, M.H., et al. Human cortical networks for new and familiar sequences of saccades. *Cereb. Cortex* 11:936–945, 2001.

Grüsser, O.-J., et al. Vestibular neurones in the parieto-insular cortex of monkeys (*Macaca fascicularis*): visual and neck receptor responses. *J. Physiol.* 430:559–583, 1990.

Grüsser, O.-J., et al. Cortical representation of head-in-space movement and some psychophysical experiments on head movement. In: Berthoz, A., et al. (Eds.), *The head-neck sensory motor system* (pp. 497–509). Oxford: Oxford University Press, 1992.

Horn, A.K.E., et al. Brainstem and cerebellar structures for eye movement generation. In: Büttner, U. (Ed.), *Vestibular dysfunction and its therapy* (pp. 1–25). Basel: Karger, 1999.

Ilg, U.J. Slow eye movements. *Prog. Neurobiol.* 53:293–329, 1997.

Ito, M. *The cerebellum and neural control.* New York: Raven Press, 1984.

Kawano, K. Ocular tracking: behavior and neurophysiology. *Curr. Opin. Neurobiol.* 9:467–473, 1999.

Kennard, C., Clifford Rose F. *Physiological aspects of clinical neuro-ophthalmology.* New York: Chapman & Hall, 1988.

Lempert, T., et al. Effect of otolith dysfunction: impairment of visual acuity during linear head motion in labyrinthine defective subjects. *Brain* 120:1005–1013, 1997.

Lisberger, S.G., et al. Visual motion processing and sensory-motor integration of smooth pursuit eye movements. *Annu. Rev. Neurosci.* 10:97–129, 1987.

Martinez-Conde, S., et al. The role of fixational eye movements in visual perception. *Nat. Rev. Neurosci.* 5:229–240, 2004.

Müri, R.M. MRI and fMRI analysis of oculomotor function. *Prog. Brain Res.* 151:503–526, 2006.

Quaia, C., et al. Model for the control of saccades by superior colliculus and cerebellum. *J. Neurophysiol.* 82:999–1018, 1999.

Raphan, T., Cohen, B. The vestibulo-ocular reflex in three dimensions. *Exp. Brain Res.* 145:1–27, 2002.

Robinson, F.R. The role of the cerebellum in voluntary eye movements. *Annu. Rev. Neurosci.* 24:981–1004, 2001.

Rüb, U., et al. Functional neuroanatomy of human premotor oculomotor brainstem nuclei: insights from postmortem and advanced in vivo imaging studies. *Exp. Brain Res.* 187:167–180, 2008.

Scudder, C.A., et al. The brainstem burst generator for saccadic eye movements: a modern synthesis. *Exp. Brain Res.* 142:439–462, 2002.

Shinoda, Y., et al. Neural circuits for triggering saccades in the brainstem. *Prog. Brain Res.* 171:79–85, 2008.

Sparks, D.L. Conceptual issues related to the role of the superior colliculus in the control of gaze. *Curr. Opin. Neurobiol.* 9: 698–707, 1999.

Suzuki, D.A., et al. Smooth-pursuit eye movement deficits with chemical lesions in macaque nucleus reticularis tegmenti pontis. *J. Neurophysiol.* 82:1178–1186, 1999.

Their, P., Ilg, U.J. The neural basis of smooth-pursuit eye movements. *Curr. Opin. Neurobiol.* 15:645–652, 2005.

Thier, P., Möck, M. The oculomotor role of the pontine nuclei and the nucleus reticularis tegmenti pontis. *Prog. Brain Res.* 151:293–2320, 2006.

Waterston, J.A., et al. A quantitative study of eye and head movements during smooth pursuit in patients with cerebellar disease. *Brain* 115:1343–1358, 1992.

Cortical Level

Andersen, R.A., et al. Evidence for the lateral intraparietal area as the parietal eye field. *Curr. Opin. Neurobiol.* 2:840–846, 1992.

Anderson, T.J., et al. Cortical control of saccades and fixation in man: a PET study. *Brain* 117:1073–1084, 1994.

Corbetta, M., et al. A common network of functional areas for attention and eye movements. *Neuron* 71:761–773, 1998.

Heide, W., et al. Deficits of smooth pursuit eye movements after frontal and parietal lesions. *Brain* 119:1951–1969, 1996.

Hikosaka, O., Isoda, M. Brain mechanisms for switching from automatic to controlled eye movements. *Prog. Brain Res.* 171:375–382, 2008.

Krauzlis, R.J., Stone, L.S. Tracking with the mind's eye. *Trends Neurosci.* 22:544–550, 1999.

Latto, R. The role of the inferior parietal cortex and the frontal eye-fields in visuospatial discriminations in the macaque monkey. *Behav. Brain Res.* 22:41–52, 1986.

Leff, A.P., et al. The planning and guiding of reading saccades: a repetitive transcranial magnetic stimulation study. *Cereb. Cortex* 11:918–923, 2001.

Liversedge, S.P., Findlay, J.M. Saccadic eye movements and cognition. *Trends Cogn. Sci.* 4:6–14, 1999.

Rosenthal, C.R., et al. Supplementary eye field contributions to the execution of saccades to remembered target locations. *Prog. Brain Res.* 171:419–423, 2008.

Sweeney, J.A., et al. Positron emission tomography study of voluntary saccadic eye movements and spatial working memory. *J. Neurophysiol.* 75:454–468, 1996.

Zhang, M., et al. Monkey primary somatosensory cortex has a proprioceptive representation of eye position. *Prog. Brain Res.* 171:37–45, 2008.

CHAPTER 26: THE RETICULAR FORMATION: PREMOTOR NETWORKS, CONSCIOUSNESS, AND SLEEP

Structure and Physiology

Azmitia, E.C. Serotonin neurons, neuroplasticity, and homeostasis of neural tissue. *Neuropsychopharmacology* 21(Suppl.):33S–45S, 1999.

Barlow, J.S. The electroencephalogram: its patterns and origins. Cambridge, MA: MIT Press, 1993.

Brodal, A. The reticular formation of the brain stem: anatomical aspects and functional correlations. Edinburgh: Oliver & Boyd, 1957.

Dobbins, E.G., Feldman J.L. Brainstem network controlling descending drive to phrenic motoneurons in rat. *J. Comp. Neurol.* 347:64–86, 1994.

Feldman, J.L., Del Negro, C.A. Looking for inspiration: new perspectives on respiratory rhythm. *Nat. Rev. Neurosci.* 7:232–242, 2006.

Foote, S.L., Morrison, J.H. Extrathalamic modulation of cortical function. *Annu. Rev. Neurosci.* 10:67–95, 1987.

Grantyn, A., et al. Tracing premotor brain stem networks of orienting movements. *Curr. Opin. Neurobiol.* 3:973–981, 1993.

Jordan, L.M., et al. Control of functional systems in the brainstem and spinal cord. *Curr. Opin. Neurobiol.* 2:794–801, 1992.

Kerman, I. Organization of brain somatomotor-sympathetic circuits. *Exp. Brain Res.* 187:1–16, 2008.

Korn, H., Faber, D.S. Escape behavior: brainstem and spinal cord circuitry and function. *Curr. Opin. Neurobiol.* 6:826–832, 1996.

Lagercrantz, H. Neuromodulators and respiratory control during development. *Trends Neurosci.* 10:368–372, 1987.

Lund, J.P., et al. Brainstem mechanisms underlying feeding behaviors. *Curr. Opin. Neurobiol.* 8:718–724, 1998.

Miller, K.W. Are lipids or proteins the target of general anaesthetic action? *Trends Neurosci.* 9:49–51, 1986.

Mironov, S. Respiratory circuits: function, mechanisms, topology, and pathology. *Neuroscientist* 15:194–208, 2009.

Moruzzi, G., Magoun, H.W. Brain stem reticular formation and activation of the EEG. *Electroencephalogr. Clin. Neurophysiol.* 1:455–473, 1949.

Müller, C.M., et al. Structures mediating cholinergic reticular facilitation of cortical structures in the cat: effects of lesions in immunocytochemically characterized projections. *Exp. Brain Res.* 96:8–18, 1993.

Ramirez, J.-M., Richter, D.W. The neuronal mechanisms of respiratory rhythm generation. *Curr. Opin. Neurobiol.* 6:817–825, 1996.

Rho, M.-J., et al. Organization of the projection from the pericruciate cortex to the pontomedullary reticular formation of the cat: a quantitative retrograde tracing study. *J. Comp. Neurol.* 388:228–249, 1997.

Richter, D.W., Spyer, K.M. Studying rhythmogenesis of breathing: comparison of *in vivo* and *in vitro* models. *Trends Neurosci.* 24:464–472, 2002.

Scheibel, M.E., Scheibel, A.B. Structural substrates for integrative patterns in the brain stem reticular core. In: Jasper, H.H., et al. (Eds.), *Reticular formation of the brain* (pp. 31–55). Boston: Little Brown, 1958.

Simpson, K.L., et al. Projection patterns from the raphe nuclear complex to the ependymal wall of the ventricular system in the rat. *J. Comp. Neurol.* 399:61–72, 1998.

Steriade, M. Impact of network activities on neuronal properties in corticothalamic systems. *J. Neurophysiol.* 86:1–39, 2001.

Tononi, G., et al. Complexity and coherence: integrating information in the brain. *Trends Cogn. Sci.* 2:474–484, 1998.

Locus Coeruleus and Raphe Nuclei

Amat, J., et al. Medial frontal cortex determines how stressor controllability affects behavior and dorsal raphe nucleus. *Nat. Rev. Neurosci.* 8:365–371, 2005.

Aston-Jones, G., Cohen, J.D. An integrative theory of locus coeruleus-norepinephrine function: adaptive gain and optimal performance. *Ann. Rev. Neurosci.* 28:403–450, 2005.

Aston-Jones, G., et al. Role of locus coeruleus in attention and behavioral flexibility. *Biol. Psychiatry* 46:1309–1320, 1999.

Berridge, C.W., Foote, S.L. Effects of locus coeruleus activation on electroencephalographic activity in neocortex and hippocampus. *J. Neurosci.* 11:3135–3145, 1991.

Bouret, S., Sara, S.J. Network reset: a simplified overarching theory of locus coeruleus noradrenaline function. *Trends Cogn. Sci.* 28:574–582, 2005.

Cirelli, C., Tononi, G. Locus coeruleus control of state-dependent gene expression. *J. Neurosci.* 24:5410–5419, 2004.

Jacobs, B.L., Fornal, C.A. Serotonin and motor activity. *Curr. Opin. Neurobiol.* 7:820–825, 1997.

Kobayashi, K., et al. Modest neuropsychological deficits caused by reduced noradrenaline metabolism in mice heterozygous for a mutated tyrosine hydroxylase gene. *J. Neurosci.* 20:2418–2426, 2000.

Lovick, T.A. The medullary raphe nuclei: a system for integration and gain control in autonomic and somatomotor responsiveness? *Exp. Physiol.* 82:31–41, 1997.

Richerson, G.B. Serotonergic neurons as carbon dioxide sensors that maintain pH homeostasis. *Nat. Rev. Neurosci.* 5:449–461, 2004.

Saper, C.B. Function of the locus coeruleus. *Trends Neurosci.* 10:343–344, 1987.

Sara, S.J. The locus coeruleus and noradrenergic modulation of cognition. *Nat. Rev. Neurosci.* 10:211–223, 2009.

Sergeyev, V., et al. Serotonin and substance P co-exist in dorsal raphe neurons of the human brain. *NeuroReport* 10:3967–3970, 1999.

Consciousness and Attention

Baars, B.J., et al. Brain, conscious experience and the observing self. *Trends Neurosci.* 26:671–675, 2003.

Berlucchi, G. One or many arousal systems? Reflections on some of Guiseppe Moruzzi's foresights and insights about the intrinsic regulation of brain activity. *Arch. Ital. Biol.* 135:5–14, 1997.

Cattaneo, L., et al. Pathological yawning as a presenting symptom of brain stem ischaemia in two patients. *J. Neurol. Neurosurg. Psychiatry* 77:98–100, 2006.

Crick, F.C., Koch, C. Consciousness and neuroscience. *Cereb. Cortex* 8:97–107, 1998.

Dehaene, S., et al. Conscious, preconscious, and subliminal processing: a testable taxonomy. *Trends Cogn. Sci.* 10:204–211, 2006.

Franks, N.P. General anaesthesia: from molecular targets to neuronal pathways of sleep and arousal. *Nat. Rev. Neurosci.* 9:370–386, 2008.

Gazzaniga, M.S. Brain mechanisms and conscious experience. *Ciba Found. Symp.* 174:247–262, 1993.

Hesslow, G. Conscious thought as simulation of behaviour and perception. *Trends Cogn. Sci.* 6:242–247, 2002.

Jennett, B. The vegetative state. *J. Neurol. Neurosurg. Psychiatry* 73:355–357, 2002.

Kaada, B. Site of action of myanesin (mephenesin, tolserol) in the central nervous system. *J. Neurophysiol.* 13:89–104, 1950.

Kinomura, S., et al. Activation by attention of the human reticular formation and thalamic intralaminar nuclei. *Science* 271:512–515, 1996.

Knudsen, E.I. Fundamental components of attention. *Annu. Rev. Neurosci.* 30:57–78, 2007.

Koch, C., Tsuchiya, N. Attention and consciousness: two distinct brain processes. *Trends Cogn. Sci.* 11:16–22, 2006.

Kurthen, M., et al. Will there be a neuroscientific theory of consciousness? *Trends Cogn. Sci.* 2:229–234, 1998.

Laureys, S. The neural correlate of (un)awareness: lessons from the vegetative state. *Trends Cogn. Sci.* 9:556–559, 2005.

Llinas, R., Ribary, U. Consciousness and the brain: the thalamocortical dialogue in health and disease. *Ann. NY Acad. Sci.* 929:166–175, 2001.

Naccache, L. Is she conscious? *Science* 313:1395–1396, 2006.

Owen, A.M., Coleman, M.R. Functional neuroimaging of the vegetative state. *Nat. Rev. Neurosci.* 9:235–243, 2008.

Peltier, S.J., et al. Functional connectivity changes with concentration of sevoflurane anesthesia. *NeuroReport* 16:285–288, 2005.

Perry, E., et al. Acetylcholine in mind: neurotransmitter correlate of consciousness? *Trends Neurosci.* 22:273–280, 1999.

Platek, S.M., et al. Contagious yawning and the brain. *Cogn. Brain Res.* 23:448–452, 2005.

Raz, A., Buhle, J. Typologies of attentional networks. *Nat. Rev. Neurosci.* 7:367–379, 2006.

Rudolph, U., Antkowiak, B. Molecular and neuronal substrates for general anaesthetics. *Nat. Rev. Neurosci.* 5:709–720, 2004.

Sarter, M., Bruno, J.P. Cortical cholinergic inputs mediating arousal, attentional processing and dreaming: differential afferent regulation of the basal forebrain by telencephalic and brainstem afferents. *Neuroscience* 95:933–952, 2000.

Searle, J.R. Consciousness. *Annu. Rev. Neurosci.* 23:557–578, 2000.

Shipp, S. The brain circuitry of attention. *Trends Cogn. Sci.* 8:223–230, 2004.

Siegel, J.M. Do all animals sleep? *Trends Neurosci.* 31:208–213, 2008.

Singer, O.C., et al. Yawning in acute anterior circulation stroke. *J. Neurol. Neurosurg. Psychiatry* 78:1253–1254, 2007.

Singer, W. Consciousness and the binding problem. *Ann. NY Acad. Sci.* 929:123–146, 2001.

Steriade, M. Thalamocortical oscillations in the sleeping and aroused brain. *Science* 262:679–685, 1993.

Sumner, P., Husain, M. At the age of consciousness: automatic motor activation and voluntary control. *Neuroscientist* 14:474–486, 2008.

Velman, M. How to separate conceptual issues from empirical ones in the study of consciousness. *Prog. Brain Res.* 168:1–9, 2008.

Weiskrantz, L. Consciousness lost and found: a neuropsychological exploration. New York: Oxford University Press, 1997.

Womelsdorf, T., Fries, P. The role of neuronal synchronization in selective attention. *Curr. Opin. Neurobiol.* 17:154–160, 2007.

Zeki, S. The disunity of consciousness. *Prog. Brain Res.* 168:11–18, 2008.

Sleep and Dreaming

Fort, P., et al. Alternative vigilance states: new insights regarding neuronal networks and mechanisms. *Eur. J. Neurosci.* 29:1741–1753, 2009.

Geraschenko, D., et al. Identification of a population of sleep-active cerebral cortex neurons. *Proc. Natl. Acad. Sci. USA* 105:10227–10232, 2008.

Gottesmann, C. Noradrenaline involvement in basic and higher integrated REM sleep processes. *Prog. Neurobiol.* 85:237–272, 2008.

Hobson, J.A. The neuropsychology of REM sleep dreaming. *NeuroReport* 9.R1–R14, 1998.

Huber, R., et al. Local sleep and learning. *Nature* 430:78–81, 2004.

Jha, S.K., et al. Sleep-dependent plasticity requires cortical activity. *J. Neurosci.* 25:9266–9274, 2005.

Jouvet, M. Sleep and serotonin: an unfinished story. *Neuropsychopharmacology* 21(Suppl.):24S-27S, 1999.

Kavanau, J.L. Dream contents and failing memories. *Arch. Ital. Biol.* 140:109–127, 2002.

Krueger, J.M., et al. Sleep as a fundamental property of neuronal assemblies. *Nat. Rev. Neurosci.* 9:910–919, 2008.

Massimini, M., et al. Breakdown of cortical effective connectivity during sleep. *Science* 309:2228–2232, 2005.

Massimini, M., et al. Slow waves, synaptic plasticity and information processing: insights from transcranial magnetic stimulation and high-density EEG experiments. *Eur. J. Neurosci.* 29:1761–1770, 2009.

Mednick, S.C. The restorative effects of naps on perceptual deterioration. *Nat. Neurosci.* 5:677–681, 2002.

Mölle, M., Born, J. Hippocampus whispering in deep sleep to prefrontal cortex—for good memories? *Neuron* 61:496–498, 2009.

Nelson, L.E., et al. The sedative component of anesthesia is mediated by GABA$_A$ receptors in an endogenous sleep pathway. *Nat. Neurosci.* 5:979–984, 2002.

Nishino, S., Mignot, E. Neurobiology of narcolepsy. *Neuroscientist* 4:133–143, 1998.

Oishi, Y., et al. Adenosine in the tuberomammillary nucleus inhibits the histaminergic system via A1 receptors and promotes non-rapid eye movement sleep. *Proc. Natl. Acad. Sci. USA* 105:19992–19997, 2008.

Pose, I., et al. Cuneiform neurons activated during cholinergically induced active sleep in the cat. *J. Neurosci.* 20:3319–3327, 2000.

Rasch, B., et al. Odor cues during slow-wave sleep prompt declarative memory consolidation. *Science* 315:1426–1429, 2007.

Sakai, K., et al. Pontine structures and mechanisms involved in the generation of paradoxical (REM) sleep. *Arch. Ital. Biol.* 139:93–107, 2001.

Scharf, M.T., et al. The energy hypothesis of sleep revisited. *Prog. Neurobiol.* 86:264–280, 2008.

Siegel, J.M. The stuff dreams are made of: anatomical substrates of REM-sleep. *Nat. Rev. Neurosci.* 9:721–722, 2006.

Steriade, M. Sleep, epilepsy and thalamic reticular neurons. *Trends Neurosci.* 28:317–324, 2005.

Stickgold, R. Sleep: off-line memory reprocessing. *Trends Cogn. Sci.* 2:484–492, 1998.

Stickgold, R., Walker, M.P. Memory consolidation and reconsolidation: what is the role of sleep?. *Trends Neurosci.* 28:408–415, 2005.

Taheri, S., et al. The role of the hypocretins (orexins) in sleep regulation and narcolepsy. *Annu. Rev. Neurosci.* 25:283–313, 2002.

van den Pol, A.N. Narcolepsy: a neurodegenerative disease of the hypocretin system? *Neuron* 27:415–418, 2000.

Vassalli, A., Dijk, D.-J. Sleep function: current questions and new approaches. *Eur. J. Neurosci.* 29:1830–1841, 2009.

Winson, J. The meaning of dreams. *Sci. Am.* 263:42–48, 1990.

CHAPTER 27: THE CRANIAL NERVES

Amarenco, P. Hauw, J.-J. Cerebellar infarction in the territory of the anterior and inferior cerebellar artery. *Brain* 113:139–155, 1990.

Combarros, O., et. al. Isolated unilateral hypoglossal nerve palsy: nine cases. *J. Neurol.* 245:98–100, 1998.

Craig, A.D. How do you feel? Interoception: the sense of the physiological condition of the body. *Nat. Rev. Neurosci.* 3:655–666, 2002.

Farkas, E., et al. Periaqueductal gray matter projection to vagal preganglionic neurons and the nucleus tractus solitarius. *Brain Res.* 764:257–261, 1997.

Fay, R.A., Norgren, R. Identification of rat brainstem multisynaptic connections to the oral motor nuclei using pseudorabies virus. II. Facial muscle motor system. *Brain Res. Rev.* 25:276–290, 1997.

Goadsby, P.J., et al. Stimulation of the greater occipital nerve increases metabolic activity in the trigeminal nucleus caudalis and cervical drosal horn of the cat. *Pain* 73:23–28, 1997.

Haxhiu, M.A., Loewy, A.D. Central connections of the motor and sensory vagal systems innervating the trachea. *J. Auton. Nerv. Syst.* 57:49–56, 1996.

Kameda, W., et al. Lateral and medial medullary infarction. A comparative analysis of 214 patients. *Stroke* 35:694–702, 2004.

Knox, A.P., et al. The central connections of the vagus nerve in the ferret. *Brain Res. Bull.* 33:49–63, 1994.

Kubota, K., et al. Central projection of proprioceptive afferents arising from maxillo-facial regions in some animals studied by HRP-labeling technique. *Anat. Anz.* 165:229–251, 1988.

Kumral, E., et al. Clinical spectrum of pontine infarction. Clinical-MRI correlations. *J. Neurol.* 249:1659–1670, 2003.

Lawrence, A.J., Jarrott, B. Neurochemical modulation of cardiovascular control in the nucleus tractus solitarius. *Prog. Neurobiol.* 48:21–53, 1996.

Lazarov, N.E. Neurobiology of orofacial proprioception. *Brain Res. Rev.* 56:362–383, 2007.

Lee, B.H., et al. Calcitonin gene-related peptide in nucleus ambiguous motoneurons in rat: viscerotopic organization. *J. Comp. Neurol.* 320:531–543, 1992.

Love, S., Coakham, H.B. Trigeminal neuralgia: pathology and pathogenesis. *Brain* 124:2347–2360, 2001.

Monrad-Krohn, G.H. *The clinical examination of the nervous system*, 10th ed. London: H. K. Lewis, 1954.

Mumenthaler, M. *Neurologie*, 6th ed. Stuttgart: Thieme Verlag, 1979.

Oliveri, R.L., et al. Pontine lesion of the abducens fasciculus producing so-called posterior internuclear ophthalmoplegia. *Eur. J. Neurol.* 37:67–69, 1997.

Réthelyi, M., et al. Distribution of neurons expressing calcitonin gene-related peptide mRNAs in the brain stem, spinal cord and dorsal root ganglia of rat and guinea-pig. *Neuroscience* 29: 225–239, 1989.

Reynolds, S.M., et al. The pharmacology of couch. *Trends Pharmacol. Sci.* 25:569–576, 2004.

Samii, M., Janetta, P.J. The cranial nerves: anatomy, pathology, pathophysiology, diagnosis, treatment. New York: Springer-Verlag, 1981.

Silverman, I.E., et al. The crossed paralyses: the original brain-stem syndromes of Millard-Gubler, Foville, Weber, and Raymond-Cestan. *Arch. Neurol.* 52:635–638, 1995.

Strominger, N.L., et al. The connectivity of the area postrema in the ferret. *Brain Res. Bull.* 33:33–47, 1994.

Urban, P.P., et al. The course of corticofacial projections in the human brainstem. *Brain* 124:1866–1876, 2001.

Uzawa, A., et al. Laryngeal abductor paralysis can be a solitary manifestation of multiple system atrophy. *J. Neurol. Neurosurg. Psychiatry* 76:1739–1741, 2005.

Zhuo, H., et al. Neurochemistry of the nodose ganglion. *Prog. Neurobiol.* 52:79–107, 1997.

CHAPTER 28: VISCERAL EFFERENT NEURONS: THE SYMPATHETIC AND PARASYMPATHETIC DIVISIONS

Sympathetic and Parasympathetic Systems

Andrew, J., Nathan, P.W. Lesions of the anterior frontal lobes and disturbances of micturition and defaecation. *Brain* 87:233–262, 1964.

Appel, N.M., Elde, R.P. The intermediolateral cell column of the thoracic spinal cord is comprised of target-specific subnuclei: evidence from retrograde transport studies and immunohistochemistry. *J. Neurosci.* 8:1767–1775, 1988.

Appenzeller, O. The autonomic nervous system: an introduction to basic and clinical concepts. Philadelphia: Elsevier, 1990.

Appenzeller, O., et al. *The autonomic nervous system.* Part II. *Dysfunctions.* Philadelphia: Elsevier, 2001.

Berntson, G.G., et al. Autonomic space and psychophysical response. *Psychophysiology* 31:44–61, 1994.

Blok, B.F., et al. Brain activation during micturition in women. *Brain* 121:2033–2042, 1998.

Burnstock, G. The changing face of autonomic neurotransmission. *Acta Physiol. Scand.* 126:67–91, 1986.

Cheng, Z., Powley, T.L. Nucleus ambiguus projections to cardiac ganglia of rat atria: an anterograde tracing study. *J. Comp. Neurol.* 424:588–606, 2000.

Elfvin, L.-G., et al. The chemical neuroanatomy of sympathetic ganglia. *Annu. Rev. Neurosci.* 16:471–504, 1993.

Farkas, E., et al. Periaqueductal gray matter input to cardiac-related sympathetic premotor neurons. *Brain Res.* 792:179–192, 1998.

Fowler, C.J. Neurological disorders of micturition and their treatment. *Brain* 122:1213–1231, 1999.

Gabella, G. *Structure of the autonomic nervous system.* New York: Chapman & Hall, 1976.

Giuliano, F., Rampin, O. Central regulation of penile erection. *Neurosci. Biobehav. Rev.* 24:517–533, 2000.

Goldstein, D.S. The autonomic nervous system in health and disease. New York: Marcel Dekker, 2001.

Gourine, A.V., et al. Purinergic signaling in autonomic control. *Trends Neurosci.* 32:241–248, 2009.

Guyenet, P.G. The sympathetic control of blood pressure. *Nat. Rev. Neurosci.* 7:335–346, 2006.

Hakusui, S., et al. Postprandial hypotension: microneurographic analysis and treatment with vasopressin. *Neurology* 41:712–715, 1991.

Haymaker, W., Woodhall, B. *Peripheral nerve injuries. Principles of diagnosis.* Philadelphia: W.B. Saunders, 1945.

Hirst, G.D.S., Edwards, F.R. Sympathetic neuroeffector transmission in arteries and arterioles. *Physiol. Rev.* 69:546–604, 1989.

Jänig, W. The integrative action of the autonomic nervous system. Neurobiology of homeostasis. Cambridge, UK: Cambridge University Press, 2006.

Jänig, W., McLachlan, E.M. Characteristics of function-specific pathways in the sympathetic nervous system. *Trends Neurosci.* 15:475–481, 1992.

Kaufmann, H., et al. Vestibular control of sympathetic activity: an otolith-sympathetic reflex in humans. *Exp. Brain Res.* 143: 463–469, 2002.

Kellogg, D.L., Jr. In vivo mechanisms of cutaneous vasodilation and vasoconstriction in humans during thermoregulatory challenges. *J. Appl. Physiol.* 100:1709–1718, 2006.

Kerman, I. Organization of brain somatomotor-sympathetic circuits. *Exp. Brain Res.* 187:1–16, 2008.

Laskey, W., Polosa, C. Characteristics of the sympathetic preganglionic neuron and its synaptic input. *Prog. Neurobiol.* 31:47–84, 1988.

Miolan, J.P., Niel, J.P. The mammalian sympathetic prevertebral ganglia: integrative properties and role in the nervous control of digestive tract motility. *J. Auton. Nerv. Syst.* 58:125–138, 1996.

Nour, S., et al. Cerebral activation during micturition in normal men. *Brain* 123:781–789, 2000.

Paton, J.F.R., et al. The yin and yang of cardiac autonomic control: vago-sympathetic interactions revisited. *Brain Res. Rev.* 49: 555–565, 2005.

Pick, J. The autonomic nervous system: morphological, comparative, clinical and surgical aspects. Philadelphia: Lippincott, 1970.

Pyner, S., Coote, J.H. Evidence that sympathetic preganglionic neurones are arranged in target-specific columns in the thoracic spinal cord of the rat. *J. Comp. Neurol.* 342:15–22, 1994.

Rossi, P., et al. Stomach distension increases efferent muscle sympathetic nerve activity and blood pressure in healthy humans. *J. Neurol. Sci.* 161:148–155, 1998.

Sartor, D.M., Verberne, A.J.M. Abdominal vagal signalling: a novel role for cholecystokinin in circulatory control? *Brain Res. Rev.* 59:140–154, 2008.

Simmons, M.A. The complexity and diversity of synaptic transmission in the prevertebral sympathetic ganglia. *Prog. Neurobiol.* 24:43–93, 1985.

Spalteholz, W. *Handatlas der Anatomie des Menschen. III.* 13. Auflage, Stuttgart: Hirzel Verlag, 1933.

Standish, A., et al. Central neuronal circuit innervating the rat heart defined by transneuronal transport of pseudorabies virus. *J. Neurosci.* 15:1998–2012, 1995.

Travagli, R.A., et al. Brainstem circuits regulating gastric function. *Annu. Rev. Physiol.* 68:279–305, 2006.

Wallin, B.G., Fagius, J. The sympathetic nervous system in man: aspects derived from microelectrode recordings. *Trends Neurosci.* 9:63–67, 1986.

Wallin, B.G., et al. Coherence between the sympathetic drives to relaxed and contracting muscles of different limbs of human subjects. *J. Physiol.* 455:219–233, 1992.

Zhuo, H., et al. Neurochemistry of the nodose ganglion. *Prog. Neurobiol.* 52:79–107, 1997.

The Enteric Nervous System

Furness, J.B., et al. Roles of peptides in transmission in the enteric nervous system. *Trends Neurosci.* 15:66–71, 1992.

Goyal, R.K., Hirano, I. The enteric nervous system. *N. Engl. J. Med.* 334:1106–1115, 1996.

Grundy, D., Schemann, M. Enteric nervous system. *Curr. Opin. Gastroenterol.* 23:121–126, 2007.

Holst, M.C., et al. Vagal preganglionic projections to the enteric nervous system characterized with *Phaseolus vulgaris* leucoagglutinin. *J. Comp. Neurol.* 381:81–100, 1997.

Kunze, W.A.A., Furness, J.B. The enteric nervous system and regulation of intestinal motility. *Annu. Rev. Physiol.* 61:117–142, 1999.

McLean, P.G., et al. 5–HT in the enteric nervous system: gut function and neuropharmacology. *Trends Neurosci.* 30:9–13, 2007.

Wood, J.D. Application of classification schemes to the enteric nervous system. *J. Auton. Nerv. Syst.* 48:17–19, 1994.

CHAPTER 29: SENSORY VISCERAL NEURONS AND VISCERAL REFLEXES

Arendt-Nielsen, L., et al. Referred pain as an indicator for neural plasticity. *Prog. Brain Res.* 129:343–356, 2000.

Argiolas, A., Melis, M.R. Central control of penile erection: role of the paraventricular nucleus of the hypothalamus. *Prog. Neurobiol.* 76:1–21, 2005.

Bajaj, P., et al. Osteoarthritis and its association with muscle hyperalgesia: an experimental controlled study. *Pain* 93:107–114, 2001.

Bernard, J.F., et al. The parabrachial area: electrophysiological evidence for an involvement in visceral nociceptive processes. *J. Neurophysiol.* 71:1646–1660, 1994.

Blackshaw, L.A., et al. Sensory transmission in the gastrointestinal tract. *Neurogastroenterol. Motil.* 19 (Suppl. 1):1–19, 2007.

Carro-Juárez, M., Rodriguez-Manzo, G. The spinal pattern generator for ejaculation. *Brain Res. Rev.* 58:106–120, 2008.

Cervero, F. Visceral pain: mechanisms of peripheral and central sensitization. *Ann. Med.* 27:235–239, 1995.

Cope, Z. *The early diagnosis of the acute abdomen.* New York: Oxford University Press, 1968.

Davis, K.D., et al. Visceral pain evoked by thalamic microstimulation in humans. *NeuroReport* 6:369–374, 1995.

Dunckley, P., et al. A comparison of visceral and somatic pain processing in the human brainstem using functional magnetic resonance imaging. *J. Neurosci.* 25:7333–741, 2005.

Fowler, C.J., et al. The neural control of micturition. *Nat. Rev. Neurosci.* 9:453–466, 2008.

Fugère, F., Lewis, G. Coeliac plexus block for chronic pain syndromes. *Can. J. Anaesth.* 40:954–963, 1993.

Gybels, J.M., Sweet, W.H. Neurosurgical treatment of persistent pain: physiological and pathological mechanisms of human pain. Basel: Karger, 1989.

Hubscher, C.H. Ascending spinal pathways from sexual organs: effects of chronic spinal lesions. *Prog. Brain Res.* 152:401–420, 2006.

Jänig, W. Neurobiology of visceral afferent neurons: neuroanatomy, functions, organ regulations and sensations. *Biol. Psychol.* 42:29–51, 1996.

Karlsson, A.-K. Autonomic dysfunction in spinal cord injury: clinical presentation of symptoms. *Prog. Brain Res.* 152:1–8, 2006.

Knowles, C.H., Aziz, Q. Basic and clinical aspects of gastrointestinal pain. *Pain* 141:191–209, 2009.

Mayer, E.A., et al. Differences in brain responses to visceral pain between patients with irritable bowel syndrome and ulcerative colitis. *Pain* 115:398–409, 2005.

McMahon, S.B. Are there fundamental differences in the peripheral mechanisms of visceral and somatic pain? *Behav. Brain Sci.* 20:381–391, 1997.

Meller, S.T., Gebhart, G.F. A critical review of afferent pathways and the potential chemical mediators involved in cardiac pain. *Neuroscience* 48:501–524, 1992.

Palaček, J. The role of the dorsal column pathway in visceral pain. *Physiol. Res.* 53 (Suppl. 1):S125–S130, 2004.

Raj, H., et al. How does lobeline injected intravenously produce a couch? *Respir. Physiol. Neurobiol.* 145:79–90, 2005.

Russo, A., Conte, B. Afferent and efferent branching axons from the rat lumbo-sacral spinal cord project both to the urinary bladder and the urethra as demonstrated by double retrograde neuronal labeling. *Neurosci. Lett.* 219:155–158, 1996.

Sartor, D.M., Verberne, A.J.M. Abdominal vagal signalling: a novel role for cholecystokinin in circulatory control? *Brain Res. Rev.* 59:140–154, 2008.

Treede, R.-D., et al. The plasticity of cutaneous hyperalgesia during sympathetic ganglion blockade in patients with neuropathic pain. *Brain* 115:607–621, 1992.

CHAPTER 30: THE CENTRAL AUTONOMIC SYSTEM: HYPOTHALAMUS

Structure, Connections, General Organization

Bandler, R., Shipley, M.T. Columnar organization in the periaqueductal gray: modules for emotional expression? *Trends Neurosci.* 17:379–389, 1994.

Blessing, W.W. *Lower brain stem and bodily homeostasis.* New York: Oxford University Press, 1997.

Cameron, A.A., et al. The efferent projections of the periaqueductal gray in the rat: a *Phaseolus vulgaris*–leucoagglutinin study. II. Descending projections. *J. Comp. Neurol.* 351:585–601, 1995.

Clark, Le Gros, W.E., et al. The hypothalamus. Morphological, functional, clinical, and surgical aspects. London: Oliver and Boyd, 1936.

Giesler, G.J., et al. Direct spinal pathways to the limbic system for nociceptive information. *Trends Neurosci.* 17:244–250, 1994.

Kostarczyk, E., et al. Spinohypothalamic tract neurons in the cervical enlargement of rats: locations of antidromically identified ascending axons and their collateral branches in the contralateral brain. *J. Neurophysiol.* 77:435–451, 1997.

Mtui, E.P., et al. Medullary visceral reflex circuits: local afferents to nucleus tractus solitarii synthesize catecholamines and project to thoracic spinal cord. *J. Comp. Neurol.* 351:5–26, 1995.

Risold, P.Y., et al. The structural organization of connections between hypothalamus and cerebral cortex. *Brain Res. Rev.* 24:197–254, 1997.

Saper, C.B. The central autonomic nervous system: conscious visceral perception and autonomic pattern generation. *Annu. Rev. Neurosci.* 25:433–469, 2002.

Saper, C.B. The hypothalamus. In: Paxinos, G., Mai, J.K. (Eds.), *The human nervous system*, 2nd ed. (pp. 513–550). Philadelphia: Elsevier Academic Press, 2004.

Smith, O., DeVito, J.L. Central neural integration for the control of autonomic responses associated with emotion. *Annu. Rev. Neurosci.* 7:43–65, 1984.

Swanson, L.W. The neural basis of motivated behavior. *Acta Morphol. Neerl. Scand.* 26:165–176. 1989.

Vann, S.D., Aggleton, J.P. The mammillary bodies: two memory systems in one? *Nat. Rev. Neurosci.* 5:35–44, 2004.

Westerhaus, M.J., Loewy, A.D. Central representation of the sympathetic nervous system in the cerebral cortex. *Brain Res.* 903:117–127, 2001.

Hypothalamus and the Endocrine System

Brunton, P.J., Russel, J.A. The expectant brain: adapting for motherhood. *Nat. Rev. Neurosci.* 9:11–25, 2008.

De Kloet, E.R., et al. Stress and cognition: are corticosteroids good or bad guys? *Trends Neurosci.* 22:422–426, 1999

De Voogd, T.J. Androgens can affect the morphology of mammalian CNS neurons in adulthood. *Trends Neurosci.* 10:341–342, 1987.

Donaldson, Z.R., Young, L.J. Oxytocin, vasopressin, and the neurogenetic of sociality. *Science* 322.900–904, 2008.

Ericsson, A., et al. A functional anatomical analysis of central pathways subserving effects of interleukin-1 on stress-related neuroendocrine neurons. *J. Neurosci.* 14:897–913, 1994.

Herman, J.P., Cullinan, W.E. Neurocircuitry of stress: central control of the hypothalamo-pituitary-adrenocortical axis. *Trends Neurosci.* 20:78–84, 1997.

Landgraf, R., Neumann, I.D. Vasopressin and oxytocin release within the brain: a dynamic concept of multiple and variable modes of neuropeptide communication. *Front. Neuroendocrinol.* 25:150–176, 2004.

Lee, H.-J., et al. Oxytocin: the great facilitator of life. *Prog. Neurobiol.* 88:127–151, 2009.

Ludwig, M., Leng G. Dendritic peptide release and peptide-dependent behaviors. *Nat. Rev. Neurosci.* 7:127–136, 2006.

Park, C.R. Cognitive effects of insulin in the central nervous system. *Neurosci. Biobehav. Rev.* 25:311–323, 2001.

Ulrich-Lai, Y.M., Herman, J.P. Neural regulation of endocrine and autonomic stress responses. *Nat. Rev. Neurosci.* 10:397–409, 2009.

Yoshimura, F., Gorbman, A. Pars distalis of the pituitary gland: structure, function and regulation. Philadelphia: Elsevier, 1986.

Thermoregulation, Sleep, and Circadian Rhythms

Aston-Jones, G., et al. A neural circuit for circadian regulation of arousal. *Nat. Neurosci.* 4:732–738, 2001.

Buijs, R.M., et al. Organization of circadian functions: interaction with the body. *Prog. Brain Res.* 153:341–350, 2006.

Falcon, J. Cellular circadian clocks in the pineal. *Prog. Neurobiol.* 58:121–162, 1999.

Foster, R.G. Shedding light on the biological clock. *Neuron* 20:829–832, 1998.

Haas, H., Panula P. The role of histamine and the tuberomammillary nucleus in the nervous system. *Nat. Rev. Neurosci.* 4:121–130, 2003.

Ibata, Y., et al. The suprachiasmatic nucleus: a circadian oscillator. *Neuroscientist* 3:215–225, 1997.

Maywood, E.S. Circadian timing in health and disease. *Prog. Brain Res.* 253–266, 2006.

Moore, R.Y., et al. The retinohypothalamic tract originates from a distinct subset of retinal ganglion cells. *J. Comp. Neurol.* 352:351–366, 1995.

Morin, L.P. The circadian visual system. *Brain Res. Rev.* 67:102–127, 1994.

Nagashima, K., et al. Neuronal circuitries involved in thermoregulation. *Auton. Neurosci.* 85:18–25, 2000.

Nakamura, K., Morrison, S.F. A thermosensory pathway that controls body temperature. *Nat. Rev. Neurosci.* 11:62–71, 2008.

Pandi-Perumal, S.R., et al. Physiological effects of melatonin: role of melatonin receptors and signal transduction pathways. *Prog. Neurobiol.* 85:335–353, 2008.

Romanovsky, A.A. Thermoregulation: some concepts have changed. Functional architecture of the thermoregulatory system. *Am. J. Physiol. Regul. Integr. Comp. Physiol.* 292:R37–R46, 2007.

Sakurai, T. The neural circuit of orexin (hypocretin): maintaining sleep and wakefulness. *Nat. Rev. Neurosci.* 8:171–181, 2007.

Saper, C.B., et al. The sleep switch: hypothalamic control of sleep and wakefulness. *Trends Neurosci.* 24:726–731, 2002.

Vanecek, J. Cellular mechanisms of melatonin action. *Physiol. Rev.* 78:687–721, 1998.

Osmoregulation, Feeding, and Energy Balance

Beaver, J.D., et al. Individual differences in reward drive predict neural responses to images of food. *J. Neurosci.* 26:5160–5166, 2006.

Bergh, C., Söderström, P. Anorexia nervosa, self-starvation and the reward of stress. *Nat. Med.* 2:21–22, 1996.

Bourque, C.W. Central mechanisms of osmosensation and systemic osmoregulation. *Nat. Rev. Neurosci.* 9:519–531, 2008.

Diano, S., et al. Ghrelin controls hippocampal spine synapse density and memory performance. *Nature Neurosci.* 9:381–388. 2006.

Elmquist, J.K., et al. From lesions to leptin: hypothalamic control of food intake and body weight. *Neuron* 22:221–232, 1999.

Inui, A. Feeding and body-weight regulation by hypothalamic neuropeptides: mediation of the actions of leptin. *Trends Neurosci.* 22:62–67, 1999.

Jobst, E.E., et al. The electrophysiology of feeding circuits. *Trends Endocrinol. Metab.* 15:497–499, 2004.

Knecht, S., et al. Obesity in neurobiology. *Prog. Neurobiol.* 84:85–103, 2008.

Lawrence, C.B. Hypothalamic control of feeding. *Curr. Opin. Neurobiol.* 9:778–783, 1999.

Saper, C.B., et al. The need to feed: homeostatic and hedonic control of eating. *Neuron* 36:199–211, 2002.

Seeley, R.J., Woods S.C. Monitoring of stored and available fuel by the CNS: implications for obesity. *Nat. Rev. Neurosci.* 4:901–909, 2003.

Uher, R., Treasure, J. Brain lesions and eating disorders. *J. Neurol. Neurosurg. Psychiatry* 76:852–857, 2005.

van den Top, M., Spanswick, D. Integration of metabolic stimuli in the hypothalamic arcuate nucleus. *Prog. Brain Res.* 153:141–152, 2006.

Willie, J.T. To eat or sleep? Orexin in the regulation of feeding and wakefulness. *Annu. Rev. Neurosci.* 24:429–458, 2001.

Sexual Behavior and Sex Differences

Arnold, A.P., Gorski R.A. Gonadal steroid induction of structural sex differences in the central nervous system. *Annu. Rev. Neurosci.* 7:413–442, 1984.

Cooke, B.M., et al. A brain sexual dimorphism controlled by adult circulating androgens. *Proc. Natl. Acad. Sci. USA* 96:7538–7540, 1999.

DeVoogd, T.J. Androgens can affect the morphology of mammalian CNS neurons in adulthood. *Trends Neurosci.* 10:341–342, 1987.

De Vries, G.J. Sex differences in vasopressin and oxytocin innervation of the brain. *Prog. Brain Res.* 170:17–27, 2008.

Federman, D.D. The biology of human sex differences. *N. Engl. J. Med.* 354:1507–1514, 2006.

Lasco, M.S., et al. A lack of dimorphism of sex or sexual orientation in the human anterior commissure. *Brain Res.* 936:95–98, 2002.

McEwen, B.S. Permanence of brain sex differences and structural plasticity of the adult brain. *Proc. Natl. Acad. Sci. USA* 96:7128–7130, 1999.

Morgan, M.A., et al. Estrogens and non-reproductive behaviors related to activity and fear. *Neurosci. Biobehav. Rev.* 28:55–63, 2004.

Morris, J.A., et al. Sexual differences of the vertebrate nervous system. *Nat. Neurosci.* 7:1034–1039, 2004.

Pfaus, J.G. Neurobiology of sexual behavior. *Curr. Opin. Neurobiol.* 9:751–758, 1999.

Schwaab, D.F., et al. Structural and functional sex differences in the human hypothalamus. *Horm. Behav.* 40:93–98, 2001.

Simerly, R.B. Wired for reproduction: organization and development of sexually dimorphic circuits in the mammalian forebrain. *Annu. Rev. Neurosci.* 25:507–536, 2002.

Sisk, C.L., Foster D.L. The neural basis of puberty and adolescence. *Nat. Rev. Neurosci.* 7:1040–1047, 2004.

Van Furth, W.R., et al. Regulation of masculine sexual behavior: involvement of brain opioids and dopamine. *Brain Res. Rev.* 21:162–184, 1995.

Hypothalamus and the Immune System

Banks, W.A., et al. Passage of cytokines across the blood–brain barrier. *Neuroimmunomodulation* 2:241–248, 1995.

Borsody, M.K., Weiss, J.M. The subdiaphragmatic vagus nerves mediate activation of locus coeruleus neurons by peripherally administered microbial substances. *Neuroscience* 131:235–245, 2005.

Cohen, N. The uses and abuses of psychoneuroimmunology: a global overview. *Brain Behav. Immunol.* 20:99–112, 2006.

Cohen, S., Herbert, T.B. Health psychology: psychological factors and physical disease from the perspective of human psychoneuroimmunology. *Annu. Rev. Psychol.* 47:113–142, 1996.

Dantzer, R., Kelley, K.W. Twenty years of research on cytokine-induced sickness behavior. *Brain Behav. Immun.* 21:153–160, 2007.

Dantzer, R., et al. From inflammation to sickness and depression: when the immune system subjugates the brain. *Nat. Rev. Neurosci.* 9:46–57, 2008.

Felten, D.L. Direct innervation of lymphoid organs: substrate for neurotransmitter signaling of cells of the immune system. *Neuropsychobiology* 28:110–112, 1993.

Goehler, L.E., et al. Interleukin-1b in immune cells of the abdominal vagus nerve: a link between the immune and nervous system? *J. Neurosci.* 19:2799–2806, 1999.

Hori, T., et al. The autonomic nervous system as a communication channel between the brain and the immune system. *Neuroimmunomodulation* 2:203–215, 1995.

Kavelaars, A., Heijnen, C.B. Stress, genetics and immunity. *Brain Behav. Immun.* 20:313–316, 2006.

Kemeny, M.E. Psychobiological responses to social threat: evolution of a psychological model in psychoneuroimmunology. *Brain Behav. Immun.* 23:1–9, 2009.

Koh, K.B., et al. Counter-stress effects of relaxation on pro-inflammatory and anti-inflammatory cytokines. *Brain Behav. Immun.* 22:1130–1137, 2008.

Konsman, J.P., et al. Cytokine-induced sickness behaviour: mechanisms and implications. *Trends Neurosci.* 25:117–127, 2001.

LaCroix, S., Rivest, S. Functional circuitry in the brain of immune-challenged rats: partial involvement of prostaglandins. *J. Comp. Neurol.* 387:307–324, 1997.

Lagercrantz, H. Neuromodulators and respiratory control during development. *Trends Neurosci.* 10:368–372, 1987.

Madden, K.S., et al. Sympathetic nervous system modulation of the immune system. *J. Neuroimmunol.* 49:77–87, 1994.

Marazziti, D., et al. Immune cell imbalance in major depressive and panic disorders. *Neuropsychobiology* 26:23–26, 1992.

Pariante, C.M. Chronic fatigue syndrome and the immune system: "findings in search of meanings." *Brain Behav. Immun.* 23:325–326, 2009.

Pavlov, V.A., Tracey, K.J. The cholinergic anti-inflammatory pathway. *Brain Behav. Immun.* 19:493–499, 2005.

Rinner, I., Schauenstein, K. The parasympathetic nervous system takes part in the immuno-neuroendocrine dialogue. *J. Neuroimmunol.* 34:165–172, 1991.

Salzet, M., et al. Crosstalk between nervous and immune systems through the animal kingdom: focus on opioids. *Trends Neurosci.* 23:550–555, 2000.

Sanders, V.M. Interdisciplinary research: noradrenergic regulation of adaptive immunity. *Brain Behav. Immun.* 20:1–8, 2006.

Sloan, E.K., et al. Social stress enhances sympathetic innervation of primate lymph nodes: mechanisms for viral pathogenesis. *J. Neurosci.* 27:8857–8865, 2007.

Steptoe, A., et al. Positive affect and health-related neuroendocrine, cardiovascular and inflammatory processes. *Proc. Natl. Acad. Sci. USA* 102:6508–6512, 2005.

Sundgren-Andersson, A.K., et al. Neurobiological mechanisms of fever. *Neuroscientist* 4:113–121, 1998.

Watkins, L., Maier S.F. Implications of immune-to-brain communication for sickness and pain. *Proc. Natl. Acad. Sci. USA* 96:7710–7713, 1999.

Stress and Psychosomatic Relations

Amat, J., et al. Medial prefrontal cortex determines how stressor controllability affects behavior and dorsal raphe nucleus. *Nat. Neurosci.* 8:365–371, 2005.

Arnsten, A.F.T. Stress signalling pathways that impair prefrontal cortex structure and function. *Nat. Rev. Neurosci.* 10:410–422, 2009.

Dantzer, R. Somatization: a psychoneuroimmune perspective. *Psychoneuroendocrinology* 30:947–952, 2005.

de Kloet, E.R., et al. Stress and the brain: from adaptation ot disease. *Nat. Rev. Neurosci.* 6:463–475, 2005.

Ekman, P. Expression and the nature of emotion. In: Scherer, K.R., Ekman, P. (Eds.), *Approaches to emotion.* Mahwah, NJ: Lawrence Erlbaum, 1984.

Feder, A., et al. Psychobiology and molecular genetics of resilience. *Nat. Rev. Neurosci.* 10:446–457, 2009.

Friedman, H.S. The multiple linkages of personality and disease. *Brain Behav. Immun.* 22:668–675, 2008.

Gunnar, M., Quevedo, K. The neurobiology of stress and development. *Annu. Rev. Psychol.* 58:145–173, 2007.

Joëls, M., Baram, T.Z. The neuro-symphony of stress. *Nat. Rev. Neurosci.* 10:459–466, 2009.

Joëls, M., et al. Learning under stress: how does it work? *Trends Cogn. Sci.* 10:152–158, 2006.

Kellner, R. Psychosomatic syndromes, somatization and somatoform disorders. *Psychother. Psychosom.* 61:4–24, 1994.

Liston, C., et al. Stress-induced alterations in prefrontal cortical dendritic morphology predict selective impairments in attentional set-shifting. *J. Neurosci.* 26:7870–7874, 2006.

Liston, C., et al. Psychosocial stress reversibly disrupts prefrontal processing and attentional control. *Proc. Natl. Acad. Sci. USA* 106:912–917, 2009.

Miller, G., et al. Health psychology: developing biologically plausible models linking the social world and physical health. *Annu. Rev. Psychol.* 60:501–524, 2009.

Rief, W., Barsky, A.J. Psychobiological perspectives on somatoform disorders. *Psychoneuroendocrinology* 30:996–1002, 2005.

Segerstrom, S.Z. Optimism and immunity: do positive thoughts always lead to positive effects? *Brain Behav. Immun.* 19:195–200, 2005.

Steptoe, A., et al. Positive affect and health-related neuroendocrine, cardiovascular, and inflammatory processes. *Proc. Natl. Acad. Sci. USA* 102:6508–6512, 2005.

Thayler, J.F., Brosschat, J.F. Psychosomatics and psychopathology: looking up and down from the brain. *Psychoneuroendocrinology.* 30:1050–1058, 2005.

Ursin, H., Eriksen, H.R. The cognitive activation theory of stress. *Psychoneuroendocrinology* 29:567–592, 2004.

Ursin, H., Olff, M. Psychobiology of coping and defense strategies. *Neuropsychobiology* 28:66–71, 1993.

CHAPTER 31: THE AMYGDALA, THE BASAL FOREBRAIN, AND EMOTIONS

Damasio, A. Toward a neurobiology of emotion and feeling: operational concepts and hypotheses. *Neuroscientist* 1:19–25, 1995.

Davidson, R.J., Irwin, W. The functional neuroanatomy of emotion and affective style. *Trends Cogn. Sci.* 3:11–21, 1999.

Davidson, R.J., Sutton, S.K. Affective neuroscience: the emergence of a discipline. *Curr. Opin. Neurobiol.* 5:217–224, 1995.

Grossman, S.P. Behavioral functions of the septum: a reanalysis. In: DeFrance, J.F. (Ed.), *The septal nuclei* (pp. 361–422). New York: Plenum Press, 1976.

LaBar, K.S., Cabeza R. Cognitive neuroscience of emotional memory. *Nat. Rev. Neurosci.* 7:54–64, 2006.

LeDoux, J.E. Emotion circuits in the brain. *Annu. Rev. Neurosci.* 23:155–184, 2000.

Papez, J.W. A proposed mechanism for emotion. *Arch. Neurol.* 38:725–743, 1937.

Pessoa, L. On the relationship between emotion and cognition. *Nat. Rev. Neurosci.* 9:148–158, 2008.

Phan, K.L., et al. Functional neuroanatomy of emotion: a meta-analysis of emotion activation studies in PET and fMRI. *NeuroImage* 16:331–348, 2002.

Rolls, E.T. *The brain and emotion.* Oxford: Oxford University Press, 1999.

Amygdala

Adolphs, R. Fear, faces, and the human amygdala. *Curr. Opin. Neurobiol.* 18:166–172, 2008.

Adolphs, R., et al. A mechanism for impaired fear recognition after amygdala damage. *Nature* 433:68–72, 2005.

Alvarez, R.P., et al. Contextual fear conditioning in humans: cortical-hippocampal and amygdala contributions. *J. Neurosci.* 28: 6211–6219, 2008.

Anderson, A.K., Phelps, E.A. Is the human amygdala critical for the subjective experience of emotion? Evidence of intact dispositional affect in patients with amygdala lesions. *J. Cogn. Neurosci.* 14:709–720, 2002.

Bancaud, J., et al. Anatomical origin of *déjà vu* and vivid "memories" in human temporal lobe epilepsy. *Brain* 117:71–90, 1994.

Barrett, L.F., et al. The experience of emotion. *Annu. Rev. Psychol.* 58:373–403, 2007.

Bauman, M.D., et al. The development of mother-infant interactions after neonatal amygdala lesions in rhesus monkeys. *J. Neurosci.* 21:711–721, 2004.

Bechara, A., et al. Different contributions of the human amygdala and ventromedial prefrontal cortex to decision-making. *J. Neurosci.* 19:5473–5481, 1999.

Bernard, J.F., et al. Nucleus centralis of the amygdala and the globus pallidus ventralis: electrophysiological evidence for an involvement in pain processes. *J. Neurophysiol.* 68:551–569, 1992.

Berton, O., Nestler, E.J. New approaches to antidepressant drug discovery: beyond monoamines. *Nat. Rev. Neurosci.* 7:137–151, 2006.

Buchanan, T.W., et al. Emotional autobiographical memories in amnesic patients with temporal lobe damage. *J. Neurosci.* 25:3151–3160, 2005.

Callagher, M., Schoenbaum, G. Functions of the amygdala and related forebrain areas in attention and cognition. *Ann. NY Acad. Sci.* 877:397–411, 1999.

Costafreda, S.G., et al. Predictors of amygdala activation during the processing of emotional stimuli: a meta-analysis of 385 PET and fMRI studies. *Brain Res. Rev.* 58:57–70, 2008.

Dapretto, M., et al. Understanding emotions in others: mirror neuron dysfunction in children with autism spectrum disorders. *Nat. Neurosci.* 9:28–30, 2006.

Dijksterhuis, A. Think different: the merits of unconscious thought in preference development and decision making. *J. Person. Social Psychol.* 87:586–598, 2004.

Heilig, M., et al. Corticotropin-releasing factor and neuropeptide Y: role in emotional integration. *Trends Neurosci.* 17:80–85, 1994.

Heimburger, R.F., et al. Stereotactic amygdalotomy for convulsive and behavioral disorders. *Appl. Neurophysiol.* 41:43–51, 1978.

Herry, C., et al. Switching on and off fear by distinct neuronal circuits. *Nature* 454:600–608, 2008.

Holland, P.C., Callagher, M. Amygdala circuitry in attentional and representational processes. *Trends Cogn. Sci.* 3:65–73, 1999.

Hooker, C.I., et al. Amygdala response to facial expressions reflects emotional learning. *J. Neurosci.* 26:8915–8922, 2006.

Jacobson, R. Disorders of facial recognition, social behaviour and affect after combined bilateral amygdalotomy and subcaudate tractotomy: a clinical and experimental study. *Psychol. Med.* 16:439–450, 1986.

Kalin, N.H., et al. The role of the central nucleus of the amygdala in mediating fear and anxiety in the primate. *J. Neurosci.* 24:5506–5515, 2004.

Korpelainen, J.T., et al. Asymmetrical skin temperature in ischemic stroke. *Stroke* 26:1543–1547, 1995.

LeDoux, J.E. Emotion: clues from the brain. *Annu. Rev. Psychol.* 46:209–235, 1995.

Machado, C.J., et al. Bilateral neurotoxic amygdala lesions in Rhesus monkeys (*Macaca mulatta*): consistent pattern of behavior across different social contexts. *Behav. Neurosci.* 122:251–266, 2008.

McDonald, A.J. Cortical pathways to the mammalian amygdala. *Prog. Neurobiol.* 55:257–332, 1998.

Murray, E.A. The amygdala, reward, and emotion. *Trends Cogn. Sci.* 11:490–497, 2007.

Narabayashi, H., et al. Stereotactic amygdalectomy for behavior disorders. *Arch. Neurol.* 9:11–26, 1963.

Ono, T., et al. Amygdala role in associative learning. *Prog. Neurobiol.* 46:401–422, 1995.

Ousdal, O.A., et al. The human amygdala is involved in general behavioral relevance detection: evidence from an event-related functional magnetic resonance imaging go-nogo task. *Neuroscience* 156:450–455, 2008.

Paton, J.J., et al. The primate amygdala represents the positive and negative value of visual stimuli during learning. *Nature* 439:865–870, 2006.

Phelps, E.A. Human emotion and memory: interactions of the amygdala and hippocampal complex. *Curr. Opin. Neurobiol.* 14:198–202, 2004.

Pitkänen, A., et al. Intrinsic connections of the rat amygdaloid complex: projections originating in the lateral nucleus. *J. Comp. Neurol.* 356:288–310, 1995.

Roozendaal, B., et al. Stress, memory, and the amygdala. *Nat. Rev. Neurosci.* 10:423–433, 2009.

Schafe, G.E., et al. Tracking the fear engram: the lateral amygdala is an essential locus of fear memory. *J. Neurosci.* 25:10010–10015, 2005.

Seymour, B., Dolan, R. Emotion, decision making, and the amygdala. *Neuron* 58:662–671, 2008.

Shaikh, M.B., et al. Basal amygdaloid facilitation of midbrain periaqueductal gray elicited defensive rage behavior in the cat mediated trough NMDA receptors. *Brain Res.* 635:187–195, 1994.

Shaw, P., et al. The impact of early and late damage to the human amygdala on 'theory of mind' reasoning. *Brain* 127:1535–1548, 2004.

Swanson, L.W., Petrovich, G.D. What is the amygdala? *Trends Neurosci.* 21:323–331, 1998.

Vuilleumier, P. How brains beware: neural mechanisms of emotional attention. *Trends Cogn. Sci.* 9:585–594, 2005.

Young, A.W., et al. Facial expression processing after amygdalotomy. *Neuropsychologia* 34:31–39, 1996.

Cortical Areas Related to Autonomic Functions and Emotions

Adolphs, R. Neural systems for recognition of emotion. *Curr. Opin. Neurobiol.* 12:169–177, 2002.

Allman, J.M., et al. The anterior cingulate cortex: the evolution of an interface between emotion and cognition. *Ann. NY Acad. Sci.* 935:107–117, 2001.

Boksem, M.A.S., Tops, M. Mental fatigue: costs and benefits. *Brain Res. Rev.* 59:125–139, 2008.

Botvinik, M.M., et al. Conflict monitoring and anterior cingulate cortex: an update. *Trends Cogn. Sci.* 8:539–546, 2004.

Bush, G., et al. Dorsal anterior cingulate cortex: a role in reward-based decision making. *Proc. Natl. Acad. Sci. USA* 99:523–528, 2002.

Calder, A.J., et al. Neurospychology of fear and loathing. *Nat. Rev. Neurosci.* 2:352–363, 2001.

Carmichael, S.T., Price, J.L. Limbic connections of the orbital and medial prefrontal cortex in macaque monkeys. *J. Comp. Neurol.* 363:615–641, 1995.

Chu, C.-C., et al. The autonomic-related cortex: pathology in Alzheimer's disease. *Cereb. Cortex* 7:86–95, 1997.

Cohen, R.A., et al. Impairments of attention after cingulotomy. *Neurology* 53:819–824, 1999.

Davis, K.D., et al. Human anterior cingulate cortex neurons encode cognitive and emotional demands. *J. Neurosci.* 25:8402–8406, 2005.

Devinsky, O., et al. Contributions of the anterior cingulate cortex to behavior. *Brain* 118:279–306, 1995.

Immordino-Yang, M.H., et al. Neural correlates of admiration and compassion. *Proc. Natl. Acad. Sci. USA* 106:8021–8026, 2009.

Izquierdo, A., et al. Comparison of the effects of bilateral orbital prefrontal cortex lesions and amygdala lesions on emotional responses in Rhesus monkeys. *J. Neurosci.* 25:8534–8542, 2005.

Kensinger, E.A. Remembering the details: effects of emotion. *Emotion Rev.* 1:99–113, 2009.

Likhtik, E., et al. Prefrontal control of the amygdala. *J. Neurosci.* 25:7429–7437, 2005.

Oppenheimer, S.M., et al. Cardiovascular effects of human insular cortex stimulation. *Neurology* 42:1727–1732, 1992.

Price, J.L. Prefrontal cortical networks related to visceral function and mood. *Ann. NY Acad. Sci.* 877:383–396, 1999.

Reekie, Y.L., et al. Uncoupling of behavioral and autonomic responses after lesions of the primate orbitofrontal cortex. *Proc. Natl. Acad. Sci. USA* 105:9787–9792, 2008.

Richter, E.O., et al. Cingulotomy for psychiatric disease: microelectrode guidance, a callosal reference system for documenting lesion location, and clinical results. *Neurosurgery* 54:622–630, 2004.

Vogt, B.A. Pain and emotion interactions in subregions of the cingulate gyrus. *Nat. Rev. Neurosci.* 6:533–544, 2005.

Wager, T.D., et al. Prefrontal-subcortical pathways mediating successful emotion regulation. *Neuron* 59:1037–1050, 2008.

The Basal Forebrain

Alheid, G.F., Heimer, L. New perspectives in basal forebrain organization of special relevance for neuropsychiatric disorders: the striatopallidal, amygdaloid, and corticopetal components of substantia innominata. *Neuroscience* 27:1–39, 1988.

Baxter, M.G., Chiba, A.A. Cognitive functions of the basal forebrain. *Curr. Opin. Neurobiol.* 9:178–183, 1999.

de Olmos, J.S., Heimer, L. The concepts of the ventral striatopallidal system and extended amygdala. *Ann. NY Acad. Sci.* 877:1–32, 1999.

Fudge, J.L., Haber, S.N. Bed nucleus of the stria terminalis and the extended amygdala inputs to dopamine subpopulations in primates. *Neuroscience* 104:807–827, 2001.

Ghashgaei, H.T., Barbas, H. Neural interaction between the basal forebrain and functionally distinct prefrontal cortices in the rhesus monkey. *Neuroscience* 103:593–614, 2001.

Gray, T.S. Functional and anatomical relationships among the amygdala, basal forebrain, ventral striatum, and cortex: an integrative discussion. *Ann. NY Acad. Sci.* 877:439–444, 1999.

Hohmann, C.F., Berger-Sweeney, J. Cholinergic regulation of cortical development and plasticity: new twists to an old story. *Perspect. Dev. Neurobiol.* 5:401–425, 1998.

Holland, P.C., Gallagher, M. Differential roles for amygdala central nucleus and substantia innominata in the surprise-induce enhancement of learning. *J. Neurosci.* 26:3791–3797, 2006.

Koob, G.F. The neurocircuitry of addiction: implications for treatment. *Clin. Neurosci. Res.* 5:89–101, 2005.

McLin, D.E. III, et al. Induction of behavioral associative memory by stimulation of the nucleus basalis. *Proc. Natl. Acad. Sci. USA* 99:4002–4007, 2002.

Mesulam, M.-M. The cholinergic innervation of the human cerebral cortex. *Origr. Brain Res.* 145:67–78, 2004.

Reynolds, S.M., Zahm, D.S. Specificity in the projections of the prefrontal and insular cortex to ventral striatopallidum and the extended amygdala. *J. Neurosci.* 25:11757–11767, 2005.

Selden, N.R., et al. Trajectories of cholinergic pathways within the cerebral hemispheres of the human brain. *Brain* 121:2249–2257, 1998.

Wright, C.I., et al. Basal amygdaloid complex afferents to the rat nucleus accumbens are compartmentally organized. *J. Neurosci.* 16:1877–1893, 1996.

Zaborsky, L., et al. The basal forebrain corticopetal system revisited. *Ann. NY Acad. Sci.* 877:339–367, 1999.

CHAPTER 32: THE HIPPOCAMPAL FORMATION: LEARNING AND MEMORY

Hippocampal Formation

Alvarez, P., et al. Damage limited to the hippocampal region produces long-lasting memory impairment in monkeys. *J. Neurosci.* 15:3796–3807, 1995.

Amaral, D.G. Emerging principles of intrinsic hippocampal organization. *Curr. Opin. Neurobiol.* 3:225–229, 1993.

Andersen, P., et al. Lamellar organization of excitatory hippocampal pathways. *Exp. Brain Res.* 13:222–238, 1971.

Andersen, P., et al. (Eds.) *The hippocampus book.* New York: Oxford University Press, 2006.

Bear, M.F., Abraham, W.C. Long-term depression in hippocampus. *Annu. Rev. Neurosci.* 19:437–462, 1996.

Bird, C.M., Burgess, N. The hippocampus and memory: insights from spatial processing. *Nat. Rev. Neurosci.* 9:182–194, 2008.

Blatt, G., Rosene D.L. Organization of direct hippocampal efferent projections to the cerebral cortex of the rhesus monkey. *J. Comp. Neurol.* 392:92–114, 1998.

Buzsáki, G. The hippocampo-neocortical dialogue. *Cereb. Cortex.* 6:81–92, 1996.

Holland, P.C., Bouton, M.E. Hippocampus and context in classical conditioning. *Curr. Opin. Neurobiol.* 9:195–202, 1999.

Ji, D.M., Wilson A. Coordinated memory replay in the visual cortex and the hippocampus during sleep. *Nat. Neurosci.* 10:100–107, 2007.

Kentros, C. Hippocampal place cells: the "where" of episodic memory? *Hippocampus* 16:743–754, 2006.

Klintsova, A.Y., Greenough, W.T. Synaptic plasticity in cortical systems. *Curr. Opin. Neurobiol.* 9:203–208, 1999.

Lim, C., et al. Connections of the hippocampal formation in humans. I. The mossy fiber pathway. *J. Comp. Neurol.* 385:325–351, 1997.

Maguire, E.A., et al. Human spatial navigation: cognitive maps, sexual dimorphism, and neuronal substrates. *Curr. Opin. Neurobiol.* 9:171–177, 1999.

Martin, S.J., Clark, R.E. The rodent hippocampus and spatial memory: from synapses to systems. *Cell. Mol. Life Sci.* 64:401–431, 2007.

Meunier, M., et al. Effects of rhinal cortex lesions combined with hippocampectomy on visual recognition memory in rhesus monkeys. *J. Neurophysiol.* 75:1190–1205, 1996.

Monteggia, L.M., et al. Essential role of brain-derived neurotrophic factor in adult hippocampal function. *Proc. Natl. Acad. Sci. USA* 101:10827–10832, 2004.

Morris, R.G.M. Elements of a neurobiological theory of hippocampal function: the role of synaptic plasticity, synaptic tagging and schemas. *Eur. J. Neurosci.* 23:2829–2846, 2006.

Moser, E.I., Paulsen, O. New excitement in cognitive space: between place cells and spatial memory *Curr. Opin. Neurobiol.* 11:745–751, 2001.

Moser, E. I., et al. Place cells, grid cells, and the brain's spatial representation system. *Annu. Rev. Neurosci.* 31:69–89, 2008.

O'Keefe, J., Nadel, L. *The hippocampus as a cognitive map.* Oxford: Clarendon Press, 1978.

Roman, F.S., et al. Correlations between electrophysiological observations of synaptic plasticity modifications and behavioral performance in mammals. *Prog. Neurobiol.* 58:61–87, 1999.

Saunders, R.C., Aggleton, J.P. Origin and topography of fibers contributing to the fornix in macaque monkeys. *Hippocampus* 17:396–411, 2007.

Suzuki, W.A., Amaral, D.G. Perirhinal and parahippocampal cortices of the macaque monkey: cortical afferents. *J. Comp. Neurol.* 350:497–533, 1994.

Van Strien, N.M., et al. The anatomy of memory: an interactive overview of the parahippocampal-hippocampal network. *Nat. Rev. Neurosci.* 10:272–282, 2009.

Vinogradova, O.S. Expression, control, and probable functional significance of the neuronal theta-rhythm. *Prog. Neurobiol.* 45:523–583, 1995.

Learning and Memory

Alain, C., et al. A distributed network for auditory sensory memory in humans. *Brain Res.* 812:23–37, 1998.

Baxter, M.G. Involvement of medial temporal lobe structures in memory and perception. *Neuron* 12:667–677, 2009.

Buckner, R.L., et al. Frontal cortex contributes to human memory formation. *Nat. Neurosci.* 2:311–314, 1999

Cabeza, R., et al. Brain regions differentially involved in remembering what and when: a PET study. *Neuron* 19:863–870, 1997.

Cabeza, R., Jacques, P.St. Functional neuroimaging of autobiographical memory. *Trends Cogn. Sci.* 11:219–227, 2007.

Costa-Mattioli, M., et al. Translational control of long-lasting synaptic plasticity and memory. *Neuron* 15:10–26, 2009.

Damasio, A.R., Tranel, D. Knowledge systems. *Curr. Opin. Neurobiol.* 2:186–190, 1992.

De Haan, M., et al. Human memory development and its dysfunction after early hippocampal injury. *Trends Neurosci.* 29:374–381, 2006.

Elgersma, Y., Silva, A.J. Molecular mechanisms of synaptic plasticity and memory. *Curr. Opin. Neurobiol.* 9:209–213, 1999.

Epstein, R.A. Parahippocampal and retrosplenial contributions to human spatial navigation. *Trends. Cogn. Sci.* 12:388–396, 2008.

Frackowiak, R.S.J. Functional mapping of verbal memory and language. *Trends Neurosci.* 17:109–114, 1994.

Gaffan, D. Widespread cortical networks underlie memory and attention. *Science* 309:2172–2173, 2005.

Gaffan, D., Parker, A. Mediodorsal thalamic function in scene memory in rhesus monkeys. *Brain* 123:816–827, 2000.

Hasselmo, M.E., McClelland, J.L. Neural models of memory. *Curr. Opin. Neurobiol.* 9:184–188, 1999.

Kim, J.J., Baxter, M.G. Multiple memory systems: the whole does not equal the sum of its parts. *Trends Neurosci.* 24:324–330, 2001.

Leutgeb, S., et al. Independent codes for spatial and episodic memory in hippocampal neuronal ensembles. *Science* 309:619–623, 2005.

Lisman, J.E. Relating hippocampal circuitry to function: recall of memory sequences by reciprocal dentate–CA3 interactions. *Neuron* 22:233–242, 1999.

Martin, S.J., et al. Synaptic plasticity and memory: an evaluation of the hypothesis. *Annu. Rev. Neurosci.* 23:649–711, 2000.

Maguire, E.A., et al. London taxi drivers and bus drivers: a structural MRI and neuropsychological analysis. *Hippocampus* 16:1091–1101, 2006.

Mottaghy, F.M., et al. Neuronal correlates of encoding and retrieval in episodic memory during a pair-word association learning task: a functional magnetic resonance imaging study. *Exp. Brain Res.* 128:332–342, 1999.

Nadel, L., Moskowitch, M. The hippocampal complex and long-term memory revisited. *Trends Cogn. Sci.* 5:228–230, 2002.

Nader, K., Hardt, O. A single standard for memory: the case for reconsolidation. *Nat. Rev. Neurosci.* 10:224–234, 2009.

Nee, D.E., et al. Neuroscientific evidence about the distinction between short- and long-term memory. *Curr. Dir. Psychol. Sci.* 17:102–106, 2008.

Neves, G., et al. Synaptic plasticity, memory, and the hippocampus: a neural network approach to causality. *Nat. Rev. Neurosci.* 9:65–75, 2008.

Polyn, S.M., Kahana, M.J. Memory search and the neural representation of context. *Trends Cogn. Sci.* 12:24–30, 2007.

Raymond, C.R. LTP forms 1, 2 and 3: different mechanisms for the 'long' in long-term potentiation. *Trends Neurosci.* 30:167–174, 2007.

Schnider, A., Ptak, R. Spontaneous confabulators fail to suppress currently irrelevant memory traces. *Nat. Neurosci.* 2:677–680, 1999.

Shastri, L. Episodic memory and cortico-hippocampal interactions. *Trends Cogn. Sci.* 6:162–168, 2002.

Shrager, Y., et al. Neural basis of the cognitive map: path integration does not require hippocampus or entorhinal cortex. *Proc. Natl. Acad. Sci. USA* 105:12034–12038, 2008.

Svoboda, E., et al. The functional neuroanatomy of autobiographical memory: a meta-analysis. *Neuropsychologia* 44:2189–2208, 2006.

Tronson, N.C., Taylor, J.R. Molecular mechanisms of memory consolidation. *Nat. Rev. Neurosci.* 8:262–275, 2007.

Tsivilis, D., et al. A disproportionate role for the fornix and mammillary bodies in recall versus recognition memory. *Nat. Neurosci.* 11:834–842, 2008.

Tulving, E., Markowitsch, H.J. Memory beyond the hippocampus. *Curr. Opin. Neurobiol.* 7:209–216, 1997.

Vargha-Khadem, F., et al. Differential effects of early hippocampal pathology on episodic and semantic memory. *Science* 277:376–380, 1997.

Woolf, N.J. A structural basis for memory storage in mammals. *Prog. Neurobiol.* 55:59–77, 1998.

Amnesia

Aggleton, J.P., et al. Differential cognitive effects of colloid cysts in the third ventricle that spare or compromise the fornix. *Brain* 123:800–815, 2000.

Alvarez, P., et al. Damage limited to the hippocampal region produces long-lasting memory impairment in monkeys. *J. Neurosci.* 15:3796–3807, 1995.

Bayley, P.J., et al. The fate of old memories after medial temporal lobe damage. *J. Neurosci.* 26:13311–13317, 2006.

Cipolotti, L., et al. Long-term retrograde amnesia: the crucial role of the hippocampus. *Neurospsychology* 39:151–172, 2001.

Dusoir, H., et al. The role of diencephalic pathology in human memory disorder. Evidence from a penetrating paranasal brain injury. *Brain* 113:1695–1706, 1990.

Gaffan, D., Gaffan, E.A. Amnesia in man following transection of the fornix. *Brain* 114:2611–2618, 1991.

Harding, A., et al. Degeneration of anterior thalamic nuclei differentiates alcoholics with amnesia. *Brain* 123:141–154, 2000.

Kopelman, M.D. The Korsakoff syndrome. *Br. J. Psychiatry* 166: 154–173, 1995.

Mishkin, M., et al. Amnesia and the organization of the hippocampal system. *Hippocampus* 8:212–216, 1998.

Morris, M.K., et al. Amnesia following a discrete basal forebrain lesion. *Brain* 115:1827–1847, 1992.

Schnider, A., Ptak, R. Spontaneous confabulators fail to suppress currently irrelevant memory traces. *Nat. Rev. Neurosci.* 2: 677–680, 1999.

Scoville, W.B., Milner, B. Loss of recent memory after bilateral hippocampal lesions. *J. Neurol. Neurosurg. Psychiatry* 20:11–21, 1957.

Zola-Morgan, S., et al. Human amnesia and the medial temporal region: enduring memory impairment following a bilateral lesion limited to field CA1 of the hippocampus. *J. Neurosci.* 6: 2950–2967, 1986.

CHAPTER 33: THE CEREBRAL CORTEX: INTRINSIC ORGANIZATION AND CONNECTIONS

Structure, Physiology, and Development

Bear, M.F., Kirkwood, A. Neocortical long-term potentiation. *Curr. Opin. Neurobiol.* 3:197–202, 1993.

Bolz, J., et al. Pharmacological analysis of cortical circuitry. *Trends Neurosci.* 12:292–296, 1989.

Brodmann, K. Vergleichende Lokalisationslehre der Grosshirnrinde. Leipzig: J.A. Barth, 1909.

Creutzfeldt, O., Creutzfeldt, M. Cortex cerebri: performance, structural and functional organisation of the cortex. Oxford: Oxford University Press, 1995.

Di Virgilio, G., et al. Cortical regions contributing to the anterior commissure in man. *Exp. Brain Res.* 124:1–7, 1999.

Egger, V., et al. Coincidence detection and changes of synaptic efficacy in spiny stellate neurons in rat barrel cortex. *Nat. Neurosci.* 2:1098–1103, 1999.

Gilbert, C.D. Horizontal integration and cortical dynamics. *Neuron* 9:1–13, 1992.

Herculana-Houzel, S., et al. The basic nonuniformity of the cerebral cortex. *Proc. Natl. Acad. Sci. USA* 105:12593–12598, 2008.

Hornung, J.-P., De Tribolet, N. Distribution of GABA-containing neurons in human frontal cortex: a quantitative immunocytochemical study. *Anat. Embryol. (Berl)* 189:139–145, 1994.

Hutsler, J.J., et al. Individual variation of cortical surface area asymmetries. *Cereb. Cortex* 8:11–17, 1998.

Jones, E.G. Anatomy of cerebral cortex: columnar input–output relations. In: *The cerebral cortex*, Schmidt, F.O. et al. eds. pp. 199–235. MIT Press, 1981.

Jones, E.G., Powell, T.P.S. An anatomical study of converging sensory pathways within the cerebral cortex of the monkey. *Brain* 93:793–820, 1970.

Klntsova, A.Y., Greeough, W.T. Synaptic plasticity in cortical systems. *Curr. Opin. Neurobiol.* 9:203–208, 1999.

Krnjević, K. Synaptic mechanisms modulated by acetylcholine in cerebral cortex. *Prog. Brain Res.* 145:81–93, 2004.

Majewska, A.K., Sur, M. Plasticity and specificity of cortical processing networks. *Trends Neurosci.* 29:323–328, 2006.

Markram, H., et al. Interneurons of the neocortical inhibitory system. *Nat. Rev. Neurosci.* 5:793–807, 2004.

Matelli, M., et al. Superior area 6 afferents from the superior parietal lobule in the macaque monkey. *J. Comp. Neurol.* 402:327–352, 1998.

McCormick, D.A., et al. Neurotransmitter control of neocortical neuronal activity and excitability. *Cereb. Cortex* 3:387–398, 1993.

Mesulam, M.-M. The cholinergic innervation of the cerebral cortex. *Prog. Brain Res.* 145:67–78, 2004.

Mountcastle, V.B. The columnar organization of the neocortex. *Brain* 120:701–722, 1997.

Parnavelas, J.G., Papadopolous, G.C. The monoaminergic innervation of the cerebral cortex is not diffuse and nonspecific. *Trends Neurosci.* 12:315–319, 1989.

Passingham, R.E., et al. The anatomical basis of functional localization in the cortex. *Nat. Rev. Neurosci.* 3:606–616, 2002.

Penfield, W., Rasmussen, T. *The cerebral cortex of man.* New York: Macmillan, 1950.

Percheron, G. Thalamus. In: Paxinos, G., Mai, J.K. (Eds.), *The human nervous system*, 2nd ed. (pp. 592–675). Philadelphia: Elsevier Academic Press, 2004.

Peters, A., Jones, E.G. *Cellular components of the cerebral cortex. Cerebral cortex.* Vol. 1 New York: Plenum Press, 1984.

Peters, A., Jones, E.G. Development and maturation of the cerebral cortex. Cerebral cortex. Vol. 7. New York: Plenum Press, 1988.

Pucak, M.L., et al. Patterns of intrinsic and associational circuitry in monkey prefrontal cortex. *J. Comp. Neurol.* 376:614–630, 1996.

Rakic, P., et al. Decision by division: making cortical maps. *Trends Neurosci.* 32:291–301, 2009.

Rakic, P., Singer, W. *Neurobiology of neocortex.* New York: John Wiley & Sons, 1988.

Ranganath, C., Rainer, G. Neural mechanisms for detecting and remembering novel events. *Nat. Rev. Neurosci.* 4:193–202, 2003.

Rockel, A.J., et al. The basic uniformity in structure of the neocortex. *Brain* 103:221–244, 1980.

Uylings, H.B.M. Consequences of large interindividual variability for human brain atlases: converging macroscopical imaging and microscopical neuroanatomy. *Anat. Embryol.* 210:423–431, 2005.

Van Hoesen, G. The modern concept of association cortex. *Curr. Opin. Neurobiol.* 3:150–154, 1993.

Wall, J.T. Variable organization in cortical maps of the skin as an indication of the lifelong adaptive capacities of the circuits in the mammalian brain. *Trends Neurosci.* 11:549–558, 1988.

West, M. Stereological methods for estimating the total number of neurons and synapses: issues of precision and bias. *Trends Neurosci.* 22:51–61, 1999.

Zador, A., Dobrunz, M. Dynamic synapses in the cortex. *Neuron* 19:1–4, 1997.

Thalamus

Briggs, F., Usrey, W.M. Emerging views of corticothalamic function. *Curr. Opin. Neurosci.* 18:403–407, 2008.

Crick, F. Function of the thalamic reticular complex: the searchlight hypothesis. *Proc. Natl. Acad. Sci. USA.* 81:4586–4590, 1984.

Ergenzinger, E.R., et al. Cortically induced thalamic plasticity in the primate somatosensory system. *Nat. Neurosci.* 1:226–229, 1998.

Grieve, K.L., et al. The primate pulvinar nuclei: vision and action. *Trends Neurosci.* 23:35–39, 2000.

Jones, E.G. *The thalamus*, 2nd ed. Cambridge, UK: Cambridge University Press 2007.

Lee Robinson, D., Petersen, S.E. The pulvinar and visual salience. *Trends Neurosci.* 15:127–132, 1992.

Llinás, R.R., et al. Temporal binding via cortical coincidence detection of specific and nonspecific thalamocortical inputs: a voltage dependent dye-imaging study in mouse brain slices. *Proc. Natl. Acad Sci. USA* 99:449–454, 2002.

Macchi, G., Bentivoglio, M. Is the "nonspecific" thalamus still "nonspecific"? *Arch. Ital. Biol.* 137:201–226, 1999.

McAlonan, K., et al. Attentional modulation of thalamic reticular neurons. *J. Neurosci.* 26:4444–4450, 2006.

Miniamimoto, T., et al. Complementary process to response bias in the centromedian nucleus of the thalamus. *Science* 308:1798–1801, 2005.

Pinault, D. The thalamic reticular nucleus: structure, function and concept. *Brain Res. Rev.* 46:1–31, 2004.

Sherman, S.M. Thalamic relays and cortical functioning. *Prog. Brain Res.* 149:107–126, 2005.

Sherman, S.M. The thalamus is more than just a relay. *Curr. Opin. Neurosci.* 17:417–422, 2007.

Sherman, S.M., Guilllery R.W. *Exploring the thalamus and its role in cortical function.* Cambridge, MA: MIT Press 2005.

Shipp, S. Pulvinar structure and circuitry in primates. In: Squire, L. (Ed.), *Encyclopedia of neuroscience* (pp. 1233–1244). Philadelphia: Elsevier, 2009.

Trageser, J.C., Keller, A. Reducing the uncertainty: gating of peripheral inputs by the Zona incerta. *J. Neurosci.* 24:8911–8915, 2004.

CHAPTER 34: FUNCTIONS OF THE NEOCORTEX

Association Areas and Higher Mental Functions

Adolphs, R. Neural systems for recognition of emotion. *Curr. Opin. Neurol.* 12:169–177, 2002.

Berlucchi, G., Aglioti, S. The body in the brain: neural bases of corporeal awareness. *Trends Neurosci.* 20:560–564, 1997.

Blood, A.J., et al. Emotional responses to pleasant and unpleasant music correlate with activity in paralimbic brain regions. *Nat. Neurosci.* 2:382–387, 1998.

Bolz, J., et al. Pharmacological analysis of cortical circuitry. *Trends Neurosci.* 12:292–296, 1989.

Bookheimer, S. Functional MRI of language: new approaches to understanding the cortical organization of semantic processing. *Annu. Rev. Neurosci.* 25:151–188, 2002.

Cloninger, C.R. Temperament and personality. *Curr. Opin. Neurobiol.* 4:266–273, 1994.

Colby, C.L. Action-oriented spatial reference frames in cortex. *Neuron* 20:15–24, 1998.

Deary, I.J. Human intelligence differences: a recent history. *Trends Cogn. Sci.* 5:127–130, 2001.

Fair, D.A., et al. The maturing architecture of the brain's default network. *Proc. Natl. Acad. Sci. USA* 105:4028–4032, 2008.

Flint, J. The genetic basis of cognition. *Brain* 122:2015–2031, 1999.

Fox, M.D., et al. The human brain is intrinsically organized into dynamic, anticorrelated functional networks. *Proc. Natl. Acad. Sci. USA* 102:9673–9678, 2005.

Friston, K. Beyond phrenology: what can neuroimaging tell us about distributed circuitry? *Annu. Rev. Neurosci.* 25:221–250, 2002.

Gaffan, D. Widespread cortical networks underlie memory and attention. *Science* 309:2172–2173, 2005.

Gauthier, I., et al. Expertise for cars and birds recruits brain areas involved in face recognition. *Nat. Neurosci.* 3:191–197, 2000.

Gisiger, T., et al. Computational models of association cortex. *Curr. Opin. Neurobiol.* 10:250–259, 2000.

Goldman-Rakic, P.S. Topography of cognition: parallel and distributed networks in primate association cortex. *Annu. Rev. Neurosci.* 11:137–156, 1988.

Gross, C.G., Graziano, M.S.A. Multiple representations of space in the brain. *Neuroscientist* 1:43–50, 1995.

Halder, B., McCormick, D.A. Rapid neocortical dynamics: cellular and network mechanisms. *Neuron* 62:171–189, 2009.

Harrison, B.J., et al. Consistency and functional specialization in the default mode brain network. *Proc. Natl. Acad. Sci. USA* 105: 9781–9786, 2008.

Haynes, J.-D., Rees, G. Decoding mental states from brain activity in humans. *Nat. Rev. Neurosci.* 7:523–534, 2006.

Heeger, D.J., Ress, D. What does fMRI tell us about neuronal activity? *Nat. Rev. Neurosci.* 3:142–151, 2002.

Horwitz, B., et al. Neural modeling, functional brain imaging, and cognition. *Trends Cogn. Sci.* 3:91–98, 1999.

Hummel, F., Gerloff, C. Larger interregional synchrony is associated with greater behavioral success in a complex sensory integration task in humans. *Cereb. Cortex* 15:670–678, 2005.

Libet, B., et al. Control of the transition from sensory detection to sensory awareness in man by the duration of a thalamic stimulus: the cerebral "time-on" factor. *Brain* 114:1731–1757, 1991.

Marois, R., Ivanoff, J. Capacity limits of information processing in the brain. *Trends Cogn. Sci.* 9:296–305, 2005.

Mesulam, M.-M. From sensation to cognition. *Brain* 121:1013–1052, 1998.

Norman, K.A., et al. Beyond mind-reading: multi-voxel pattern analysis of fMRI data. *Trends Cogn. Sci.* 10:424–430, 2006

Ojeman, G.A., et al. Lessons from the human brain: neuronal activity related to cognition. *Neuroscientist* 4:285–300, 1998.

Owen, A.M. Cognitive planning in humans: neuropsychological, neuroanatomical and neuropharmacological perspectives. *Prog. Neurobiol.* 53:431–450, 1997.

Poldrack, R.A. Can cognitive processes be inferred from neuroimaging data? *Trends Cogn. Sci.* 10:59–63, 2006.

Posner, M.I., Dehaene, S. Attentional networks. *Trends Neurosci.* 17:75–79, 1994.

Rauschecker, J.P., Korte, M. Auditory compensation for early blindness in cat cerebral cortex. *J. Neurosci.* 13:4538–4548, 1993.

Sacks, O. *An anthropologist on Mars. To see and not see* (pp. 102–144). New York: Picador, 1995.

Singer, W. Neuronal synchrony: a versatile code for the definition of relations? *Neuron* 24:111–125, 1999.

Tovée, M.J. Is face processing special? *Neuron* 21:1239–1242, 1993.

Varela, F., et al. The brainweb: phase synchronization and large scale integration. *Nat. Rev. Neurosci.* 2:251–262, 2001.

Parietal Cortex

Andersen, R.A., Bueno, C.A. Intentional maps in posterior parietal cortex. *Annu. Rev. Neurosci.* 25:189–220, 2002.

Brannon, E.M. The representation of numerical magnitude. *Curr. Opin. Neurobiol.* 16:222–229, 2006.

Critchley, M. *The parietal lobes.* London: Edward Arnold, 1953.

Desmurget, M., et al. Movement intention after parietal cortex stimulation in humans. *Science* 324:811–813, 2009.

Fogassi, L., et al. Parietal lobe: from action organization to intention understanding. *Science* 308:662–666, 2005.

Gottlieb, J. From thought to action: the parietal cortex as a bridge between perception, action, and cognition. *Neuron* 53:9–16, 2007.

Husain, M., Nachev, P. Space and the parietal cortex. *Trends Cogn. Sci.* 11:30–36, 2006.

Hyvärinen, J. *The parietal cortex of monkey and man*. New York: Springer-Verlag, 1982.

Iriki, A. The neural origins and implications of imitation, mirror neurons ans tool use. *Curr. Opin. Neurobiol.* 16:660–667, 2006.

Rizzolatti, G., Fabbri-Destro, M. The mirror system and its role in social cognition. *Curr. Opin. Neurobiol.* 18:179–184, 2008.

Sack, A.T. Parietal cortex and spatial cognition. *Behav. Brain Res.* 202:153–161, 2009.

Shadlen, M.N., Newsome, W.T. Neural basis of a perceptual decision in the parietal cortex (area LIP) of the Rhesus monkey. *J. Neurophysiol.* 86:1916–1936, 2001.

Vandeberghe, R., Gillebert, C.R. Parcellation of parietal cortex: convergence between lesion-symptom mapping and mapping of the intact functioning brain. *Behav. Brain Res.* 199:171–182, 2009.

Wheaton, L., et al. Synchronization of parietal and premotor areas during preparation and execution of praxis hand movements. *Clin. Neurophysiol.* 116:1382–1390, 2005.

Prefrontal Cortex

Amodio, D.M., Frith C.D. Meeting of minds: the medial frontal cortex and social cognition. *Nat. Rev. Neurosci.* 7:268–277, 2006.

Anderson, S.W., et al. Impairment of social and moral behavior related to early damage in human prefrontal cortex. *Nat. Neurosci.* 2:1032–1037, 1999.

Badre, D. Cognitive control, hierarchy, and the rostro-caudal organization of the frontal lobes. *Trends Cogn. Sci.* 12:193–200, 2008.

Brass, M., Haggard, P. The what, when, whether model of intentional action. *Neuroscientist* 14:319–325, 2008.

Fletcher, P.C., Henson, R.N.A. Frontal lobes and human memory: insights from functional neuroimaging. *Brain* 124:849–881, 2001.

Frith, C.D., Frith, U. Implicit and explicit processes in social cognition. *Neuron* 60:503–510, 2008.

Gray, J.R., Thompson, P.M. Neurobiology of intelligence: science and ethics. *Nat. Rev. Neurosci.* 5:471–482, 2004.

Hein, G., Singer, T. I feel how you feel but not always: the emphatic brain and its modulation. *Curr. Opin. Neurobiol.* 18:153–158, 2008.

Hauser, M.D. Perseveration, inhibition and the prefrontal cortex: a new look. *Curr. Opin. Neurobiol.* 9:214–222, 1999.

Mansouri, F.A., et al. Conflict-induced behavioural adjustment: a clue to the executive functions of the prefrontal cortex. *Nat. Rev. Neurosci.* 10:141–152, 2009.

Miller, E.K. The prefrontal cortex: complex neural properties for complex behavior. *Neuron* 22:15–17, 1999.

Procyk, E., Goldman-Rakic, P.M. Modulation of dorsolateral prefrontal delay activity during self-organized behavior. *J. Neurosci.* 26:11313–1323, 2006.

Ramnani, N., Owen, A.M. Anterior prefrontal cortex: insights into function from anatomy and neuroimaging, *Nat. Rev. Neurosci.* 5:184–194, 2004.

Roberts, A.C. Primate orbitofrontal cortex and adaptive behaviour. *Trends Cogn. Sci.* 10:83–90, 2006.

Rolls, E.T., Grabenhorst, F. The orbitofrontal cortex: from affect to decision-making. *Prog. Neurobiol.* 86:216–244, 2008.

Rossi, A.F., et al. The prefrontal cortex and the executive control of attention. *Exp. Brain Res.* 192:489–497, 2009.

Sakagami, M., Pan, X. Functional role of the ventrolateral prefrontal cortex in decision making. *Curr. Opin. Neurobiol.* 17:228–233, 2007.

Seitz, R.J., et al. Value judgment and self-control of action: the role of the medial frontal action. *Brain Res. Rev.* 60:368–378, 2009.

Shammi, P., Stuss, D.T. Humor appreciation: a role of the right frontal lobe. *Brain* 122:657–666, 1999.

Stoet, G., Snyder, L.H. Neural correlates of executive control functions in the monkey. *Trends Cogn. Sci.* 13:228–234, 2009.

Thompson-Schill, S.L., et al. The frontal lobes and the regulation of mental activity. *Curr. Opin. Neurobiol.* 15:219–224, 2005.

Wallis, J.D., et al. Single neurons in prefrontal cortex encode abstract rules. *Nature* 411:953–956, 2001.

White, I.M., Wise, S.P. Rule-dependent neuronal activity in the prefrontal cortex. *Exp. Brain Res.* 126:315–335, 1999.

Temporal Cortex and Insula

Augustine, J.R. Circuitry and functional aspects of the insular lobe in primates including humans. *Brain Res. Rev.* 22:229–244, 1996.

Barnes, C.L., Pandya, D.N. Efferent cortical connections of multimodal cortex of the superior temporal sulcus in the rhesus monkey. *J. Comp. Neur.* 318:222–244, 1992.

Baumgärtner, U., et al., Laser-evoked potentials are graded and somatotopically organized anteroposteriorly in the operculoinsular cortex of anesthetized monkeys. *J. Neurophysiol.* 96:2802–2808, 2006.

Beachamp, M.S. See me, hear me, touch me: multisensory integration in lateral occipital-temporal cortex. *Curr. Opin. Neurobiol.* 15:145–153, 2005.

Carr, L., et al. Neural mechanisms for empathy in humans: a relay from neural systems for imitation to limbic areas. *Proc. Natl. Acad. Sci. USA* 100:5497–5501, 2003.

Craig, A.D. Interoception: the sense of the physiological condition of the body. *Curr. Opin. Neurobiol.* 13:500–505, 2003.

Craig, A.D. How do you feelnow? The anterior insula and human awareness. *Nat. Rev. Neurosci.* 10:59–70, 2009.

Farrer, C., et al. Modulating the experience of agency: a positron emission tomographic study. *NeuroImage* 18:324–333, 2003.

Critchley, H.D., et al. Neural systems supporting interoceptive awareness. *Nat. Rev. Neurosci.* 7:189–195, 2004.

Gauthier, I., et al. Expertise for cars and birds recruits brain areas involved in face recognition. *Nat. Neurosci.* 3:191–197, 2000.

Haxby, J.V., et al. Distributed and overlapping representations of faces and objects in ventral temporal cortex. *Science* 293:2425–2430, 2001.

Karnath, H.O., et al. Awareness of the functioning of one's own limbs mediated by the insular cortex? *J. Neurosci.* 25:7134–7138, 2005.

Klüver, H., Bucy, P.C. Psychic blindness and other symptoms following bilateral temporal lobectomy in rhesus monkeys. *Am. J. Physiol.* 119:352–353, 1937.

Levy, D.A., et al. The anatomy of semantic knowledge: medial vs. lateral temporal lobe. *Proc. Natl. Acad. Sci. USA* 101:6710–6715, 2004.

Lovero, K.L., et al. Anterior insular cortex anticipates impending stimulus significance. *NeuroImage* 45:976–983, 2009.

Messinger, A., et al. Neuronal representations of stimulus associations develop in the temporal lobe during learning. *Proc. Natl. Acad. Sci. USA* 98:12239–12244, 2001.

Naqvi, N.H., et al. Damage to the insula disrupts addiction to cigarette smoking. *Science* 315:531–534, 2007.

Olson, I.R., et al. The enigmatic temporal pole: a review of findings on social and emotional processing. *Brain* 130:1718–1731, 2007.

Ostrowsky, K., et al. Representation of pain and somatic sensation in the human insula: a study of responses to direct electrical cortical stimulation, *Cereb. Cortex* 12:376–385, 2002.

Schwarzlose, R.F., et al. Separate face and body selectivity on the fusiform gyrus. *J. Neurosci.* 23:11055–11059, 2005.

Tovée, M.J. Is face processing special? *Neuron* 21:1239–1242, 1998.

Symptoms after Damage to Association Areas

Committeri, G., et al. Neural bases of personal and extrapersonal neglect in humans. *Brain* 130:431–441, 2007.

Coslett, H.B. Neglect in vision and visual imagery: a double dissociation. *Brain* 120:1163–1171, 1997.

Farah, M.J. Agnosia. *Curr. Opin. Neurobiol.* 2:162–164, 1992.

Greene, J.D.W. Apraxia, agnosias, and higher visual function abnormalities. *J. Neurol. Neurosurg. Psychiatry* 76 (Suppl V):v25–v34, 2005.

Halligan, P.W., et al. Spatial cognition: evidence from visual neglect. *Trends Cogn. Sci.* 7:125–133, 2003.

Orfei, M.D., et al. Unawareness of illness in neuropsychiatric disorders: phenomenological certainty versus etiopathogenic vagueness. *Neuroscientist* 14:203–222, 2008.

Petreska, B., et al. Apraxia: a review. *Prog. Brain Res.* 164:61–83, 2007.

Pouget, A., Driver, J. Relating unilateral neglect to the neural coding of space. *Curr. Opin. Neurobiol.* 10:242–249, 2000.

Rafal, R.D. Neglect. *Curr. Opin. Neurobiol.* 4:231–235, 1994.

Schindler, I., et al. Neck muscle vibration induces lasting recovery in spatial neglect. *J. Neurol. Neurosurg. Psychiatry* 73:412–419, 2002.

Zadikoff, C., Lang, A.E. Apraxia in movement disorders. *Brain* 128:1489–1497, 2005.

Language and Music

Bavelier, D., et al. Brain and language: a perspective from sign language. *Neuron* 21:275–278, 1998.

Belin, P., et al. Recovery from nonfluent aphasia after melodic intonation therapy: a PET study. *Neurology* 47:1504–1511, 1996.

Bookheimer, S. Functional MRI of language: new approaches to understanding the cortical organization of semantic processing. *Annu. Rev. Neurosci.* 25:151–188, 2002.

Brust, J.C.M. Music and language: musical alexia and agraphia. *Brain* 103:367–392, 1980.

Crinion, J., et al. Language control in the bilingual brain. *Science* 312:1537–1540, 2006.

Dehaene-Lambertz, G., et al. Nature and nurture in language acquisition: anatomical and functional brain-imaging studies in infants. *Trends Neurosci.* 29:367–373, 2006.

Evers, S., et al. The cerebral haemodynamics of music perception: a transcranial Doppler sonography study. *Brain* 122:75–85, 1999.

Fiez, J.A. Sound and meaning: how native language affects reading strategies. *Nat. Rev. Neurosci.* 3:3–5, 2000.

Frost, J.A., et al. Language processing is strongly left lateralized in both sexes. *Brain* 122:199–208, 1999.

Greenfield, P.M. Language, tools and brain: the ontogeny and phylogeny of hierarchially organized sequential behavior. *Behav. Brain Sci.* 14:531–595, 1991.

Hagoort, P. On Broca, brain, and binding: a new framework. *Trends Cogn. Sci.* 9:416–423, 2005.

Halpern, A.R., Zatorre, R.J. When that tune runs through your head: a PET investigation of auditory imagery for familiar melodies. *Cereb. Cortex* 9:697–704, 1999.

Hannon, E.E., Trainor, L.J. Music acquisition: effects of enculturation and formal training on development. *Trends Cogn. Sci.* 11:466–472, 2007.

Hickok, G., Poeppel, D. The cortical organization of speech processing. *Nat. Rev. Neurosci.* 8:393–402, 2007.

Hinke, R.M., et al. Functional magnetic resonance imaging of Broca's area during internal speech. *NeuroReport* 4:675–678, 1993.

Howard, D., et al. The cortical localization of the lexicons: positron emission tomography evidence. *Brain* 115:1769–1782, 1992.

Koelsch, S., Siebel, W.A. Towards a neural basis of music perception. *Trends Cogn. Sci.* 9:578–584, 2005.

Kuhl, P.K. Early language acquisition: cracking the speech code. *Nat. Rev. Neurosci.* 5:831–843, 2004.

Lecours, A.R., et al. *Aphasiology.* London: Bailliere Tindall, 1983.

Lotto, A.J., et al. Reflections on mirror neurons and speech perception. *Trends Cogn. Sci.* 13:110–114, 2008.

Nobre, A.C., Plunkett, K. The neural system of language: structure and development. *Curr. Opin. Neurobiol.* 7:262–268, 1997.

Onishi, T., et al. Functional anatomy of musical perception in musicians. *Cereb. Cortex* 11:754–760, 2001.

Patterson, K., Ralph, M.A.L. Selective disorders of reading? *Curr. Opin. Neurobiol.* 9:235–239, 1999.

Pell, M.D. Judging emotion and attitudes from prosody following brain damage. *Prog. Brain Res.* 156:303–315, 2006.

Penfield, W., Roberts, L. *Speech and brain mechanisms.* Princeton, NJ: Princeton University Press, 1959.

Price, C.J. The functional anatomy of word comprehension and production. *Trends Cogn. Sci.* 2:281–288, 1998.

Pulvermüller, F. Brain mechanisms linking language and action. *Nat. Rev. Neurosci.* 6:576–582, 2005.

Schirmer, A., Kotz, S.A. Beyond the right hemisphere: brain mechanisms mediating vocal emotional processing. *Trends Cogn. Sci.* 10:24–30, 2006.

Schuppert, M., et al. Receptive amusia: evidence for cross-hemispheric networks underlying music processing strategies. *Brain* 123:546–559, 2000.

Sergent, J. Music, the brain and Ravel. *Trends Neurosci.* 16:168–172, 1993.

Shalom, D.B., Poeppel, D. Functional anatomic models of language: assembling the pieces. *Neuroscientist* 14:119–127, 2008.

Springer, J.A., et al. Language dominance in neurologically normal and epilepsy subjects: a functional MI study. *Brain* 122:2033–2045, 1999.

Stewart, L., et al. Music and the brain: disorder of musical listening. *Brain* 129:2533–2553, 2006.

Weiskrantz, L. *Thought without language.* Oxford: Oxford University Press, 1988.

Willems, R.M., Hagoort, P. Neural evidence for the interplay between language, gesture, and action: a review. *Brain. Lang.* 101:278–289, 2007.

Willmes, K., Poeck, K. To what extent can aphasic syndromes be localized? *Brain* 116:1527–1540, 1993.

Lateralization

Annett, M. Cerebral asymmetry in twins: predictions of the right shift theory. *Neuropsychology* 41:469–479, 2003.

Bryden, M.P., et al. Handedness is not related to self-reported disease incidence. *Cortex* 27:605–611, 1991.

Canli, T. Hemispheric asymmetry in the experience of emotion: a perspective from functional imaging. *Neuroscientist* 5:201–207, 1999.

Catani, M., ffytche, D.H. The rises and falls of disconnection syndromes. *Brain* 128:2224–2239, 2005.

Corballis, M.C. Cerebral asymmetry: motoring on. *Trends Cogn. Sci.* 2:152–157, 1998.

Davidson, R.J. Hemispheric asymmetry and emotion. In: Scherer, K.R., Ekman, P. (Eds.), *Approaches to emotion* (pp. 39–57). Mahwah, J: Lawrence Erlbaum, 1984.

Gazzaniga, M.S. Principles of human brain organization derived from split-brain studies. *Neuron* 14:217–228, 1995.

Glass, A. Individual differences in hemispheric specialization. New York: Plenum Press, 1987.

Jäncke, L., et al. The relationship between corpus callosum size and forebrain volume. *Cereb. Cortex* 7:48–56, 1997.

Kim, S.-G., et al. Functional magnetic resonance imaging of motor cortex: hemispheric asymmetry and handedness. *Science* 261: 615–617, 1993.

Kotz, S.A., et al. Lateralization of emotional prosody in the brain: an overview and synopsis on the impact of study design. *Prog. Brain Res.* 156:285–294, 2006.

Lent, R., Schmidt, S.L. The ontogenesis of the forebrain commissures and the determination of brain asymmetries. *Prog. Neurobiol.* 40:249–276, 1993.

Moffat, S.D., et al. Morphology of the planum temporale and corpus callosum in left handers with evidence of left and right hemisphere speech representation. *Brain* 121:2369–2379, 1998.

Myers, R.E. Phylogenetic studies of commissural connexions. In: Ettinger, E.G. et al. (Eds.), *Functions of the corpus callosum*. (pp. 138–142). New York: Churchill Livingstone, 1965.

Paul, L.K., et al. Agenesis of the corpus callosum: genetic, developmental and functional aspects of connectivity. *Nat. Rev. Neurosci.* 8:287–299, 2007.

Pujol, J., et al. Cerebral lateralization of language in normal left-handed people studied by functional MRI. *Neurology* 52:1038–1043, 1999.

Sperry, R.W. Lateral specialization in the surgically separated hemispheres. In: Schmidt, F.O., Worden, F.G. (Eds.), *The neurosciences. Third study program* (pp. 5–19). Cambridge, MA: MIT Press, 1974.

Springer, S.P., Deutsch, G. *Left brain, right brain: perspectives from cognitive neuroscience*, 5th. ed. New York: W.H. Freeman, 1997.

Stone, V.E., et al. Left hemisphere representations of emotional facial expressions. *Neuropsychologia* 34:23–29, 1996.

Sun, T., Walsh, C.A. Molecular approaches to brain asymmetry and handedness. *Nat. Rev. Neurosci.* 7:655–662, 2006.

Toga, A.W., Thompson, P.M. Mapping brain asymmetry. *Nat. Rev. Neurosci.* 4:37–48, 2003.

Woods, B.T. Is the left hemisphere specialized for language at birth? *Trends Neurosci.* 6:115–117, 1983.

Cognitive Sex Differences; Nature and Nurture

Aboitiz, F., et al. Morphometry of the sylvian fissure and the corpus callosum, with emphasis on sex differences. *Brain* 115: 1521–1541, 1992.

Allen, J.S., et al. Sexual dimorphism and asymmetries in the gray-white composition of the human cerebrum. *NeuroImage* 18:880–894, 2003.

Baron-Cohen, S., et al. Sex differences in the brain: implications for explaining autism. *Science* 310:819–823, 2005.

Benbow, C.P. Sex differences in mathematical reasoning ability in intellectually talented preadolescents: their nature, effects, and possible causes. *Behav. Brain Sci.* 11:169–232, 1988.

Bleier, R., et al. Can the corpus callosum predict gender, handedness, or cognitive differences? *Trends Neurosci.* 9:391–394, 1986.

Cooke, B.M., Woolley, C.S. Sexually dimorphic synaptic organization of the medial amygdala. *J. Neurosci.* 16:10759–10767, 2005.

de Courten-Myers, G.M. The human cerebral cortex: gender differences in structure and function. *J. Neuropathol. Exp. Neurol.* 58:217–226, 1999.

Federman, D.D. The biology of human sex differences. *N. Engl. J. Med.* 354:1507–1514, 2006.

Grön, G., et al. Brain activation during human navigation: gender different neural networks as substrate of performance. *Nat. Neurosci.* 3:404–408, 2000.

Holden, C. Parsing the genetics of behavior. *Science* 322:892–895, 2008.

Janowsky, J.S. Thinking with your gonads: testosterone and cognition. *Trends Cogn. Sci.* 10:77–82, 2006.

Kimura, D. Sex, sexual orientation and sex hormones influence human cognitive function. *Curr. Opin. Neurobiol.* 6:259–263, 1996.

Landis, S., Insel, T.R. The "neuro" in neurogenetics. *Science* 322:821, 2008.

McCarthy, M.M., Konkle, A.T.M. When is a sex difference not a sex difference? *Front. Neuroendocrinol.* 26:85–102, 2005.

Moffat, S.D., et al. Navigation in a "virtual" maze: sex differences and correlation with psychometric measures of spatial abilities. *Evol. Hum. Behav.* 9:73–87, 1999.

Mohr, C., et al. Brain state-dependent functional hemispheric specialization in men but not in women. *Cereb. Cortex* 15:1451–1458, 2005.

Shors, T.J. Stress and sex effects on associative learning: for better or for worse. *Neuroscientist* 4:353–364, 1998.

Sowell, E., et al. Sex differences in cortical thickness mapped in 176 healthy individuals between 7 and 87 years of age. *Cereb. Cortex* 17:1550–1560, 2007.

Sullivan, E.V., et al. Sex differences in corpus callosum size: relationship to age and intracranial size. *Neurobiol. Aging* 22:603–611, 2001.

Watson, N.V. Sex differences in throwing: monkeys having a fling. *Trends Cogn. Sci.* 5:98–99, 2001.

The Cerebral Cortex and Mental Illness

Abi-Dargam, A., et al. Prefrontal dopamine D1 receptors and working memory in schizophrenia. *J. Neurosci.* 22:3708–3719, 2002.

Altar, C.A. Neurotrophins and depression. *Trends Pharmacol. Sci.* 20:59–62, 1999.

Belzung, C., et al. Neuropeptides in psychiatric diseases: an overview with particular focus on depression and anxiety disorders. *CNS Neurol. Disord. Drug Targets* 5:135–145, 2006.

Beneyto, M., et al. Abnormal glutamate receptor expression in the medial temporal lobe in schizophrenia and mood disorders. *Neuropsychopharmacology* Advance online publication 14 February, 2007.

Castrén, E. Is mood chemistry? *Nat. Rev. Newurosci.* 6:251–246, 2005.

Cotter, D., et al. Reduced neuronal size and glial cell density in area 9 of the dorsolateral prefrontal cortex in subjects with major depressive disorder. *Cereb. Cortex* 12:386–394, 2002.

Drzyzga, L., et al. Cytokines in schizophrenia and the effects of antipsychotic drugs. *Brain Behav. Immun.* 20:532–545, 2006.

Egan, M.F., Weinberger, D. Neurobiology of schizophrenia. *Curr. Opin. Neurobiol.* 7:701–707, 1997.

Fallon, J.H., et al. The neuroanatomy of schizophrenia: circuitry and neurotransmitter systems. *Clin. Neurosci. Res.* 3:77–107, 2003.

Goodwin, F.K. Neurobiology of manic-depressive illness. *Clin. Neurosci.* 1:157–162, 1993.

Hahn, C.-G., et al. Altered neuregulin 1–erbB4 signaling contributes to NMDA receptor hypofunction in schizophrenia. *Nat. Med.* 12:824–828, 2006.

Hariri, A.R., Holmes, A. Genetics of emotional regulation: the role of the serotonin transporter in neural function. *Trends Cogn. Neurosci.* 10:182–191, 2006.

Harrison, P.J. The neuropathology of schizophrenia: a critical review of the data and their interpretation. *Brain* 122:593–624, 1999.

Henn, F.A. Animal models of depression. *Clin. Neurosci.* 1:152–156, 1993.

Kristiansen, L.V., et al. Changes in NMDA receptor subunits and interacting PSD proteins in dorsolateral prefrontal and anterior cingulated cortex indicate abnormal regional expression in schizophrenia. *Mol. Psychiatry* 11:737–747, 2006.

Kuperberg, G., Heckers, S. Schizophrenia and cognitive function. *Curr. Opin. Neurobiol.* 10:205–210, 2000.

Lewis, D.A., et al. Cortical inhibitory neurons and schizophrenia. *Nat. Rev. Neurosci.* 6:312–324, 2005.

Marx, C.E., et al. Neuroactive steroids are altered in schizophrenia and bipolar disorder: relevance to pathophysiology and therapeutics. *Neuropsychopharmacology* 31:1249–1263, 2006.

Narr, K.L., et al. Mapping cortical thickness and gray matter concentrations in first episode of schizophrenia. *Cereb. Cortex* 15:708–719, 2005.

Rolls, E.T., et al. Computational models of schizophrenia and dopamine modulation in the prefrontal cortex. *Nat. Rev. Neurosci.* 9:696–709, 2008.

Scarr, E., et al. Cortical glutamatergic markers in schizophrenia. *Neuropsychopharmacology* 30:1521–1531, 2005.

Sharp, F.R. Psychosis: pathological activation of limbic thalamocortical circuits by psychomimetics and schizophrenia? *Trends Neurosci.* 24:330–334, 2001.

Sheline, Y.I. Neuroanatomical changes with unipolar major depression. *Neuroscientist* 4:331–334, 1998

Styner, M., et al. Morphometric analysis of lateral ventricles in schizophrenia and healthy controls regarding genetic and disease-specific factors. *Proc. Natl. Acad. Sci. USA* 102:4872–4877, 2005.

Vaidya, V.A., Duman, R.S. Depression: emerging insights from neurobiology. *Br. Med. Bull.* 57:61–79, 2001.

Weinberger, D., et al. Evidence for dysfunction of the prefrontal-limbic network in schizophrenia: a magnetic resonance imaging and regional blood flow study of discordant monozygotic twins. *Am. J. Psychiatry* 149:890–897, 1992.

Index